004
NEO

Neonatal Emergencies

Neonatal Emergencies

A Practical Guide for Resuscitation, Transport
and Critical Care of Newborn Infants

Edited by

Georg Hansmann

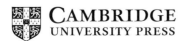

CAMBRIDGE UNIVERSITY PRESS
Cambridge, New York, Melbourne, Madrid, Cape Town, Singapore,
São Paulo, Delhi

Cambridge University Press
The Edinburgh Building, Cambridge CB2 8RU, UK

Published in the United States of America by
Cambridge University Press, New York

www.cambridge.org
Information on this title: www.cambridge.org/9780521701433

First published by Georg Thieme Verlag (2004)
This edition published 2009

Printed in the United Kingdom at the University Press, Cambridge

A catalog record for this publication is available from the British Library

Library of Congress Cataloging-in-Publication Data

Neonatal emergencies : a practical guide for resuscitation, transport,
and critical care of newborn infants / edited by Georg Hansmann.
   p. ; cm.
  Includes bibliographical references and index.
  ISBN 978-0-521-70143-3 (pbk.)
  1. Neonatal emergencies. 2. Neonatal intensive care. I. Hansmann,
Georg, 1972–
  [DNLM: 1. Infant, Newborn, Diseases. 2. Intensive Care, Neonatal–
methods. 3. Infant, Newborn. 4. Intensive Care Units, Neonatal.
5. Resuscitation. 6. Transportation of Patients. WS 421 N4373 2009]
  RJ253.5.N457 2009
  618.92′01–dc22

                                         2009013052

ISBN 978-0-521-70143-3 Paperback

This book is dedicated to my family.

Wherever you go, go with all your heart.

Confucius, 551–479 BC, China

Contents

Contents

Section 3–Classic and rare scenarios in the neonatal period

Contents

Section 4–Transport

Section 5–Appendix

Contributors

John H. Arnold, MD
Department of Anesthesia, Perioperative
and Pain Medicine
Division of Critical Care Medicine
Children's Hospital Boston
Harvard Medical School
Boston, MA
USA

Christoph Bührer, MD, PhD
Department of Neonatology
Charité University Medical Center
Berlin
Germany

Alan C. Fenton, MD, MRCP(UK)
Newcastle Neonatal Service
Royal Victoria Infirmary
Queen Victoria Road
Newcastle upon Tyne
UK

Shannon E. G. Hamrick, MD
Department of Pediatrics
Division of Neonatology
Emory University
Atlanta, GA
USA

Georg Hansmann, MD, PhD
Department of Cardiology
Children's Hospital Boston
Harvard Medical School
Boston, MA
USA

Tilman Humpl, MD, PhD
Department of Critical Care Medicine
Hospital for Sick Children
Toronto, ON
Canada

Juan C. Ibla, MD
Department of Anesthesia, Perioperative
and Pain Medicine
Division of Cardiac Anesthesia
Children's Hospital Boston
Harvard Medical School
Boston, MA
USA

Sam Richmond, MBBS, FRCP
Neonatal Service
Sunderland Royal Hospital
Sunderland
Tyne and Wear
UK

Andrea Zimmermann, MD
Division of Neonatology
Children's Hospital Munich-Schwabing/
Klinikum rechts der Isar
Technical University Munich
Munich
Germany

Foreword (1)

In many ways neonatology is synonymous with emergency. Many of us in the field chose neonatology because of the potential for complex, medically and ethically challenging scenarios to arise anytime we are called to the delivery room and the opportunity to care for critically ill newborns while working under intense time pressure in the neonatal intensive care unit. *Neonatal Emergencies*, edited by Georg Hansmann, MD, PhD, is a welcome addition to our field of medicine. One of the most unique and valuable aspects of this text is its focus on emergency and critical care of the newborn. Unlike other textbooks of neonatology that attempt to cover all aspects of neonatal care, and because of this tend to become too unwieldy to serve as a source of rapidly accessible information, *Neonatal Emergencies* presents pertinent information in a concise, easy-to-read manner. Figures, tables, and algorithms convey information clearly and succinctly. There are many examples of practical advice for the health care professional at the bedside including topics such as what questions to ask when on the phone with a colleague who wishes to refer a patient to you for transport, and lists of appropriate procedures to perform, equipment to use, and medications to deliver when caring for a sick neonate. Key points are emphasized by positioning in a box where the text is preceded by an exclamation mark or is shaded. Pertinent questions are also included so that the reader may perform a self-assessment after reviewing the material in a particular section or chapter.

The practical nature of the content of this text is also plainly evident in its emphasis on physical examination skills and what can be learned about the neonatal patient using one's eyes, ears, and hands. Other important topics covered in the following pages but rarely found in other references include decision-making, training issues, and the importance of effective communication with fellow health care professionals (between and among the obstetric and neonatology team members) and with parents. Although not a comprehensive resource on the ethical challenges inherent in neonatal care, this text does touch upon them in a sensitive and compassionate manner.

Simulation-based training is finding its way into the formal preparation and assessment of multidisciplinary teams of health care professionals charged with caring for newborns. Indeed the Neonatal Resuscitation Program (NRP) of the American Academy of Pediatrics will be evolving into a career-long learning program with simulation-based training at its core. In a way *Neonatal Emergencies* serves as a primer for those looking to develop realistic immersive scenarios for their training programs; thus its publication is timely, indeed.

Neonatal Emergencies presents an evidence-based approach to care of the critically ill newborn with contributions from an international panel of experts and supported by multiple contemporary references. It will serve as a readily accessible resource to a broad group of users including established pediatric/neonatal and obstetric physicians, anesthesiologists, nurses, nurse practitioners, midwives, and transport specialists as well as trainees in these domains. Mastery of the content knowledge written in this book as well as the technical skills described in its pages will prepare one well for the emergencies that are sure to arise when caring for newborns in the delivery room and intensive care unit.

Louis P. Halamek, MD, FAAP
Division of Neonatal and Developmental Medicine
Stanford University, California

Foreword (2)

Emergencies constitute a fundamental part of newborn medicine. I learned this the hard way shortly after I had finished medical school 35 years ago. As a research fellow in perinatal medicine I was offered to work for a week now and then in the neonatal intensive care unit, in spite of no formal training. After one or two days I had my first call and had to run to the obstetrical department, where a severely asphyxiated boy had been delivered. I have to admit that I did not know what to do. The insufficiency I felt and the incompetence of my handlings made me decide that this would not happen again. The fascination of dealing with and handling acute events in a satisfactory way has been an important part of my life ever since. However, I have never forgotten this boy at my first call, in spite of the fact that I, during the past 35 years, have dealt with thousands of severely ill newborn infants.

Today we talk about the first "golden minutes" of life: these precious minutes when it is so important to do everything as correctly as possible. We know today that newborn babies should not be ventilated with too high or too low tidal volumes and we know that we should avoid excessive oxygen even briefly. And so many acute events may occur in the nursery in the time following these first "golden minutes" after birth. For many of the most immature and vulnerable infants even small deviations from normality for a brief period may be catastrophic. It is a huge burden for health personnel to carry the future of the whole life of a human being during these important minutes – and not only the life of the newborn but also implications for their family.

There is a need for evidence-based guidelines for everyone involved in emergencies in the neonatal period. Georg Hansmann and his colleagues have written an impressive comprehensive volume in *Neonatal Emergencies*. Here we find the most recent and modern views on a wide specter of emergencies in neonatal medicine summarized in a clear and didactic manner. This is simply a book for the future. Every pediatric resident and fellow and every neonatologist would benefit from reading this book. Experienced or not, *Neonatal Emergencies* will be a great help in the daily and often stressful life of everyone dealing with sick and fragile newborn infants.

Ola Didrik Saugstad, MD, PhD, FRCPE
Department of Pediatric Research
Rikshospitalet University Hospital
Oslo, Norway

Preface

Over the past decades, evidence-based medicine has become an international endeavor. In neonatal intensive care, however, well-designed randomized controlled trials (RCTs) are quite rare, and clinical decision-making – especially in time-sensitive emergency situations (delivery room, NICU) – may be challenging and mainly based on the providers' expertise and experience. Since the approaches to key issues in neonatal intensive care often differ significantly between countries, I found it was now time to bring together the best and most current clinical evidence available, and the broadest experience possible. The challenge of this new handbook *Neonatal Emergencies* therefore was to find a group of internationally distinguished experts, not only among different institutions but also across countries, continents, and disciplines. I am pleased to have gathered a group of accomplished neonatologists, pediatric cardiologists, anesthesiologists, and critical care physicians from all over the world. We learned a lot from each other while writing the chapters that will follow this Preface.

The book is written for an interdisciplinary readership, i.e., pediatric residents, fellows and junior faculty, NICU nurses and nurse practitioners, obstetricians, midwifes, anesthesiologists, physicians in emergency medicine, and specialized paramedics. It can be used for emergency situations as well as a guide for mock codes or clinical workshops. Our goals were straightforward: this handbook should be comprehensive but practical and easy to use so that the information provided may actually help health care providers with different levels of experience to save newborn lives and prevent disability. Thus, we added multiple illustrations and tables, and developed several flow sheets (algorithms), many of which are based on the ILCOR/AAP/AHA/ERC guidelines 2005 (neonatal and pediatric life support), RCTs, and meta-analyses such as Cochrane systematic reviews. More than 2000 original and review articles were screened, and about 600 of those are now cited in the final text. Where evidence-based data are not available, sparse or ambiguous, the authors pass on their clinical experience in several neonatal, pediatric, and cardiac intensive care units, and neonatal emergency transport to the reader.

Briefly, this handbook is divided in five major sections: Section 1 covers history and reality of neonatal transport services. Section 2 describes the essential "basics" in neonatal resuscitation and critical care, including two separate chapters on mechanical ventilation and ethics. In Section 3, about 30 clinical scenarios are subdivided in etiology/pathophysiology, epidemiology, clinical presentation, differential diagnosis, diagnostics and treatment in multiple (often subsequent) clinical settings. Both our patients and pediatric cardiology are close to our hearts so cardiovascular diseases are more extensively described than in most other handbooks on neonatal intensive care. The book covers, for the first time to our knowledge, the management of critically ill newborns from the first minute of life (i.e., the delivery room), during transport and in the first days on the intensive care unit. By focusing on the first 72 hours of life, the text goes beyond the National Resuscitation Program (NRP) and its excellent handbook, published in 2006 by the American Academy of Pediatrics (AAP) and the American Heart Association (AHA). Section 4 outlines the fundamentals and challenges of neonatal transport. Section 5 gives recommendations for the clinical training of transport and delivery room staff, and offers several normograms (laboratory, etc.).

Neonatal emergency and critical care medicine is constantly developing towards new or modified treatments that should be based on the principle "do no harm." Good examples of ongoing controversies are the current discussions about oxygen toxicity, therapeutic hypothermia, and the perinatal management of babies born out of meconium-stained amniotic fluid. The authors and Cambridge University Press have done their best to provide the reader with the most current, accurate, evidence-based diagnostic, and therapeutic recommendations. However, when data from well-designed RCTs were not available, our recommendations are based on "expert opinion" only. Therefore, we highly encourage the readers to use additional standard textbooks as well as online resources, and to utilize their own experience and updated knowledge when caring for critically ill newborn infants. Particularly for drug dosing, drug–drug interactions, drug adverse effects, and non-pharmacological interventions, the reader needs to follow the instructions and warnings provided by the manufacturers (i.e., package insert) and the Food and Drug Administration (FDA, and its equivalents in countries outside the United States of America) before administering these medications or performing the procedures described. Realizing that more than one approach to the clinical problem may be right, we nevertheless aimed to give precise and detailed treatment recommendations. However, in the individual emergency situation, certain treatment options may need to be added, changed or omitted by the critical care provider.

Although we might have achieved our goal of internationality to some extent already, we hope to broaden our range. Hence, the authors would very much appreciate your comments and suggestions on this first English edition of *Neonatal Emergencies* (neonatal.emergencies@ gmail.com).

Georg Hansmann
Boston
July 2009

Acknowledgments

I am indebted to my dedicated co-authors and many of my colleagues for being an invaluable resource while writing this book:

Proofreading, suggestions, and comments by:

Agnes Bartha (UCSF; seizures)

Carlos Botas (UCSF; several scenario chapters)

Ronald Clyman (UCSF; PDA)

Robert Lustig (UCSF; hypoglycemia)

Douglas Miniati (UCSF Pediatric Surgery; GI malformations, birth trauma)

Colin Partridge (UCSF; ethics, TTTS, hydrops fetalis, GI malformations, PPHN)

Rod Phibbs (UCSF; history of neonatal transport services)

Ted Ruel (UCSF; HIV)

Sarah Scarpace (UCSF Pharmacy; drug dosing)

Thomas Shimotake (UCSF; basics, PPHN)

Yao Sun (UCSF; basics)

H. William Taeusch (UCSF; ethics)

Jay Tureen (UCSF; sepsis)

I appreciate the support I have received from ICU and transport staff, faculty, and trainees with whom I have had the pleasure of working over the years.

Moreover, I would like to thank Dr Michelle Lazaro and the editorial staff at Cambridge University Press for their tremendous help and patience with the translation, editing, and layout of this new handbook.

The authors would very much appreciate your comments and suggestions on this first English edition of *Neonatal Emergencies*: Please send an email with your comments and suggestions to neonatal.emergencies@gmail.com.

Georg Hansmann
Boston
July 2009

Organization of neonatal transport

History and challenges of neonatal emergency transport services (NETS)

Alan C. Fenton and Georg Hansmann

History of neonatal emergency transport services

Services for neonatal transport have evolved alongside in-hospital services for neonatal care. Early portable incubators were used to transport infants to hospitals that were designated to provide neonatal care, from either home or maternity hospitals. The treatments offered during transfer were limited to thermal support and supplemental oxygen, although interestingly early reports acknowledged the need for accompanying staff (invariably nurses) to have expertise in handling sick infants and administering emergency treatment while in transit.

The development of specialized neonatal intensive care units (NICUs) providing an evolving "package" of care began in **North America, Europe, and Australia in the late 1960s**. Regionalization of care[1,2] that paralleled the establishment of tertiary centers influenced the pattern of infants transported, with increases in the number of in-utero transfers, particularly in North America. The majority of these are for fetal rather than maternal reasons. It is as yet uncertain whether the more recent development of formal neonatal networks in other countries such as the UK will have similar effects on the profile of postnatal transfers. What is clear, however, is that neonatal transport services will remain an essential component of perinatal care.

In 1966, the first newborn with respiratory distress syndrome was transported to University of California San Francisco by its NICU staff, and the first recorded transport of a mother in preterm labor from another city was undertaken in 1969. Several other centers such as Phoenix, Utah, Wisconsin, and Toronto were instrumental in developing transport opportunities for newborn infants. In 1970, the Stanford/Lucile Packard Children's Hospital Neonatal Transport Program began with the development of a regional perinatal access program that initially covered several counties of **Northern California**. Transport of critically ill infants for longer than 30 minutes was not feasible because of the inability to provide life support and an adequate thermal environment. At the same time, there was clinical evidence that the transport of such infants led to a significant reduction in morbidity and mortality. A perinatal outreach program was created with the main goal of training health care providers in community hospitals in neonatal resuscitation and the pretransport early care of critically ill infants. A resource management (dispatch/communications) center was created and connected to newly formed networks of NICUs. The program expanded and a mutual relationship with a similar program in Paris, **France**,

Neonatal Emergencies: A Practical Guide for Resuscitation, Transport and Critical Care, ed. Georg Hansmann. Published by Cambridge University Press. © Cambridge University Press 2009.

led to advances in both, ultimately leading to the creation of the *California Perinatal Transport System* (http://www.perinatal.org, accessed 13 October 2008).

Neonatal intensive care practices in **Europe** – especially for very preterm infants[3,4] – vary widely, and the majority of transfer services have evolved in an ad hoc way. For example, neonatal transport services in the **northern region of the UK** developed in parallel with the establishment of the Northern Neonatal Network (1991), a collaborative consortium of tertiary-level NICUs, from an initial single regional center in Newcastle (1972) over a 20-year period. The consortium oversees that intensive care beds (UK: cots) are utilized appropriately and that return transfers are suitable. Staffing for this transfer service is a mixture of neonatal nurses and either neonatologists or pediatric/neonatal trainees. More recently paramedic neonatal transport practitioners (similar to the British Columbia model in **Canada**) have been introduced.

In 1978 a local neonatal emergency transport service (NETS) was established at the German Heart Center **Munich** in cooperation with the city's local fire department. Other cities followed so that NETS became available 24 hours a day, 7 days a week in many, but not all, regions of Germany. In the last 30 years, survival rates and outcome of critically ill neonates – not least because of NETS – have considerably improved: 3 years after the establishment of NETS in Munich, the perinatal mortality rate in the region had decreased by 50%. A more recent study from **Toronto** showed that dedicated neonatal retrieval teams significantly improve delivery room resuscitation of outborn preterm infants[5]. Such success and high quality of neonatal care can only be guaranteed by a 24-h on-call service provided by well-trained nurse practitioners (NP), nurses (RN), paramedics, midwives, and doctors (pediatricians, emergency physicians, obstetricians, and anesthesiologists). The frequency of annual NETS calls, however, is dependent on many factors, including: (1) term and preterm birth rates; (2) early antepartum transports for high-risk pregnancies; and (3) the establishment of small neonatal units in hospitals with obstetric departments (counteracting earlier efforts to centralize neonatal intensive care in tertiary centers). Hence, both limited clinical exposure and increasing requests for retrievals, such as in the UK, underline the need for ongoing training of NETS health care providers.

In the US, hospitals are classified by the **level of NICU care** available:

- No NICU: level I
- Intermediate NICU: level II
- Expanded intermediate NICU: level II+
- Tertiary NICU: level III

The American Academy of Pediatrics recommends that deliveries that occur before 32 weeks of gestation take place in level III (i.e., highly specialized) units[6], and most European countries have passed laws or issued recommendations based on this premise. However, no consensus exists in Europe about size or other criteria for NICUs[7].

- There is an abundance of literature showing a decrease in infant morbidity and mortality by maternal (i.e., prenatal) transport of high-risk pregnancies when compared to emergency transport of sick newborn infants. Hence, the best transport incubator is the uterus.
- In a recent Californian study (2007)[2], mortality among very-low-birth-weight (VLBW) infants was lowest for deliveries that occurred in hospitals with NICUs that had both a high level of care and a high volume of such patients. Increased use of such facilities most likely reduces mortality among VLBW infants[2].

- In contrast, a study from the UK (1999)[8] showed that actual survival rates for infants ≤32 weeks' gestation and for the group of babies ≤28 weeks' gestation fell within the 95% confidence interval of the rate predicted by the clinical risk index for babies (CRIB) score (see Table 2.5, page 146) for both the larger referral units and the smaller district units[8]. Given the improved levels of specialist medical and nursing input since 1987, the authors of this study feel it is plausible that differences in survival should have disappeared between both types of NICUs. However, they do see such a new structure as a potential threat to the teaching, training, and research base of the neonatal service as a whole.

Challenges of neonatal emergency transport services

For those infants requiring intensive care, the members of a transport team should be able to provide intensive care during that transfer at a quality that is similar to that in the receiving intensive care unit itself. Developments in equipment now enable the majority of intensive therapeutic measures (for example inhaled nitric oxide or extracorporeal membrane oxygenation (ECMO)) and intensive monitoring (including blood gas analysis) used within the NICU setting to be delivered during transfer. It is however important to appreciate that caring for sick infants in the transport environment poses numerous additional challenges compared to working within the NICU setting[9]. These include movement, noise, vibration, temperature, and (in the case of air transfer) changes in atmospheric pressure, all of which may adversely affect both the patient and the transport team. Access to the patient may also be poor, lighting less than optimal, and equipment relatively unfamiliar. In summary the environment is extremely stressful and potentially hostile.

For the above reasons it should be recognized that individuals who function well within the NICU environment may not function as effectively within the transport setting where additional support is not immediately available. Skills highly desirable in the transport environment therefore include both the ability to act decisively and independently in addition to solving problems in acutely stressful situations within a team setting.

Neonatal transport units may be staffed by a variety of health care professionals including physicians, nurse practitioners (NP), neonatal-trained nurses, respiratory therapists, and specialized paramedics. Paramedics have the advantage of being familiar with working in a moving environment, though they require additional training to be able to assist in delivering "hands on" care to the infant. Acutely sick infants should be transported by a minimum of two trained personnel. There are potential advantages and disadvantages with each combination of personnel: the final choice should be dictated by the clinical problems that an individual patient presents, although in reality availability and cost are also major factors. While highly specialized NP used to run neonatal transport units in North America and the UK, it is commonly medical doctors certified in neonatal emergency medicine in continental Europe.

Whatever team composition is used, its members must work effectively to:

- Deliver appropriate neonatal care within both the hospital and the transport environment
- Manage the range of anticipated problems for the types of transport undertaken
- Manage emergencies appropriately as they arise
- Communicate effectively with each other, with referring and receiving unit staff, and with the infant's family

Expectations and demands placed upon neonatal transport teams cannot be exactly the same as those experienced by NICU teams. The transport team and the obstetric staff, as well as the difficulties of individual transport situations, vary greatly in quality and quantity (e.g., equipment, transport distance). However, the priority (and challenge) for the NETS team should be to transport the neonate in optimum condition to the nearest appropriate intensive care unit.

> **!** Blood gas, blood glucose, body temperature, and transportation time – among other criteria – document the quality of care provided by the neonatal emergency transport service (NETS).

Successes in some areas of neonatal care have resulted in new problems. The improvements in survival rates have had an impact on resources, particularly intensive care bed (cot) availability, and no area of medicine is currently free from budget constraints. For example, the cost-effectiveness of senior medical personnel during "routine" neonatal transfer has been questioned. These problems are compounded by heightened public expectation of a favorable outcome for even the sickest and extreme preterm infants. It is therefore essential that neonatal transfer services continually assess the quality of service that they deliver and strive to improve. This process must include appropriate support for those who access those services.

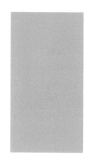

Interdisciplinary approach for neonatal emergencies

Georg Hansmann

Team work of paramedics, nurse practitioners, and neonatologists in the neonatal emergency transport service

In the neonatal emergency transport service (NETS), effective coordination between paramedics, highly specialized neonatal intensive care unit (NICU) nurses or nurse practitioners (NP), and neonatal emergency doctors (NETS-MD) is essential. The NETS-MD – especially in the first weeks in service – is well advised to take advantage of the experience of paramedics and NP, particularly in terms of transport logistics. That said, the NETS-MD, preferably with a minimum of 12 months of NICU experience, should lead the initial care/ neonatal resuscitation and subsequent transport (i.e., runs code and transport). Depending on their experience level, two paramedics or one experienced NICU nurse or NP may go with the NETS-MD to the emergency site, in order to perform initial care/neonatal resuscitation. This particularly applies to emergent deliveries of extremely premature or sick infants, or preterm twins (32 + 0/7 till 35 + 0/7 weeks' gestation), who need simultaneous initial care (see Table 1.1).

- In uncomplicated cases, the common goal is for active initial care (including neonatal resuscitation) to be provided by the least experienced paramedic, RN, NP or doctor under the supervision of highly qualified and experienced health care providers. Nobody gets better just by watching, and there is no learning by osmosis.
- If problems occur at the emergency site, e.g., after a cesarean (c-section) section of twins, the NETS-MD should either call the anesthesiologist on service for help, or, if available, additional neonatal or pediatric emergency transport services.

Team work of obstetricians, midwives, anesthesiologists, neonatal intensive care unit nurses and nurse practitioners, and neonatologists

With an increasing number of emergency calls, the new NETS team members get to know the obstetricians, midwives, and NP/RN working in each local district and county.

However, since NETS personnel may change frequently, established care providers may need to rely on their own expertise, risk aversion, and stress tolerance during decision making.

Neonatal Emergencies: A Practical Guide for Resuscitation, Transport and Critical Care, ed. Georg Hansmann.
Published by Cambridge University Press. © Cambridge University Press 2009.

Table 1.1 Suggestions on how to coordinate a neonatal transport right after an emergency call.

Gestational age (weeks p.m.)/birth weight	Emergency transport of pregnant women	Personnel needed in the delivery room/OR	Take with you from NICU (plus standard equipment)	Admitting unit
<28+0/7 or <1000 g	Yes, if possible	1 (–2) pediatrician(s) (call for additional NETS, if needed!) + 2 experienced Peds-MD (alternative: 1 PARAM + 1 RN/NP)	1 vial of surfactant, straight blades (size 00), ET tubes (size 2.0 and 2.5), preterm ECG electrodes	NICU
<28+0/7 or <1000 g, and twins	Yes, if possible	2 (–4) pediatricians (ask for additional NETS) + 2 experienced Peds-MD (alternative: 1 PARAM + 1 RN/NP)	2 vials of surfactant, 2 straight blades (size 00), ET tubes (size 2.0 and 2.5), preterm ECG electrodes	NICU
28+0/7 to 32+0/7 or 1000–1500 g	Yes, if possible	2 pediatricians (or: 1 pediatrician and 1 RN/NP) + 1 senior PARAM (alternative: 1 RN)	1 vial of surfactant, straight blades (size 00), ET tubes (size 2.5), preterm ECG electrodes	NICU
28+0/7 to 32+0/7 or 1000–1500 g and twins	Yes, if possible	2 (–4) pediatricians (eventually call for NETS-MD) + 1 senior PARAM/NP/RN + 1 PARAM (or: 1 PARAM + 1 RN/NP)	2 vials of surfactant, straight blades (size 00), ET tubes (size 2.5), preterm ECG electrodes	NICU
32+0/7 to 35+0/7 or 1500–2500 g	If applicable	1 pediatrician + 1 PARAM (or + 1 RN/NP)	Preterm ECG electrodes	see p. 179
32+0/7 to 35+0/7 or 1500–2500 g and twins	If applicable	1 pediatrician and 1 senior PARAM/NP/RN + 1 PARAM (or 1 pediatrician + 1 RN/NP + 1 PARAM; optimum 2 pediatricians + 2 PARAM/NP/RN)	Preterm ECG electrodes	see p. 179
>35+0/7 or >2500 g	Normally no	When indicated (see p. 179): 1 pediatrician/MD + 1 PARAM (or: 1 NP/RN)	Standard equipment	see p. 179
>35+0/7 or >2500 g and twins	Normally no	1 (–2) pediatrician/MD, 2 senior PARAM (or: 1 pediatrician + 1 NP/RN + 1 PARAM; optimum: 2 pediatricians + 2 PARAM/RN/NP)	Standard equipment	see p. 179

Suspected congenital heart disease	Yes (elective)	1 pediatrician + 2 PARAM/NP/RN (or: 1 PARAM + 1 NP/RN)	1 vial PGE$_1$	Pediatric Heart Center
Suspected hemorrhage/asphyxia	No	1 pediatrician and 1 senior PARAM + 1 PARAM (or 1 pediatrician and 1 NP/RN; optimum: 2 pediatricians + 1 PARAM/NP/RN)	Type O rhesus-negative blood, as indicated; prepare 50 ml volume (NS, human albumin 5%) with tubing and store in an incubator (37°C)	NICU
Anticipated hypoxic ischemic encephalopathy	No	1 pediatrician and 1 senior PARAM + 1 PARAM (or 1 pediatrician and 1 NP/RN; optimum: 2 pediatricians + 1 PARAM/NP/RN)	Eventually cooling device (cap or blanket); safety and efficacy data on cooling during transport limited	NICU

Estimated birth weight and calculated weeks of gestational age post menstruation (p.m.) may be inaccurate. Hence, the birth weight range given in the table is between the 10th and 50th percentile of the corresponding gestational age. Always assume that the NETS-MD emergency bag is incomplete (e.g. surfactant, ET tubes 2.0 for birth weights <750 g and small larynx, straight blades 00; preterm ECG electrodes, plastic wrap/bag), and take drugs you might need with you in a cooling mini case (e.g. surfactant, PGE$_1$). While 2 pediatricians would be favorable for the management of singletons of 28–32 weeks' gestation in the delivery room, this is rarely achieved in a real-life NETS emergency call. Resuscitations of those preterm and SGA infants are generally well manageable by a team of 1 pediatrician plus 1 experienced NP, RN or PARAM. However, depending on the status of the neonate and additional risk factors, the attendance of a second pediatrician may be indicated, regardless of the birth weight and gestational age, and even in the absence of multiple gestations. MD, medical doctor; NP, nurse practitioner; PARAM, paramedic; RN, registered nurse; PGE$_1$, prostaglandin E$_1$; peds-MD, pediatrician.

The in-patient doctor in charge is responsible for clinical assessment and urgent treatment of the fetus or newborn in the delivery room. When the newborn shows signs of postnatal deterioration, the midwife or nurse informs the obstetrician (or pediatrician – if available), who must then decide whether to notify the NETS team.

! General guidelines
- Call the NETS with your initial concerns (don't wait until the fetal heart sounds or SpO_2 and blood gas are really bad). Call too early rather than too late!.
- Immediate and appropriate neonatal resuscitation by obstetricians, anesthesiologists, NP, RN, and midwives is essential for a good outcome of the neonate. The obstetrician or anesthesiologist on service carries full responsibility while awaiting the NETS.
- Pregnant women in labor with additional risk factors must be transported immediately to a tertiary perinatal center. If prepartal transport is no longer possible, call the pediatrician/ NETS as soon as possible.

Interdisciplinary training workshops, unlike the less hands-on neonatal emergency seminars, are still rare (e.g., Center for Advanced Pediatric and Perinatal Education at www.lpch.org/cape/, and American Academy of Pediatrics at www.aap.org/nrp). This handbook has an interdisciplinary approach (obstetrics, anesthesiology, neonatology, emergency medicine). Its overall goals include maximizing efficiency and optimal care for just-delivered infants prior to and after arrival of the NETS (see pp. 9–15, pp. 124–72, and p. 511).

Principles of crisis resource management (CRM)

1. Know your environment
2. Anticipate and plan for crises
3. Assume a leadership role
4. Communicate effectively
5. Call for help early enough
6. Distribute workload optimally
7. Allocate attention wisely
8. Utilize all available resources
9. Utilize all available information
10. Maintain professional behavior

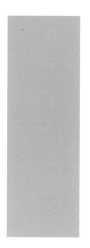

Neonatal emergency call: what the neonatology team would like to know from obstetricians and midwives

Georg Hansmann

Important information for the neonatal emergency transport service

- Name and role of the person calling doctor, midwife, nurse practitioner, neonatal intensive care unit nurse
- Name and location of referring hospital
- Indication for referral (i.e., emergency call), for example:
  - "Emergency cesarean section (C-section) due to pathological cardiotocogram/fetal heart sounds," or
  - "Transfer of newborn for evaluation of nasal flaring and gray skin color, etc."
- Time and place of birth, for example:
  - "Plan urgent C-section in 30 min, operating room (OR) no. 3, second floor," or
  - "C-section in delivery room 2, first floor"
- Gestational age in postmenstrual weeks
- Estimate of lung maturity
- Antenatal corticosteroids given? Yes/no, when, how many doses, how far apart?
- Birth weight (prenatal estimation or postnatal weight), small/large for gestational age (SGA/LGA)
- Rupture of membranes (ROM) (≥ 18 hours before birth?), mother with signs of infection (high white blood cell count, C-reactive protein, fever, fetal tachycardia, uterine tenderness)? Bacterial smears, blood cultures taken? Antibiotic treatment – yes/no, when started, how many doses? Color/smell of the amniotic fluid? Maternal risk factors (group B streptococcus status, antibiotic coverage $> 4\,h$, ROM $> 18\,h$, herpes simplex virus lesions, etc.)
- High-risk pregnancy (see p. 231, pp. 504–5)?, e.g. impending preterm delivery:
  - Can the pregnant woman be transferred to a hospital with a tertiary neonatal intensive care unit?
  - Arterial hypertension/preeclampsia/HELLP syndrome (hemolysis, elevated liver enzymes plus low platelet count)
  - Diabetes mellitus?

Neonatal Emergencies: A Practical Guide for Resuscitation, Transport and Critical Care, ed. Georg Hansmann.
Published by Cambridge University Press. © Cambridge University Press 2009.

- - Vaginal bleeding/placental anomaly?
  - Pathological cardiotocogram/fetal heart sounds?
  - Fetus SGA?
  - Previous miscarriages or premature births?
  - Prenatal diagnosis (malformations, amniocentesis/chromosomes)?
- If the birth has taken place:
  - Grunting, retractions, nasal flaring?
  - Skin color?
  - SO_2 per pulse oximeter (S_pO_2)?
  - Oxygen requirement (F_iO_2)?
  - Blood gases (arterial, capillary, venous, umbilical arterial pH)?
  - Blood glucose?
  - Body temperature?
  - Malformations/deformities?
- In case of life-threatening neonatal condition:
  - Who is currently performing the resuscitation of the newborn infant?
  - Is a pediatrician or anesthesiologist at the bedside or readily available?
- Is any incubator or cot with radiant warmer organized in the NICU?

! If the complete information has not been obtained at the time of the emergency call, the NETS-MD/-NP should be provided with all necessary information on arrival. If the midwife does not have enough time to gather all relevant data (e.g., due to an approaching C-section), help must be provided by the midwife/nursery staff to: (1) obtain all birth-related information; and (2) to check on or even prepare the resuscitation unit for immediate use (e.g., running suctioning, oxygen source, and radiant warmer "on"; see checklist p. 136). Information can often be obtained by a transport operator/clerk while the team is being dispatched. The resuscitation unit should be functional at all times; daily checks by the staff in charge of the delivery room are mandatory.

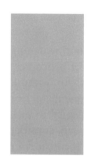

Coordinating health care providers after a neonatal emergency call

Georg Hansmann

Questions that need to be clarified by the neonatologist after an emergency call include (see Table 1.1):

- Is this a life-threatening situation for the newborn infant?
  - yes/no/likely/possibly
- Is one physician/NP sufficient to manage the initial care/resuscitation of the preterm or term infant?

This decision depends on the following:

- Training and experience of the NETS-MD/-NP
- Possible presence of a pediatrician/neonatologist at the site
- Assembly of the NETS team members (NP, paramedic, RN, MD)
- Clinical presentation (prematurity, multiple gestation, ongoing advanced resuscitation?)

In the case of preterm infants <1000 g or <28 weeks' gestation, as well as preterm twins <1500 g or <32 weeks' gestation, generally two NETS-MD highly experienced in neonatal intensive care should be present in the delivery room or operating room. At night, during weekends and holidays, however, it is unlikely that a second pediatrician/NETS-MD is readily available. In this case, the physician in charge should request either a second NETS-MD or a second pediatric emergency MD from the emergency call center/dispatcher. If necessary, an ambulance equipped with a transport incubator or – if available – a specially equipped NETS ambulance should be sent directly to the referring hospital. Twins without ventilatory support may be transported in one incubator. In the case of twin births with an (estimated) birth weight of 1500–2500 g or twins of full 32 weeks' to 35 weeks' gestation, the NETS-MD may consider taking a NETS-NP or an experienced NICU nurse on this particular neonatal transport (based on the experience and training of the local paramedics). Depending on the clinical presentation and perinatal risk factors, even infants in this "weight/immaturity class" may need the attendance of a second pediatrician/neonatologist, regardless of the multiplicity of gestation.

Information sharing in perinatal emergencies

- "Name of caller" (i.e., usually the MD in charge), then "… needs NETS ambulance urgently/as soon as possible to pick up the NETS-MD/-NP from hospital A, to proceed to the birth hospital B in XX (location)," eventually "NICU bed at YY hospital is available"
- If indicated (see above): request a second NETS-MD, pediatric ambulance or second ambulance with a portable incubator

Neonatal Emergencies: A Practical Guide for Resuscitation, Transport and Critical Care, ed. Georg Hansmann.
Published by Cambridge University Press. © Cambridge University Press 2009.

- If the estimated transportation time is longer than 30 min *and* a life-threatening condition exists for the newborn, consider airborne emergency transport (jet/helicopter) (see p. 501); i.e., helicopter with or without a transport incubator, with or without MD/paramedic/RN/NP. If the ambulance (equipped with the transport incubator) or the NETS ambulance is not available, hindered or cannot arrive at the hospital to pick up the NETS-MD/-NP within a maximum of 15 min after the emergency call, consider picking up the NETS-MD/-NP with a standard ambulance (i.e., without incubator) or with a helicopter (without incubator, e.g., helicopter from police or fire department). The helicopter or ambulance without MD/NP then meets the NETS team/NETS-MD/-NP at the site of the emergency ("rendezvous-system"). Fixed-wing (aeroplane) transport is an alternative, however, it usually takes considerably longer because of the hospital-to-airport journey.

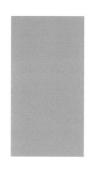

What the neonatologist would like to find in the delivery room

Georg Hansmann

The 4 "S" of a prepared resuscitation unit: **S**uctioning, **S**upplemental oxygen, **S**pecified temperature, and **S**afety

The NETS team expects a well organized and functional resuscitation unit (p. 13 and pp. 25–40), i.e.:

- **Suction** running (at -200 mbar ≈ -2.9 psi ≈ -80 in H_2O), catheter size usually Ch 10 = 10 F; for preemies use: Ch 8 (= 8 F) or Ch 6 (= 6 F)
- **Oxygen**:
  - Flow 5 l/min for self-inflating bags, 8–10 l/min for flow-inflating bags (= "floppy anesthesia bags"); free-flowing O_2 delivery may be less reliable with self-inflating bags
  - Oxygen blender must be available: begin with room air (F_iO_2 0.21) (increase in 20 percent-point increments up to 100% = F_iO_2 1.0, as needed)
  - Pressure manometer is needed to monitor and avoid inadvertently high peak inspiratory pressures and tidal volumes
- **Connected and tested bag-and-mask-system**, i.e., self-inflating bag with reservoir (e.g., "model infant," 250-ml bag, Laerdal), positive end-expiratory pressure (PEEP) and pop-off valves (maximum PIP $\approx$ 40 cmH$_2$O); round silicon ventilation masks (e.g., sizes 00 or 01; preemies/SGA 00)
  - Alternatives: (1) flow-inflating bags (also called anesthesia bags, or Kuhn systems) with PEEP valve; or (2) T-piece/continuous positive airway pressure (CPAP)/ positive pressure ventilation (PPV) equipment (e.g., "Tom-Thumb," "Perivent," "Neo-Puff")
- **Intubation equipment** (laryngoscope with straight blade size 0–1, endotracheal tube (ETT) size 2.0–3.5, stylets)
- **Radiant warmers**, set to "maximum" prior to NETS arrival (adjust after delivery), six to eight prewarmed soft cotton blankets/towels (two under the radiant warmer on the resuscitation unit, four to six blankets/towels within reach, but stored in a closed cabinet at 37°C (98.6°F). Resuscitation units are unfortunately often placed in rooms that facilitate rapid heat loss (due to repeated opening and closing of doors, the presence of tiles and windows, or a room temperature <25°C, 77°F). Warm soft cotton blankets/ towels are preferred

Neonatal Emergencies: A Practical Guide for Resuscitation, Transport and Critical Care, ed. Georg Hansmann.
Published by Cambridge University Press. © Cambridge University Press 2009.

- A well-secured **resuscitation unit** with side walls and light, equipped with enough compressed-air, an oxygen blender and an oxygen supply (wall outlet or O_2 cylinder), and an efficient (i.e., leak-proof) bag-and-mask system, various sizes of **suction catheters**, UV/UA catheter kit, peripheral intravenous (PIV) access kits
- Functional **monitoring** (S_pO_2, ECG, blood pressure cuffs, temperature probe)
- Rapid access to O-Rhesus-negative, lysine-free, packed red blood cells (PRBC, 200-ml bag) and one vial of surfactant (most surfactant drugs come in liquid form and must be refrigerated)
- Good documentation by the midwife of the birth hospital: partly filled out transfer protocol of the referring hospital providing the following information:
    - Name of mother, correct family name of the newborn infant
    - Exact date and time of birth (if delivery has already occurred)
    - Health insurance
    - Gestational age
    - Estimated fetal weight
    - Fetal position
    - Diagnoses of mother and additional risk factors (e.g., drug abuse, methadone program)
    - Maternal blood type and prenatal labs such as HBSAg (if known: human immuno-deficiency virus (HIV), cytomegalovirus (CMV) status etc.)
    - Indication for induced/surgical delivery

! An obstetric department without rapid access to O-rhesus-negative PRBCs and without surfactant is like a football team without any players on the bench … one will not make it through the season without disasters.

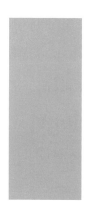

What the neonatologist does not want to find in the delivery room

Georg Hansmann

- A resuscitation unit that does not work
- An obstetrician who continues discussing the "1-min Apgar score" at 3 a.m. despite efficient and successful delivery and newborn care
- A nursery lacking a device for measuring blood glucose (Dextrostix)
- A hypothermic and hypoxic infant without oxygen supplementation but large amounts of fluid in the oropharynx (caution: 4 "S", p. 14).
- A pale neonate (±grayish skin color) that is tachypneic, has nasal flaring or subcostal retractions for hours is probably dehydrated, and supplemented with oxygen but without adequate monitoring (pulse oximetry for S_pO_2 and heart rate monitoring, blood glucose and blood gas sampling, blood pressure)

> **!** Blood gas, blood glucose, body temperature, and transportation time document severity of illness and quality of care provided by the NETS and the obstetric team.

Neonatal Emergencies: A Practical Guide for Resuscitation, Transport and Critical Care, ed. Georg Hansmann.
Published by Cambridge University Press. © Cambridge University Press 2009.

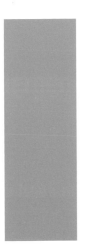

Definitions and abbreviations in neonatology, pediatric cardiology, neonatal emergency transport service (NETS), and obstetrics

Georg Hansmann

Table 1.2 Definitions and abbreviations in evidence-based medicine, neonatology, pediatric cardiology, neonatal emergency transport service, and obstetrics

Evidence-based medicine

COR, Class	Class of Recommendation:
	Class I: *absolutely indicated* (always acceptable, proven safe, definitely useful)
	Class IIa: *standard* of care or intervention of choice (acceptable, safe, useful)
	Class IIb: within the standard of care or an *optional* or alternative intervention (acceptable, safe, useful)
	Class indeterminate: *preliminary* research stage with promising results but insufficient evidence available
	Class III: *unacceptable* (no documented evidence, may be harmful)
LOE, Level	Level of Evidence:
	LOE 1: *Randomized clinical trials* or meta-analyses of multiple clinical trials with substantial treatment effects
	LOE 2: *Randomized clinical trials* with smaller or fewer significant treatment effects
	LOE 3: *Prospective*, controlled, non-randomized cohort studies
	LOE 4: *Historic*, non-randomized, cohort or case-control studies
	LOE 5: *Case series*: patients compiled in series fashion, lacking a control group
	LOE 6: Animal studies or mechanical model studies
	LOE 7: Extrapolations from existing data collected for other purposes, theoretical analyses
	LOE 8: Rational conjecture (*common sense*); common practices accepted before evidence-based guidelines
RCT	Randomized controlled trial

Abbreviations in clinical scenarios

Def.	Definition
Syn.	Synonyms

Neonatal Emergencies: A Practical Guide for Resuscitation, Transport and Critical Care, ed. Georg Hansmann.
Published by Cambridge University Press. © Cambridge University Press 2009.

Table 1.2 (cont.)

Epidem.	Epidemiology
Etiol.	Etiology, cause
PPh.	Pathophysiology
Clin. pres.	Clinical presentations (i.e., signs, symptoms)
DDx	Differential diagnosis
$t_{1/2}$	Pharmacokinetic half-life of drugs
Proc.	Procedure
Neonatology	
Asphyxia	"Pulselessness" (Greek). Diagnosis: • Clinical presentation: extremely abnormal postnatal transition with cardiac arrest or severe bradycardia, apnea, cyanosis or pallor, and unconsciousness (5-min Apgar score: 0–3) AND • Severe umbilical artery acidosis: pH <7.00 AND • Organ damage with possible sequelae: renal failure, seizures, hypoxic-ischemic encephalopathy (HIE) (definition by Carter et al., 1993)[10] Some neonatologists avoid the term "asphyxia"
Neonatal period	The first 28 days of life
Perinatal period	28 + 0 gestational weeks up to the completed 7th day of life (several definitions exist: range 20 + 0 gestational weeks to 7th or 28th day of life)
Live birth	Bearing signs of life: spontaneous breathing, heart beat, pulsation of umbilical cord or active movement of muscles
Still birth	The CDC definition of "fetal death" is based on the definition promulgated by the WHO in 1950: "Fetal death means death prior to the complete expulsion or extraction from its mother of a product of human conception, irrespective of the duration of pregnancy and which is not an induced termination of pregnancy. The death is indicated by the fact that after such expulsion or extraction, the fetus does not breathe or show any other evidence of life, such as beating of the heart, pulsation of the umbilical cord, or definite movement of voluntary muscles. Heart beats are to be distinguished from transient cardiac contractions; respirations are to be distinguished from fleeting respiratory efforts or gasps." Both miscarriage and stillbirth are terms describing pregnancy loss (fetal death), but they differ according to when the loss occurs. The distinction between both is arbitrary. The dividing line is variously set at 20–24 weeks of gestation. Before that time it is a miscarriage (also called a spontaneous abortion). After that time it is a stillbirth. UK: The Stillbirth Definition Act (1992) requires that any "child" expelled or issued forth from its mother after the 24th week of pregnancy that did not breathe or show any other signs of life be registered as a stillbirth USA: A miscarriage (or spontaneous abortion) usually refers to a pregnancy loss before 20 weeks of gestation, and a stillbirth refers to a loss after 20 weeks. If the age is not known, then a baby weighing 350 g or more is considered a stillbirth. Stillbirths are further classified as early, late, term, or post-term (CDC definition) Canada: In 2001, most provinces and all three territories required a stillbirth with a gestational age of at least 20 weeks or a birth weight of at least 500 g to be registered In Australia any stillborn fetus weighing more than 400 g, or being more than 20 weeks in gestation, must have its birth registered
Perinatal mortality	Still birth and death during the first 7 days of life in 1000 live births
Gestational age (GA)	Duration of pregnancy, calculated from the date of last menstrual period in complete weeks of gestation plus days
Term neonate (FT)	Gestational age 37 0/7 weeks to 41 6/7 weeks
Preterm neonate (PT)	Gestational age <37 0/7 weeks
Post term neonate	Gestational age ≥42 0/7 weeks

17

Table 1.2 (cont.)

Large for gestational age (LGA)	Birth weight >90th percentile
Appropriate for gestational age (APA)	Birth weight between 10th and 90th percentile
Small for gestational age (SGA)	Birth weight <10th percentile
Low-birth-weight infant (LBW)	Birth weight <2500 g
Very-low-birth-weight infant (VLBW)	Birth weight <1500 g
Extremely-low-birth-weight infant (ELBW)	Birth weight <1000 g
aEEG	Amplitude-integrated electroencephalography (also called cerebral functioning monitoring)
BP	Blood pressure
BG (ABG, CBG, VBG)	Blood gases (A arterial, C capillary, V venous)
BPD	Bronchopulmonary dysplasia (see CLD)
BW, BWt	Birth weight
DIC	Disseminated intravascular coagulation
PIV	Peripheral intravenous (access)
CLD	Chronic lung disease
ET or ETT	Endotracheal tube
TTTS (syn. FFTS)	Twin-twin (= feto-fetal) transfusion syndrome
PRBC	Packed red blood cells
FIRS	Fetal inflammatory response syndrome
HR	Heart rate
HIE	Hypoxic-ischemic encephalopathy
UTI	Urinary tract infection
PVL	Periventricular leukomalacia
ICH	Intracranial hemorrhage: germinal-matrix hemorrhage (GMH) or intraventricular hemorrhage (IVH) or parenchymal hemorrhage
GMH	Germinal-matrix hemorrhage
IVH	Intraventricular hemorrhage
ICU	Intensive care unit
SEH	Subependymal hemorrhage (IVH grade I)
LP	Lumbar puncture
MAP	Mean arterial pressure (Pāw)
MAS	Meconium aspiration syndrome
NEC	Necrotizing enterocolitis
NICU	Neonatal intensive care unit US hospitals are ranked as follows: • No NICU: level I • Intermediate NICU: level II • Expanded intermediate NICU: level II+ • Tertiary NICU: level III In some countries, level I indicates the highest level of care

Table 1.2 (*cont.*)

NSVD	Normal spontaneous vaginal delivery
UAC	Umbilical artery catheter
UVC	Umbilical vein catheter
AE	Adverse effects
O.I.	Oxygenation index; O.I. $= (F_iO_2 \times \bar{P}_{aw} \times 100) \div P_aO_2$ ($\bar{P}_{aw}$ = mean airway pressure). An O.I. value of >40 over 2 h brings a mortality risk rate of $>80\%$ and is an indication for ECMO treatment. Use P_aO_2 in mmHg not kPa
F_iO_2	Fraction of inspired oxygen = the percentage of oxygen in the inspired gas in decimals
PEEP	Positive end-expiratory pressure
PIP	Peak inspiratory pressure
CPAP, N-CPAP	Continuous positive airway pressure; nasal CPAP
PTT	Partial thromboplastin time
AT III	Antithrombin III
INR	International Normalized Ratio
PIE	Pulmonary interstitial emphysema
RDS	Respiratory distress syndrome
CXR	Chest X-ray
ROP	Retinopathy of prematurity
SIRS	Septic inflammatory response syndrome
TTN	Transient tachypnea of the newborn (syn.: wet lung)
Infant	Infant (29 days to 12 months of life)
DI	Drug interactions, also: diabetes insipidus
DDH	Developmental dysplasia of the hip (formerly called congenital dysplasia of the hip)

Neonatology/Pediatric Cardiology

ALCAPA syndrome	Anomalous origin of left coronary artery from pulmonary artery (syn.: Bland – White – Garland syndrome)
AoVS (or AS)	Aortic valve stenosis
AR (AI)	Aortic regurgitation (incompetence, insufficiency)
AS	Aortic stenosis
ASD	Atrial septal defect
BAS	Balloon atrial septostomy (also called Rashkind procedure): interventional enlargement of atrial shunt (ASD, PFO)
CAVSD (also CAVC)	Complete atrioventricular septal defect, complete atrioventricular canal
CHD	Congenital heart disease (previously also congenital hip dislocation that is now called DDH or developmental dysplasia of the hip)
CHF	Congestive heart failure
CO, CI	Cardiac output (l/min), cardiac index ($l \cdot min^{-1} \cdot m^{-2}$)
CoA	Coarctation of aorta (aortic isthmus stenosis)
DORV	Double-outlet right ventricle
ECHO	Echocardiography (transthoracic), TEE – transesophageal echocardiography
ECM	External cardiac massage (terminology more common in UK than US)

Table 1.2 (*cont.*)

HLHS	Hypoplastic left heart syndrome
IAA	Interrupted aortic arch
LA	Left atrium
LAH	Left atrial hypertrophy
LV	Left ventricle
LVH	Left ventricular hypertrophy
LVOTO	Left ventricular outflow tract obstruction
MAP	Mean arterial pressure
MI	Myocardial infarction; also, mitral insufficiency
MR	Mitral regurgitation (insufficiency)
MS	Mitral stenosis
PA	Pulmonary atresia or pulmonary artery
PAP	Pulmonary artery pressure
PaVA (PA)	Pulmonary valve atresia
PaVS (PS)	Pulmonary valve stenosis
PCPC	Partial cavo-pulmonary connection (syn.: bidirectional Glenn operation)
PCWP	Pulmonary capillary wedge pressure
P-CVICU	Pediatric cardiovascular intensive care unit, i.e., pediatric unit with sufficient expertise and resources including right and left catheterization laboratory and in-house pediatric cardiovascular surgery team
PICU	Pediatric intensive care unit
PS	Pulmonary stenosis (valvar, sub- and supravalvar)
PDA	Patent ductus arteriosus, patent arterial duct
PFO	Patent foramen ovale
PR, PI	Pulmonary regurgitation (incompetence, insufficiency)
PPHN	Persistent pulmonary hypertension of the newborn (old syn.: persistent fetal circulation = PFC)
PVR	Pulmonary vascular resistance = transpulmonary pressure gradient (TPG) divided by the pulmonary blood flow (QP). The "hybrid" vascular resistance unit, the Wood unit, is defined in $mmHg \cdot l^{-1} \cdot min^{-1}$, and is used in pediatric hemodynamic calculations. Formula: $PVR = (PAP_{mean} - LAP_{mean}) \div Q_P$. The result is said to be in Wood units. The conversion to metric units is as follows: vascular resistance (dyne × s/cm^5) = Wood units × 80. In pediatric patients Wood units are indexed to body surface area ($mmHg \cdot l^{-1} \cdot min^{-1} \cdot m^{-2}$). Normal PVR in the neonatal period is <3 indexed Wood units (<240 dyne × s/cm^5)
RA	Right atrium
RAH	Right atrial hypertrophy
RV	Right ventricle
RVH	Right ventricular hypertrophy
RVOTO	Right ventricular outflow tract obstruction
SVR	Systemic vascular resistance
SVT	Supraventricular tachycardia
TA	Tricuspid atresia
TAC	Truncus arteriosus communis

Table 1.2 (*cont.*)

TAPVC	Total anomalous pulmonary venous connection
TAPVR	Total anomalous pulmonary venous return
TCPC	Total cavo-pulmonary connection (syn.: modified Fontan operation)
TGA	Transposition of the great arteries
TR, TI	Tricuspid regurgitation (incompetence, insufficiency)
ToF	Tetralogy of Fallot
TS	Tricuspid stenosis
VSD	Ventricular septal defect

Neonatal transport team on call

PETS	Pediatric emergency transport service
NETS	Neonatal emergency transport service
PARAM	Paramedic
RN	Registered nurse
NP	Nurse practitioner
NNP	Neonatal nurse practitioner
ANNP	Advanced neonatal nurse practitioner

Obstetrics

NSVD, "normal spontaneous vaginal delivery"	Anticipate delivery soon if: • Spotting • Regular painful contractions every 15–20 min • Premature rupture of membranes
Stage of dilatation = first stage of labor	Begins with regular contractions (every 3–6 min) and ends with the complete dilatation of the opening of uterus. Woman has no urge to push • Length: nulliparae 12 ± 4 hours, multiparae 7 ± 4 hours • C-section should be considered when there is no progress (i.e., no active phase of activity with cervix dilatation of 1.5 cm/h) even under induced labor (with oxytocin drip)
Stage of expulsion (delivery) = second stage of labor	Begins with the full dilation of the cervix (approx. 10 cm) and ends with the birth of the child. Pushing contractions for 1 min every 2–3 min Active pushing in accordance with contractions is supportive for the mother • Length: nulliparae 30–60 min, multiparae (rarely only 5 min) 20–30 min. The stage of expulsion is often prolonged in case of lumbar epidural anesthesia • If labor takes longer than 60 min (max. 120 min for nulliparae) → re-evaluate for an operative delivery • The second stage of labor is the period during which the baby is at greatest risk for hypoxia
Afterbirth = third stage of labor	Begins after the birth of the child and ends with the birth of the placenta. The placental detachment is induced by contraction of the empty uterus • Physiologic blood loss: 200–400 ml • Length: 10–30 min. Eventually manual support (e.g., Credé maneuver) and careful tugging of umbilical cord by an experienced midwife • Oxytocin to prevent bleeding in at-risk pregnancies • Prostaglandins or methylergometrin to treat uterine atony and uterine bleeding
EDC or EDD	Estimated date of confinement (delivery)
EFM	Electronic fetal heart rate monitoring (*see* CTG)
FBS	Fetal blood sample, also: fasting blood sugar

Table 1.2 (*cont.*)

FHR	Fetal heart rate
FHT	Fetal heart tones
CTG	Cardiotocogram (fetal heart rate recording)
Silent CTG	Absent oscillation of fetal heart rate • Warning signs!
Decelerations, early (also called Dip 1)	*Early decelerations* in the CTG (electronic fetal monitoring, EFM): • Short contractions which are synchronized with decrease of fetal heart rate • Not pathognomic for fetal risk
Decelerations, late (also called Dip 2)	*Late decelerations* in the CTG (electronic fetal monitoring, EFM): • Decrease of fetal heart rate, which occurs with the beginning of contractions and has its lowest point after the peak of contractions • Suspected utero-placental insufficiency • Warning signs!
Variable decelerations	Combination of Dip 1 and Dip 2 in the CTG • Suspected: complication of umbilical cord • Warning signs!
Prolonged decelerations	Continuous deep decelerations over minutes, e.g., maternal hypotension, continuous contractions, etc.
FBG	Fetal blood pH and gases: micro blood samples obtained from the fetal presenting part: pathologic pH <7.20 (in some references pathologic pH <7.25)
FBS, MBU	Fetal blood sample, micro blood sampling (usually the fetal scalp), *see* FBG; pathologic pH <7.20 (in some references pathologic pH <7.25)
PUBS	Percutaneous umbilical cord blood sampling
CO	Cervical opening; also: cardiac output
SVD	Spontaneous vaginal delivery
UC pH	Umbilical cord blood pH value: • Obtained from the umbilical artery (if from umbilical vein, then pH falsely high!) • Pathologic UA pH value <7.15 or <7.20 (depending on literature)
UA pH	Umbilical arterial pH value: • Pathologic if <7.15 or 7.20 (depending on reference literature)
GA	Gestational age in weeks after the first day of the last menstrual period
U/S	Ultrasound
BW, BWt	Birth weight
IAP	Intrapartum antimicrobial prophylaxis
IUGR	Intrauterine growth retardation (expected weight by U/S <10th percentile)
SGA	Small for gestational age: <10th percentile
LGA	Large for gestational age: >90th percentile
LBW	Low birth weight <2500 g
VLBW	Very low birth weight: <1500 g
ELBW	Extremely low birth weight: <1000 g
Full-term, term infant	Full-term/ near-term neonate, 37–42 completed gestational weeks (37+0 to 42+0 weeks p.m.)
PB	Preterm baby, i.e., preterm newborn infant <37+0 GA in weeks
AIS	Amniotic infection syndrome (also: intra-amniotic infection, amniotic fluid infection syndrome) syn. chorioamnionitis

Table 1.2 (*cont.*)

OCT	Oxytocin challenge test
ROM	Rupture of membranes: • Classical def. of premature ROM: rupture of membranes without uterine contractions • Prolonged rupture of membranes >18 h (and >24 h) before birth. If ROM occurs >18 h before birth, the risk for GBS sepsis increases. Neonatologists refer to the time interval mentioned above. The term *early* rupture of the membranes means ROM under contractions but cervical dilatation <10 cm, i.e., before complete dilation of the cervix (another definition: ROM at dilation of cervix <6 cm)
PROM	Premature rupture of membranes: rupture of membranes without uterine contractions
PPROM	Prolonged premature rupture of membranes
AF	Amniotic fluid
MSAF	Meconium-stained amniotic fluid
GBS	Group B streptococci
HBsAg	Hepatitis B surface antigen
HELLP syndrome	Hemolysis, elevated liver enzymes, low platelet count, proteinuria, with hypertension in 90%, eventually renal insufficiency and DIC
VE	Vacuum extraction
FD	Forceps delivery
C-section	Cesarean section
SinciP	Sinciput presentation
VertexP	Vertex presentation
BreechP	Breech presentation, pelvic presentation

Table 1.2 is compiled from:

Rennie JM, Robertson NRC. *Robertson's Textbook of Neonatology*, 4th Edn. Edinburgh, Churchill Livingstone, 2005.

Gomella T. *Management, Procedures, On-Call Problems, Diseases and Drugs*, 5th edn. New York, Lange Medical Books/McGraw-Hill, 2004.

Niermeyer S, Kattwinkel J, Van Reempts P, *et al.* International Guidelines for Neonatal Resuscitation: An Excerpt from the Guidelines 2000 for Cardiopulmonary Resuscitation and Emergency Cardiovascular Care: International Consensus on Science. *Pediatrics* 2000; *106*(3): E29 (http://pediatrics.aappublications.org/cgi/reprint/106/3/e29, accessed 21 October 2008).

2005 International Consensus on Cardiopulmonary Resuscitation and Emergency Cardiovascular Care Science with Treatment Recommendations. Part 1: introduction. *Resuscitation* 2005; *67*(2–3): 181–6.

2005 International Consensus on Cardiopulmonary Resuscitation and Emergency Cardiovascular Care Science with Treatment Recommendations. Part 7: Neonatal resuscitation. *Resuscitation* 2005; *67*(2–3): 293–303.

References (Section 1)

1. Lucey JF. Why we should regionalize perinatal care. *Pediatrics* 1973; **52**(4): 488–91.

2. Phibbs CS, Baker LC, Caughey AB, Danielsen B, Schmitt SK, Phibbs RH. Level and volume of neonatal intensive care and mortality in very-low-birth-weight infants. *N Engl J Med* 2007; **356**(21): 2165–75.

3. European Network for Perinatal Transport. Maternal and Neonatal Transport in Europe. Report of the European Network for Perinatal Transport (EUROPET). *Prenat Neonatal Med* 1999; **4** (Suppl 1).

4. Zeitlin J, Papiernik E, Breart G. Regionalization of perinatal care in Europe. *Semin Neonatol* 2004; **9**(2): 99–110.

5. McNamara PJ, Mak W, Whyte HE. Dedicated neonatal retrieval teams improve delivery room resuscitation of outborn premature infants. *J Perinatol* 2005; **25**(5): 309–14.

6. Stark AR. Levels of neonatal care. *Pediatrics* 2004; **114**(5): 1341–7.

7. Van Reempts P, Gortner L, Milligan D, *et al.* Characteristics of neonatal units that care for very preterm infants in Europe: results from the MOSAIC study. *Pediatrics* 2007; **120**(4): e815–25.

8. Field D, Draper ES. Survival and place of delivery following preterm birth: 1994–96. *Arch Dis Child Fetal Neonatal Ed* 1999; **80**(2): F111–14.

9. Woodward GA, Insoft RM, Kleinman ME, Alexander SN. *Guidelines for Air and Ground Transport of Neonatal and Pediatric Patients*, 3rd edn. Elk Grove Village, Section on Transport Medicine, American Academy of Pediatrics, 2007.

10. Carter BS, Haverkamp AD, Merenstein GB. The definition of acute perinatal asphyxia. *Clin Perinatol* 1993; **20**(2): 287–304.

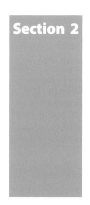

Basics in cardiopulmonary resuscitation of newborn infants
Basic equipment setup for initial neonatal care and resuscitation

Georg Hansmann

Resuscitation unit

Figures 2.1–2.3 show a resuscitation unit that is fully operational and "ready to use" (4S: suction, supplemental oxygen, specified temperature, and safety).

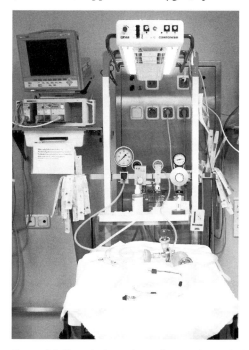

Figure 2.1 Resuscitation unit: a well-secured resuscitation table with side guards (down in the picture), covered with soft cotton blankets, with radiant warmer (here on stand-by), stethoscope, bag-mask-ventilation system (here self-inflating bag manufactured by Laerdal, model "infant," 250 ml) with PEEP-valve, pressure gauge (manomometer for PIP monitoring), oxygen blender and flowmeter (both regulate inspiratory gas), mechanical suction with manometer (measured here in bar), suction catheters in various sizes (5–14 F, 5–18 Ch), Apgar timer, thermometer, sterile gauze, disinfectant solution, cardiopulmonary monitor (SpO_2, respiratory rate, heart rate, BP-NIBP or BP-arterial, CVP, ECG), oxygen and compressed-air wall supply.

Not shown: heating pad (K-pad), drawers with additional face masks, bulb syringe, meconium aspirator (ET tube adapter), intubation kit (laryngoscope, straight blades nos. 0 and 1, Magill forceps), endotracheal tubes (2.0–4.0), stylet (optional), laryngeal mask airway (optional), tape, scissors, extra bulb and battery for laryngoscope, oropharyngeal airways (Guedel sizes: 0, 00, 000 or 20-, 40-, and 50-mm lengths), CO_2 detector (colorimetric) or

Neonatal Emergencies: A Practical Guide for Resuscitation, Transport and Critical Care, ed. Georg Hansmann.
Published by Cambridge University Press. © Cambridge University Press 2009.

Caption for Figure 2.1 (*cont.*)

capnograph, umbilical vein/artery catheter equipment, alcohol sponges/swabs, angiocaths (24 G, 26 G) plus utensils for peripheral venous access, butterfly (22 G, 24 G), plastic wrap or reclosable, food-grade plastic bag (1-gallon size for preterms babies or abdominal wall defects), emergency drugs, normal saline, sodium bicarbonate 4.2% (5 mEq/10 ml = 5 mmol/10 ml), dextrose 10%, utensils for blood draw (blood gases, blood glucose and other labs, blood culture) and smears. Transport incubator to maintain baby's temperature on transport to the nursery. CVP, central venous pressure; ET, endotracheal tube; LMA, laryngeal mask airway; NIBP, non-invasive blood pressure; PEEP, positive end-expiratory pressure; PIP, peak inspiratory pressure. See color plate section for full color version.

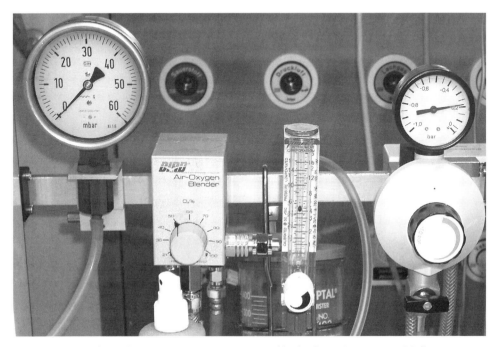

Figure 2.2 From left to right: pressure manometer, air-oxygen blender (here F_iO_2 0.5 = 50% O_2), flow meter (here 5 l O_2/air mix per minute for self-inflating bag), mechanical suction (with negative pressure, here −0.2 bar). At the back: additional wall supply for oxygen and compressed air.

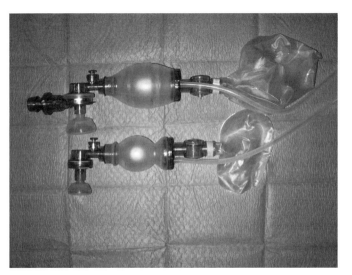

Figure 2.3 Two self-inflating bag-and-mask systems (Laerdal): upper device = model "child" (500 ml, with PEEP valve); and lower device model: "infant" (250 ml, here suboptimally without a PEEP valve). Safety pop-off valves make overinflation less likely. Refills even if not attached to compressed air source, but also refills if there is not a good seal between the mask and the patient's face. Can deliver PEEP if PEEP valve is added. See color plate section for full color version.

Resuscitation supplies and equipment for the delivery room and NETS-ambulance
Recommended equipment for delivery room resuscitation of newborn infants (preterm, term) (Figures 2.1–2.9)

- Apgar timer
- Stethoscope with neonatal head
- Resuscitation unit (as described in Figure 2.1)
- Warm temperature:
  - Four to eight preheated, dry, absorbent blankets (cotton blankets are better than terry clothes)
  - Radiant warmer (is part of the resuscitation unit in the delivery room); a heating pad may be used (K-pad) ($37.0°C = 98.6°F$)
  - For preterm infants: plastic wrap (e.g., Saran wrap) or 4-l (i.e., 1-gallon) plastic bag (also useful for abdominal wall defects)
- Suction device (see p. 66)
  - One fully operational/pneumatically driven suction device connected to a waste container
  - One portable suction device during delivery (when the head is born); only use mouth suction device, if no better device is available in an emergency
  - Bulb syringe
- Suction catheters
  - Meconium aspirator (Meconium Aspirator™ = ET tube adapter, by Neotech; compare with Vital Signs Meconium Suction Device™): for thick meconium increase suction negative pressure
  - Alternative (second choice): one large and rigid suction catheter (Yankauer catheter), when suspecting meconium in oropharynx and airways,
  - 18 F (= Ch 18): in suspected meconium aspiration (alternative to Yankauer catheter)
  - 10 F (= Ch 10): standard for oropharyngeal suctioning of term neonates, fits through 4.0 ET tube
  - 8 F (= Ch 8): for oral/nasal suctioning of preterm infants/small for gestational age (SGA), fits through 3.0–3.5 ET tube
  - 5/6 F (= Ch 5/6): for nasal suctioning of preterm infants/SGA, fits through 2.5 and 2.0 ET tube
  - 5 F (= Ch 5): fits through a 2.0 ET tube
  - Soft, flexible tip similar to a bulb syringe (e.g., Neotech Little Sucker™ in standard and premiere size), connectible to the suction device, for both oral and nasal suctioning

> When using suction catheters by Mallinckrodt (beige = 10 F = Ch 10), suction can run continuously.

Ventilatory support and assisted-ventilation devices (Figures 2.3, 2.4, 2.5 and 2.6, p. 26, pp. 70–80)[1–3]:

27

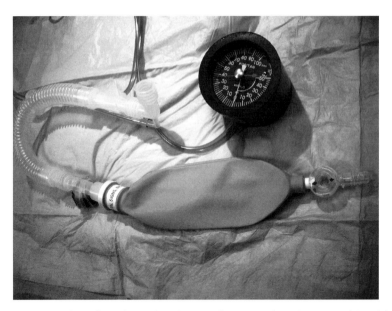

Figure 2.4 Flow-inflating bag-and-mask system (floppy "anesthesia bag"), 400 ml. Can deliver CPAP and PEEP (regulate PEEP with flow-control valve). Disadvantages: requires a compressed air source. Requires a tight seal between the mask and the patient's face to remain inflated. Usually does not have a safety pop-off valve and therefore carries the risk of overinflation (check the connected pressure gauge frequently!). Note: flow-inflating bag systems need higher flow (8–10 ml/min) and better seal than those with self-inflating bags. CPAP, continuous positive airway pressure; PEEP, peak end-expiratory pressure. See color plate section for full color version.

Self-inflating bag-and-mask systems (see legend of Figure 2.3; for advantages/disadvantages):

- A bag-and-mask system must be tested (seal, PIP, pop-off valve, PEEP valve?) and connected to the oxygen flow meter (5 l/min for self-inflating bags, e.g., by Laerdal infant = 250 ml or Laerdal child = 450–500 ml; Figure 2.5a–d) with:
    - PEEP valve (turn to +3 to +6 mbar)
    - Pop-off valve (most often set to open for PIP >30 or 40 mbar)
    - Reservoir for self-inflating bag-and-mask systems enables 90%–100% O_2 delivery (when disconnected from device, approx. 40% oxygen is delivered (F_iO_2 0.4). Alternative (second choice): pipe instead of reservoir
    - Oxygen source and tubing system without leakage and kinking
- At all times, use a compressed air source and an oxygen blender. Set the blender initially to 21% oxygen (i.e., start with room air) and 5 (−8) l/min gas flow). If the newborn is not responding after 60–90 s positive pressure ventilation (PPV), you may increase F_iO_2 by 20-percentage-point increments. If oxygen blenders are not available, disconnect the reservoir bag from the self-inflating bag-and-mask system in order to supply oxygen concentrations ≪100% (i.e., approx. 40%). Use 100% oxygen only if clearly indicated[4].
- High-quality manometer (mask seal, PEEP and PIP monitoring) connected to the ventilation device, in order to minimize baro- and volutrauma
- Face masks with soft margins, sizes: 00 and 01

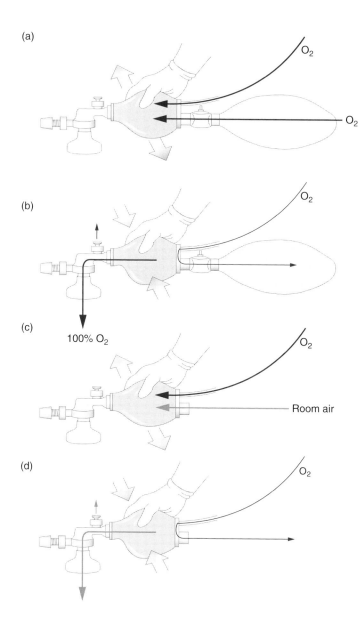

(a)

(b)

(c)

100% O₂

(d)

Room air

O₂

O₂

O₂

O₂

O₂

Figure 2.5a–d (a) Self-inflating bag-and-mask system with oxygen tubing, pop-off valve and PEEP valve. The gas mixture exhaled by the patient ends up in the atmosphere (a, c). (a) Bag re-expansion: O_2 flows from the source and the reservoir to the ventilation bag (ca. 100% O_2). (b) Bag compression: with a reservoir, almost 100% O_2 is delivered to the patient. (c) Re-expansion of the bag without a reservoir: with 5 l pure O_2/min flow → approx. 40%–50% O_2 in the bag. (d) Compression of bag without a reservoir: with a flow of 5 l pure O_2/min flow → ca. 40% O_2 will reach the patient. Modified from Ralston et al. (2006). *PALS Provider Manual.* American Heart Association and American Academy of Pediatrics. See color plate section for full color version.

Alternative devices

- **Flow-inflating bag-and-mask systems** (see legend of Figure 2.4 for advantages/disadvantages)
- **"T-piece resuscitators"** allow PPV with T-piece and continuous PEEP (e.g., *Neopuff; Neonatal Resuscitator*™ = *Neovent*™, Figure 2.6a; and *Tom Thumb*™ Figure 2.6b). They are as effective as conventional bag-and-mask systems. Some neonatologists argue that "T-piece resuscitators" are easier to handle, and deliver continuous PEEP and more accurate PIP than any bag-and-mask device
- **"Bubble CPAP"** = simple CPAP with water seal (Figure 2.7).

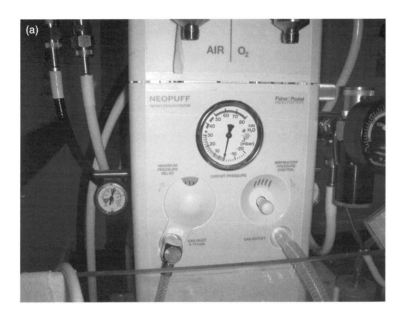

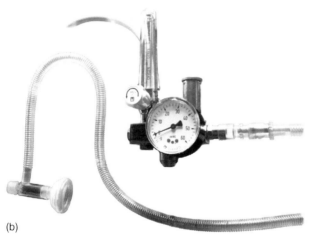

Figure 2.6a, b "T-piece resuscitator": PPV option with T-piece and continous PEEP. (a) "Neopuff Neonatal Resuscitator™" = "Perivent™". (b) "Tom Thumb™". T-piece resuscitators can deliver oxygen concentrations from 21% to 100% from a flow meter or a blender. The patient T-piece connects to neonatal masks or endotracheal tubes. When the PEEP cap (air outlet) in the T-piece is closed with the index finger or thumb, the pre-set PIP is delivered. The built-in manometer provides confirmation of mask seal and delivered PIP and PEEP. Consistent CPAP and PEEP can be delivered to assist with breathing in the delivery room, during transport or ventilator circuit change. The experience, training, concentration, and fatigue level of the operator do not affect the pressures delivered. T-piece resuscitators facilitate the consistent delivery of the desired airway pressure while maximizing the operator's ability to obtain and maintain a patent airway (one hand free). T-piece resuscitators facilitate the delivery of prolonged lung inflation (ventilation) which can also be achieved with a flow-inflating bag ("floppy anesthesia bag"), but is more difficult with an infant-sized self-inflating bag (250 ml). Disadvantages of T-pieces: require gas supply; lung compliance cannot be "felt"; changing the pre-set PIP during resuscitation is more difficult.

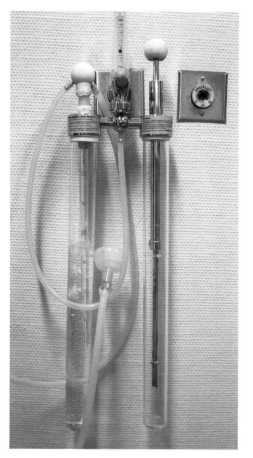

Figure 2.7 "Bubble CPAP." Basic but similar alternative to more modern "T-piece resuscitators." A flow of 5 l/min creates an airway pressure of about 20 cmH$_2$O (=20 mbar), when mask-to-face seal is tight.

For an analysis of different volume bag-and-mask systems for infants, see p. 73 and further literature[8–10].

Intubation kit

- Endotracheal tubes (Table 2.2) by: Vygon® = green; Mallinckrodt® = transparent; Portex® = light blue. Sizes: 2.0 (rarely needed), 2.5, 3.0, and 3.5 inner diameter. Vygon tubes with black-colored tip, Mallinckrodt tube with 3 line markings. For preterm infants <35 weeks' gestation, consider ET tubes with built-in surfactant application tube. (Dual-lumen ET tubes are designed for surfactant delivery. Second lumen delivers surfactant directly to the tip of the tube. This may maximize the delivery efficiency of the surfactant. The second lumen can also be used for saline instillation or CO$_2$ sampling.) Consider cuffed ET tubes only for special clinical conditions or procedures (inner diameter of cuffed ET tubes should be chosen approx. 0.5 mm smaller than uncuffed ET tubes)
- Laryngoscope (functional) with straight blades (by: Miller®, Foregger®, Negus®): sizes #0 for preterm infants and #1 for term infants (#00 blade optional for extremely low birth weight infants); spare batteries
- Small and large Magill's forceps for nasal intubation (commonly performed in Europe)
- Optional: flexible stylet may help guide the ET tube while intubating orally. (Be sure the stylet is shorter than the tube! It is controversial whether a stylet is really mandatory, especially in preterm infants at risk for hypopharyngeal and tracheal injuries)
- CO$_2$ detector (colorimetric, disposable; e.g. Pedicap™ turns yellow when end-tidal CO$_2$ is adequate: "Yellow for Yes")[11] or capnograph

Chest tube placement set (here standard equipment listed). More advanced safety systems are provided by Argyle, or Intra Special Catheters, see p. 410):

- Sterile drapes
- Disinfectant solution appropriate for neonatal use
- Chest tubes with trochar: 10 F (<2 kg), 12 F (>2 kg) (see pp. 413–14)
- 22 G butterfly or 22 G angiocath for emergency decompression
- Stopcock
- 2- or 3-ml and 20-ml syringes
- 22 G and 25 G needle

- 1% lidocaine for local anesthesia
- Curved hemostat clamps
- Gauze pads
- 3–0 or 4–0 silk suture, sterile scissors and needleholder
- Sharp scalpel (no. 15)
- Sterile gloves, mask, cap
- Suction drainage system. In the NICU: water container, e.g., Tyco Healthcare Kendall Argyle

Cord clamping (see p. 121)
- Cord clamps (plastic) or umbilical tape (strong)
- Scissors
- Sterile gauze pads

Monitoring (see p. 131, see Figures 2.2, 2.8, 2.9, 2.10)
- Pulse oximeter (may need disposable hand/foot warmers)
- Oscillometric sphygmomanometer
- Cuffs for BP (<1000 g: size 1, 1000–3000 g: size 2, >3000 g: size 3)
- Monitor showing heart rate, respiratory rate, BP and SpO_2
- If applicable, protocol to document vital parameters, measures, and procedures

Hygiene (see p. 133)
- Gloves (disposable), sterile gloves for procedures
- Hand disinfectant (e.g., Purell™)
- If necessary, a face mask and cap
- If necessary, a sterile gown (disposable)
- Alcohol solution (e.g., by Kodan™) for venous puncture and placement of catheters (caution: harmful to immature skin). May use disinfectant for soft tissue, i.e., 2% 2-phenoxyethanol and 0.1% octenidine, a soft tissue disinfectant (wait 2 min/until dried, more skin friendly), although not approved for such use[12]

Peripheral venous or arterial puncture and blood draw
(see Figures 2.28, 2.29a–c and 2.34, see p. 104):
- Glucometer/Dextrostix with test stripes (should be air tight, check expiry date!)
- Falsely high values often in low (<40 mg/dl) or low–normal (40–50 mg/dl) range for newborns
- Capillaries, tubes, and needles for blood gases and hematocrit
- Tubes (EDTA, serum/plasma/heparin/citrate) for collection of blood samples, (pre-warmed) blood cultures bottles (aerobe)
- Angiocatheters sizes 24 G and 26 G, connection line, stopcock, syringes for pump (continuous infusion), pump lines, syringe pump (see Figure 2.8)

Umbilical vein and artery catheter sets (Figure 2.29a–c)
- Umbilical vessel catheters (flushed with normal saline and connected to 3-way stopcock umbilical artery: use size Ch 5 = 5 F in infants >1500 g; use Ch 2.5–3.5 = 2.5–3.5 F in infants <1500 g. Umbilical vein: use 5 Ch = 5 F in infants >1500 g; use 3.5 Ch = 3.5 F umbilical vein catheter for infants <1500 g (have two catheters of each size available)
- Sterile anatomical forceps, sterile scalpel

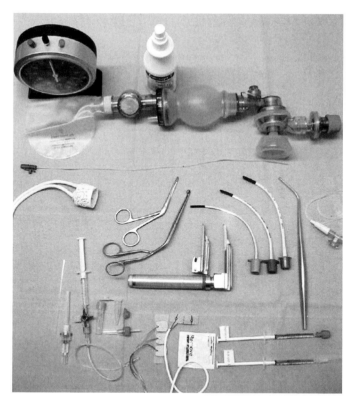

Figure 2.8 Ready-to-use equipment for initial care and resuscitation of neonates: timer, suction catheters, Yankauer suction catheter (not shown: meconium aspirator = tube adapter, Figure 2.16), bag-and-mask-system with inflatable reservoir and PEEP valve, intubation set [laryngoscope, straight blades (nos. 0 and 1), ET tubes (ETT shown here by Vygon) and Magill's forceps for nasal intubation (here two sizes: nasal intubation frequently performed in Europe), stylets for oral intubation (not shown; stylet optional; caution especially in preterm infants]. Oral intubation is standard technique in North America), two 1-ml syringes with epinephrine 1:10 000 (0.1 ml = 0.01 mg), gastric tube, utensils for blood workup: arterial blood gases, blood sugar, and chemistry (optional: blood cultures, smears), sphygmomanometer, ECG electrodes (here for preterm infants). See color plate section for full color version.

- Gauze pads
- Disinfectant solution
- Sterile band for cord
- Sterile powder-free gloves, cap and mask
- Tape and sewing material

Complete set for intraosseous access and infusion (see Figure 2.34)
- Disinfectant
- Intraosseous needle, e.g., Cook 18–20 G
- Connecting tubing prefilled with normal saline, stopcock
- 50–60 ml normal saline in syringe (inject at least 20 ml for confirmation of correct placement)
- Gauze, tape

Drugs (see Table 2.1, see p. 41)
- Epinephrine (= adrenaline; standard ampulles 1:10 000, i.e., 0.1 ml = 10 µg = 0.01 mg): for high-risk deliveries prepare epinephrine 1:10 000 solution in 3 × 1-ml syringes

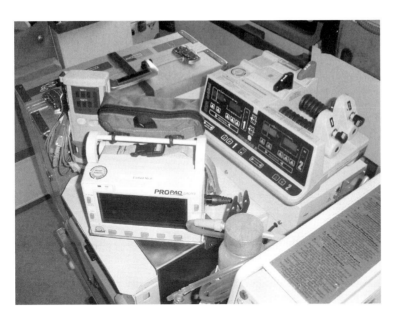

Figure 2.9
Neonatal emergency transport service (NETS) equipment attached to the portable transport incubator: monitor for pulse oximetry (SpO_2) and heart rate, ECG respiratory rate and blood pressure (standard: oscillometric; arterial BP measurement, e.g., on NICU-to-NICU transport, is possible), two syringe pumps for continuous IV infusion, suction device, emergency case. Monitor, pulse oximeter, and syringe pumps can be removed quickly.

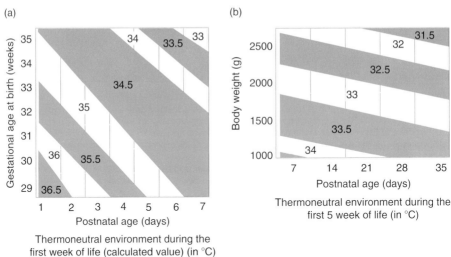

Figure 2.10 Neutral thermal environment for preterm and term infants. The range of temperatures needed in the incubator is based on gestational age (a) rather than body weight (b). Portable incubators must be thermo-adjusted to the infant's incubator – depending on the external temperature. In the portable incubator the temperature should be set higher, than in the stationary incubator of the referring hospital, at least until the infant has been transferred to the transport incubator and its doors are closed. Avoid hypo- and hyperthermia.

(if only 1:1000 solution available, prepare 1 ml epinephrine plus 9 ml normal saline; draw mix in 3 × 1-ml syringes and label). Single standard dose is 10 (–30) µg/kg IV = 0.01 (–0.03) mg/kg IV = 0.1 (–0.3) ml/kg IV. May give 30–100 µg/kg/dose (=0.3–1 ml/kg/dose) via ET tube

- Rarely: sodium bicarbonate 4.2% (1 ml = 0.5 mEq = 0.5 mmol) or 8.4% stock solution to be diluted 1:1 (1 ml = 1 mEq = 1 mmol, mix 1:1 solution with distilled water in 10-, 1-, 20- or 50-ml syringe). Aim to give a continuous IV infusion over 30–120 min!

Consider THAM (tris-hydroxymethyl-aminomethane) solution if repetitive sodium bicarbonate was given and hypernatremia is expected/present
- Sterile water
- On the NICU: naloxone 0.1 mg/kg (second choice: IM or ET). Note: this naloxone dose is *not* evidence-based. Naloxone is rarely used and only used for clear indications. A secured airway (ETT, LMA) always comes first. The International Liaison Committee on Resuscitation (ILCOR) guidelines 2005 no longer recommend naloxone administration for respiratory depressed newborn infants in the delivery room!

Volume therapy (see p. 173)
- Normal saline (NS; NaCl 0.9%) or Ringer's lactate (RL) solution for hypovolemia (bolus and continuous infusion; for volume expansion prepare, if needed)
- Human albumin 5% (HA 5%) for bolus and continuous IV infusion (second choice compared to normal saline or Ringer's lactate solution)
- Prepare syringe with 50 ml volume (normal saline, RL) if hypovolemia is expected (e.g., placental disruption)
- Note: The ILCOR guidelines 2005 no longer recommend colloid solutions (e.g., HA 5%) for the resuscitation of newborn infants!
- Sodium bicarbonate 4.2% (1 ml = 0.5 mEq = 0.5 mmol) or 8.4% (1 ml = 1 mEq = 1 mmol, mix 1:1 solution with distilled water in 10-, 1-, 20- or 50-ml syringe). Aim to give a continuous IV infusion over 30 min to 2 h! Consider THAM solution if repetitive sodium bicarbonate was given and hypernatremia is expected/present
- Sterile water
- Dextrose 10% ($D_{10}W$), for bolus (2–3 ml/kg/bolus) in hypoglycemia and continuous IV infusion (maintenance/transport)
- Dextrose 5% (D_5W) (for maintenance/transport of neonates with high – normal or increased blood glucose, e.g., after resuscitation/epinephrine administration)
- Three syringe IV pumps (two belong to the portable NETS incubator, but can be moved to the bedside)

Miscellaneous
- Gastric tube (orogastric or nasogastric): size 5 F for infants <2500 g, 8 F for infants >2500 g
- 1-ml, 2- or 3-ml, 10-ml and 20- or 30-ml syringes. IV pump syringes (20–50 ml) with line
- Have at least one ampoule of surfactant in the refrigerator
- Have one reserved emergency packed red blood cells unit (100–250 ml, blood type O, Rhesus negative) in the blood bank or (even better) in the resuscitation room at 37.0 °C

> *!* Everyday: Check if the equipment is operational and ready to use. Be prepared for emergencies. Assign duties for routine daily checks.

Incubators with mechanical ventilator
Transport incubator (Figure 2.11)
Operation of the transport incubator
- Connect oxygen and compressed air outlets
- Turn on heater, and set initial temperature at 37.0°C (98.6°F) (Figure 2.10)
- Connect ventilation tubing to portable ventilation unit

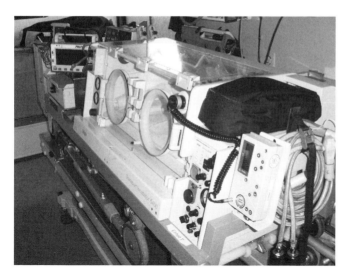

Figure 2.11 Incubator 5400, by Dräger. Weight including chassis, monitor station, drawer, catheter holder, gas cylinders, Babylog 2000 ventilator, and oxygen analyzer (by Oxydig, on the right): 90–130 kg. Preheating time approx. 30 min.

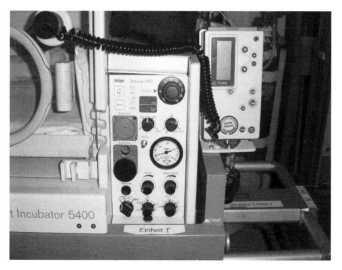

Figure 2.12 Babylog 2000 (mechanical ventilation unit), by Dräger.

- Preset ventilator: do the test run
  - Setting: 21%–100 % (FiO_2 0.21–1.0)
  - Ventilator rate depending on the child's condition (20–60 breaths/min)
  - PEEP 3–4 mmHg
  - PIP, depending on the child's condition 16–20 ($\leq$30) mbar
- Keep bag-and-mask ventilator assembled, even if neonate is intubated and mechanically ventilated by a respirator
- Open compressed air and oxygen tank shortly before decoupling oxygen and compressed air from the wall outlet

Figures 2.9 and 2.11 illustrate transport incubators and equipment. The Babylog 2000 ventilator, used during the transport of neonates, is illustrated in Figure 2.12 and instructions for the use of ventilators during transport are given in Figures 2.13a–c. Figure 2.14 illustrates a transport incubator with an integrated mechanical ventilator.

(a)

Front panel

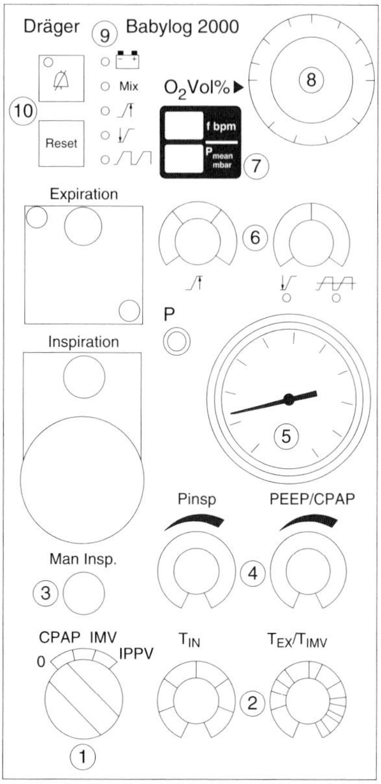

(1) Rotary switch: To set up the mode
    CPAP/IMV/IPPV 0 = OFF

(2) Two rotary knobs for setting the time: T_{IN}
    (inspiration time) and T_{EX} (expiration time)/T_{IMV}

(3) Button for manual inspiration

(4) Rotary knobs for setting P_{insp} and PEEP/CPAP

(5) Analog mechanical pressure gauge of inspiratory
    and expiratory airway pressure

(6) Two rotary knobs for setting alarm limits of
    airway pressure: left–upper alarm limit,
    right–lower alarm limit

(7) Display for: frequency (f) and mean pressure (P_{mean}).
    CPAP mode: display for (f) = "_ _"

(8) Rotary knob for setting of inspiratory O_2 concentration
    of 21%–100%

(9) LED

    Power supply
    (power requirement/power supply system)
    green = operation
    red = (operating / supply / working voltage) –
          low – alarm

    ／│ Airway pressure – upper limit

    ↓／ Airway pressure – lower limit

    ／∨／ Fail-to-Cycle-Alarm

    Green = recognized inspiration phase in IMV/IPPV mode

    Red = not recognized inspiration phase in IMV/IPPV mode (Fail-to-Cycle-Alarm)

(10) (Canceled bell) button: turns off alarm tone for 2 minutes

    Reset "Reset" button: resets the alarm after the problem has been remedied

Supply:

Gas supply with O_2 and air from the central gas supply or from gas cylinder with compressed
air regulator

Electrical supply with electrical supply unit 1 (with battery) or electrical supply with electrical unit 2
(with battery and mains adapter), eventually with external power supply

Figure 2.13 Instructions for the use of ventilators during transport, for example Babylog 2000, by Dräger, Part 1–4.
(a) Instructions, Babylog 2000 (Part 1); (b) instructions, Babylog 2000 (Part 2); (c) Instructions, Babylog 2000 (Part 3);
(d) Instructions, Babylog 2000 (Part 4). Front panel

37

(b)

IPPV (intermittent positive-pressure ventilation, controlled ventilation)

$$\text{Respiratory frequency } (f) = \frac{60}{T_{IN} + T_{EX}} = \frac{\text{Ventilation rate}}{\text{min}} = \text{breaths per min}$$

(1) Set required oxygen concentration monitor oxygen sensor (Oxydig)!
Read instructions for use!
● Controlled ventilation (IPPV)

(2) Turn rotary switch on IPPV mode

(3) Yellow LED lights up

(4) Turn rotary knob to "green dots," the apparatus
will work now with the following parameters:

T_{IN} = 0.8 s too long for neonates
T_{EX} = 1.2 s
f = 30 bpm
I : E = 1 : 1.5
PEEP = 2 mbar
P_{insp} = 20 mbar

Or always better:
Set ventilation parameters as follows:
● Standard values: T_{IN} = 0.4 s T_{EX} = 0.8 –1.4, f = 35–50
● PEEP = +3 to +5 mbar, PIP = P_{insp} = 20 + 4 mbar
● Connect patient
● Set alarm limits of pressure control

Ventilation with plateau:
Pressure limits:

(5) Set the desired inspiratory pressure plateau with P_{insp} rotary knob
(according to display), with incremental increases until plateau
and sufficient chest rise is achieved

(6) Set PEEP/CPAP rotary knob

The ventilation pattern with plateau and moderate P_{insp}
prevents barotrauma to the lungs

Dräger Babylog 2000

Dräger Babylog 2000

(c) Alarm limits for IPPV

Lower limit

(1) Turn rotary knob to approx. 5 mbar above the end-expiratory pressure

(2) The green LED blinks at the beginning of every inspiration = the correct setting of alarm limit

Upper limit

(3) Set P_{max} by turning rotary knob to approx. 10 mbar above the maximum pressure

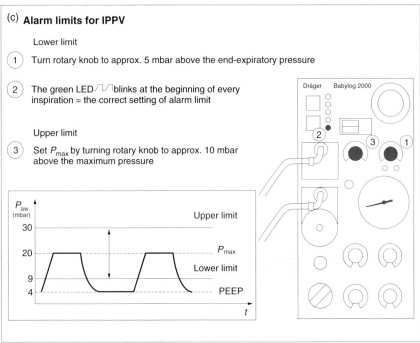

(d) Spontaneous breathing under CPAP

The apparatus maintains a continuous flow of 8.5 l/min
The end-expiratory pressure is adjusted with the expiration valve

Alarm limits

(1) Turn rotary switch to CPAP mode

(2) The yellow LED ↓ will light up

(3) Set positive airway pressure with the PEEP/CPAP rotary knob. Set lower alarm limit Figure 2.13c

(4) The mean pressure P_{mean} showed on the display must coincide with the adjusted PEEP/CPAP

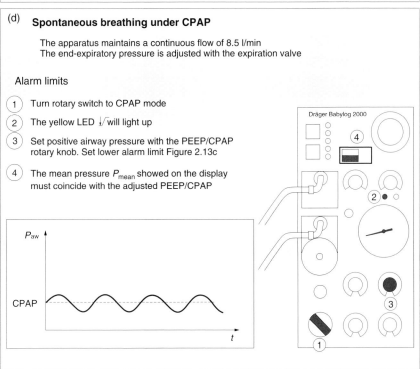

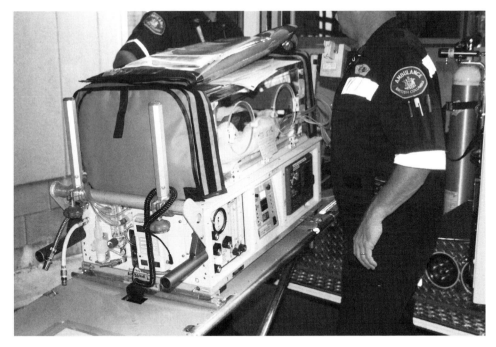

Figure 2.14 Transport incubator with integrated mechanical ventilator and monitoring.

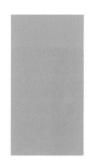

Drugs for neonatal emergencies

Georg Hansmann

Dosing intervals for commonly used antibiotics (see Table 2.1[13])

Gestational age (weeks p.m.)	Postnatal age (days)	Interval				
		1	2	3	4	5
≤29 (or <1200 g)	0–28	q 12 h	q 12 h	q 12 h	q 48 h	q 18 h
	>28	q 8 h	q 8 h	q 8 h	q 24 h	q 12 h
30–36 (≈1200–2700 g)	0–14	q 12 h	q 12 h	q 12 h	q 24 h	q 12 h
	>14	q 8 h	q 8 h	q 8 h	q 12 h	q 8 h
37–44	0–7	q 8 h	q 12 h	q 12 h	q 12 h	q 12 h
	>7	q 6 h	q 8 h	q 8 h	q 8 h	q 8 h
≥45	All	q 6 h	q 6 h	q 8 h	q 8 h	q 8 h

Dosing of gentamicin and tobramycin (aminoglycosides)
Dosing chart A

Birth to 1 month of age

Gestational age (weeks p.m.)	Dose	Interval[a]
<35	3.5 mg/kg/dose	q 24 h
≥35	5 mg/kg/dose	q 24 h

Dosing chart B

>1 month postnatal

Corrected gestational age (weeks p.m.)	Dose	Interval[a]
<35	2.5 mg/kgdose	q 12 h
≥35	2.5 mg/kg/dose	q 12 h

[a]Special circumstances require modified aminoglycoside dosing:
1. In infants >1 month of age with renal or cardiac dysfunction (e.g., s/p asphyxia, large patent ductus arteriosus, left ventricular outflow tract obstruction such as hypoplastic left heart syndrome), use 2.5 mg/kg/dose IV q 12 to 24 h.
2. For preterm infants ≤29 weeks postmenstrual age (= corrected gestational age p.m.), some recommend the following dosing regimen[13]: postnatal day 0–7 → 5 mg/kg/dose q 48 h IV, postnatal day 8–28 → 4 mg/kg/dose q 36 h IV, postnatal day ≥29 days → 4 mg/kg/dose q 24 h IV.
3. Avoid aminoglycosides while treating PDA with indomethacin (use ampicillin and cefotaxime).
4. If preterm infants ≤26 weeks GA need to receive aminoglycosides, extend the dosing interval to 36 h to avoid renal failure.

Neonatal Emergencies: A Practical Guide for Resuscitation, Transport and Critical Care, ed. Georg Hansmann.
Published by Cambridge University Press. © Cambridge University Press 2009.

Emergency drugs for initial neonatal care and resuscitation are summarized in Table 2.1.

Warning

1. You MUST check whether your individual stock solution has the same concentration as that given in the emergency drug table (Table 2.1, first column). If the stock solutions are different, you can only use mg per kg body weight dosing.
2. We greatly encourage individual, weight-based emergency drug cards (code cards) for infants in intensive care or step-down units!

Table 2.1 Drugs for neonatal emergencies

Drug class	Preparation (immediate use)	Application/dosage	Indication
Adenosine[*] (Adenocard®) (vial 6 mg/2 ml) 2 ml = 6 mg 1 ml = 3 mg 0.1 ml = 0.3 mg Antiarrhythmic → transient total heart block (third-degree AV block) Do NOT refrigerate (may precipitate)! Solutions must be clear at the time of use	3 × 1-ml syringes, 5-ml syringe, and 20-ml syringe filled with saline Dilution: 1 ml adenosine (3 mg/ml) + 4 ml saline in 5-ml syringe, then 1:5 dilution → 1 ml = 0.6 mg; 0.1 ml = 0.06 mg Then: → Draw single first dose in 1-ml syringe (1:5). Start with 0.15 ml/kg/dose (see inset table, second dose), flush, prepare second dose adenosine undiluted (i.e., pure, without saline) in 1-ml syringe → Always flush rapidly with 5–10 ml normal saline IV	*PIV (right arm)/central IV line/IO:* first dose 0.1 mg/kg/dose rapid IV push, second dose 0.2 mg/kg/dose rapid IV push (PALS 2006). Adenosine always followed by rapid flush with 5–10 ml normal saline. $t_{1/2}$ adenosine = 1–5 s. Use central IV line if available. *Adenosine – emergency dosing chart* | BW	First Dose	Second Dose	Third Dose
1.5–2.5 kg	0.2 mg ≅0.3 ml (1:5)	0.3 mg ≅ 0.5 ml (1:5)	0.45 mg ≅0.75 ml (1:5)
2.5–3.5 kg	0.3 mg ≅0.5 ml (1:5)	0.45 mg ≅0.75 ml (1:5)	0.6 mg ≅ 1 ml (1:5)	 Legend: ml doses for adenosine (stock = 3 mg/ml), diluted 1:5 (then 0.1 ml = 60 μg), see inset table above. If adenosine unsuccessful or only with transient effect: repeat single dose after 2 min and increase dose by 0.05 mg/kg/dose (see inset table above). Usual maximum single dose is 0.25 mg/kg *Rule of thumb:* Perform synchronized cardioversion (DCCV) if patient unstable or 3 doses of adenosine IV unsuccessful • Use central IV line if available • PIV should be as close as possible to the heart (right arm preferred) • ECG monitoring + documentation • Have defibrillator/cardioverter at the bedside	• Supraventricular-(re-entry)-tachycardia • To unmask atrial tachycardia *Contraindication:* AV Block II°/ III°, sick-sinus syndrome without a pacemaker, known WPW syndrome Careful in patients with sinus and AV node dysfunction, and in patients on digoxin, digitoxin or verapamil (VFib possible) *Adverse effects (AE):* dyspnea (bronchospasm), hypotension, flushing *Antidote:* Theophylline (adenosine-receptor antagonist, in case of bronchospasm); shock: epinephrine IV
Adrenaline[*] *See Epinephrine*			
Amiodarone[*] *Antiarrhythmic [III]* 150 mg/3 ml or 250 mg/5 ml ampoule (glass), i.e., 1 ml = 50 mg Amiodarone HCl contains 37% iodine and may cause hypo- and hyperthyroidism.	Dilute 250 mg/125 ml D$_5$W or 150 mg/75 ml D$_5$W, i.e., 2 mg/ml (=2000 μg/ml) Dilute in D$_5$W NOT in normal saline! Kinetics: complex rapid uptake by adipose tissue, slow uptake by myocardium, concentrates in both. $t_{1/2}$ biphasic, first 50% reduction of	*IV (IO):* 5 mg/kg/loading dose (= 2.5 ml/kg/loading dose), in cardiac arrest as rapid IV/IO bolus, give in 20–30 min IV for perfusing tachycardias. Central IV line preferred. Maintenance dose ca. 5–10 (–15–20) μg/kg/min. (≈10–20 mg/kg/day; glass bottle, central line, volumetric infusion device). Consult electrophysiologist. Amiodarone is not listed in the NLS guidelines (ILCOR 2005), but in the PALS guidelines 2005.	• Frequently recurrent VFib or VFlu • Unstable VTach unresponsive to other therapy (i.e., synchronized cardioversion) • SVT unresponsive to other therapy

43

Table 2.1 (cont.)

Drug class	Preparation (immediate use)	Application/dosage	Indication
Amiodarone (cont.) Benzyl alcohol-free solution under development Prepare fresh drug q 24 h, consider PO therapy within 24–48 h Irritating to peripheral vein: for infusions >1 h, concentration should not exceed 2 mg/ml unless using central line	single IV dose after ≈ 20–30 days. Elimination $t_{1/2}$ about 30 days with chronic oral therapy (range 8–107 days). Levels detectable 9 months after stopping treatment. Therapeutic effect seen 1–3 h after IV dose. Peak serum level at 5 h after oral dose	Rarely used in neonates without congenital heart disease. Hardly ever given in the delivery room *Drug interactions (CytP450 inhibitor):* may increase plasma levels of digoxin, phenytoin, warfarin, etc. (reduce those drug doses by ≈50%) *Drug levels:* Therapeutic >1.0 µg/ml. Toxicity common at >2.5 µg/ml. Very limited safety data on its use in pediatric population	• Cardiac arrest with pulseless VTach or VFib (unresponsive to defibrillation, CPR, and epinephrine) • JET s/p cardiosurgery *Adverse effects:* hypotension/CHF and arrhythmias common, LFT elevation, thyroid dysfunction, pulmonary fibrosis Do not use with drugs that prolong QT interval

Drug class	Preparation (immediate use)	Application/dosage	Indication
Ampicillin 500 mg* (See also p. 41) (powder with compatible solution) β-lactam antibiotic. Especially effective against ampicillin-sensitive strains of: Enterococci, Streptococci (GBS) Listeria, Haemophilus influenzae → always prepare solution just for immediate use! Alternative: Piperacillin (common combination is piperacillin + netilmicin)	5-ml syringe, dilute powder in 5 ml sterile water or normal saline, then 1 ml = 100 mg	*IV:* initial dose 100 mg/kg/dose = 1 ml/kg/dose in 5 min slow IV push • daily dose: 200 mg/kg/day divided in 2–4 single doses slow IV push; divided daily dose see interval 2 below • In severe infections (e.g., suspected meningitis), some recommend 100 mg/kg/dose q 6 h to 12 h IV, then usually in combination with cefotaxime 150–200 mg/kg/day divided in 3–4 single doses IV (see below) and aminglycoside (e.g., gentamicin, see below) See dosing table below. • Alternatives: piperacillin (150–300 mg/kg/day in 2–4 single doses IV) → Septic work-up including blood culture and LP, as indicated!	Suspected neonatal sepsis *Effective against:* β-Streptococci (GBS) (combine with aminoglycoside), *Listeria,* some Enterococci, some *E. coli, Haemophilus influenzae* Not active against: *Staphylococcus aureus* (β-lactamase +)! *Adverse effects:* diarrhea, rarely pseudomembranous colitis *Remember:* 1. Cephalosporins do not cover *Listeria* and *Enterococci* 2. Gram-negative pathogens are more and more resistant to ampicillin and its derivatives

GA (weeks p.m.)	Postnatal Days	Interval (no. 2)
≤29 (or <1200 g)	0–28	q 12 h
	>28	q 8 h
30–36 (≈1200–2700 g)	0–14	q 12 h
	>14	q 8 h
37–44	0–7	q 12 h
	>7	q 8 h
≥45	All	q 6 h

Contains 0.3 mmol sodium/ 100 mg

Atropine*

1 ml = 0.5 mg 0.1 ml = 0.05 mg
Parasympatholytic, chronotropic, dromotropic. Atropine is not listed in the International Neonatal Resuscitation Guidelines 2005 (ILCOR)

1-ml syringe: (1) undiluted (0.1 ml = 0.05 mg) or (2) 0.2 ml atropine + 0.8 ml saline (1:5 solution: 0.1 ml = 0.01 mg)

IV, ET: 0.02 mg/kg minimum IV single dose is 0.1 mg = 0.2 ml (undiluted)

- Second- and third-degree heart (AV) block
- Bradycardia with arterial hypotension after epinephrine IV and volume expansion
- May be given prior to (elective or semi-elective) intubation together with analgesia and sedation (0.01–0.02 mg/kg IV)

Bicarbonate, see Sodium bicarbonate

Calcium chloride 10%

10-ml vials, 100 mg/ml
270 mg elemental calcium per 1000 mg Calcium chloride, i.e., 27 mg elemental calcium/ml, 1 ml = 27 mg elemental calcium 1 ml = 1.36 mEq Ca 1 ml = 0.68 mmol elemental calcium
Not listed in the ILCOR recommendations for neonatal resuscitation (2005). Not an evidence-based drug

10-ml syringe dilute 1:10 in D_5W or NS (1 ml + 9 ml) so that 10 mg calcium chloride per ml

IV/IO, PIV, UVC/central IV line (preferred): 20 mg/kg/dose = 2 ml/kg/dose as slow IV push (5 min). May infuse up to 70 mg/kg in 30 min IV. Central IV line preferred. Always flush slowly IV with NS. Stop slow IV push or infusion if HR <100 bpm. Do not give calcium intra-arterially!
Max. total daily dose for neonates = 1000 mg/day
Exchange transfusion: Give 33 mg calcium chloride per 100 ml citrated blood exchanged in 10 min IV (equals 0.33 ml per 100 ml blood exchanged)

- Hyperkalemia
- Electromechanical dissociation (rarely)
- Hypotension due to cardiac insufficiency (→ short-term increase of BP)
- Hypocalcemia (+ seizures)
Adverse effects: arrhythmia/AV block, myocardial necrosis, skin necrosis due to extravasation. Do not give IV to digitalized patients!

Calcium gluconate 10%*

100 mg/ml 90 mg elemental calcium per 1000 mg calcium gluconate. 9 mg elemental calcium/ml
1 ml = 9 mg elemental calcium
1 ml = 0.46 mEq elemental calcium
1 ml = 0.22 mmol calcium

10-ml syringe

IV/IO, PIV, UVC/central IV line (preferred): 100 mg/kg/dose = 1 ml/kg/dose as slow IV push (5 min) Central IV line preferred. Always flush slowly IV with NS
Some dilute 1:1 in D_5W or $D_{10}W$, and give 2 ml/kg/single dose. Do not give calcium intra-arterially! *Maintenance dose:* 200–800 mg/kg/day IV/PO (2–8 ml/kg/day)
Max. 400 mg/kg cumulative dose. Max. total daily dose for neonates = 3000 mg/day

- Hyperkalemia
- Electromechanical dissociation (rarely)
- Hypotension due to cardiac insufficiency (→ short-term increase of BP)
- Hypocalcemia (+ seizures)

Table 2.1 (cont.)

Drug class	Preparation (immediate use)	Application/dosage	Indication
Calcium gluconate (cont.) Not listed in the ILCOR recommendations for neonatal resuscitation (2005). Not an evidence-based drug		*Exchange transfusion:* Give 100 mg calcium gluconate per 100 ml citrated blood exchanged in 10 min IV (equals 1 ml per 100 ml blood exchanged)	*Adverse effects:* arrhythmia/AV block, myocardial necrosis, skin necrosis due to extravasations Do not give IV to digitalized patients!

Cefotaxime* 500 mg (See also p. 41) (powder) Third-generation cephalosporin, β-lactam-antibiotic, broad-spectrum. When compared to first-generation cephalosporins and ampicillin, less active against → Keep solution at room temperature (only stable for 24 h) 0.22 mmol sodium/100 mg Do NOT use ceftriaxone in the first 2 months of life (see page 300).

Preparation: 5-ml syringe, dilute powder in 5 ml sterile water or normal saline, then 1 ml = 100 mg

IV: 50 mg/kg/dose = 0.5 ml/kg/dose in 5 min slow IV push

GA (weeks p.m.)	Postnatal days	Interval (no. 2)
≤29 (or <1200 g)	0–28	q 12 h
	>28	q 8 h
30–36 (≈1200–2700 g)	0–14	q 12 h
	>14	q 8 h
37–44	0–7	q 12 h
	>7	q 8 h
≥45	All	q 6 h

For meningitis, subtract one dosing interval stated in the table (i.e., q 6 h instead of q 8 h; q 8 h instead of q 12 h). Meningitis dose for infants >1 month old is 50 mg/kg/dose q 6 h IV Others recommend the use of 50 mg/kg/dose q 8 h IV for all newborn infants >2000 g without meningitis → Septic work-up incl. blood culture and LP, as indicated!

Indication (Cefotaxime):
• Suspected neonatal sepsis *Especially active against:* Gram-negative organisms and sensitive strains of *Staphylococcus aureus. Not active against:* MRSA, *Enterococci, Listeria, Pseudomonas aeruginosa!*

Remember:
1. Cephalosporins do not cover *Listeria* and *Enterococci*
2. Gram-negative pathogens are increasingly resistant against ampicillin and its derivatives
Adverse effects: Rare: leukopenia/granulocytopenia, diarrhea

Clindamycin 75 mg
(See p. 41)
(powder). Bactericidal activity by inhibiting protein synthesis

Dilute 75 mg powder in 5 ml sterile water, then 1 ml = 25 mg

IV: 5–7.5 mg/kg/dose, 30 min IV infusion (or PO)

GA (weeks p.m.)	Postnatal days	Interval (no. 1)
≤29 (or <1200 g)	0–28	q 12 h
	>28	q 8 h
30–36 (≈1200–2700 g)	0–14	q 12 h
	>14	q 8 h
37–44	0–7	q 8 h
	>7	q 6 h
≥45	All	q 6 h

Increase dosing interval in significant liver dysfunction.
→ Septic work-up incl. blood culture and LP, as indicated!

- *Especially active against:* aerobic and anaerobic streptococci (except enterococci), most staphylococci (not all MRSA), *Bacteroides* spp., *Fusobacterium varium*, *Actinomyces israelii*, *Clostridium perfringens* and *C. tetani*
Not active against: Enterococci, some MRSA, Gram-negative organisms, many clostridial species
Remember: If MRSA is reported as having susceptibility to clindamycin, a D-test should be performed to look for inducible macrolide-lincosamide-streptogamin (MLS$_B$) resistance. If the D-test is positive, consider using vancomycin
Adverse effects: pseudomembranous colitis (common)

Diazepam*
(Valium®, Stesolid®)
1 ml = 5 mg
Benzodiazepines: Sedative, Antiepileptic
The clear solution contains benzyl alcohol!
Alternative benzodiazepines: lorazepam, clonazepam, midazolam

1-ml syringe: undiluted

IV: (0.25–) 0.5 mg/kg = (0.05–) – 0.1 ml/kg slow IV push. Max. total dose = 2 mg (= 0.4 ml)
rectal: 0.5 mg/kg/dose (approved for infants >6 months). 5 mg/ml rectal gel; enema, Diastat®) available in 2.5 mg, 5 mg and 10 mg strengths; give ≈half of a 2.5-mg enema if there is no IV access (3-kg infant). The IV solution can be given per rectum. Onset of action: IV 1–2 min, rectal: 2–10 min (peak 1 h). $t_{1/2}$ = 50–100 h

- Sedation
- Seizures (third choice)
Adverse effects: hypotension, apnea, severe myoclonus in preterm infants *Neurotoxicity described for chronic exposure to benzodiazepines!*

Table 2.1 (cont.)

Drug class	Preparation (immediate use)	Application/dosage	Indication
Dobutamine (Dobutrex®) Careful, multiple stock solutions available! 1 mg/ml, 2 mg/ml (vial 250 mg/125 ml), 4 mg/ml, 25 mg/ml (vial 250 mg/10ml) *Inochronotropic → Caution: incompatible, with furosemide, heparin, potassium and calcium*	2 ml- or 5-ml syringe, pump syringe for continous IV infusion. **a.** Dilute 0.8 ml/kg Dobutamine (25 mg/ml stock solution) in total of 30 ml D$_5$W or NS, then 1 ml = 0.66 mg/kg OR **b.** Use standard solution, ie., final conc. = 2 mg/ml, i.e. final conc. = 1.6 mg/ml. Use either premixed final solution (2 mg/ml) or add 250 mg (=10 ml of stock vial 250 mg/10ml) to 115 ml D$_5$W or NS	*UVC/central venous line* (in emergency also PIV): initial dose: 3–10 (–20) µg/kg/min, according to effect **a.** Solution with 1 ml = 0.66 mg/kg 	3	5	11	≅µg/kg/min
0.3	0.5	1.0	≅ml/h | → Onset of action: 1–10 min, serum half-life ca. 2 min, tolerance begins after ca. 72 h OR **b.** Final conc. = 2 mg/ml (body weight) | 3	5	10	≅µg/kg/min
0.09	0.15	1.3	≅ml/h (1 kg)
			≅ml/h (…kg)	 *Correct hypovolemia with volume before giving dobutamine! Consider combination of dopamine + dobutamine. Consider milrinone or combination of milrinone + dopamine instead of dobutamine. Do not give sole dobutamine in sepsis*	• Cardiogenic shock. Dobutamine increases CO without increase of SVR *Do not give in:* significant pericardial effusion, LVOTO, hypovolemia sepsis *Adverse effects:* tachyarrhythmia, decreased diastolic BP
Dopamine* Careful, multiple stock solutions available! e.g. 0.8 mg/ml, 1.6 mg/ml, 3.2 mg/ml, 10 mg/ml, 40 mg/ml *Inochronotropic*	2 ml- or 5-ml syringe, pump syringe for continous IV infusion. **a.** Dilute 2 ml/kg dopamine (10 mg/ml stock solution) in total of 30 ml D$_5$W or NS, then 1 ml = 0.66 mg/kg OR **b.** Use standard solution, i.e. final conc. = 1.6 mg/ml. Use either premixed final solution (1.6 mg/ml) or add 200 mg (=5 ml of stock vial 40 mg/ml) to 120 ml D$_5$W or NS	*UVC or CVC (in emergency also PIV):* initial dose: (2–) 5–10 (–20) µg/kg/min, according to effect: **a.** solution with 1 ml = 0.66 mg/kg 	3	5	11	≅µg/kg/min
0.3	0.5	1.0	≅ml/h | → Onset of action: after 5–10 min, $t_{1/2}$ = 2 min OR **b.** Final conc. = 1.6 mg/ml (body weight) | 3	5	10	≅µg/kg/min
0.11	0.19	1.38	≅ml/h (1 kg)
			≅ml/h (…kg)		• CHF • Renal failure/oliguria. Increases CO, mesenteric and renal perfusion. Dosing >(3–) 5 µg/kg/min increases SVR and PVR *Adverse effects:* pulmonary right–left shunts, arrhythmias (more common with dobutamine!)

Dopamine* (cont.)

Correct hypovolemia with volume before giving dopamine. Consider combination of milrinone + dopamine

The "diuretic dopamine dose" is ≈2–3 µg/kg/min. In low urine output s/p cardiac surgery, consider fenoldopam (0.1–0.3 µg/kg/min), a selective dopamine-1 receptor agonist that causes systemic vasodilation and increased renal blood flow and tubular sodium excretion

Epinephrine* 1:10 000

= Adrenaline (1:10 000)
1 ml = 0.1 mg 0.1 ml = 0.01 mg
0.1 ml = 10 µg *Inochronotropic with high dosage: vasoconstriction. bronchodilatation. Drug of choice for neonatal resuscitation.* Rarely needed for successful neonatal resuscitation

First choice: epinephrine 1:10 000 stock solution (e.g., in emergency kits, code cart), 1-ml syringe or *dilute 1:1000 solution (second choice):* first 10-ml syringe: dilution: 1 ml epinephrine 1:1000 plus 9 ml saline. Then draw 1 ml each in two 1-ml syringes (0.1 ml = 0.01 mg)

Cardiac arrest, bradycardia, CPR. Max. single dose during resuscitation: 0.03 mg/kg/dose (=0.3 ml/kg/dose) IV. Max. ET dose is unclear: aim for max. 0.1 mg/kg/dose (=1 ml/kg/dose) ET

PIV/IO/UVC/central IV line: 10 µg/kg/dose = 0.01 (–0.02–0.03) mg/kg/dose = 0.1 (–0.2–0.3) ml/kg/dose
→ Repeat after 1–5 min depending on effect (check pulses+HR!). Higher single doses without proven benefit. Always flush with 5–10 ml NS. Give volume (10 ml/kg NS) after second epinephrine dose
ET (if no IV access): 30–100 µg/kg/dose = 0.03–0.1 mg/kg/dose = 0.3–1.0 ml/kg/dose, repeat q 1–5 min if indicated (i.e., still no IV/IO access)

Epinephrine 1:1000*

= Adrenaline (1:1000) i.e., without dilution: 1 ml = 1 mg use 1:1000 solution to prepare IV infusion. Do not use 1:1000 solution for IV or ET bolus in newborn infants *Inochronotropic. with high dosage: vasoconstriction, bronchodilatation*

1- and 50-ml syringe for pump (do not use 1:1000 solution for individual doses)
a. Add 0.2 ml/kg to total of 30 ml D_5W or NS, then 1 ml = 6.6 µg/kg

OR

b. Use standard solution, i.e., add 1 ml (1000 µg) of stock vial (1 mg/ml, i.e., 1:1000) to 124 ml D_5W or NS, then final concentration 8 µg/ml *inhalation:* pure (undiluted) or diluted in 3 ml saline

Indication hypotension in acute low cardiac output despite volume IV
Low dose: increase of cardiac output, HR, systolic BP. MAP remains constant. Decrease of SVR
High dose: increases also diastolic BP, MAP and SVR
Inhalation: stridor

Start IV infusion at: (0.05–) 0.1 µg/kg/min, then depending on effect (max. 1–2 µg/kg/min)

a. Solution with 1 ml = 6.6 µg/kg

0.05	0.11	0.5	≅µg/kg/min
0.5	1.0	4.5	≅ml/h

OR

b. Final conc. 8 µg/ml (body weight)

0.05	0.1	0.5	≅µg/kg/min
0.38	0.75	3.75	≅ml/h (1 kg)
			≅ml/h (...kg)

ET, IV bolus: may dilute to 1:10 000 solution, start with 0.01 mg/kg/dose IV. Max. single dose during resuscitation: 0.1 mg/kg = 1 ml/kg ET, and 0.03 mg/kg/dose (=0.3 ml/kg/dose) IV

Table 2.1 (cont.)

Drug class	Preparation (immediate use)	Application/dosage	Indication
Epinephrine* 1:1000 (cont.)		*Inhalation for stridor:* 0.5 mg/kg/dose = 0.5 ml/kg/dose (max. 6 mg/dose = 6 ml/dose), may dilute in 3 ml NS, give per nebulizer. May use *racemic epinephrine 2.25%* → 0.5 ml/dose in 3 ml NS per nebulizer	• Analgesia (e.g., before "elective" intubations) *Adverse effects:* respiratory depression, hypotension, bradycardia, muscular chest wall rigidity with reduced pulmonary compliance (rare when injected slowly), constipation
Fentanyl 1 ml = 50 µg 0.1 ml = 5 µg *Caution:* Several stock solutions available *Opioid, analgetic Protect from light. Incompatible with azithromycin, pentobarbital, phenytoin*	**1-ml syringe:** pure *For infants <2000 g, a 10 µg/ml solution may be prepared by adding 1 ml (50 µg) of 50 µg/ml solution to 4 ml normal saline (total volume 5 ml), then give 0.2–0.5 ml/kg/dose (2–5 µg/ kg/dose) SLOWLY IV* *To prepare IV drip:* Add 5 ml (250 µg) of stock vial (50 µg/ml) to 45 ml D₅W or NS, so that final concentration is 0.005 mg/ml (5 µg/ml).	*IV:* 2–5 µg/kg/dose = 0.04–0.1 ml/kg/dose SLOW IV push (minimum is 1 min), repeat ≈2–4 h → Onset of action in 30 s, peak of action after 1 min, serum half-life ca. 4–5 h. Biological (effective) half-life for first single dose ≈10 min (neonates?), second dose ≈ 2–4 h (neonates?). Effect of first single dose lasts ≈20–30 min (in neonates?) → *Caution:* adjust dose and dose interval to renal function! *Continuous IV infusion, e.g., s/p surgery (see adverse effects):* initial bolus 1–3 µg/kg/dose SLOW IV push (≥1 min), then	

Analgesia	1–2	µg/kg/h
Sedation/analgesia	1–5 (–10)	µg/kg/h
Fentanyl 5 µg/ml	1	ml/h (1 kg)
	0.2	ml/h (…kg)

Drug class	Preparation (immediate use)	Application/dosage	Indication
Fosphenytoin 1 ml = 50 mg PE, available in 2- and 10-ml vials *Antiepileptic, antiarrhythmic [lb]* Fosphenytoin is a water-soluble prodrug of phenytoin that is rapidly converted by phosphatases in blood and tissue. Conversion half-life fosphenytoin (inactive) → phenytoin (active) ≈7 min 1.5 mg fosphenytoin is equivalent to 1 mg phenytoin sodium which is equivalent to fosphenytoin 1 mg PE. $t_{1/2} \approx 18$–60 h	Administer IV diluted after diluting in NS or D₅W or D₁₀W to a concentration of 1.5–25 mg PE/ml, e.g., add 2 ml (100 mg) PE to 3 ml NS, then final concentration 20 mg/ml, give 1 ml/kg/loading dose in 15 min IV Administer Fosphenytoin IM undiluted (second choice)	Fosphenytoin dosing is expressed in phenytoin equivalents (PE). (Fosphenytoin 1 mg PE = phenytoin 1 mg) *IV: loading dose:* 20 mg PE /kg SLOWLY, i.e., max. rate is 2 mg PE/kg/min (rule of thumb for neonates: give loading dose in ≈15 min IV). Flush with saline before and after administration. If seizures continue → give 5–10 mg/kg/dose boluses until phenytoin level is 20 mcg/ml For non-emergent loading use 10–15 mg PE/kg/dose in 30 min IV (the older drug, phenytoin, has to be given even slower: 15–20 mg/kg/loading dose in two single doses over 15 min each) → *Give only under ECG monitoring* → *Monitor BP closely during infusion* → *Remember high pH of solution*	• Phenytoin, but not fosphenytoin is FDA approved for neonates • Drug of second choice for neonatal seizures *Contraindication:* sinus bradycardia, second- and third-degree heart (AV) block *Adverse effects:* arrhythmia, hypotension (especially with rapid IV push), interaction with other drugs (CytP450). *Use with caution in neonates with hyperbilirubinemia:* both fosphenytoin and bilirubin displace phenytoin from

Fosphenytoin (cont.)

Store unopened vials in refrigerator. Do not use vials containing precipitate.
Incompatible with midazolam.
1 mg PE contains 0.0037 mmol phosphate, pH is 8.6–9.0
To be stored at 4–8°C

Maintenance IV dosing: 3–5 mg PE/kg q 12 h (or q 24 h)
SLOW IV push (maximum rate 1.5 mg PE/kg/min)
Phenytoin (not fosphenytoin) levels: trough levels 48 h after loading dose: therapeutic goal is 6–15 µg/ml (up to 10–20 µg/ml)
Reduce dose in renal and hepatic insufficiency and hypoalbuminemia
For recurrent, prolonged seizures, many also recommend a concurrent phenobarbital level ≥40 µg/ml while treating with fosphenytoin

protein-binding sites, resulting in increased free phenytoin concentration.
Neurotoxicity described for chronic exposure to phenytoin!
Fosphenytoin drug interactions as for phenytoin (cytochrome P450 substrate): see package inserts.
Drugs that are highly protein-bound compete with phenytoin and may increase phenytoin levels.

Furosemide*

(Lasix®) 1 ml = 10 mg
Loop diuretic
Alkaline solution: pH = 8–9.3

1-ml syringe: continuous IV infusion:
50 mg in 50 ml NS (Alternative: D₅W) then 1 ml = 1 mg

IV: 0.5 (–1–max. 2) mg/kg = 0.05 (–0.1–0.2) ml/kg over 5 min q 8 h or q 12 h
Continuous IV infusion: 5–10 mg/kg/day, i.e., initially IV bolus 0.1 mg/kg followed by IV infusion 0.1 mg/kg/h, doubled every 2 h (titrate to effect) to a max. of 0.4 mg/kg/h
Consider furosemide 1–2 mg/kg per dose in 2 ml NS inhalation (nebulizer) for preterm infants with BPD/CLD undergoing mechanical ventilation
Adjust dose in renal and hepatic impairment

● Hydrops
● CHF with pulmonary edema
Adverse effects: hypokalemia, Na↓, Cl↓, Ca↓, Mg↓, alkalosis, nephrocalcinosis, interstitial nephritis, ototoxicity. Do not give together with aminoglycoside and cephalosporin (stack dosing).
Can increase PGE production:
caution: Preterm infant with PDA

Gentamicin* (See also p. 41)

2 ml = 10 mg (pediatric)
1 ml = 5 mg *Aminoglycoside; additive effect with β-lactam antibiotic (esp. cephalosporin)*
Alternatives:
● Tobramycin
● Netilmicin

1-ml syringe: undiluted

IV: 3.5–5 mg/kg/first dose = 0.7–1 ml/kg/dose over 10 min, or better as 30-min IV infusion
Serum trough level: 30–60 min before the third dose: 0.5–1 (–2) µg/ml (mg/l), check level. Hold medication until drug level is known and in goal (non-toxic) range. It might be useful to draw trough levels 60 min prior to next dose in order to get the results back in time.
Serum peak level: 30 min after end of infusion of second dose (preterm, renal impairment) or third dose (term neonates): 6–12 µg/ml (mg/l)
Half-life is 3–11.5 h (<1 week), 3–6 h (1 week to 1 month)
Precaution: in preterm infants or renal insufficiency, optional to reduce dose or extend dosing interval. Consider starting empiric therapy with ampicillin/cefotaxim instead of ampicillin/gentamicin in preterm infants <26 weeks' GA and

● Suspected neonatal sepsis:
Active esp. against Gram-negative bacilli (except N. gonorrhoea, Salmonella) and Gram-positive bacilli (partly against *Staphylococcus aureus*, but not against *Pneumococci*).
Use of aminoglycosides with β-lactam antibiotics when B-Streptococci (GBS) is suspected (synergism).
Adverse effects: Ototoxicity and nephrotoxicity: do NOT give aminoglycosides together with cephalosporins and/or

Table 2.1 (cont.)

Drug class	Preparation (immediate use)	Application/dosage	Indication
Gentamicin* (cont.)		those on indomethacin as well as newborns s/p severe hypotension → *Septic work-up before use: obtain blood culture, optionally LP*	furosemide (Lasix®) → stack dosing
Lidocaine 1%* 1 ml = 10 mg *Local anesthetic, antiarrhythmic [Ib] Careful: do not use combi drug: lidocaine+epinephrine (for local anesthesia)*	1-ml, 2-ml or 20-ml syringe: pure	*IV:* initial dose 1 mg/kg/dose = 0.1 ml/kg/dose, then IV *infusion:* 1–1.5 mg/kg/h = 0.1–0.15 ml/kg/h Decreased efficacy when hypokalemia is present *Local anesthesia:* infiltrate approx. 0.5 ml/kg 1% lidocaine prior to procedure (e.g., chest tube) *Caution:* no IV application	• Ventricular tachycardia • Ventricular flutter (very rare indication and controversial) • Local anesthesia (chest tube placement in non-depressed neonates) *Adverse effects:* Sinus arrest, heart (AV) block, seizures, breathing problems
Lorazepam* (Ativan®) 1 ml = 2 mg *Benzodiazepine: sedative, antiepileptic IV solution contains 2% benzyl alcohol Refrigerate, protect from light. Alternative benzodiazepines:* clonazepam, diazepam, midazolam	2-ml- or 3-ml syringe. Dilute 1:1 in D5W or NS prior to use, i.e., 1 ml + 1 ml D5W or NS, then 1 ml = 1 mg. Use 1-ml syringe for IV administration	*IV:* 0.05 (–0.1) mg/kg/dose = 0.05 (–0.1) ml/kg/dose slow IV push (in 2–5 min). Optional to repeat single doses once or twice No sufficient data on multiple dosing (solution contains benzyl alcohol and propylene glycol) Onset of action 15–30 min, duration 8–12 h (sedation)	• Sedation • Seizures (third choice) *Adverse effects:* hypotension, apnea, severe myoclonus in preterm infants *Neurotoxicity described for chronic exposure to benzodiazepines*
Meropenem (See also p. 41) *Antibiotic, carbapenem* Minimal data on the safety and efficacy in infants <3 months of age. When reconstituted, stable for 1 h at room temperature and for 4 h in refrigerator	To be reconstituted with sterile water or normal saline	*IV:* <36 weeks' GA: 20 mg/kg/dose q 12 h ≥36 weeks' GA: 20 mg/kg/dose q 8 h Some use q 12 h interval dosing regardless of GA on day 0–7 or if <2000 g Meningitis dose is 30–40 mg/kg/dose q 8 h IV Half-life is 2–3 h, the drug cleared by the kidneys	• Neonatal sepsis. Used as primary combination together with vancomycin in sick VLBW preterm infants with suspected sepsis • Treatment of multi-drug-resistant Gram-negative and Gram-positive aerobic and anaerobic pathogens documented or suspected to be susceptible to meropenem • Treatment of meningitis, pneumonia, UTI, intra-abdominal infections (e.g., necrotizing enterocolitis) *Active against susceptible S. aureus, S. pyogenes, S. agalactiae (GBS), H. influenzae, N. meningitidis,*

Midazolam

(Versed®, Dormicum®)
1 ml = 1 mg preservative-free solution (caution also 1 mg/ml and 5 mg/ml in 1% benzyl alcohol available)
Benzodiazepine: sedative, antiepileptic solution contains 1% benzyl alcohol
Refrigerate, protect from light
Alternative benzodiazepines: clonazepam, diazepam, midazolam

1-ml syringe

To prepare IV drip: add 2.5 ml (12.5 mg) of stock vial (5 mg/ml) to 47.2 ml D₅W or NS, so that final concentration is 0.25 mg/ml (250 µg/ml)

IV: 0.05 (–0.1) mg/kg/dose = 0.05 (–0.1) ml/kg/dose slow IV push (in 2–5 min). Optional to repeat single doses once or twice
No sufficient data on multiple dosing (solution contains benzyl alcohol). Onset of action 1–5 min, duration 20–30 min (variable)
Conscious sedation during mechanical ventilation (see Adverse effects) by continuous IV infusion (e.g., s/p surgery): initial dosing (250 µg/ml):

Midazolam 250 µg/ml (body weight)

≥32 weeks' gestation	0.03	≈mg/kg/h
	0.12	≈ml/h (1 kg)
		≈ml/h (...kg)

Midazolam 250 µg/ml (body weight)

<32 weeks' gestation	0.06	≈mg/kg/h
	0.24	≈ml/h (1 kg)
		≈ml/h (...kg)

Use lowest dose possible

M. catarrhalis, E. coli, Klebsiella, Enterobacter, Serratiae, P. aeruginosa, B. cepacia, B. fragilis

• Sedation
• Seizures (third choice)
Adverse effects: hypotension, apnea, severe myoclonus in preterm infants. Paradoxical reactions appear to be common with midazolam. Continuous IV infusions prolong time on ventilator and in ICU (Cochrane)
Neurotoxicity described for chronic exposure to benzodiazepines
A recent Cochrane analysis (2003) argues against the use of midazolam in the NICU

Milrinone

Primacor® 10mg/10ml
vial 1 ml = 1 mg 1 mg/ml
(1000 µg/ml) Caution: Premixed Primacor® (in D₅W) as 200 µg/ml stock solution available.
Phosphodiesterase II inhibitor inodilatator incompatible with fursosemide, sodium bicarbonate

5-ml or 10-ml syringe

a. Dilute 1.8 ml/kg (1 mg/ml solution) Milrinone in total volume of 30 ml D₅W or NS, then 1 ml = 60 µg/kg

Loading dose via central line/UVC: loading dose (optional): initially 25 µg/kg/dose (=0.75 ml/kg/dose) IV or 50 µg/kg/dose (=1.5 ml/kg/dose) IV SLOWLY in 30 (–60) min, then IV infusion start at 0.5 µg/kg/min, and titrate to dose effect
Maintenance IV infusion: 0.25–0.5–0.75 µg/kg/min

a. Solution with 1 ml = 60 µg/kg

0.25	0.5	0.75	≈µg/kg/min
0.25	0.5	0.75	≅ml/h

Continuous IV infusion should be given on (cardiac) ICU

OR

Indication: short term treatment (<72 h) of low cardiac output s/p cardiac surgery or due to septic shock
• Decreases pre- and afterload
• Improves systolic and diastolic ventricular function
• Improves RV function
• Improves outcome after cardiac surgery

Table 2.1 (cont.)

Drug class	Preparation (immediate use)	Application/dosage	Indication

Milrinone (cont.)

Preparation:
b Use standard solution, i.e., add 10 ml (10 mg) of stock vial (1 mg/1 ml) to 90 ml D$_5$W or NS, then final concentration = 100 µg/ml *Usual final concentration ≤200 µg/ml*

Application/dosage:
b. Final conc. 100 µg/ml (body weight)

0.25	0.5	0.75	≈µg/kg/min
0.15	0.30	0.6	≅ml/h (1 kg)
			≅ml/h (...kg)

Serum $t_{1/2}$ after cardiac surgery = 1–5 h. Hemodynamic effects can still be present 3–5 h after infusion ceases. Elimination in urine as unchanged drug (83%) and glucuronide metabolite (12%) → reduce dose in patients with renal insufficiency

Indication:
• See above
Adverse effects: ventricular arrhythmias (12%, VTach 1%, VFib 0.2%), SVT (3.8%), hypokalemia, LFT elevation
Contraindications: severe obstructive aortic or pulmonic valvular disease, LVOTO (HOCM). Use with caution in patients with history of ventricular arrhythmias

---

Morphine
1 ml = 10 mg
0.1 ml = 1 mg
Opioid, analgetic

Preparation:
1 ml syringe: add 0.1 ml morphine (10 mg/ml) to 0.9 ml saline, so that final conc. 0.1 mg/0.1 ml (1 mg/ml)
To prepare IV drip: add 2.5 ml (2.5 mg) of stock vial (1 mg/ml) to 47.5 ml D$_5$W or NS, so that final concentration is 0.05 mg/ml (50 µg/ml)

Application/dosage:
IV: 0.05–0.1 mg/kg/dose = 0.05–0.1 ml/kg/dose (1 mg/ml solution)
→ Onset of action after 1 min, max. effect after ca. 30 min, serum half-life ca. 3–5 h, biological (effective) half-life after the first single dose ca. 4 h, after the second single dose >4 h
Continuous IV infusion, e.g. s/p surgery (see Adverse effects): 0.02–0.1 mg/kg/h IV

Morphine 50 µg/ml (weight in kg)

0.02	0.05	0.1	≈mg/kg/h
20	50	100	≅µg/kg/h
0.2	0.5	1	≅ml/h (1 kg)
			≅ml/h (...kg)

Indication:
• Analgesia or sedation
• Decrease of pulmonary resistance (PVR)
Adverse effects: respiratory depression, histamine release, hypotension, constipation

---

Nafcillin
(See also p. 41)
Semi-synthetic penicillinase-resistant penicillin
Drug of choice for MSSA

Application/dosage:
IV: 25 mg/kg/dose q 6 to 12 h, see interval 2
For treatment of meningitis of a nafcillin-sensitive pathogen: 50 mg/kg/dose, see interval 2

Naloxone
1 ml = 0.4 mg
0.1 ml = 0.04 mg
Opioid antagonist Caution:

Preparation:
1-ml syringe: undiluted

Application/dosage:
IV: 0.1 mg/kg/dose. This dose in not evidence-based. In the absence of an emergency, many intensivists use lower doses, such as 0.01–0.05 mg/kg/dose (IM, SC and ET possible, but second choice)

Indication:
• Opioid overdose
• May be considered when mothers have been treated with opioids (e.g. fentanyl, tramadol,

Naloxone (cont.)

Narcan®, Narcanti® come in different stock solutions
Naloxon is not listed in the ILCOR resuscitation guidelines 2005.
If indicated, give naloxone in NICU (not in delivery room)

1-ml and 50-ml or 60-ml syringe for IV infusion

→ *Onset of action: seconds to 2 min*
Peak of effect after 2–3 min
Effective half-life: much shorter than of opioids; serum half-life: for neonates 1–3 h
Duration of action: first single dose 10–30 min, therefore, repeat dose every 10–30 min, optional to begin with IV Infusion in the NICU

pethidin) in the 4 h prior to delivery
Contraindication: heroin- or methadone- addicted mothers and mothers suspected of drug abuse (→ acute withdrawal syndrome). Hence, DO NOT use naloxone in the delivery room

Norepinephrine

(= noradrenaline) 1 ml = 1 mg
Vasoconstrictor, inochronotropic

a. Add 0.2 ml/kg (1 mg/ml stock solution) to total of 30 ml D_5W or NS, then 1 ml = 6.6 µg/kg

OR

b. Use standard solution, i.e., add 1 ml (1000 µg) of stock solution (1 mg/ml) to 124 ml D_5W or NS, then final concentration 8 µg/ml

Start IV infusion at: 0.05–0.1 µg/kg/min, then titrate to desired effect (max IV rate 1–2 µg/kg/min). Infuse via central IV line

a. Solution with 1 ml = 6.6 µg/kg

0.05	0.11	0.5	≅µg/kg/min
0.5	1.0	4.5	≅ml/h

OR

b. Final conc. 8 µg/ml (body weight)

0.05	0.11	0.5	≅µg/kg/min.
0.38	0.75	3.75	≅ml/h (1 kg)
			≅ml/h (...kg)

- Arterial hypotension despite volume IV (e.g., TGA with poor S_aO_2 prior to Rashkind procedure, septic shock)
- Increases SVR and PVR, BP (diastolic > systolic), may increase pulmonary perfusion in case of large PDA
- *Caution:* may provoke vagus-induced bradycardia

Phenobarbital*

1 ml = 200 mg
barbiturate, antiepileptic
neurotoxicity described for chronic exposure to phenobarbital

1 ml phenobarbital + 9 ml saline:
1 ml = 20 mg

IV: Loading dose: ca. 20 mg/kg in 2–4 doses IV over a total period of 20 min (or IV infusion over 20 min). If necessary, may re-load with an additional 20 mg/kg in aliquots of 5–10 mg/kg until level is ≥40 µg/ml.
→ Give no faster than 1 mg/kg/min IV
Maintenance IV dose: ca. 3–5 mg/kg/dose q 12 h or 4–6 mg/kg/dose q 24 h
Serum half-life: 37 h up to over 150 h. Serum concentration: "therapeutic" ≥40 µg/ml

- Neonatal seizures (first choice)
DO NOT give as prophylaxis without initial symptoms
DO NOT give as an initial sedation drug
Adverse effects: drug interaction, hypotension, serum concentration

Table 2.1 (cont.)

Drug class	Preparation (immediate use)	Application/dosage	Indication
Phenylephrine (phenylephrine hydrochloride 1%) 10 mg/ml (1 ml and 5 ml vial) *Peripheral vasoconstrictor (mainly α₁-adrenoreceptor agonist)* *Do not use if solution turns brown or contains a precipitate*	1- and 50-ml syringe for pump Use standard solution, i.e., add 0.5 ml (5000 μg) of stock solution (10 mg/ml) to 124.5 ml D₅W or NS, then final concentration 40 μg/ml	*IV:* 5–20 μg/kg/dose q 10–15 min IV. *Start IV infusion at:* 0.1 (–0.5) μg/kg/min, titrate to desired effect (max. usually 2 μg/kg/min)	*Indication:* treatment of hypotension and vascular failure in shock Increases diastolic > systolic BP, MAP and systemic vascular resistance

Final conc. 40 μg/ml (body weight)

				$\cong$μg/kg/min
0.1	0.3	0.5		$\cong$ml/h (1 kg)
0.15	0.45	0.75		$\cong$ml/h (...kg)

Epinephrine but not phenylephrine is the drug of choice for neonatal resuscitation

Drug class	Indication
Phenytoin see Fosphenytoin	
Piperacillin (See also p. 41) *Semi-synthetic extended-spectrum penicillin (spectrum as for mezlocillin). Primarily excreted renally (hardly any hepatic metabolism). CSF penetration similar to that of other penicillins*	Gram-positive spectrum as for other β-lactam penicillins. Generally also effective against Gram-negative organisms including *Hemophilus influenzae, Klebsiella pneumoniae, Proteus mirabilis, E. coli, Pseudomonas aeruginosa, some Serratia,* and many anaerobes

IV: 80 mg/kg/dose, see interval 2

GA (weeks p.m.)	Postnatal days	Interval (no. 2)
≤29 (or <1200 g)	0–28	q 12 h
	>28	q 8 h
30–36 (≅1200–2700 g)	0–14	q 12 h
	>14	q 8 h
37–44	0–7	q 12 h
	>7	q 8 h
≥45	All	q 6 h

Piperacillin-Tazobactam

(Zosyn®) (See also p. 41)
Semi-synthetic extended-spectrum penicillin. Zosyn® combines the extended-spectrum antibiotic piperacillin with the β-lactamase inhibitor tazobactam in an 8:1 ratio. Tazobactam undergoes significant hepatic metabolism. CNS penetration is modest (limited data)

Treatment of non-CNS infections. Gram-positive spectrum as for other β-lactam penicillins. Generally also effective against Gram-negative organisms including *Hemophilus influenzae, Klebsiella pneumoniae, Proteus mirabilis, E. coli, Pseudomonas aeruginosa,* some *Serratia,* and many anaerobes

IV: 80 mg/kg/dose, see interval 2

GA (weeks p.m.)	Postnatal days	Interval (no. 2)
≤29 (or <1200 g)	0–28	q 12 h
	>28	q 8 h
30–36 (≈1200–2700 g)	0–14	q 12 h
	>14	q 8 h
37–44	0–7	q 12 h
	>7	q 8 h
≥45	All	q 6 h

Prostaglandin E_1*

(Alprostadil®)
1 ml (ampoul) = 500 μg
Vasodilatator Alternative: PGE_2; however, PGE_2 is not approved for neonatal use

• Suspected duct-dependent congenital heart disease
Adverse effects: apnea, hypotension, seizures, pulmonary hypersecretion, fever, jitteriness; steal effect via PDA (CNS, abdomen)
Many centers leave patients NPO while on PGE_1

IV infusion start: 50 (–max. 100) ng/kg/min (= 0.05–0.1 μg/kg/min) IV infusion maintenance: according to infant's response and ECHO, aim for lowest rate (rule of thumb for transport: minimal dose ≅10 ng/kg/min)

a. PGE_1 solution with 1 ml = 1 μg/kg

10	50	100	≅ng/kg/min
0.01	0.05	0.1	≅μg/kg/h
0.6	3.0	6.0	≅μg/kg/h
0.6	3.0	6.0	≅ml/h

OR

b. PGE_1 final conc. 5 μg/ml

10	50	100	≅ng/kg/min
0.01	0.05	0.1	≅μg/kg/min
0.6	3.0	6.0	≅μg/kg/h
0.12	0.6	1.2	≅ml/h (1 kg)
			≅ml/h (...kg)

Sample dilution:
a. Add 1 ml PGE_1 stock solution (500 μg) + 9 ml NS, then concentration 50 μg/ml, then dilute further 1 ml/kg (50 μg/kg) in total of 50 ml D_5W or NS, then final concentration 1 ml = 1 μg/kg

OR

b. Add 0.5 ml (250 μg) of stock solution (500 μg/ml) to 49.5 ml D_5W or NS, then final conc. 5 μg/ml

Table 2.1 (cont.)

Drug class	Preparation (immediate use)	Application/dosage	Indication
Rocuronium* 5 ml = 50 mg 1 ml = 10 mg 0.1 ml = 1 mg *Non-depolarizing neuromuscular blocker. Alternatives:* 1. *cis-Atracurium (0.1 mg/kg/ dose IV); advantage: Hoffman elimination independent of renal and hepatic function* 2. *Vecuronium 0.1–0.2 mg/kg/ dose*	1-ml syringe: undiluted	IV: 0.6–1.2 mg/kg/dose = 0.06–0.12 ml/kg/dose, eventually repeat single dose. Always flush with 5–10 ml NS Continuous infusion: 5–10 (–15) µg/kg/min = 0.3–0.6 (–0.7) mg/kg/h (alternative: pancuronium 0.1 mg/kg/dose q 1–2 h) Onset and maximum effect after 30–60 s (intubation) *Duration of effect: 30–60 min, longer with hepatic and renal dysfunction, as well as bile duct diseases* → *Primarily biliary excretion (70%); ≈30% excreted unchanged in urine* → *Refrigerate! Can be stored at room temperature for 3 months*	• Difficult intubations despite analgesia and sedative • Bad lung compliance under PPV to avoid barotrauma (adjust PIP afterwards) *Adverse effects: histamine release* → *rarely anaphylaxis, hypotension; for more* *Adverse effects and drug interactions see package insert*
Sildenafil 20 mg (Revatio®) or 50 mg (Viagra®) tablets *Phosphodiesterase (PDE) 5 inhibitor (may also inhibit other PDE isoforms)* *Suspension is stable for one month at 4–8°C*	To prepare an oral suspension, thoroughly crush one tablet into fine powder and add enough Ora-Plus to make a final concentration of 2 mg/ml *Use in neonates should be considered experimental since clinical data are still very limited*	NG/PO: 0.3–1 mg/kg/dose q 6 to q 8 h per oro- or nasogastric tube. Some authors have succesfully used doses of 2 mg/kg/ dose IV: IV solution not yet approved for neonatal use *Oral absorption is rapid with approx. 40% bioavailability* *Initiate sildenafil treatment on ICU. Continuous monitoring of BP and oxygenation (pre- and postductal SpO₂, PaO₂) mandatory*	• PPHN refractory to iNO and other conventional therapies • Neonates who are unable to be weaned off iNO • Situation where iNO is indicated but unavailable *Adverse effects: Worsening oxygenation, systemic hypotension. May increase the risk of retinopathy of prematurity in preterm infants*
Sodium bicarbonate 8.4%* 1 ml = 1 mmol = 1 mEq *Indication: correction of metabolic acidosis Rare indications:* • hyperkalemia • hypermagnesemia • symptomatic intoxication with tricyclic antidepressant *Sodium bicarbonate should not be infused with catecholamine, calcium, magnesium, serum protein solutions, human*	20ml- or 50-ml pump syringe always dilute 1:1 in Aqua dest. (or glucose 5%); e.g., 10 ml sodium bicarbonate + 10 ml Aqua dest. Alternatively, use premade sodium bicarbonate 4.2% solution	After PPV, administer by IV when metabolic acidosis is established and IV is secure For sodium bicarbonate 8.4%, 1 mmol = 1 mEq *Desired sodium bicarbonate in mEq (= mmol) = (base deficit × kg body weight) ÷ 3* Dilute sodium bicarbonate 1:1 with sterile water and administer via continuous IV infusion over (15–) 30–60 (–120) min Maximum IV INFUSION rate: 0.1 mEq/kg/min = 6 mEq/kg/h (= 12 ml of 1:1 dilution/kg/h); always do blood gas analysis before and after buffer treatment → *Avoid IV bolus: "blind" treatment only in emergency cases (e.g., when blood gas apparatus is out of order or child*	• Metabolic acidosis (pH <7.15; base excess below –10 and PCO₂ <60 mmHg) in spite volume expansion. *Do not administer sodium bicarbonate when:* • Respiratory acidosis overweighs (PCO₂ more than 60 mmHg and up to base excess-9) • Metabolic acidosis plus hypoventilation (especially during respiratory insufficiency)

Sodium bicarbonate 8.4%* (cont.)

albumin, diverse antibiotics, amino acids, fentanyl, pancuronium, phenobarbital, vitamin B_1 or vitamin B_6 (see package insert)

Surfactant*

Take 2–3 ampoules in cooled mini bag on transport

1. Poractant (Curosurf®, porcine surfactant) available in 1.5-ml (120 mg phospholipid) and 3-ml (240 mg phospholipid) vials
2. Beractant (Survanta®, bovine surfactant) available in 4-ml (100 mg phospholipid) and 8-ml (200 mg phospholipid) vials
3. Alveofact® (bovine surfactant; 50 mg/1.2 ml), available in Europe but not in US: 50–100 mg/kg/dose ET
4. Calfactant (Infasurf®, calf surfactant, 35 mg phospholipid/ml. 3 ml/kg/dose)

Most surfactant preparations must be stored at 4–8°C. Do NOT use 1 ml "insulin" syringes with plunger because this inactivates surfactant. Do NOT "clean" surface of ampoule with alcohol solution. Used vials with residual drug should be discarded

Kit: no dilution for Curosurf and Alveofact: draw the total dose from several vials in one (or two) 5-ml or 6-ml syringe

Give total dose in 2–4 single doses. May administer total dose in divided single doses (2–4), thereby changing head or body positions to the right and left with each administration

Curosurf®, Survanta® and Infasurf® must be refrigerated and protected from light. Alveofact® powder is stable at room temperature

homebirth), after 10 min of ineffective resuscitation 2 (–4)ml/kg IV of the 1:1 mixture over 10 min

→ *Restrictive indication for buffer treatment, particularly in preterm and both preterm/term infants without vital indication*

Curosurf: 100–200 mg/kg/dose ET, e.g., 2.5 ml/kg/dose (=200 mg/kg/dose) in 1–2 aliquots, followed by up to 2 subsequent doses of 1.25 ml/kg/dose (=100 mg/kg/dose) at 12-h intervals if needed. No clear evidence from literature that 200 mg/kg is superior to 100 mg/kg as first dose ET. *May gently turn vial upside down (→ suspension), but do not shake Curosurf*

Survanta: 100 mg/kg in 4 doses = 4 ml/kg in 4 doses = 1 ml/kg × 4 (caution: high volume ET), up to 3 additional doses q6 in first 48 h after birth if indicated. *Swirl vial, but do not shake Survanta*

Alveofact®: 100 mg/kg = 2.4 ml/kg for the first single dose, 50 mg/kg for the second single dose 2–12 h interval after the last dose, eventually the third single dose (20–) 50 mg/kg, 12 h after last the last dose

Surfactant application; a word of caution: verify the position of ET tube (clinically and/or chest X-ray) before giving surfactant. Check on S_pO_2 and tidal volume and reduce F_iO_2 ventilatory rate and PIP (often in this order) after ET surfactant instillation in the NICU

→ Surfactant application, 4 options: (1) via 5 F end-hole catheter; (2) via inbuilt application tubing; (3) through large IV catheter (e.g. 17 G/45 mm), which is shorter than the ET tube; (4) surfactant instillation is also possible over a shortened suction catheter or gastric tube

Surfactant and neonatal transport: Necessary ventilator changes and lung compliance are poorly controlled during transport using mobile ventilators/transport incubators, i.e.,

Do not administer sodium bicarbonate when:

- short cardiopulmonary resuscitation (<10 min)
- Resuscitation and (still) inadequate ventilation and circulation are present
- Hypernatremia (then use TRIS (Tris-hydroxymethyl aminomethane) buffer (=THAM)
- PIV not definitely in the vein (extravasation → necrosis)

- *Prophylactic administration* of intubated preterm infants at risk for RDS in the delivery room in the first 30–60 min of life:i.e., preterm infant <30 0/7 (–32 0/7) weeks' GA
- *Early therapeutic administration* to preterm infants <28 0/7 weeks' GA with severe RDS (intubated) and high oxygen requirement in the delivery room
- *Rescue treatment* for preterm infants (intubated or on CPAP) with RDS by chest X-ray and F_iO_2 >0.4 (for P_aO_2 goal ≈60–70 mmHg) in the NICU
- *Secondary RDS due to meconium aspiration* DO NOT aim for P_aO_2 >80 mmHg in VLBW infants. Surfactant therapy prior to transport without initial chest X-ray (verification of ET tube) is justified when the neonate is unstable for transport or already on high ventilatory support and F_iO_2 and chest

Table 2.1 *(cont.)*

60

Drug class	Preparation (immediate use)	Application/dosage	Indication
Surfactant* *(cont.)*		adjust ventilator settings on NICU or re-evaluate whether surfactant is indicated prior to neonatal transport	X-ray is not readily available. When FRC and compliance improve with surfactant ET, adjust the following rapidly: $F_iO_2(\downarrow)$, $T_{in}(\downarrow)$ and $T_{exp}(\uparrow)$, then adjust PIP and eventually PEEP

THAM
= Tris bufffer = Tromethamine
= Tris-hydroxymethyl
aminomethane
0.3 mol/ml = 0.3 M = 0.3 Eq/ml
(caution: some stock solutions come as 3 mmol/ml; required THAM (3 M) in ml = (BE × kg body weight) : 10
THAM = Tris buffer = should not run with catecholamine, serum protein solutions, human albumin, cephalosporin, vancomycin, opioids, pancuronium, tolazoline, vitamin B_1 and vitamin B_6 (see package insert)

	Preparation (immediate use)	Application/dosage	Indication
THAM	• Dilute 0.3 M solution 1:1 in $D_{10}W$ (1 ml Tris 0.3 M : 1 ml $D_{10}W$, then peripheral THAM infusion possible • Better: THAM can run up to maximum of 3 M with $D_{10}W$ via UVC/central line • If only THAM 3 mmol/l (=3 M) available: *dilute Tris (=THAM) 3 M 1:10 with sterile water, then 0.3 M solution*	• Very rarely indicated: required THAM (0.3 M) in ml = base deficit × kg body weight. Dilute 1:1 in $D_{10}W$ and replace initially only half of the required amount over 30 min (in asphyxia)–60–(–120) min IV	*Indication: correction of metabolic acidosis* Advantage of THAM = Tris buffer (versus sodium bicarbonate): no increase of PCO_2 and sodium. *Adverse effects:* hypertonic, volume burden, hypoglycemia (dilute in $D_{10}W$), apnea, liver cell necrosis, etc. *Contraindication:* uremia/anuria

Vancomycin (See also
pp. 300–1)

• Neonatal sepsis
Active against most
Gram-positive pathogens, such as coagulase-negative, oxacillin-resistant *Staphylococci (Staphylococcus epidermidis), Staphylococcus aureus* (including MRSA) and *Enterococci (Enterococcus faecalis > Enterococcus faecium)*, and also against a few anaerobic pathogens (clostridia and actinomyces)

IV: 15 mg/kg/dose q 8 to q 18 h IV infusion over 60 min

GA (weeks p.m.)	Postnatal days	Interval (no. 5)
≤29 (or <1200 g)	0–28	q 18 h
	>28	q 12 h
30–36 (≈1200–2700 g)	0–14	q 12 h
	>14	q 8 h
37–44	0–7	q 12 h
	>7	q 8 h
≥45	All	q 8 h

Vancomycin* (cont.)

Serum trough level: 5–10 (–15) µg/ml (mg/l), depending on the severity of the infection. Sample to be obtained 30 (–60) min before the third (or second) dose
In preterm neonates or renal impairment: determine serum levels before/after the second dose; some experts still recommend serum peak levels when treating meningitis (goal: 30–40 µg/ml), to be obtained 30 min after the end of the 60-min infusion. However, many centers no longer determine peak levels (time-dependent killing)
Interval and dosage must be individually adjusted to the serum trough level! Serum half-life is 6–10 h

- Difficult intubations despite analgesia and sedation
- Bad lung compliance under PPV to avoid barotrauma (adjust PIP afterwards!)
- *Adverse effects*: histamine release
  → rarely anaphylaxis, hypotension, for more *Adverse effects*: and drug interactions see package insert

Vecuronium

Non-depolarizing neuromuscular blocker
Contains benzyl alcohol and bromide
Alternatives:
1. Rocuronium (0.6–1.2 mg/kg/dose IV)
2. *cis*-atracurium (0.1 mg/kg/dose IV)

1-ml syringe
Dilute with NS or sterile water to max. concentration of 2 mg/ml

IV: 0.1 mg/kg/dose. Repeat q 1 h as needed
Onset of action: within 1–3 min (i.e., slower than rocuronium, but similar to *cis*-atracurium)
Duration (dose dependent): 30–40 min
Rate of elimination is appreciably reduced with hepatic but not with renal dysfunction

Vitamin K1*

(Phytonadione 10 mg/ml
0.1 ml = 1 mg
Contains 0.9% benzyl alcohol and bromide

Prophylaxis:
IM: 1 mg/dose (US)
SQ (=SC): 1 mg/dose to correct high INR
IV: 0.2 mg/kg or 1 mg/dose SLOW IV push (anaphylaxis reported)
PO: 2 mg/dose (PO route not recommended in US): 3 doses: first at birth, then at 1 week and 4 weeks of life); intestinal absorption not completely reliable, plasma levels not always at target level (especially with underlying biliary atresia)
Treatment (high INR):
SQ (SC): 1–2 mg/day
IV: 1–2 mg/day

- Prophylaxis of hemorrhagic disease (*M. hemorrhagicus neonatorum*)
- Correction of abnormal coagulation i.e., high INR (e.g. in sepsis)

*Medications marked with an asterisk should be found in every neonatal emergency bag (NETS). Have prostaglandin E, only one muscle relaxant, one benzodiazepine, two antibiotics and at least one vial surfactant and prostaglandin refrigerated (i.e., separate mini bag with cooling pads).

Abbreviations:

$t_{1/2}$ = serum half-life
AE, adverse effects
BP, blood pressure
BPD, bronchopulmonary dysplasia
CLD, chronic lung disease
CHF, congestive heart failure
CPR, cardiopulmonary resuscitation
ET, endotracheal
GA, gestational age
HR, heart rate
IM, intramuscular(ly)
IO, intraosseous(ly)
IV, intravenous(ly)
JET, junctional ectopic tachycardia
LFT, liver function tests
LP, lumbar puncture
LVOTO, left ventricular outflow tract obstruction
Aqua dest. = aqua destillata (sterile water)

MRSA, methicillin-resistant *S. aureus*
NLS, neonatal life support
PALS, pediatric advanced life support
PDA, patent ductus arteriosus
PIV, peripheral intravenous access
SC, subcutaneous(ly)
SQ, subcutaneous(ly)
SVR, systemic vascular resistance
SVT, supraventricular tachycardia
UTI, urinary tract infection
VFib, ventricular fibrillation
VFlu, ventricular flutter
VTach, ventricular tachycardia
WPW, Wolf–Parkinson–White syndrome
Solvents:
D_5W = glucose 5% solution
$D_{10}W$ = glucose 10% solution
NS = normal saline = NaCl 0.9% (isotonic)

Drip calculation: $\dfrac{\mu g/kg/min \times kg \times (60\,min/h)}{conc.\ (mg/ml) \times (1000\,\mu g/mg)}$ = rate (ml/h)

Table 2.1 is compiled from: Neofax 2007[1], Lexicomp 2006[2], RedBook 2006[3], ILCOR Recommendations On Neonatal Resuscitation 2005[4], Park MK 2008[5]. www.pedialink.org

[1]Young TE, Mangum B. *Neofax 2007, 20th edn., London: Thomson PDR, 2007.*

[2]Taketomo CK, Hodding JH, Kraus DM. *Lexi Comp's Pediatric Dosage Handbook with International Index.* 13th edn. Hudson: Lexicomp, 2006.

[3]Pickering LK. *Red Book:* 2006 Report of the *Committee on Infectious Diseases,* 27th edn: Washington, DC: American Academy of Pediatrics, 2006.

[4]ILCOR. International consensus on cardiopulmonary resuscitation and emergency cardiovascular care science with treatment recommendations. Part 7. Neonatal resuscitation. *Resuscitation* 2005;67:293–303.

[5]Park MK. *Pediatric Cardiology for Practitioners,* 5th edn. St. Louis: Mosby, 2008.

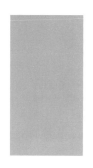

Postnatal cardiopulmonary adaptation

Georg Hansmann

An extensive description of perinatal physiological changes is beyond the scope of this handbook. However, for a better understanding, essential key points are listed below[14–19].

- The fetal alveoli are filled with fluid, the pulmonary vessels are constricted and the pulmonary vascular resistance (PVR) is high. With the first breath, the alveoli are filled with air, leading to establishment of functional residual capacity (FRC), adequate gas exchange and a rapid fall in PVR. During spontaneous breathing, inspiratory airway pressure can initially reach values up to $-80\,cmH_2O$ (where $1\,cmH_2O$ roughly equates to 1 mbar). Under mechanical ventilation, FRC is largely determined by the positive end-expiratory pressure (PEEP) rather than the peak inspiratory pressure (PIP)

- Surfactant improves alveolar stability and lung compliance by decreasing surface tension within each alveolus. Surfactant is produced by alveolar type II cells, which are evident in the lung by approximately 24 weeks of gestation. In addition to adequate surfactant production and function, fluid remaining within the alveoli must be cleared by transepithelial transport. Endogenous surfactant production is – in the absence of risk factors – sufficient at the beginning of 35 weeks' gestation. Besides prematurity, lack of functional surfactant is frequently caused by excessive amniotic fluid remaining in the alveoli, e.g., after C-sections, when lungs are not compressed in the small pelvis prior to the first breath and alveolar fluid clearance is delayed

- The main stimulus that drives breathing in babies born at 40 weeks' gestation is the P_aCO_2. The P_aO_2 response is relatively minor. Oxygen delivery to tissues is initially impaired by high hematocrit levels and the leftward shift of the oxygen – hemoglobin dissociation curve (due to high amounts of fetal hemoglobin, prematurity, hypothermia, alkalosis, hypocapnia, and a decrease of 2,3-diphosphoglycerate)

- The fetal circulation has the following shunts: right-to-left shunt through the ductus arteriosus (pulmonary artery $\rightarrow$ aorta), the foramen ovale [superior vena cava and inferior vena cava $\rightarrow$ right atrium (RA) $\rightarrow$ left atrium (LA) $\rightarrow$ left ventricle (LV) $\rightarrow$ aorta] and intrapulmonary shunts (Figure 2.15). Pulmonary blood flow, systemic arterial PO_2 (P_aO_2) and SO_2 (S_aO_2) are low (25–35 mmHg and 60%, respectively), whereas pulmonary arterial pressure is high (40–60 mmHg)

- Regulation of pulmonary vascular tone (arterioles) is different from that of systemic arteries: PVR drops when postnatal levels of P_aO_2 and S_aO_2 increase (oxygenation), P_aCO_2 decreases (ventilation) and the arterial pH rises. The decrease in mechanical resistance upon alveolar inflation further improves this postnatal transition. The sum of these postnatal changes leads to a remarkable increase in pulmonary blood flow, which

Neonatal Emergencies: A Practical Guide for Resuscitation, Transport and Critical Care, ed. Georg Hansmann. Published by Cambridge University Press. © Cambridge University Press 2009.

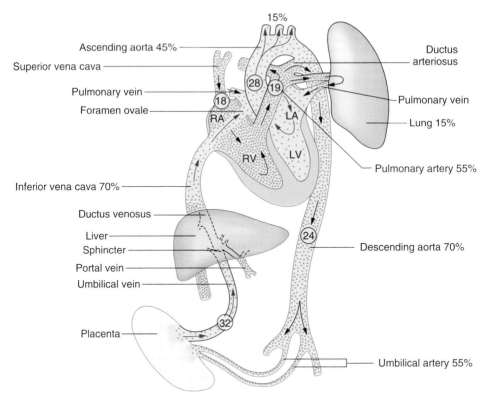

Figure 2.15 Fetal circulation with the four shunts: placenta, ductus venosus, foramen ovale, ductus arteriosus. The density of the dots is inversely proportional to the oxygen saturation: the less dense, the higher the oxygen partial pressure (PO_2). The numbers marked in the heart chambers and vessels correspond with the PO_2 in mmHg (circles). The percentages outside the cardiovascular structures stand for the relative flow in the main in-flow and outflow tracts of both heart chambers. The output of both ventricles adds up to 100%. VCI = V. cava inferior, LA = left atrium, LV = left ventricle, RA = right atrium, RV = right ventricle, VCS = V. cava superior. Modified from: Guntheroth WG et al. (1983) Physiology of the circulation: fetus, neonate and child. In: Kelly VC (ed.) *Practice of Pediatrics*, Vol. 8. Philadelphia: Harper & Row. See color plate section for full color version.

in turn improves gas exchange (given that cardiovascular anatomy and function are normal)

- With the postnatal rapid fall in PVR and the rise of systemic arterial resistance after clamping the umbilical cord, the foramen ovale closes functionally (left atrium pressure exceeds right atrium pressure), so that within 6 h the prenatal right-to-left-shunt of 90% is reduced to approx. 20%. The ductus arteriosus remains open for hours or days after birth, but mainly shunts left-to-right (aorta → PA, so-called *transitory perinatal circulation*) because of the dramatic postnatal changes in the pulmonary and systemic vascular resistance. The rise in P_aO_2 leads to vasoconstriction and functional closure of the ductus arteriosus. Therefore, duct-dependent congenital heart disease usually becomes symptomatic during the first week of life; newborns with coarctation of the aorta (CoA) may develop symptoms later in life, e.g., at 2–6 weeks of age (see p. 356). IV fluid boluses for neonatal resuscitation of ≫10 ml/kg in the delivery room are often associated with a greater ductal flow, and eventually persistent patent ductus arteriosus (PDA) (murmur may be louder in the NICU than in the delivery room). Low systemic pressure (e.g., continuous hypovolemia, low output, septic shock) and high PVR (pulmonary hypertension) may result in right-to-left shunt through the ductus (PA $\rightarrow$ aorta) and subsequently to a reduction of arterial oxygen saturation. With predominant ductal right-to-left-shunting, a significant S_aO_2 difference between the preductal (right arm or right ear lobe) and postductal (lower extremities, umibilical artery) oxygen saturation is common (e.g. 8–10 percentage points in S_pO_2; represent a so-called **ductal-split; caution: persistent pulmonary hypertension of the newborn!**, see p. 392). A ductal split may be absent if the atrial right-to-left shunt is much larger than the ductal shunt, or if an aberrant left subclavian artery is present (in the latter case, preductal S_pO_2 can only be measured accurately at the right ear lobe)

- The PVR of a healthy neonate decreases to normal values (<3 indexed Wood units or 1/5 of SVR) during the first 7 weeks of life, associated with a fall in pulmonary artery pressure. At this age (approx. 4th to 6th weeks after birth), large intra- or extracardiac left-to-right shunts [e.g., large ventricular septal defect (VSD), complete atrioventricular septal defect = CAVSD = CAVC, wide-open PDA, truncus arteriosus, complex heart disease without obstruction between ventricle and pulmonary artery] may become symptomatic, due to heightened shunt volume ($\rightarrow$ pulmonary artery $\rightarrow$ left atrium $\rightarrow$ left ventricle). The same is true for preterm infants: When respiratory distress syndrome and bronchopulmonary dysplasia ($\rightarrow$ chronic lung disease) improve, pH and P_aO_2 increase, thus, leading to a significant fall of PVR and pulmonary artery pressure. Generally, the decrease of PVR in preterm infants (especially in preterm infants $<1000\,g$, due to the "immaturity" of vascular smooth muscle cells) occurs earlier and faster than in term infants. Depending on the severity of the newborn's lung disease that is accompanied by high PVR, a significant fall of PVR may be observed either during the first week of life (e.g., improvement of respiratory distress syndrome in preterm infants) or later after mechanical ventilation for several weeks due to chronic lung disease. If the pulmonary blood flow is unrestricted (i.e., no right ventricular outflow tract obstruction/no pulmonary stenosis), this will cause enhanced left-to-right-shunting (e.g. VSD, large patent foramen ovale, PDA) and may lead to volume overload, pulmonary edema and congestive heart failure. Extremely low and very low birth weight infants often have moderate to severe myocardial insufficiency that may be associated with a significant ductal steal phenomenon (aorta $\rightarrow$ ductus arteriosus $\rightarrow$ pulmonary artery $\approx$ functional aortic regurgitation), leading to worsening systemic perfusion (caution: cardiac shock)

- In perinatal shock (birth asphyxia: prenatal, intrapartal, postnatal; e.g., meconium aspiration syndrome), PVR is elevated and may prevent both ductal shunt reversal and functional closure of the foramen ovale ($\rightarrow$ PPHN, "persistent pulmonary hypertension of the newborn," characterized by high PVR and remaining right-to-left shunts in ductus arteriosus and atria; see p. 392). Neonates with PPHN may initially show only signs of poor postnatal adaptation (e.g., tachypnea, pallor) but then gradually develop moderate to severe central cyanosis a few hours later

- For physiology of perinatal hypoxia ("birth asphyxia") see also p. 310

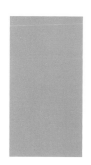

ABC techniques and procedures
Suctioning

Georg Hansmann

The following techniques and procedures are described in this subsection: suctioning, stimulation, oxygen supplementation, bag-and-mask ventilation, pharyngeal and bi-nasal continuous positive airway pressure (CPAP), pharyngeal positive pressure ventilation, endotracheal intubation, gastric tube placement, laryngeal mask airway (LMA) placement, chest compressions, peripheral venous access, umbilical vein/artery catheterization, central venous access (IJ), intraosseous access, and cord clamping. *For chest tube placement see chapter entitled "Pneumothorax."*

> A vigorous newborn infant born out of clear amniotic fluid who begins to cry within 5–10 s after birth does not need to be suctioned.

Unnecessary suctioning is uncomfortable for the infant and may cause lesions in the mucous membrane and occasionally a vagal reflex with subsequent bradycardia, laryngeal spasm and apnea[20].

Indications for suctioning of the upper respiratory tract
- Excessive amount of amniotic fluid in the oropharynx (e.g., after C-section)
- Green-stained, bloody or smelly fluid
- Prematurity (i.e., preterm newborn infants usually need suctioning)
- Abnormal adaptation, respiratory distress or apnea
- Polyhydramnion
- Visualization of vocal cords during intubation

> The **A** of the ABCD measures stands for **A**irways: term or preterm infants with respiratory distress, apnea or bradycardia need rapid clearing of their airways by suctioning.

Rule of thumb for the suctioning of newborn infants (Figure 2.16 and 2.17)
- *Always suction the mouth/throat before the nose:* Nasal suctioning is a strong stimulus that may lead to aspiration of fluid that is still in the hypopharynx

Neonatal Emergencies: A Practical Guide for Resuscitation, Transport and Critical Care, ed. Georg Hansmann.
Published by Cambridge University Press. © Cambridge University Press 2009.

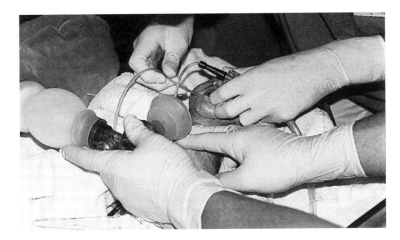

Figure 2.16 Oropharyngeal suctioning of amniotic fluid (here with simultaneous oxygen supplementation). See color plate section for full color version.

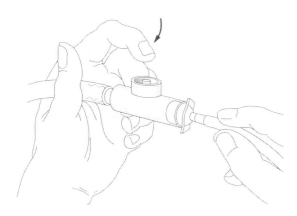

Figure 2.17 Adapter for tracheal suctioning of meconium (Meconium aspirator). From: Hansmann G, Neugeborenen-Notälle 2004, Thieme Stuttgart New York.

- *Avoid deep (i.e., hypopharyngeal or esophagogastric) suctioning in the first 5 min after birth:* Vagal reflex resulting in bradycardia, laryngeal spasm and apnea is possible. Suction only as needed (see above)!
- *A vigorous, active, and healthy neonate should be dried, wrapped up and then given to the mother.* Attempt to pass naso- or orogastric tube through the esophagus into the stomach 10–30 min after birth (i.e., before the first feeding)
- *Suctioning technique*
- Use vaccum suctioning with negative pressure of –0.2 bar (= –200 mbar = –150 mmHg) for standard suctioning and –0.4 bar (= –400 mbar = –300 mmHg) when trying to remove thick secretions. Thick green-stained or bloody amniotic fluid should be removed quickly by oral, oropharyngeal/hypopharyngeal suctioning with Yankauer's or other large-bore diameter catheter (12 Ch = 12 F). Laryngoscopy: eventually endotracheal suctioning, either with meconium aspirator (= ET tube adapter for suction hose, needs higher negative pressure; Figure 2.17) or Yankauer's suction catheter (shown in Figure 2.8)
- Generally, yellow-and-green-stained or bloody amniotic fluid, blood or secretions must be removed from the airways by oropharyngeal/hypopharyngeal suctioning as soon as

possible (initially by the obstetrician, then by the neonatal care team), i.e., after the head is delivered and prior to the first breath (large-diameter catheter), as any aspiration (blood, meconium) can lead to a secondary respiratory distress syndrome (RDS). It should be noted that – on the basis of one randomized-controlled trial[21] – this procedure is no longer recommended in the most recent ILCOR guidelines (2005) anymore[22]. However, intrapartum suctioning of meconium-stained infants does not seem to be harmful[21], is a minimally invasive procedure, and may prevent postnatal meconium aspiration. *The authors of this handbook therefore continue to recommend intrapartum suctioning of infants with meconium-stained amniotic fluid (MSAF) until additional data become available*

- After complete birth of a meconium-stained newborn infant:
  - Place the neonate on the resuscitation table
  - Visualize the larynx (if it is unclear whether the infant is vigorous)
  - Suction the hypopharynx and, if necessary, the trachea (see below); continue with esophagogastric and nasal suctioning!
- *"Thick green-stained fluid" does not always mean meconium aspiration or meconium aspiration syndrome*
  - With a "vigorous infant" (i.e., good chest excursions/normal breathing pattern with respiratory rate of approx. 40–50 breaths/min, heart rate >100 bpm, adequate muscle tone[9]), if the upper respiratory tract is free of meconium (see larynx inspection mentioned above), there is no indication for intubation, endotracheal suctioning or lavage[23,24]. If an infant born through meconium-stained amniotic fluid is vigorous, the AAP/AHA/ILCOR guidelines underline that there is no need for inspection of the larynx[22,25]. *However, this assessment ("vigorous?") can be difficult in the first seconds of life, so we recommend performing laryngoscopy in any newborn born through MSAF when neonatal depression cannot be excluded.* Approximately one-third of meconium-stained neonates who had intrapartum supraglottal suctioning have meconium in the trachea[24].
- *When meconium-stained infants are already well adapted and vigorous:*
  - Suction the mouth and hypopharynx
  - Suction the stomach (careful with deep suctioning in the first minutes of life)
  - Monitor S_aO_2 and heart rate with pulse oximeter. If postductal S_pO_2 <90% (foot), need to check preductal S_pO_2
  - If newborn is stable, give the baby, with pulse oximeter attached, to the mother
  - Standard diagnostics (blood gases, blood glucose, body temperature) within the first 20 min postnatally
  - Assess second blood gas and blood sugar approximately 30 min after birth
- *Rapid perinatal airway management is mandatory when amniotic fluid is stained (e.g., green, bloody), AND there is suspicion of meconium aspiration with neonatal depression (see p. 269, Figure 3.6)*
  - Use a large-bore diameter suctioning catheter (Ch 10–18 = 10–18 F or Yankauer's catheter) to clear the oro-/hypopharynx of viscous amniotic fluid, as soon as the head is born (near the perineum) or in the OR (C-section) = intrapartum suctioning
  - Clamp the umbilical cord immediately
  - Place the neonate on a prewarmed resuscitation table as soon as possible

- No respiratory stimulation by any health care provider
- Prevent the first breath (by avoiding any stimulation; some recommend cautious compression of the chest by a member of the resuscitation team)
- No bag-and-mask ventilation (PPV)
- Rapid and brief oro-/hypopharyngeal suctioning
- Visualize the glottis with a laryngoscope (by experienced resuscitator)
- *Then*
    - If the neonate is depressed and/or meconium is seen in the larynx/trachea, then intubate orally (stylet optional), suction the trachea for 3–5 s with a tube adapter (Meconium Aspirator™) while gradually withdrawing the ET tube (best with meconium aspirator and high negative pressure, e.g., –0.4 bar = 400 mbar = 300 mmHg; Figure 2.17).
    - Second choice is tracheal suctioning with a large-bore catheter, i.e., Yankauer's catheter (caution: vocal cords), or through an ET tube with a regular suctioning catheter: 10 F = 10 Ch only fits through 4.0 ET tube; 8 F = Ch 8 fits through a tube of inner diameter 3.0 mm; 6 F = Ch 6 fits through a tube of inner diameter 2.5 mm. Repeat if necessary.
- *When large amounts of meconium-stained fluid are in the lower airways and severe meconium aspiration syndrome/persistent pulmonary hypertension of the newborn is expected to develop rapidly:*
    - Consider endotracheal surfactant lavage and eventually ET surfactant instillation for neonates with severe respiratory depression in the delivery room (caution: tube too deep? PIP adjusted to the improving lung compliance). However, surfactant lavage has not been proven to improve the outcome of newborns with meconium aspiration syndrome[26,27]
    - When meconium is removed, but spontaneous breathing is insufficient: reintubate and provide PPV. Choose PIP to be as low as possible (high F_iO_2 and respiratory rate are often needed). Choose expiration time (T_{exp}) >0.5 s for term and post-term neonates. Remember: suction tube ≠ ventilation tube (i.e., reintubate for PPV). Minimal handling! Consider the use of sedation and muscle relaxants to avoid pulmonary hypertensive crises and to lower mechanical airway resistance (caution: hypotension). Always place a gastric tube and leave open to gravity!
- *When the meconium-stained neonate is depressed:*
    - During suctioning: watch for heart rate and S_aO_2
    - If unstable (e.g., severe bradycardia with HR <60–80 bpm, severe hypoxia): stop ET suctioning, reintubate immediately (stylet optional), and provide PPV

- When meconium aspiration is suspected, avoid any stimulation and initial bag-and-mask ventilation. Suction orpharynx and trachea, and provide positive pressure ventilation
- Anticipate pneumothorax and be prepared to place a chest tube
- Standard monitoring should include pre- and postductal S_pO_2 and arterial BP measurement
- Consider early high-frequency oscillatory ventilation or extracorporeal membrane oxygenation in severe meconium aspiration syndrome

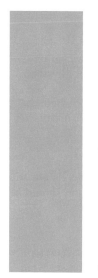

Stimulation, oxygen supplementation, bag-and-mask ventilation (M-PPV), pharyngeal/ bi-nasal CPAP, and pharyngeal positive pressure ventilation

Georg Hansmann

Rapid initial assessment (0–30 s after birth) and stimulation

After birth, assessment of breathing and heart rate is done rapidly (see p. 131, pp. 142–9, pp. 150–3), as follows:

- Palpate the umbilical cord or auscultate the heart: HR >100 bpm? Assistant may tap out HR for other resuscitators
- Is meconium visible? (Check in particular for staining of cord stump and nail beds)
- Suction (first mouth, then nose), if needed (see pp. 66–9)
- Dry and thereby stimulate breathing/keep warm (certain exceptions may apply)
- If still pale/cyanotic/insufficient breathing, proceed to stimulation (with four fingers while drying the back, may also rub the soles of the feet and sternum)
- O_2 supplementation as needed if S_pO_2 <85%–90% (F_iO_2 0.21–1.0, flow 5 l/min)

If there are signs of severe neonatal compromise/terminal (aka: secondary) apnea present, perform PPV (see below)

Oxygen supplementation

Postnatally administered oxygen (via hood, mask, phargngeal-CPAP, intubation/PPV) is a very effective "drug" (oxygen decreases PVR, increases pulmonary blood flow and oxygenation, and induces ductus constriction).

! If the S_pO_2 is rapidly improving during initial newborn care, oxygen supplementation must be continuously reduced or stopped, since high P_aO_2 levels/oxygen radicals reduce cerebral blood flow[28], induce myocardial and renal tubular damage[7], and promote the development of retinopathy of prematurity (ROP) and bronchopulmonary dysplasia (BPD) in preterm infants.

Neonatal Emergencies: A Practical Guide for Resuscitation, Transport and Critical Care, ed. Georg Hansmann.
Published by Cambridge University Press. © Cambridge University Press 2009.

> ▌In most cases, there is no need to provide a newly born infant with additional oxygen in the
> • delivery room if preductal S_pO_2 is reliably >85%–90%[3,4,29] (i.e., no meconium aspiration,
> sepsis/pneumonia, CDH or other causes of impaired lung function and PPHN).
>   At 5 min of life, approximately half of newborns in room air have S_aO_2 of 90%[30]. Preductal
> S_pO_2 values are approx. 9 percent points higher than postductal S_pO_2 in the first 10 min of life,
> and lower in preterm infants and status post (s/p) surgical deliveries (c-sections).[30]

Excess supplemental oxygen can lead to apnea, especially when P_aCO_2 levels are still high (>80 mmHg), i.e., in the first minutes of life. Hyper- and hypoventilation should be avoided (caution: cerebral hemorrhage)[31,32].

> ▌There is no sufficient evidence on the optimum S_aO_2, P_aO_2 and P_aCO_2 in preterm and term
> • infants in the delivery room and in the NICU. However, recent studies have suggested that
> long-accepted targets of oxygen saturation for preterm infants in their first weeks of life
> most likely are too high[31,33,34].
> ▌There is the future need for immediate and continuous monitoring of oxygen saturation
> • (S_pO_2) and heart rate via pulse oximetry in the delivery room[35], and the need to vary
> inspired oxygen concentrations based on the individual status of newly born infants
> ("tailored oxygen resuscitation-). When providing additional oxygen, health care providers
> should keep in mind that S_pO_2, if kept above 92%, is not reliable at detecting hyperoxia[36].
> ▌The preductal S_aO_2 of a spontaneously breathing term infant with normal cardiovascular
> • anatomy, but in need of supplementary oxygen ($F_iO_2 > 0.21$), should be approx. 90%–96%
> in most cases (i.e., no meconium aspiration, sepsis/pneumonia, CDH or other causes of
> impaired lung function and PPHN). Measure postductal S_pO_2 to detect ductal split.

Avoid oxygen supplementation during and after the initial care of newborns particularly in neonates with congenital heart defects *and* duct-dependent systemic perfusion (e.g., left ventricular outflow tract obstruction (LVOTO), interrupted aortic arch (IAA), coarctation of the aorta (CoA), hypoplastic left heart syndrome (HLHS)). Oxygen increases pulmonary blood flow and thus impairs systemic blood flow even more in these conditions. A high P_aO_2 would also induce or accelerate the postnatal closure of the ductus arteriosus (caution in duct-dependent heart disease, e.g., d-TGA). The common practice of providing excess oxygen to every newborn infant (by free-flow PPV) regardless of the underlying disease or presence of vital depression can be harmful to the newborn, especially when confronted with the duct-dependent left heart obstructions mentioned above.

Reassess after 30 s

- Adequate chest movements/crying?
- HR >100 bpm?
- Skin color? (The ILCOR algorithm 2005 no longer contains "pink" as a "neonatal vital sign"[22])
- If there is persistent pallor/cyanosis, respiratory distress/apnea and/or HR <100 bpm, perform bag-and-mask ventilation (if not contraindicated) or immediate intubation and PPV

Bag-and-mask ventilation (M-PPV)
Indications for bag-and-mask ventilation
See p. 156.

Bag-and-mask ventilation with 21%, 30%–50% or 100% oxygen?

Considerable limitations to the current data on the short- and long-term outcome of resuscitated newborn infants preclude generalizations and demand caution when applying the new findings, but the following tentative considerations seem reasonable[4]: Since 100% oxygen is not more effective than room air[37] and most likely harmful in newborn resuscitation (i.e., higher neonatal mortality in two meta-analyses[5,6], excessive oxidative stress in two prospective trials,[38,39] prolongation of PPV and therefore barotrauma,[40] and induction of myocardial and renal tubular damage in a small randomized controlled trial[7]), there is no reason to use 100% oxygen as first-line and initial gas in the delivery room.

> **!** **It is time to turn down the oxygen tanks for neonatal resuscitation**[4–7].

According to a worldwide survey from 2004, 20 of 40 centers still use 100% oxygen at the resuscitation of all babies at delivery, whereas the remaining centers have already changed their standards and use lower oxygen concentrations[41]. Caution should be exercised when using high F_iO_2 in *preterm* infants at greatest risk of detrimental oxyen effects; however, data on resuscitated infants <35 weeks' gestation remain limited[6]. Furthermore, we do not know whether ventilation with 30%, 40% or 50% oxygen as opposed to 100% oxygen (1) might prevent treatment failure in the moderately depressed (near-term) newborns initially ventilated with air or (2) might increase neonatal mortality as seen in the pooled study groups treated with 100% oxygen[4–6].

Out of the most recent international recommendations on neonatal resuscitation (ILCOR 2005)[22]:

> *There is currently insufficient evidence to specify the concentration of oxygen to be used at initiation of resuscitation. After initial steps at birth, if respiratory efforts are absent or inadequate, lung inflation/ventilation should be the priority. …Supplementary oxygen should be considered for babies with persistent central cyanosis. Some have advocated adjusting the oxygen supply according to pulse oximetry measurements to avoid hyperoxia, but there is insufficient evidence to determine the appropriate oximetry goal…. Excessive tissue oxygen may cause oxidant injury and should be avoided, especially in the premature infant.*

> **!** Standard equipment for neonatal resuscitation should include pressure gauge (manometer) for monitoring of PIP, adjustable PEEP, oxygen blender (adjustable F_iO_2 0.21–1.0), and pulse oximeter (S_pO_2 monitoring)[4,35].
>
> **!** *The authors of this handbook suggest* commencing resuscitation with room air independendly of gestational age and adjusting the inspiratory oxygen concentration thereafter on clinical grounds ("tailored oxygen resuscitation – using oxygen blenders). When bradycardia and/or central cyanosis/pallor persist up to 90 s after birth despite adequate ventilation, then the inspiratory oxygen concentration may be increased up to 100% (F_iO_2 1.0); the gas flow may be increased as well. Certain conditions such as congenital diaphragmatic hernia may require higher oxygen concentrations immediately after birth[4] (see p. 71).

How to provide oxygen supplementation and ventilatory support with a face mask

There are three options (see equipment pp. 25–40):

1. **Self-inflating bag-and-mask systems** (Figures 2.3 and 2.5, see pp. 26–29 and legends for advantages/disadvantages)

2. **Flow-inflating bag-and-mask systems** (Figure 2.4, see p. 28 and legend for advantages/disadvantages)

3. **"T-piece resuscitators** (pp. 29–31)," which allow PPV with T-piece and continuous PEEP (e.g., *Neopuff Neonatal Resuscitator*™, Figure 2.6a; *Tom Thumb*™ Figure 2.6b) and are as effective as conventional bag-and-mask systems, but do not allow the user to "feel" lung compliance. A very simple ventilatory assist device similar to the T-piece resuscitator is the **"Bubble CPAP,"** i.e., a simple CPAP construction with water seal (Figure 2.7).

Bag-and-mask system (Figures 2.3–2.6)

- Examples include self-inflating bag-and-mask systems, e.g., Laerdal, model "infant" (250 ml)™ or "child" (second choice, 450–500 ml)™ with a self-inflating reservoir, pop-off valve, pressure gauge (if possible), PEEP valve set at +3 to +5 mbar

- Oxygen mixed gas flow 5 l/min

- O_2 blender, if available, set to 21% (default), or higher values if indicated

- Test mask (seal mask on palm of hand and set PEEP by adjusting PEEP valve or pop-off valve), circular seal membrane and tubing system (see below). Basic rule of thumb for 250-ml bags: for adequate PIP, use thumb plus one finger per kilogram body weight (e.g., only thumb and index finger at the bag for ventilation of a 1000-g baby). Initially, PIP of 25–40 cmH$_2$O may be needed to establish the functional residual capacity (FRC). Monitor PIP via pressure gauge (manometer). Note that PIP does not necessarily reflect tidal volumes!

- Ventilatory rate 30–60 breaths/min (initially, prolonged inspiratory time and tidal volumes may be needed to establish FRC and achieve visible chest rise)

Studies from the 1980s showed that the small bag-and-mask ventilator for neonates (e.g., Laerdal, model "infant," 250 ml™) may not be sufficient for term neonates and older infants to reach adequate tidal volumes and inspiration time to establish FRC. Some recommended the use of larger bag-and-mask systems (e.g., Laerdal, model "child", 450–500 ml). However, the authors of this handbook have had excellent experience with the use of "smaller" bag-and-mask (250 ml) and other ventilatory systems (e.g., flow-inflating bags and T-piece resuscitators), in neonatal resuscitation. Hence, we consider larger self-inflating bags only as an alternative for large, term newborn infants (>3500 g) and older infants (>1 month, >3500 g). When using the larger (450–500 ml) bag-and-mask systems (450–500 ml), "felt" PIP and tidal volumes have to be "adjusted" to the chest movements and PIP indicated at the manometer. Do NOT apply the rule of thumb (thumb plus one finger per kilogram body weight at the 250-ml bag) for a larger self-inflating bag (e.g., 450–500 ml)!

Bag-and-mask systems with an open-end "tube-like oxygen reservoir" (second choice) instead of a "closed-end oxygen reservoir" (=bag, first choice) do not allow supplementation or ventilation with 90% – 100% oxygen and tend to fall off at inconvenient moments. If 40% oxygen supplementation is intended, one may take the open-end tube-like or closed reservoir off the self-inflating system (e.g., if no oxygen blender available).

> ! When the lung expansion is poor and bag-and-mask ventilation is needed initially, the (adjustable) pressure control valve of the bag-mask system may be pushed downwards in order to achieve notable chest rise requiring PIP levels of over 25 mbar (approx. 25–40 mbar = 25–40 cmH$_2$O). A PEEP valve (set to approx. 3–5 mbar) should be attached to the self-inflating bag-and-mask system (it's not "optional" but rather "standard of care")

Unfortunately, pressure gauge (manometer), PEEP valve and oxygen blenders are not yet standard equipment in many delivery rooms[35]. However, there is a worldwide trend to improve such monitoring and treatment in the delivery room[3].

Resuscitation unit with T-piece resuscitators (Neopuff, Neovent; Figure 2.6) or simple mechanical ventilators

Getting started – all set?

- First (routine set-up):
  - Check whether the parts of the T-piece resuscitator are correctly assembled
  - Connect the test lung, adjust the flow meter (5–15 l/min), ensure proper gas supply
  - Connect the oxygen blender (default 21% oxygen)
  - Pre-set the maximum circuit pressure by occluding the PEEP cap (the hole in the T-piece) with your finger and adjusting the relief dial to a selected value (40 cm H$_2$O = 40 mbar recommended as default)
- Second:
  - Connect proper mask for estimated birth weight (size 00–01)
  - Check and adjust the oxygen blender (default 21% oxygen)
  - Place mask sealed onto the palm of your hand, then set the desired PIP (20–30 cm H$_2$O = 20–30 mbar) by occluding the PEEP cap with your finger, and adjusting the inspiratory pressure control to a selected PIP
  - Pre-set PEEP: (0 to) +3 to +5 cmH$_2$O = mbar
  - Set and adjust rate manually per T-piece when resuscitating the baby
  - In PPV mode hold the mask tightly, close to the palm of one's own hand and do a test run of a few cycles (T-piece resuscitator or simple mechanical ventilator)
  - Rarely set rate: 30–50 breaths/min at mechanical ventilator (T_{in} : T_{ext} = 0.40 s/0.9 s)
- During resuscitation: adjust PIP, PEEP and F_iO_2 to patient's clinical status (i.e., chest rise, spontaneous breathing, heart rate) and monitoring (heart rate and S_pO_2): PIP in particular should be reduced to 16–25 mbar if possible. If necessary (insufficient chest rise), inflate the lungs for 5 s (to a maximum of 10 s) and/or consider early endotracheal intubation

> When having trouble achieving sufficient pressure between a face mask and one's own palm while testing the bag-and-mask or T-piece system (PIP test), it is most likely that: (1) the circular seal membrane of the self-inflating bag (above the mask) is flipped over, or (2) the tubing system or flow-inflating bag is disconnected, blocked or leaking.
>
> When adequate pressure cannot be achieved with a mechanical ventilator, then the expiration valve may be blocked (e.g., Babylog 2™, by Dräger). Pushing the manual ventilation button several times often releases the valve. When lung expansion is poor and mechanical ventilation is needed initially, switch the ventilator to "manual" mode and set higher PIP levels (approx. 25–40 mbar).

"Bubble CPAP" = CPAP with water-seal/surge tank or chamber (Figure 2.7)

A flow of 5 l/min can build up an inspiratory pressure of approximately 20 cmH$_2$O (mbar) when a tight mask seal is achieved at the same time.

The advantage of using T-pieces (Neopuff/Neovent or "bubble CPAP") lies in one's ability to hold the "sealed" mask and ventilate the lungs (cover the hole in the T-piece or "bubble CPAP" with your finger) with one hand, while the other hand is still able to stimulate or auscultate the neonate. However, one cannot "feel" the lung compliance and instead is left with observation of chest excursions, S$_p$O$_2$, heart rate and skin color.

The technique of bag-and-mask ventilation (M-PPV)
Procedure
- *Ventilatory system and gas supply is checked* (see above)
    - Flow 5 l/min
    - Pre-set inspiratory gas/oxygen blender to room air ($F_iO_2 = 0.21$) in most cases
    - Connect monitoring devices (S$_p$O$_2$, pressure gauge, etc.)
- Usually *round silicon masks* with soft cushion are used
    - Mask size depends on birth weight
        - Preterm infants <1000 g: size 00
        - Term/preterm infants up to 2500 g: sizes 00–01
        - Term/preterm infants >2500 g: size 01
- *Head is placed in the sniffing position* (Figure 2.18; i.e., minimal neck extension; tip of nose = highest point):
    - Put one thin diaper/towel under the shoulders
    - "Jaw thrust (= Esmarch's grip)" is sometimes necessary, i.e., lift up/pull forward the lower jaw/mandible with the medial part of one's index finger (without exerting force on the lower jaw, which would cause the tongue to fall back)
- *Ventilation*
    - Mask and PEEP valve (and reservoir if applicable) are connected to the bag-mask system
    - Left thumb and index finger hold the mask in a "figure of C" (Figure 2.19) and place the mask cautiously, but tightly, over the mouth and nose
    - Left middle and ring finger lift the chin and the prominent mandible (don't grap the submandibular soft tissue) and hold them forward/up (like a mini jaw thrust/ Esmarch's grip; moderate extension of head)
    - Left small (fifth) finger is free, the right hand holds the bag ($\approx$ thumb plus one finger per kilogram of body weight at the 250-ml bag; Figure 2.20)
    - If initially a PIP of 25–40 mbar (cmH$_2$O) is needed, push down (i.e., close) the pop-off valve (= pressure release valve) with the right thumb (usually set to 40 cmH$_2$O = 40 mbar by default)
    - PPV rate is 40–60 breaths/min
    - While performing resuscitation with external chest compression (CPR): keep the ratio chest compressions:PPV = 3:1, i.e., 30 bag squeezes/min, 90 chest compressions/ min (= 120 events per minute)

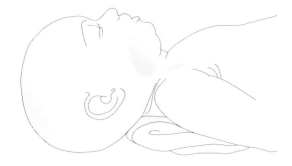

Figure 2.18 So called sniffing position of the head for bag-and-mask ventilation, pharyngeal tube ventilation and intubation. Note that the tip of the nose is the highest point in the lateral view. Modified from Ralston *et al.* (2006). *PALS Provider Manual.* American Heart Association and American Academy of Pediatrics. See color plate section for full color version.

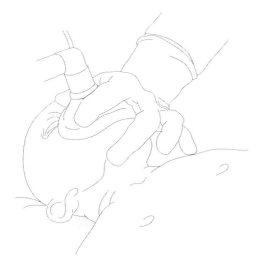

Figure 2.19 C-grip: left thumb and index finger hold the mask in a "figure of C" and the mask is cautiously, but tightly, placed over the mouth and nose ("sealed"); left middle and ring finger lift the chin and the prominent mandible (without the soft tissue) and hold it forward/up (moderate extension of head). Modified from: Hansmann G (2004) *Neugeborenen-Notfälle.* Thieme, Stuttgart, New York. See color plate section for full color version.

- *Reassess after 15–30 s PPV*
    - If the newborn infant is (still) depressed, re-evaluate one's own handling (effective PPV performed?), eventually increase PIP, gas flow and F_iO_2; consider rapid intubation, CPR and epinephrine
    - When spontaneous breathing is present, adjust the rate and PIP of bag-and-mask ventilation to the baby's spontaneous breathing
- *Reassess after 15–30 s*
    - See above
    - Gastric distension?
    - Bag-and-mask ventilation or intubation followed by PPV for more than 2 min requires placement of a naso- or orogastric tube and removal of gastric air
- *Poor clinical response*
    - Place head and mask in optimum ("sniffing") position (tip of the nose = highest point)
    - Open mouth slightly
    - Suction, if needed

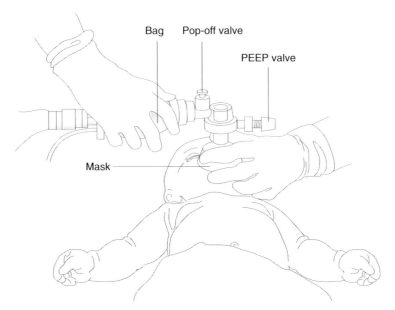

Bag   Pop-off valve

PEEP valve

Mask

Figure 2.20 Bag-and-mask ventilation of a neonate. The head is turned to the resuscitator, who performs M-PPV. The right hand holds a bag (e.g., Laerdal bag 250 ml) equipped with a PEEP valve, and connected to a reservoir and oxygen tubing. In addition to the thumb, use one finger per kilogram birth weight to squeeze the bag (applies only to 250-ml self-inflating bags). Left hand with C-grip ("figure of C"). Initially, a PIP as high as 25–45 cmH$_2$O may be needed (then, press down/close the pop-off valve with right thumb); respiratory rate = 40–60 breaths per minute. During resuscitation: 30 PPV breaths/min, 90 chest compressions/min, chest compressions: PPV = 3:1 ratio (=120 events/min). Modified from Ralston *et al.* (2006) *PALS Provider Manual.* American Heart Association and American Academy of Pediatrics.

- If necessary, place oral airway (Guedel tube; size 00 (or 000); length ≈ distance between the gum line and angle of the jaw)
- Check gas supply/F_iO_2 (i.e., Still connected? Is someone standing on the tubing?)
- In case bag-and-mask ventilation is still insufficient → consider pharyngeal CPAP. ventilation, laryngeal mask airway (LMA) placement or intubation followed by PPV.
- *Poor lung expansion or resuscitation failure*
  - Apply two to four PPV bag squeezes with prolonged inspiration time (T_{in} = 3–5 s up to a maximum of 10 s), higher PIP (approx. 25–40 mbar) and PEEP (e.g., +5 mbar) with a tightly placed ("sealed") mask in order to achieve sufficient tidal volumes. A long inspiration time ("inflating" for 3–5 s or a maximum of 10 s) is difficult to achieve with a 250-ml bag-and-mask system (neonates weighing >3500 g would eventually benefit from a bigger bag; i.e., Laerdal model "child," 450–500 ml™ vs. "Laerdal model infant, 250 ml™"). T-piece systems (see below) can provide long T_{in}
  - An alternative would be high-frequency ventilation with a self-inflating bag- and-mask system; if necessary, with a disabled pop-off valve (press down with the right thumb), closed reservoir and PEEP valve (→ attempt to achieve almost continuous flow and plateau PIP; caution: uncontrolled tidal volumes; monitor PIP via pressure gauge)
  - Another option is to use a respirator ("manual" mode), T-piece system (Neopuff = Neovent, Tom-Thumb or Bubble CPAP) with controlled PIP and PEEP. With the

long inspiration time (approx. 5 s) and PEEP, FRC and adequate gas exchange will be established, which might prevent "*atelectrauma*"; see below) and persistent pulmonary hypertension of the newborn (see p. 392). Adequate FRC is most easily achieved by intubation/PPV[17] with the disadvantage of possible *barotrauma*, especially in VLBW preterm infants.

- Early intubation of preterm infants is associated with enhanced pulmonary inflammation and a higher incidence of chronic oxygen requirement/BPD compared to those with initial CPAP treatment[42–45]. Higher P_aCO_2 in preterm infants <28 weeks' gestation treated with CPAP versus intubation does not seem to increase the risk of intraventricular hemorrhage[46]. However, many questions on the optimal (i.e., tailored) use of CPAP and non-invasive ventilation in the delivery room yet have to be answered[47,48]. It is preferable to avoid intubation (and PPV)[49], when arterial blood gases are acceptable, and early surfactant treatment is not indicated. The sequence of early intubation, surfactant administration, and early extubation followed by CPAP ("*InSurE*") comprises another approach to limit lung injury[50,51]. A group from Cologne, Germany, performed combined early nasal CPAP (ENCAPAP) with early administration of surfactant in spontaneously breathing ELBW preterm infants (23 0/7 to 27 0/7 weeks of gestation) using a thin intratracheal catheter (feeding tube; injection time 1–2 min)[52,53]. This approach appeared feasible for a skilled level-III NICU team and required secondary intubation in only about one-fifth (VLBW) to one-third (ELBW) of preterm infants[52,53].

- PPV with low PEEP (<3 mbar) or high tidal volumes (approx. >7 ml/kg) may cause *atelectrauma* or *volutrauma*. If FRC is established early by lung inflation (long T_{in} = 3–5 s) (± surfactant), and maintained with sufficient PEEP, the risk of volutrauma under PPV is significantly lower[54]

- Lung inflation (e.g., mask-CPAP, T-piece, etc.) is often necessary after c-sections, when large amounts of alveolar and interstitial amniotic fluid remain within the alveolar space. Even spontaneously delivered neonates with persistent "grunting" often benefit from prolonged initial inflations (two to three times) followed by CPAP

- However, one must remember that prolonged lung inflation (with partial over-inflation of some but not all distal airways and alveoli) may facilitate the development of bronchopulmonary dysplasia/chronic lung disease, and may worsen the outcome of preterm infants in particular (animal models[42,43,55–57]). Therefore, long and continuous lung inflations (i.e., T_{in} >5 s) and, if possible, mechanical ventilation should be avoided, especially in very preterm newborn infants

---

! If FRC and chest rise are insufficient, lung inflation (long T_{in}) may be warranted and then should be performed as early as possible: two to four PPV breaths with a tight mask, sufficient PIP (approx. 20–40 cmH$_2$O = mbar) and a PEEP (+3 to +5 mbar) over 3–5 s. After inflation and lung expansion (sufficient FRC), PIP should be reduced, if possible to 20 ± 4 mbar in order to avoid barotrauma (i.e., overinflation, pneumothorax). In preterm infants, PIP levels of 16–18 mbar are advisable and sufficient if chest rise, S_pO_2, and HR are stable. However, higher PIP may be needed initially when FRC is not yet established. Adjust ventilatory rate and PIP to the spontaneous breathing pattern of the neonate.

> **!** Hyperventilation and excessive supplemental oxygen should be prevented: low P_aCO_2 and a high P_aO_2 reduce cerebral perfusion thereby increasing the risk for intracranial hemorrhage (ICH) and later cerebral palsy, particularly in preterm infants.

> **!** Poor response to bag-and-mask ventilation requires reassessment of one's own handling. Depending on your own skills and the clinical condition of the baby, you may decide to switch to pharyngeal ventilation (P-PPV; useful in ELBW infants and poor mask seal) or rapid endotracheal intubation.

Nasal CPAP/nasopharyngeal CPAP/ventilation (pharyngeal CPAP with assisted ventilation, pharyngeal-PPV; also called NIV, non-invasive ventilation)

Technique

- Moisten the ET tube and pass it into one nostril with twisting motions. Advance the tip of the tube to the level of the uvula (approx. 4–7 cm from the nostril), i.e., beyond the soft palate
- Keep ET tube in position and connect to the PPV system (bag-and-mask, T-piece)
- Close mouth and second nostril
- Ventilate/oxygenate with bag over the tube
- If newborn improves, secure the nasopharyngeal tube with tape
- Adjust PPV breaths to spontaneous breathing pattern/rate
- Please note: pharyngeal PPV is only a temporary alternative used to overcome transitory respiratory distress (caution: gastric distension, etc.)

Comments

Some neonates may respond better to ventilation with *nasal prongs* or a *nasal mask* (vs. pharyngeal tube or standard masks), which may prevent endotracheal intubation and PPV (the goal, especially in preterm infants). Nasal CPAP is a very useful technique for avoiding endotracheal intubation in preterm infants. Careful sedation (e.g., morphine, benzodiazepine), if needed, may be helpful during neonatal transport. If long-term mechanical ventilation is indicated, a well-trained team may perform intubation, while continuing pharyngeal PPV (by an assistant standing to the right side of the provider performing the intubation). By insufflating the pharyngeal tube, ventilation/oxygenation is established and causes the closed glottis to open (see Figure 2.42). If the need for respiratory support of a preterm infant is anticipated, advance the tip of the ET tube to the level of the uvula (i.e., behind the soft palate, approx. 4–7 cm from nostril). Shorten the ET tube prior to placement (to reduce airway resistance/dead space; the optimal ET tube length for term neonates to be intubated nasally is 13–14 cm). Tape the ET tube properly. The (supporting) ventilatory rate should be adjusted to the spontaneous breathing rate and pattern at a range between 0 (nasophargngeal (NP-CPAP) CPAP delivered via nasal mask or nose prongs) and 40 breaths/min (pharyngeal PPV (P-PPV), also called NIV, achieved with nasopharyngeal

ETT or laryngeal mask airway (LMA)). PEEP in NP-CPAP should not exceed 5 mbar, the PIP in P-PPV may not be greater than 12–15 mbar (approx. opening pressure for upper and lower esophageal sphincters of term neonates). However, P-PPV is not a permanent solution (consider intubation if no improvement is seen after a few hours). Always place a gastric tube to decompress the abdomen and verify its position.

> **!** Place an oro- or nasogastric tube approx. 2 min after the beginning of PPV (mask ventilation or NP-CPAP/P-PPV). Verify both ET and gastric tube positions clinically and by chest X-ray (see pp. 81–94)

One of the most difficult on-call problems for the NETS-team is to decide whether a neonate with moderate respiratory distress and grunting (delivery room) or a neonate with suboptimal S_pO_2 (e.g., 75%–85%) and borderline blood gases should be either intubated or transported with NP-CPAP/P-PPV $\pm$ supplementary oxygen (see Silverman's respiratory distress assessment score scheme, Table 2.6, p. 147). In addition to the newborn's clinical condition, this decision depends to a great extent on the estimated transport time: if transport time is likely greater than 30 min, the leading NETS-MD/NP may perform an "elective" or a "semi"elective- intubation at the referring hospital or in the field (see below).

> **!** It is faster and more effective to supplement oxygen with a bag-and-mask system with attached reservoir than filling the whole transport incubator with oxygen, as the oxygen concentration drops every time the incubator's doors are opened. Prior to any transport, a bag-and-mask-system with oxygen tubing should be properly connected and readily available.

Contraindications for M-PPV, NP-CPAP and P-PPV (NIV)
See contraindications for mask ventilation (p. 156).
    e.g.,:
- (Suspected) diaphragmatic hernia
- (Suspected) aspiration of meconium, viscous mucus or blood
- Abdominal wall defects (omphalocele, gastroschisis)
- Esophageal atresia
- Strong suspicion of pneumothorax

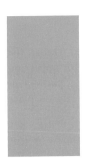

Endotracheal intubation and gastric tube placement

Georg Hansmann

Both endotracheal intubation and gastric tube placement will be discussed here together, as intubation always requires gastric tube placement to enable gastric decompression (after bag-and-mask ventilation) and drainage of air and fluid. Gastric air removal consequently improves the excursion of the diaphragm. Moreover, esophageal atresia may be diagnosed clinically by this procedure, when the tube cannot be placed into the stomach, and instead rolls up in the oropharynx (if in doubt, inject 10 ml of air into the gastric tube and auscultate simultaneously over the gastric area).

Indication
See p. 158.

Urgency for intubation – decision making based on the clinical presentation of the neonate
- Elective intubation
- Semi-elective ("semi-urgent to urgent") intubation
- Emergency intubation

Elective and semi-elective intubation
Elective intubation
- Clinical presentation: stable, spontaneously breathing neonate with adequate S_pO_2 and blood gas
- For premedication see p. 83
- Nasotracheal intubation is preferred by many centers because of the more secure ET fixation (lower accidental extubation rates); alternative: oral intubation
- Indication: e.g., a spontaneously breathing neonate, receiving continuous prostaglandin E_1 (PGE_1) intravenous (IV) infusion prior to a long distant transport (e.g., TGA, HLH)

Semi-elective intubation
- Clinical presentation: neonate with acceptable S_pO_2 and heart rate under bag-and-mask ventilation or NP-CPAP
- For premedication see p. 83
- Nasotracheal intubation or oral intubation
- Indication: e.g., a neonate with poor lung expansion/respiratory distress syndrome with CO_2 retention prior to respiratory failure

Neonatal Emergencies: A Practical Guide for Resuscitation, Transport and Critical Care, ed. Georg Hansmann.
Published by Cambridge University Press. © Cambridge University Press 2009.

Premedication

We acknowledge that premedication for neonatal intubation with centrally active drugs (opioids, benzodiazepines, N-methyl D-aspartate (NMDA) receptor antagonists, γ-aminobutyric acid (GABA) receptor agonists, barbiturates) with or without muscle relaxants is a controversial topic. There are concerns about neurotoxicity with the (long-term) use of these agents, demonstrated in cell and animal studies[58], and lack of longitudinal clinical outcome data. Despite the potential advantages (i.e., better intubation conditions, smaller trauma risk), premedication for non-emergent intubations is still not routinely used in many NICU. Reasons why premedication has not been widely adopted may include lack of familiarity with the medications, fear of adverse effects, insufficient evidence for efficacy and safety, or lack of consensus on the optimal combination of medications[59]. This section represents the author's opinion based on clinical experience and the (limited) data currently available.

Premedication in elective and semi-elective intubation[60]

- Atropine (0.5 mg/ml; optional): 0.02 mg/kg/dose IV = 0.4 ml/kg/dose of a 1:10 solution IV (in case of vagal reaction 2 ml of 1:10 solution = 0.1 mg IV)
- Fentanyl (50 μg/ml): 2–5 μg/kg IV = 0.4–1 ml of a 1:10 solution/kg/dose SLOWLY in 1–5 min IV. (Immediate onset of action. Caution: hypotension and chest wall rigidity is a rare side-effect and more common with rapid IV application and high dosages)
- Diazepam (5 mg/ml): 0.25 (−0.5) mg/kg/dose IV = 0.05 (−0.1) ml/kg IV (advantage: onset in 1–2 min, disadvantage: long half-life of metabolites; caution: hypotension!). Alternative: lorazepam 0.1 mg/kg/dose IV. May use fentanyl as only sedative
- Rocuronium (10 mg/ml; optional): 0.6 mg/kg IV = 0.06 ml/kg/dose IV (maximum effect in 30–60 s; repeat dose, if needed (caution: hypotension!). Alternatives: vecuronium (0.1 mg/kg/dose IV) or mivacurium (0.2 mg/kg/dose IV)
- Give prophylactic volume bolus, NS 10 ml/kg IV, in borderline hypotensive patients, or in drug-induced hypotension

What you need to know for premedication/ET intubation

1. Dilute all agents so that slow application is feasible. Always flush with 2–5 ml normal saline
2. Give prophylactic volume bolus (NS 10 ml/kg IV) in borderline hypotensive patients, or in drug-induced (opioid, benzodiazepine, muscle relaxant) systemic hypotension
3. *Morphine* (0.05–0.1 mg/kg/dose IV), *piritramid* (opioid; 25–50 μg/kg/dose IV) and *lorazepam* (0.05–0.1 mg/kg/dose IV) all have a prolonged onset of action (10–15 min), and therefore are feasible in elective rather than semi-elective or emergent intubations
4. *Fentanyl* has a rapid onset of action but chest wall rigidity occurs as an adverse effect. The frequency of chest wall rigidity with fentanyl is quite low (1%–2%), can be minimized by SLOW injection (1–5 min), and reversed by muscle relaxing agents. When a muscle relaxant is given prior to fentanyl, the rate of chest wall rigidity may even be lower[61]. Fentanyl seems to have less of a hypotensive adverse effect than morphine[62,63].
5. *Midazolam* IV use is associated with severe hypotension and decreased cerebral perfusion especially in preterm infants[64], and therefore cannot be recommended for IV bolus application to critically ill newborn infants
6. A single dose of the sedative *propofol* (2.5 mg/kg/dose IV) was successfully used in a small randomized controlled trial of non-emergency neonatal intubations of preterm infants[65]. However, the lack of neonatal and pediatric outcome data (not approved for neonatal use) and the absence of analgesia currently prevent its widespread use

Comments

- An elective intubation of a vigorous (vital and active) infant requires sedation and analgesia. The vocal cords are strongly innervated, and with an intermittently closing glottis, the newborn is at substantial risk of trauma during intubation (especially when stylets are used). Prior to elective intubation, the tip of the ET tube can be moistened with sterile 1% lidocaine gel. Lidocaine spray (1%) may cautiously be applied to the epiglottis, vocal cords and surrounding mucosa (under laryngoscopic view)
- Unconscious or extremely depressed neonates/preterm infants do not need to be pre-medicated (and mostly do not have IV access yet)
- Atropine: some neonatologists recommend having atropine at the bedside in case of a vagal reaction (bradycardia, laryngospasm), but do not use it as a premedication for neonatal intubation
- With sufficient analgesia, sedation, and experience in neonatal intubation, a muscle relaxant is rarely needed (e.g., when the glottis is permanently closed). However, muscle relaxants do improve intubation conditions and increase the success rate especially in trainees with limited experience[59,61]
- Keep in mind that opioids are not available in NETS emergency bags, but should be used for analgesia

Alternative drugs for intubation (drugs not approved for neonatal use)

- S-Ketamine: 1(–2) mg/kg/dose IV (less analgetic in neonates) plus benzodiazepine such as diazepam 0.25–0.5 mg/kg/dose or lorazepam (0.05–0.1 mg/kg/dose) IV

or

- Etomidate: 0.3 mg/kg/dose IV (rapid onset of action in 30–60 s, duration of effect approx. 2–10 min, not analgetic) plus fentanyl 2–5 µg/kg/dose IV. Give fentanyl IV first

Comments

Etomidate and S-*ketamine* (contraindications: especially high intracranial or intraocular pressure, hypertension) barely cause any significant hemodynamic depression. There are limited published data on the use of these drugs in newborn infants[66], and they are not approved for neonatal use. There are animal and in vitro data demonstrating neurotoxic, dose-dependent effects of ketamine[66], but clinical data on side-effects with single and repetitive dosing are currently not available. For adverse effects and contraindications see package insert!

Emergency intubation

- Clinical presentation of neonate: hemodynamic and respiratory instability
- If neonate is unconscious or Apgar <4: usually, immediate intubation (first minute) *without* premedication (orally or nasally)
- If intubation is difficult or neonate is apneic *and* meconium aspiration is suspected, usually oral intubation is performed. Oral and nasal emergent intubation are both usually carried out without premedication (e.g., in secondary apnea that can have several causes: extreme immaturity, resuscitation, etc.)

Premedication

- Atropine (0.5 mg/ml; optional): 0.02 mg/kg/dose IV = 0.4 ml/kg/dose of a 1:10 solution IV (in case of vagal reaction 2 ml of 1:10 solution = 0.1 mg IV)
- Fentanyl (50 μg/ml): 2–5 μg/kg IV = 0.4–1 ml of a 1:10 solution/kg/dose SLOWLY in 1–5 min IV (immediate onset of action). Caution: hypotension and chest wall rigidity are rare side-effects and more common with rapid IV application and high dosages)
- Diazepam (5 mg/ml): 0.25 (−0.5) mg/kg/dose IV = 0.05 (−0.1) ml/kg IV (advantage: onset in 1–2 min, disadvantage: long half-life of metabolites; caution: hypotension). Alternative: lorazepam 0.1 mg/kg/dose IV. May use fentanyl as only sedative
- Rocuronium (10 mg/ml; optional): 0.6 mg/kg IV = 0.06 ml/kg per dose IV (maximum effect in 30–60 s; repeat dose, if needed) (caution: hypotension). Alternatives: vecuronium (0.1 mg/kg/dose IV) or mivacurium (0.2 mg/kg/dose IV)
- Give prophylactic volume bolus, NS 10 ml/kg IV, in borderline hypotensive patients, or in drug-induced hypotension. A muscle relaxant is indicated when the glottis is closed (vocal cords side by side)
- Give volume bolus, NS 10 ml/kg bolus IV, in borderline hypotensive patients, or in drug-induced hypotension prior to intubation attempts
- If bradycardia <60 bpm persists after intubation and 30 s of PPV, perform chest compressions and give epinephrine ET/IV after 30 s of chest compressions if HR is not >60/min. If HR is not above 60 after another 30 s of chest compressions, give second epinephrine dose and volume (NS 10 ml/kg/bolus IV), and search for cause of depression (see standard algorithm, p. 157)

A muscle relaxant is indicated when the glottis is permanently closed and should only be administered if person with skills in intubating newborns is available. Flush with 2–5 ml NS.

- S-Ketamine: 1(−2) mg/kg/dose IV (less analgetic in neonates) plus benzodiazepine such as diazepam 0.25–0.5 mg/kg/dose or lorazepam (0.05–0.1 mg/kg/dose) IV

or

- Etomidate: 0.3 mg/kg/dose IV (rapid onset of action in 30–60 s, duration of effect approx. 2–10 min, not analgetic) plus fentanyl 2–5 μg/kg/dose IV. Give fentanyl IV first

Comments

Etomidate and *S-ketamine* (contraindications: especially high intracranial or intraocular pressure, hypertension) hardly cause significant hemodynamic depression but are not approved for neonatal use! There are very limited published data on the use of these drugs in newborn infants.[66] There are animal and in vitro data demonstrating neurotoxic, dose-dependent effects of ketamine,[66] but clinical data on side-effects with single and repetitive dosing are lacking. For adverse effects and contraindications see package insert! For further comments see above.

Table 2.2 Endotracheal tubes (non-cuffed)

Weight (g)	Inner diameter of ET tube (mm)	Nasal tube, insertion length from nose (cm)	Oral tube, insertion length from upper lip (cm)
<750	2.0 or 2.5	6.5–7.5	6.0–7.0
750–1500	2.5	7.0–9.0	6.5–7.5
1500–2000	3.0 (2.5)	8.5–10.0	7.5–8.0
2000–3000	3.0	9.5–11.0	8.0–9.0
3000–3500	3.0 (3.5)	10.5–12.0	9.0–11.0
>3500	3.5	11.0–12.5	9.0–11.0

Choice of adequate ET tube size and position. The specifications refer to ET tubes by Vygon® (green) and Mallinckrodt® (transparent). ET tubes by Portex® (light blue) have a larger internal, but a smaller external, diameter (→ may choose by 0.5 mm bigger size). Portex®-ET tubes are also less flexible, which is not necessarily a disadvantage. The visual control of the tube's position is more reliable than the length of insertion indicated above (Vygon®: black mark just visible by 2 mm. Mallinckrodt®: vocal cords at second black line). After intubation, it is mandatory to verify the position of the endotracheal tube: (1) clinically (auscultation, chest rise, increase of HR and SpO_2), (2) with a CO_2 detector or end-tidal CO_2, and (3) with a chest X-ray.

Equipment
(Table 2.2, Figure 2.7)

- Laryngoscope with straight, narrow blade (term: size no. 1; preterm <2500 g: size no. 0, consider size no. 00 for infants <1000 g; e.g., Miller®), check bulb and batteries
- Magill's forceps for nasal or difficult oral intubations (different sizes; for VLBW/ELBW you may use ENT "Weil–Blakesley" forceps)
- Endotracheal tube (Table 2.2), with or without surfactant application canal (e.g., by Vygon) and flexible stylet for oral intubations (optional; be very careful especially in BW preterm infants; some experts consider stylets contraindicated in neonates!),
- Suction catheters ready to use (Ch 8 = 8 F fits through 3.0 tube), suction set to negative pressure −0.2 bar = −200 mbar
- Bag-and-mask system with a minimum gas flow set at 5 l/min. Use 10 l/min gas flow for flow-inflating bags. Mask sizes 00 and 01
- Infant stethoscope
- Three strips of tape for securing nasally inserted ET tube (approx. 4–5 cm long, with double/slanted cut), or more sophisticated fixation device for orally inserted ET tubes
- A safety pin or anti-sliding circular tape is used by some centers to prevent downsliding of a nasally inserted ET tube (safety pin orthogonally through the outer part of the ET tube, just above the nostrils)

Anatomical features of neonates
The larynx is higher in neonates than in adults (especially in preterm infants: it is always surprising to see how far anterior and cranial the entrance of the larynx is when visualized by laryngoscopy). Particularly in preterm infants, the upper airways are unstable/flexible as collagen tissue is still underdeveloped. The epiglottis is narrow and soft. Hyperextension (reclination) of the head tightens the trachea and lifts up both the glottis and the (still prominent) prevertebral soft tissue, which makes it difficult to visualize the vestibulum of the larynx. By declining the head towards the thorax, one will see the dorsal pharyngeal wall but unable to visualize the glottis by laryngoscopy. The ideal head position for

bag-and-mask ventilation and intubation is therefore the so-called sniffing position (i.e., nose is the highest point) with slight extension of the head (Figure 2.18).

> **!** If the NETS-team is called to a neonate who is already intubated, then it is not only permissible, but absolutely essential to verify, by using a laryngoscope or auscultation, whether the ET tube is in the correct position (obtain chest X-ray if possible)

If you know the ET tube is in the correct position (i.e., not too deep), you would interpret "decreased breath sounds on the left" as a likely pneumothorax rather than as right bronchial main stem intubation. The intubation of a neonate is not trivial ... and not magic. Unsuccessful (i.e., esophageal) intubations, however, are common among unexperienced health care providers[67,68]. In a USA-based study, none of the participating pediatric residents met the authors' definition of procedural competence for intubation (successful at the first or second attempt 80% of the time) over a 2-year period[68]. The following pages should help one to reach this minimal goal. However, elective hands-on training in pediatric anesthesia and neonatal intensive care is highly recommended.

Nasotracheal intubation (Figure 2.21a-c)
Technique
- Place the head and nose in the median and sniffing position (slight extension); an assistant may also hold the head in the correct position. Moisten the ET tube and advance it towards the lower nasal cavity (winding movements may help) up to the 5- to 6-cm mark, so that the tip is behind the uvula.
- Hold the laryngoscope with the left hand using the thumb, index and middle fingers, while, with the ring and little fingers, slightly raise the lower jaw with a gentle grip on the bony ridge of the chin (not the soft tissue). If necessary, open the mouth with the right index finger (but do not waste time on this). Pass the laryngoscope's blade (preferred: Miller® no. 0 or 1) along the right side of the mouth, gently pushing the tongue to the left side towards the floor of the mouth (be careful of the maxillary alveolar ridge → future teeth). Advance the blade until the epiglottis is visualized. Improve your view by suctioning carefully, if needed. Insert the tip of the blade in the vallecula, which is the space between the base of the tongue and epiglottis (be sure to insert the blade *beneath* the epiglottis). Gently lift the entire blade vertically (i.e., pull the laryngoscope's handle upwards and forward along the axis of the handle ≈ top left corner of the room or the edge of the ceiling) to elevate the epiglottis and to visualize the glottis (Figures 2.21 and 2.23). Alternatively (and preferred by many), insert the blade down to the hypopharynx (then the esophagus can be visualized) and while slowly withdrawing the blade, the epiglottis falls down into the visual field. Then insert the blade into the vallecula and carefully lift up the epiglottis. Do not rock the tip of the blade by pulling the handle towards you, and avoid hyperextension of the neck.
- If only the posterior commissure of the glottis is visible, applying external, downward pressure to the cricoid may help you to fully see the glottis (use your own little finger or get help from an assistant). Note, however, that too much cricoid pressure can occlude the airway and prevent easy passage of the ET tube. Seize the tip of the tube with the Magill's (or ENT) forceps and insert it gently into the trachea (be careful of the uvula and vocal cords). Often the ET tube has then to be advanced manually by a few

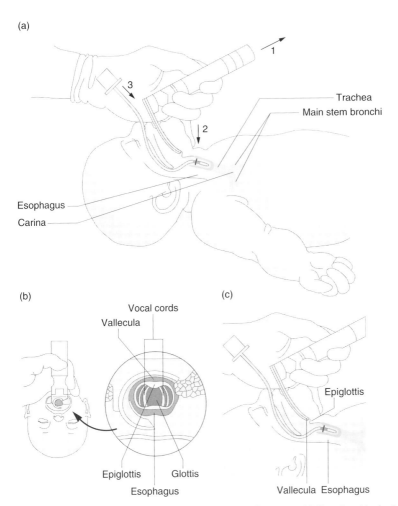

(a)

Trachea
Main stem bronchi

Esophagus
Carina

(b)

Vocal cords
Vallecula

Epiglottis   Glottis
Esophagus

(c)

Epiglottis

Vallecula Esophagus

Figure 2.21a–c Technique of nasotracheal intubation of neonates. (a) Place head in the "sniffing" position, advance the tube into the nose up to the 5- to 6-cm mark, hold the laryngoscope with the left hand and pass the blade along the right side of the mouth. Insert blade until the epiglottis is visualized (suction, if indicated). Insert the tip of the blade in the vallecula. By gently pulling the laryngoscope (along the axis of the handle) (1), the epiglottis is elevated and the glottis visualized (do not rock the tip of the blade). If necessary, apply external downward pressure appropriately to the cricoid to fully see the glottis, i.e., anterior and posterior commissure (2). Subsequently, position the ET tube with the Magill's forceps until the black mark (or second black line) is just about visible between the vocal cords (3). (b) Ideally visualized glottis: anterior and posterior commissure are visible, vocal cords (white) are almost parallel to each other. Then, position the tube with the Magill's forceps. (c) Correctly positioned endotracheal tube: black mark is just about visible between the vocal cords. Modified from: Kattwinkel J, 2006. *Neonatal Resuscitation*, 5th edn. Elk Grove Village, IL: American Academy of Pediatrics and American Heart Association. See color plate section for full color version.

millimeters (by oneself or the assistant; rotate the tube by up to 180° if unable to advance), until the black mark (or second black line) is just about visible (approx. 2 mm) between the vocal cords. If the sliding of the tube into the trachea is felt with the left little finger, then it is very likely that the ET tube is correctly positioned. *Visual control of the tube's position* is always more important than the specifications about the length shown in Table 2.2. Those who are very experienced in endotracheal intubation may be able to intubate nasally without the use of a forceps

- Then hold the tube tight with the right index finger and thumb on the maxillary ridge, cautiously remove the laryngoscope and provide PPV with the bag (do not compress the ET tube lumen). Verbally note the tube's position (insertion length measured at the nostril).
- Insert gastric tube.

Confirmation of *tracheal* intubation

Rapid increase in HR and S_pO_2 with PPV, expiratory mist (condensation) visible at the proximal end of transparent ET tubes (Mallinckrodt®), symmetrical chest rise and breath sounds, a CO_2 detector (most turn yellow), and absence of loud inspiratory sounds in the epigastric area confirm the correct position of the ET tube (obtain chest X-ray, e.g., in the NICU)

- In most cases, it is NOT necessary and NOT recommended to place the tip of the blade directly on the epiglottis and pressing the epiglottis against the base of the tongue. This procedure may cause edema of the epiglottis and subsequent problems when extubating the baby
- The advantages of nasal versus oral intubation are better fixation (fewer spontaneous extubations) and easier oropharyngeal hygiene

For technique of orotracheal intubation please see further details on p. 9 and Figure 2.22a–d.

Troubleshooting during nasotracheal intubation (Figures 2.21, 2.23)
ET tube cannot be inserted through the nose
Solutions
- Suction nasally (if not yet done)
- Moisten tube once more and insert with rotating movements, if necessary reposition the head (always pass the tube through the lower nasal cavity and advance it towards the pharynx/floor of the mouth and not towards the ethmoid bone)
- Use the other nostril
- Apply 1% lidocaine gel to the lower third of the tube
- If birth weight is <1000 g, you may "thread" a small suction catheter (Ch 6 = 8 F) through the 2.5 (2.0) ET tube, and advance the "catheter-guided" ET tube through the nose and into the trachea
- Choose a smaller ET tube: if possible, use ET tube size ≥3.0 for term infants and ≥2.5 for preterm infants
- If still unsuccessful at this point, interrupt the procedure, ventilate (until oxygen saturation and HR are sufficient) and perform oral intubation

Epiglottis or glottis cannot be visualized
Solutions
- Blade may be advanced too far, so that the esophagus is seen. Slowly withdraw the blade while gently pulling the laryngoscope (upwards and forward) in line with the handle.

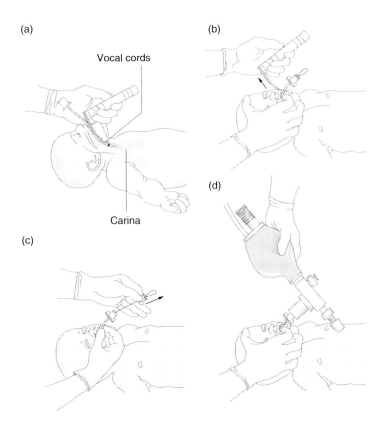

Figure 2.22a–d Technique of orotracheal intubation of neonates. (**a**) Place head in "sniffing" position, hold the laryngoscope with the left hand and pass the blade along the right side of the mouth. Insert blade until epiglottis is visualized (suction, if indicated). Insert the tip of the blade in the vallecula. By gently pulling the laryngoscope (along the axis of the handle) (step 1), the epiglottis is elevated and the glottis visualized (do not rock the tip of the blade). If necessary, apply external downward pressure appropriately to the cricoid to fully see the glottis, i.e., anterior and posterior commissure (step 2). Subsequently, advance the ET tube through the glottis until the black mark (or second black line) is just about visible between the vocal cords (step 3). (**b**) Hold the tube firmly with the right index finger against the maxillary ridge, then remove the laryngoscope. (**c**) Still holding the tube tightly with the right index finger, carefully remove the stylet from the tube. (**d**) PPV through the endotracheal tube (which is not yet taped) and always confirm correct ET tube position. (Are the chest movements sufficient and symmetrical? Are lungs equally ventilated? Is skin color more rosy? Rise of HR and SaO_2?). Then tape tube securely. Modified from: Kattwinkel J (2006) *Neonatal Resuscitation*. 5th edn. Elk Grove Village, IL: American Academy of Pediatrics and American Heart Association. See color plate section for full color version.

Apply external pressure to the cricoid so that the arytenoid cartilage and vocal cords become visible (do not occlude the trachea by applying too much cricoid pressure). Do not rock the tip of the blade and avoid hyperextension of the neck

- Blade may not be inserted far enough such that only the root of the tongue is seen. Advance blade further, and place the tip of the blade in the vallecula
- Only parts of the glottis are clearly visible (e.g., one vocal cord), because the blade is not properly positioned in the midline. Cautiously reposition the blade and apply external cricoid pressure until the vocal cords and glottis are completely visualized
- Head is not in the correct position and must be placed back at the midline and "sniffing" position

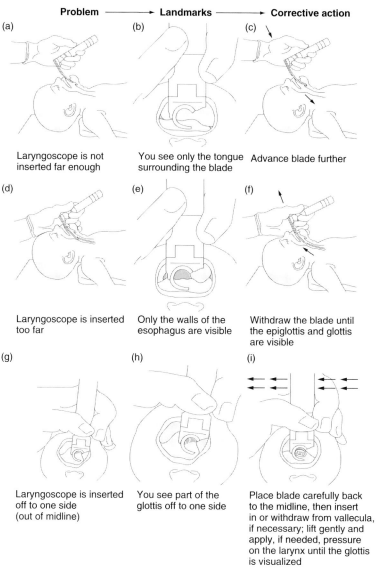

Figure 2.23 Troubleshooting during the endotracheal intubation of a neonate. Modified from: Kattwinkel J (2006) *Neonatal Resuscitation*, 5th edn. Elk Grove Village, IL: American Academy of Pediatrics and American Heart Association. See color plate section for full color version.

Glottis is visualized, the tip of the tube lies between the vocal cords, but cannot be advanced

Solutions

- Rotate the ET tube (up to 180°) and advance carefully according to ET tube markings
- If the vocal cords lie side by side such that the glottis is tightly closed, an assistant may provide mechanical breaths with the bag (pharyngeal PPV via the connected ET tube). This procedure requires an experienced team, because the tube can easily be displaced.

Alternatively, bag-and-mask ventilate, give a sedative and muscle relaxant, and try again (nasally or orally)

Intubation takes too long

> ! If an intubation attempt is unsuccessful, the procedure must be interrupted after 20–30 s or immediately if bradycardia occurs[59,67].

Prior to the next attempt, check the head position (Midline? Is the tip of the nose the highest point?), perform PPV via bag-and-mask or pharyngeal ET tube until the HR and S_pO_2 are sufficient, then give a sedative and muscle relaxant, and proceed with nasal or oral intubation.

Orotracheal intubation (Figure 2.22a–d)

Indication

Orotracheal intubation is indicated when a depressed neonate is suspected of meconium aspiration or after one to two attempts at nasal intubation have failed.

Technique

- Place the head in the midline and "sniffing" position (nose is highest point; avoid overextension!), PPV
- **Optional**: insert a stylet in the ET tube and check that it is easily movable inside. Ensure that the stylet is shorter than the ET tube and then bend it at right angles at the proximal end of the tube to prevent it from protruding out the distal end as, especially in small preterm infants, the stylet can cause fatal penetrating injuries, for example to the heart or trachea. Then bend the ET tube with the stylet inside to the correct curvature of the airway. *Many experts discourage the use of any stylets in: (1) preterm infants, (2) preterm infants <1500 g, or (3) any newborn with abnormal anatomy.*
- Insert the laryngoscope, lift the entire blade to expose the larynx and visualize the glottis (with or without external cricoid pressure), as described before. Advance the ET tube manually into the optimal position until the black mark (or second black line) is just about visible (approx. 2 mm) between the vocal cords.
- Visually checking the correct ET tube position is better than any specifications about the insertion length, as shown in Table 2.2.
- Hold the tube firmly with the right index finger and thumb against the maxillary ridge, carefully remove the laryngoscope first and then the stylet. If resistance is met while pulling back the stylet, lease the pressure on the ET tube to allow stylet removal.
- Apply PPV with bag via the ET tube. Checklist for correct tracheal intubation: rapid increase in HR and S_pO_2 with PPV, expiratory mist (condensation) visible at the proximal end of transparent ET tubes (Mallinckrodt®), symmetrical chest rise and breath sounds, a CO_2 detector (most turn yellow), and absence of loud inspiratory sounds in the epigastric area confirm the correct position of the ET tube.
- Verbally note the tube's position (insertion length measured at upper lip).

> *Rule of thumb for oral ET tube insertion length (from upper lip) by birth weight is: 1 kg → 7 cm, 2 kg → 8 cm, 3 kg → 9 cm, 4 kg → 10 cm (i.e., 6 plus weight in kg; see Table 2.2).*

- Then tape the ET tube securely in place
- Insert gastric tube
- Obtain chest X-ray, e.g., in the NICU

> **!** Advantage of orotracheal intubation: faster than nasal intubation. Important particularly in depressed newborns with suspected meconium aspiration when immediate tracheal suctioning is crucial

! T_{in} Rule of thumb for conventional mechanical ventilation of newborn infants

Inspiration time (T_{in}) in seconds $\cong$ completed weeks of gestation ÷ 100
for example, for a VLBW preterm infant born at 30 weeks of gestation → T_{in} = 0.30 seconds

Securing the endotracheal tube

There are four ways of securing the position of the tube:
- First option (after nasotracheal intubation): three strips of tape (each approx. 5 cm long) cut diagonally at 2 cm. Clean the skin with benzoin or another appropriate skin preparation. Stick most of the first strip of tape onto the bridge of the nose up as far as the glabella and stick the remainder around the proximal ET tube. Adhere the second and third strips to the cheeks, in both cases sticking most of the tape to the skin and the shorter portion around the tube
- Second option (after nasotracheal or orotracheal intubation): pre-cut three thin strips of tape: tape 1, short strip (approx. 3–4 cm) adhered to the upper lip ("moustache"); tapes 2 and 3, longer strips (approx. 7–8 cm long), each adhered to one cheek, around the tube and then onto the other cheek
- Third option: cut one strip of tape approx. 8–10 cm long and 2 cm wide. Cut the strip lengthwise into two strands, leaving 3 cm intact at one end. Adhere this end to the glabella to the nose bridge, and wrap the two strands of tape around the tube and then each strand onto one cheek
- Fourth option: for orally inserted ET tubes, more sophisticated devices than just tape are available that allow suffcent fixation and avoid skin damage

In some neonatology divisions, the ET tube (smallest internal diameter of 2.5 mm) is prevented from sliding deeper (i.e., past the carina into the right main bronchial stem) by a safety pin or circular tape. When the tube is securely in place, it may be shortened in order to minimize the ventilatory deadspace (if necessary, shorten the ET tube in the delivery room prior to a long transport or in the NICU to 13–15 cm for term neonates, shorter for preterm infants).

> **!** Remember that the ET tube is not totally fixed and dependent on the position of the head and neck. During neonatal transport in particular, keep in mind that the ET tube is in its deepest position when the head is flexed (forward), but moves upward by 1.2 cm to more than 2 cm when the head is extended, hyperextended or turned to the side

If a neonate who was properly intubated and then transferred to a transport incubator suddenly has louder breath sounds on the right side, it is likely that the ET tube has inadvertently entered the right main bronchus. In this case, the position of the head should be corrected first (extend the head and move it sidewards). If the breath sounds are still unequal, the following measures are recommended:

1. Check the length of ET tube insertion at the upper lip or nostril (was the initial length documented?)
2. Laryngoscopy:
   - If the black mark is not visible, carefully retract the tube
   - If the tube is properly placed (black mark or third black line is just about visible) and at the same time the head is in neutral position (midline and sniffing), suspect a pneumothorax and act quickly (decompression with butterfly or chest tube)!

Gastric tube placement

Equipment

See Figure 2.8: Orogastric or nasogastric tube (size Ch 5 or Ch 8 (5 F or 8 F), stylet (usually not needed), a 4-length of cm tape for securing, a urine bag (may be used to collect gastric fluid). Use a large orogastric catheter (10 F) or double-lumen gastric tube (Replogle) in cases of congenital diaphragmatic hernia, esophageal atresia or abdominal wall defects (omphalocele, gastroschisis).

Indication

- After every endotracheal intubation
- Approx. 2 min after bag-and-mask ventilation
- When ileus or esophageal atresia is suspected (then place the neonate in 20–30° upright position and on their left side, with continuous suctioning of the gastric tube)
- Omphalocele
- Gastroschisis
- Prior to the first feeding (insert gastric tube with suction catheter or tube to clinically rule out esophageal atresia)

Technique

- Measure the insertion length required: from the tip of the nose, passing behind the ear and down to the stomach
- Insert and advance the tube through the (free) nostril and the lower nasal cavity, directing it blindly towards the back of the throat. Alternatively, the gastric tube may be inserted through the mouth (i.e., orogastric tube; some neonatologists point out that this way the gastric tube interferes less with spontaneous breathing, and does not put pressure on the nasal cartilage)

- If the tube kinks in the throat, it may be helpful to gently pull the prelaryngeal soft tissue (skin) forward
- Determine the position of the gastric tube clinically by injecting 10 ml of air with a syringe or by suctioning the stomach and listening with a stethoscope under the left costal arch/xiphoid at the same time. Afterwards, decompress the stomach again via the gastric tube and syringe, or even suck out gastric secretions (litmus paper may be used: pH value <7 suggests gastric content)
- Secure the gastric tube with tape
- Verify its position by X-ray (kidney–ureter–bladder (KUB), extended chest X-ray (CXR) or CXR plus KUB in the NICU

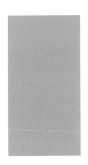

Laryngeal mask airway (LMA)

Georg Hansmann

Current evidence

Masks that fit over the laryngeal inlet (i.e., LMA) are effective for ventilating newborn full-term infants (level of evidence (LOE) 2; LOE 5). There are limited data on the use of these devices in small preterm infants (LOE 5). There is currently no evidence directly comparing LMA with bag-valve-bag-and-mask (BMV) ventilation during neonatal resuscitation. Data from two case series show that use of the LMA can provide effective ventilation in a time frame consistent with current resuscitation guidelines (LOE 5). A single randomized controlled trial found no significant difference between the LMA and tracheal intubation during resuscitation of babies by experienced providers after cesarean section (LOE 2). Case reports suggest that when ventilation via a face mask has been unsuccessful and tracheal intubation is unsuccessful or not feasible, the LMA may provide effective ventilation (LOE 5). A well-designed randomized controlled trial comparing the LMA with BMV during neonatal resuscitation is warranted[22,69].

Indication

PPV with face mask (bag or T-piece resuscitator) fails to achieve effective ventilation, and attempts at endotracheal intubation are either not feasible or unsuccessful ("can't ventilate and can't intubate"). *Examples are:*

- Congenital anomalies involving the mouth, lip, or palate, i.e., achieving a good seal with the bag and mask is difficult (head and neck cysts, cleft palate, Down syndrome, Beckwith–Wiedemann syndrome, Pierre Robin sequence, Treacher Collins syndrome, etc.)
- Anomalies of the mouth, tongue, pharynx or neck, when there is difficulty visualizing the larynx with a laryngoscope (head and neck cysts, Down syndrome, Beckwith–Wiedemann syndrome, Pierre Robin sequence, etc.)
- A very small mandible or relatively large tongue (e.g., Pierre Robin sequence, Beckwith–Wiedemann syndrome, Down syndrome, etc.)

Equipment

The LMA is an airway device that is placed "blindly" without any instruments, and can be used to provide PPV. The **size 1** LMA is a soft elliptical mask with an inflatable rim attached to a flexible airway tube (Figure 2.24). Once the LMA is fully inserted, the rim is inflated. The inflated mask covers the laryngeal inlet and the rim conforms to the contours of the hypopharynx occluding the esophagus with a low-pressure seal. The mask has bars across

Neonatal Emergencies: A Practical Guide for Resuscitation, Transport and Critical Care, ed. Georg Hansmann.
Published by Cambridge University Press. © Cambridge University Press 2009.

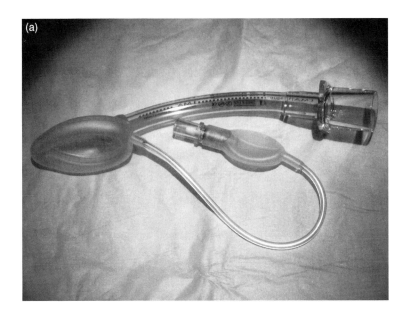

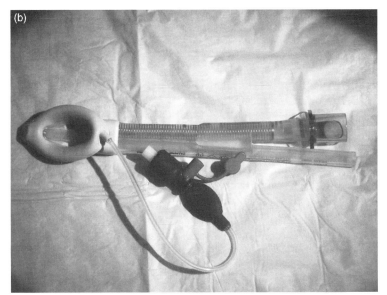

Figure 2.24a,b Laryngeal mask airways. a *Classic LMA*™ (cLMA, size 1). b *LMA-ProSeal*™ (PLMA).

the middle that prevent the epiglottis from becoming trapped within the airway tube. The airway tube has a standard 15-mm adapter that is attached to either a resuscitation bag or a ventilator. A pilot balloon attached to the rim is used to monitor the mask's inflation. Both reusable and disposable LMA versions are commercially available. The size 1 neonatal device is the only size appropriate for newborns. There is limited experience of using the LMA in infants between 1500 and 2500 g. An LMA size 1 is probably too large for babies with a birthweight <1500 g[9].

The neonatal *LMA-ProSeal*™ (PLMA; size 1) allows greater airway pressure ventilation than the *classic LMA*™ (cLMA, size 1), in a neonatal intubation manikin[70]. A small, randomized study in 2- to 20-month-old patients ($n = 30$; 5–12 kg) revealed that the size 1.5 PLMA seems to be a more suitable device for airway maintenance in infants than the same size cLMA. The ability to insert a gastric tube with the *LMA-ProSeal*™ at the same time, and a significantly greater airway leak pressure than with the cLMA (26.7 vs. 18.9 cmH$_2$O in neutral head position and 35.6 vs. 28.2 cmH$_2$O in maximum flexion) might have important implications for its use in infants in need of PPV[71]. If this is confirmed clinically in neonates, the PLMA may be of advantage during neonatal resuscitation when high airway pressures are required.

Limitations and complications of the LMA

- Cannot be used to suction meconium from the airway (use ET tube and meconium adapter instead)
- If high ventilation pressures are needed, an air leak through an insufficient seal may result in insufficient pressure to inflate the lungs and lead to gastric distension
- Insufficient evidence for effective delivery of intratracheal medications (e.g., epinephrine, surfactant)
- Insufficient evidence to recommend LMA for prolonged PPV in newborns (>8–12 h)
- Gastric tube placement may be impossible
- Complications: soft-tissue trauma, laryngospasm, gastric air distension. Lingual edema and damage to the recurrent laryngeal nerve/vocal cord paralysis may occur, particularly with prolonged use (hours or days)

What do you need for LMA placement?

- LMA size 1 (classic LMA™ or LMA-ProSeal™)
- A 5-ml syringe
- Water-soluble lubricant (optional)
- Gloves
- PPV device (self-inflating bag, flow-inflating bag, T-piece resuscitator or mechanical ventilator)
- Gastric tube (to be placed after LMA-ProSeal™ is inserted)

Technique (Figure 2.25)

Prepare the LMA

1. Wear gloves and remove the size 1 LMA from the sterile package
2. Briefly inspect the device (mask, midline aperture bars, are the airway tube and connector intact?)
3. Attach the 5-ml syringe to the pilot balloon and test the mask by inflating it with 4 ml of air. Then remove the air from the mask using the attached syringe.

Insert the LMA (here: "classic technique" of LMA placement)

4. Stand at the infant's head and position the head in the "sniffing position" (tip of the nose = highest point)
5. Hold the LMA like a pen, with your index finger placed at the junction of the cuff and the tube (Figure 2.25a). The bars in the middle of the mask must be facing forward. The flat part of the mask has no bars and will be facing the patient's palate

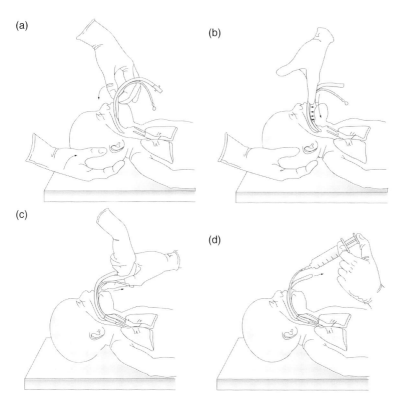

Figure 2.25 Laryngeal mask airway (LMA) placement. Here, the "classic technique" of inserting and securing the LMA is shown. The cuff should be inserted whilst deflated and then inflated after insertion. For a detailed step-by-step technique, see main text. For the common problem that the tip of the mask curls backward on itself (see classic technique, step 8), some clinicians prefer the "LMA flip technique" (i.e., LMA is inserted into the mid-pharynx upsidedown, and then turned by 180° around the axis of the tube so that the opening finally is facing forward). Modified from: Kattwinkel J (2006) *Neonatal Resuscitation*. 5th edn. Elk Grove Village, IL: American Academy of Pediatrics and American Heart Association.

6. If you decide to apply lubricant to the back of the LMA, keep the lubricant away from the apertures on the front side/inside the mask.

7. Gently open the infant's mouth and press the leading tip of the mask against the hard palate (Figure 2.25a).

8. Flatten the tip of the mask against the baby's palate with your index finger. Ensure that the tip of the mask remains flat and does not flip backward onto itself.

9. Gently guide the device along the contours of the infant's hard palate toward the back of the throat (Figure 2.25b). Do not use force! Use a smooth movement to guide the mask past the tongue and into the hypopharynx until you feel resistance.

Set the LMA in place

10. Before removing your finger, use your other hand to hold the LMA tube in place (Figure 2.25c). This prevents the device from being pulled out of place when removing your finger. At this point, the tip of the LMA should be resting near the entrance of the esophagus (upper esophageal sphincter).

11. Inflate the mask with 2–4 ml of air (Figure 2.25d). The cuff should be inflated with just enough air to achieve a seal. Do not hold the airway tube when you inflate the mask. You may notice that the tube glides slightly (1–2 cm) outward as the mask is inflated (this is a good sign and an early indicator of proper LMA placement). Never inflate the cuff of the size 1 LMA with more than 4 ml of air

Secure and ventilate through the LMA

12. Attach your resuscitation bag to the LMA adapter and begin PPV
13. Confirm proper placement by assessing rising HR, chest wall movement, audible breath sounds with the stethoscope and lack of loud inspiratory sound (leak!)
14. Secure the LMA with tape, as you would do for an orally inserted ET tube
15. You may want to check for the current airway leak pressure (e.g., elective LMA placement in an infant prior to surgery)

For the common problem that the tip of the mask curls backward on itself (see step 8), some clinicians prefer the "**LMA flip technique**" (i.e., LMA is inserted into the mid-pharynx upsidedown, and then turned through 180° so that the opening is facing forward). To achieve this, follow these steps:

1. Hold the LMA with the index finger and thumb at the proximal third of the tube, so that the mask opening is facing backward (i.e., the palate). Do not use lubricant
2. Insert the LMA this way approximately two-thirds of the distance (past the base of the tongue), then turn the LMA through 180° around the axis of the tube (now the opening is facing forward) and gently push it further into the hypopharynx until you feel resistance
3. Inflate the mask with 2–4 ml of air without holding the airway tube (see above)

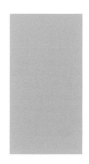

Chest compressions

Georg Hansmann

> **!** At a cardiac arrest, the first procedure is to take your own pulse[72]

Indication

Heart rate remains below 60 bpm, despite 30 s of effective PPV (F_iO_2 0.21–1.0; bag-and-mask ventilation or immediate intubation/PPV).

Goals

External cardiac massage: (1) compression of the heart muscle against the spinal column; (2) increase in intrathoracic pressure, and (3) sufficient perfusion and oxygenation of vital organs (particularly central nervous system, coronary arteries, lungs).

The indication for chest compressions (i.e., heart rate below 60 bpm) is also an indication for rapid endotracheal intubation, which helps to ensure adequate ventilation and facilitates the coordination of chest compressions with ventilation (after intubation, the ratio of chest compressions to delivered breaths remains 3:1). Moreover, epinephrine can be given via the ET tube when there is no umbilical vein catheter (UVC), peripheral intravenous (PIV) or intraosseous (IO) access.

Technique

There are two methods:
- Two-thumb (encircling hands) technique
- Two-finger technique

Two-thumb (encircling hands) technique (Figure 2.26a)

Correct application of pressure: the pressure point is at the middle third of the sternum (approx. 1 cm below the inter mammillary line). Position both thumbs on the sternum, and encircle the thorax with your palms and fingers to provide appropriate support for the back. Thumbs are adjacent to each other, either minimally superior and inferior to the pressure point, or in parallel to the sternal midline. The thumbs should be flexed at the first joint and pressure applied vertically to compress the heart between the sternum and the spine. This is the method of choice for most neonatal emergencies (it may have an advantage over the two-finger technique in that it yields greater peak systolic and coronary perfusion pressures).

Neonatal Emergencies: A Practical Guide for Resuscitation, Transport and Critical Care, ed. Georg Hansmann.
Published by Cambridge University Press. © Cambridge University Press 2009.

(a)

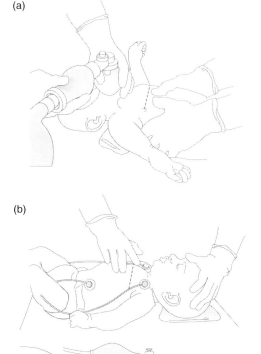

(b)

Figure 2.26 Chest compressions. (a) Two-thumb (encircling hands) technique for chest compressions. This technique is the method of choice (may have the advantage of producing greater peak systolic and coronary perfusion pressure). For small preterm infants (<1500 g): consider superimposing the thumbs (one over the other) or using the two-finger technique. (b) Two-finger technique for chest compressions. Method of second choice: it has advantages for very small preterm infants (<1000 g) and during umbilical vein catheterization. Modified from: Ralston M *et al.* (2006) *PALS. Provider Manual.* Dallas, TX: American Heart Association and American Academy of Pediatrics. See color plate section for full color version.

The two-thumb technique cannot be used, however, when your hands are small or the baby is very large. It also has the disadvantage of limiting visibility and access for other procedures.

Chest compression in small preterm infants: two-thumb technique with overlapping thumbs or two-finger technique (the latter is of particular advantage when a third neonatal life support provider places an emergency UV catheter or PIV).

Two-finger technique (Figure 2.26b)

Find the pressure point, as described above. Place two fingers (second and third or third and fourth fingers) along the sternum at 90 degrees to the chest (approx. 1 cm below the inter-mammillary line). This is the method of second choice in most instances. The other hand may be used to support the the newborn's back. The two-finger technique is advantageous in small preterm infants (<1500 g), during UV catheterization, and when one's hands are too small to perform the two-thumb technique (e.g., in a large baby). It is, however, more tiring and eventually less effective than the two-thumb technique (see above). Particular attention should be paid to the consistency and directionality of chest compressions, as the provider stands to one side of the baby.

Compressions

Pressure should be applied vertically to compress the heart between the sternum and the spine. The depth of compression is approximately one-third of the anterior – posterior diameter of the chest (i.e., 1.5–2 cm). Compressions must yield a palpable pulse (palpate

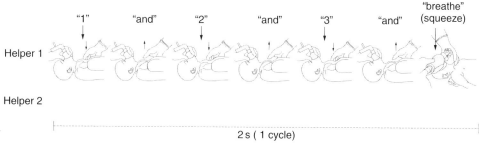

Figure 2.27 Coordination of chest compressions and ventilation (bag-and-mask PPV) in a neonate. Helper 1 performs chest compressions; helper 2 performs PPV. A 3:1 cycle takes 2 s. After three compressions deliver a PPV breath (count aloud "1-and-2-and-3-and squeeze..."). Modified from Kattwinkel J (2006) *Neonatal Resuscitation*, 5th edn. Elk Grove Village, IL: American Academy of Pediatrics and American Heart Association.

brachial or femoral artery). Do not perform staccato-like compressions. Compression-to-relaxation ratio is approximately 1:1, with a slightly shorter compression period. During the relaxation period, the thumbs or fingers remain on the sternum.

Chest compressions and PPV

A 3:1 ratio of compression to ventilation is recommended by ILCOR/AAP/AHA. A cycle with three compressions and one breath lasts 2 s, which amounts to 90 compressions and 30 breaths per min, i.e., 120 events per minute (Figure 2.27: count out loud, "1-and-2-and-3-and squeeze..."). It is important that the compressions and ventilations are well coordinated and delivered continuously (3:1 ratio even after ET intubation). During the PPV ("squeeze") phase, quickly assess whether chest rise is sufficient and symmetrical. Continue chest compression in the expiratory phase of the PPV "squeeze," so that interruption in external cardiac massage is minimal.

Chest compressions may negatively affect efficient ventilation/lung expansion. Therefore, chest compressions should not be initiated until efficient PPV has been delivered for at least 30 s (in most instances, proper PPV will lead to a rapid increase in HR). Do not perform chest compressions if HR is >60 bpm and cardiac output is generated (palpable brachial or femoral pulse).

> **! Key points when performing chest compressions**
>
> 1. Frequency (90 compressions/min, PPV 30 breaths/min, 120 events per minute)
> 2. Depth of compression (one-third of anterior – posterior diameter)
> 3. Coordination with PPV (3:1 ratio; assess chest rise during PPV phase)

After 30 s of chest compression and PPV

Assessment of heart rate (bpm) = pulse in 3 s × 20 (→ check ABCD):
- If HR <60 bpm:
  - Intubate (if not done yet) and provide PPV
  - Administer epinephrine: 0.03–0.1 mg/kg/dose intratracheally or 0.01 mg/kg/dose IV (= epinephrine 1:10 000 / 0.3–1 ml/kg/dose intracheally or 0.1 ml/kg/dose IV) after at least 30 s of chest compression and effective PPV. Use intratracheal route only if epinephrine is indicated and no UV/PIV/IO access is available. When IV access is

established, give a volume bolus (10 ml/kg/dose IV) with the second epinephrine dose (0.01–0.03 mg/kg/dose)

- If HR >60 bpm (and palpable pulse):
  - Stop chest compressions and continue PPV at a rate of 30–60 breaths per minute (faster!) with PIP and PEEP sufficient to achieve adequate and symmetrical chest rise
- When HR >100 bpm:
  - Slowly reduce PPV rate (and PIP according to chest rise) until spontaneous breathing is sufficient. Eventually continue with mask-CPAP. Continue oxygen supplementation until S_pO_2 >90% (S_pO_2 >85% in preterm infants). Note: There are currently insufficient data on the optimal S_pO_2 in the delivery room for term and preterm infants

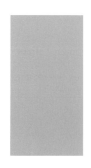

Peripheral venous access

Georg Hansmann

Indication
- When IV medication, volume expansion or dextrose is required
- Prior to any transport

Equipment
- Indwelling PIV catheters (24 gauge, 26 gauge)
- Alcohol swabs
- 2-ml syringe filled with 2–3 ml normal saline
- Three-way stopcock connected with short tubing and filled with NS flush
- Three strips of tape (2×3–4 cm, 1×6–8 cm), Tegaderm™ dressing
- Blood gas capillaries/syringe
- Glucometer/blood dextrose (glucose) stix

Technique
- Possible sites: see Figure 2.28 – PIV sites. Scalp veins, external jugular vein, internal jugular vein, subclavian vein, cubital veins, dorsal veins of hand, small saphenous vein, dorsal vein of pedis

Placement of a PIV catheter into a dorsal hand vein
Make yourself familiar with the model of the PIV catheter (24 G, 26 G) you like to place (there are several systems on the market with different inner diameters, lengths, protection systems). Flex the neonate's wrist so that the dorsal hand veins are easily visble, stretch the skin tightly with your left thumb and index finger, puncture the skin before the vein at an angle of about 20–30° (may choose "Y" branching vein), then lower the angle to 20° and advance the needle millimeter by millimeter until blood appears in the conus. The decisive moment comes when removing the introducer needle, which needs to be done without dislocating the plastic catheter or puncturing the back wall of the vein: Advance the catheter gently with the right index finger by only 1–2 mm while removing the introducer needle by approximately 3–5 mm. When blood returns into the plastic catheter, continue to advance the catheter slowly but completely while removing the needle (caution: some systems have security buttons or other devices which withdraw or protect the tip of the needle when the catheter is placed). Tape securely with a short, vertical strip. Withdraw blood for blood gases, blood glucose (dextrostix) and chemistry for work up (this is sometimes not possible

Neonatal Emergencies: A Practical Guide for Resuscitation, Transport and Critical Care, ed. Georg Hansmann.
Published by Cambridge University Press. © Cambridge University Press 2009.

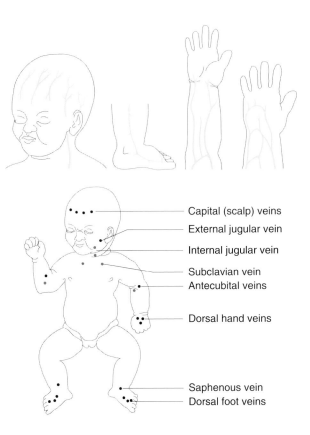

Figure 2.28 Venous access. Possible venous insertion sites in neonates and infants. Central venous access (grey), peripheral venous access (black). See color plate section for full color version.

Capital (scalp) veins
External jugular vein
Internal jugular vein
Subclavian vein
Antecubital veins
Dorsal hand veins
Saphenous vein
Dorsal foot veins

with 26 G catheters, even though they are in the proper position). Connect PIV tubing and flush with 1–3 ml normal saline; to secure the catheter: place a longer strip beneath the catheter with the sticky side facing up and tape crosswise on the dorsum of the hand, then secure looped tubing also with tape (i.e., chevron). Connect tubing to continuous IV ($D_{10}W$ 3 ml/kg/h in most instances).

> **!** 24 G and 26 G venous catheters often cannot withstand high volume boluses. Certain drugs (such as Prostaglandin E_1 (PGE$_1$), dopamine, dobutamine and also sodium bicarbonate) should run through a separate PIV in order to prevent unintentional drug boluses (e.g., "PGE$_1$ shots"), especially when volume boluses are required. Consider UV line or 22 G PIV for high volume replacement.

A quickly placed PIV is better than a central venous catheter (UV, central intrajugular or femoral line) placed under "pseudo-sterile," i.e., "non-sterile" conditions. However, if high-dose catecholamine infusions and large-volume resuscitation is needed, a UV catheter (or intrajugular or femoral venous central line) must be placed – provided that the team is well experienced (place UV line in the delivery room). Use UV catheter or central venous catheters to monitor central venous pressure in a hypovolemic neonate and those with heart failure. Central venous pressure is superior in guiding volume replacement therapy (NS, packed red blood cells, etc.) than measuring oscillometric systemic arterial pressure only.

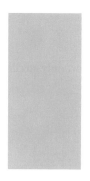

Umbilical vein/artery catheterization (UVC, UAC)

Andrea Zimmermann

Andrea Zimmermann

Indication

Umbilical vein catheter (UVC)

- During resuscitation, when peripheral venous access (PIV) is not possible
- If continuous administration of catecholamines (dopamine, epinephrine) is required

Umbilical artery catheter (UAC)

- If invasive and continuous monitoring of arterial blood pressure is required
- To obtain blood for arterial blood gas measurements
- For gentle blood sampling in preterm neonates (minimal handling)

> *I* A well-trained NETS-team should consider UVC placement in the delivery room: (1) as primary venous access and/or (2) as central venous access in an emergency or (3) in addition to peripheral IV access for further management on the NICU.

Preparation

- Two 2-ml syringes
- Three-way stopcock (one per catheter)
- Normal saline solution for flushing the catheter, sterile needles for drawing normal saline solution
- Continuous infusion (CI) with normal saline plus heparin 1 U/ml intravenous solution
- Catheters:
    - 2.5/3.5 (preterm infant) or 3.5/5 Ch (term infant)
    - Single-lumen, double-lumen or triple-lumen catheter for umbilical vein[73]
    - Single-lumen end whole catheter for umbilical artery[73,75]
    - Scalpel, umbilical tape
- Suture and tape for fixation
- Two anatomical forceps, one surgical forceps, two to three pointed anatomical forceps
- Fine probe
- Sterile gauze pads

Neonatal Emergencies: A Practical Guide for Resuscitation, Transport and Critical Care, ed. Georg Hansmann.
Published by Cambridge University Press. © Cambridge University Press 2009.

- Sterile drapes
- Sterile gown and sterile gloves, mask, cap (exeption: if child is in incubator, only sterile gloves are required)
- Make sure heat and light are adequate
- Place child in supine position (limb restraints may be required)
- Antiseptic solution (sterile gauze soaked in solution)

> **Tip:** Using *alcohol* skin disinfectants on the (very sensitive) skin of preterm/term infants can lead to toxic dermatitis and even skin necrosis. Liquid disinfectants that are antiseptic for mucous membranes and wounds are an alternative; however, they are not approved for skin disinfection. Allow 2 min for these antiseptic agents to take effect. After disinfection, the surrounding skin area must be wiped dry with sterile gauze pads. During disinfection make sure that the substance does not run down the patient's back, which may cause skin irritation or toxic dermatitis.

Technique (Figure 2.29)[74]

- Carefully clean umbilical cord and surrounding skin with antiseptic solution and cover skin with drapes
- While holding the cord clamp, extend the umbilical cord to allow the assistant to tie a piece of umbilical tie around the base of the cord and fix loosely (but tight enough to prevent significant blood loss)
- Cut off the umbilical cord with a scalpel 0.5–1.0 cm above the tape
- The umbilical cord usually contains three vessels: two smaller arteries with thickened walls, and one vein with a larger, almost oval and thinner wall
- If bleeding occurs while cutting through the umbilical cord, pull the umbilical tape tighter and cautiously swab the blood off the stump, as the stimulus may cause the arteries to contract

> Some neonatologists do not cut off the umbilical cord completely but use the excess length (i.e., the part of the umbilical cord that is nearly detached) to stabilize the whole umbilical cord by holding it upright with a forceps (left hand). One assistant can identify the vessel with forceps (if necessary, dilate gently). With the right hand the catheter can be inserted smoothly using a second anatomical forceps/tweezers.[74]

Umbilical vein catheter (UVC)

- Usually it is easier to insert a catheter into the umbilical vein than into an artery. The oval and slightly opened lumen can be dilated by an assistant with one or two fine forceps using the same procedures as described for UAC placement. The umbilical vein catheter should be flushed with normal saline solution before it is inserted. When the skin level is by passed, advance the catheter towards the patient's neck. Some neonatologists use a probe to dilate the umbilical vein (not the artery!)
- Once the calculated length is reached (Table 2.3), aspirate blood to verify the proper position in the vessel

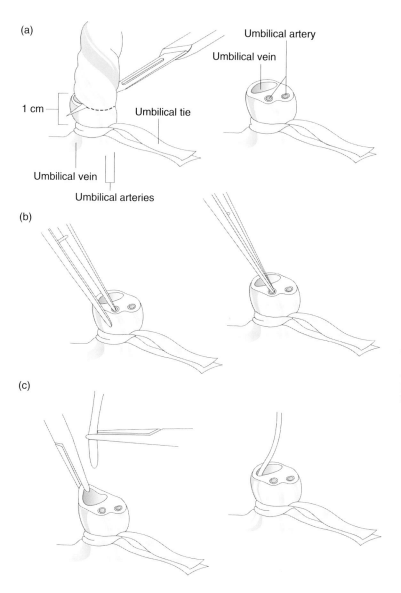

Figure 2.29 a–c
Umbilical artery
and umbilical vein
catheterization (UAC,
UVC). **(a)** Cutting the
umbilical cord. **(b)**
UAC placement: one
helper gently dilates
the umbilical artery
with forceps. Then
insert the UAC to a
depth as indicated
in Table 2.3. **(c)** UVC
placement: the helper
or physician identifies
the umbilical vein.
Next insert the UVC
to a depth as
indicated in Table 2.3.
In an emergency
(full resuscitation
including chest
compressions) with
no possibility of
immediate
radiographic control,
insert the UVC tip
only 3–5 cm until
blood can be
aspirated.[74] See color
plate section for a
full color version.

Three rules of thumb on the correct insertion depth for umbilical catheters (Table 2.3)

1.
- UVC insertion depth (in cm) from the umbilical ring to the level of T6–T8 = (2 × weight in kg) + 5 cm + stump length (in cm). Remember to add the length of the stump to the desired length of the catheter
- UAC insertion depth (in cm) from the umbilical ring to the level of T6–T8 = 1 (2 × weight in kg) + 10 cm + stump length (in cm). Remember to add the length of the stump to the desired length of the catheter

2.
- UVC insertion depth (in cm) to the level of T6–T9 = length from xiphoid to umbilicus in cm + 1 cm + stump length (in cm), OR

3.
- UVC insertion depth (in cm) from the umbilical ring to the level of T10 = (2 × weight in kg) + 5 + stump length (in cm),
- UAC insertion depth (in cm) from umbilical ring to the level of T10 = (weight in kg) + 9 + stump length (in cm)

- Obtain X-ray (combined CXR and KUB) to confirm optimal UVC placement: tip of catheter should be 1 cm above the diaphragm
- In the event of an emergency resuscitation without the possibility of immediate radiographic control, insert UVC tip only 3–5 cm below the umbilical ring until blood can be aspirated. Rationale: catheters inadvertently entering the portal system may lead to hepatic infusion of, e.g., hyperosmolaric solutions (→ necrosis).

If the catheter meets resistance, either re-enter and try again or pass a second thinner catheter alongside the first UVC in the same opening to allow the second catheter to enter the inferior vena cava through the ductus venosus.

Umbilical artery catheter (UAC)

- With straight forceps, grasp the artery wall and with one arm or a fine probe carefully dilate the lumen (for approx. 1 min)
- If an assistant is present, have the artery walls held open with two small, fine forceps
- Insert the umbilical arterial catheter – prefilled with normal saline flush solution – using fine forceps into the lumen. It may be helpful to gently pull the stump towards the head
- To control the position, aspirate blood. Proceed according to Table 2.3
- After placing the UAC, inspect the gluteal region and legs for pallor or cyanosis and carefully palpate the foot pulses
- Once no longer sterile, the catheter must not be advanced
- Confirm UAC position by X-ray in the NICU: high catheterization 1 cm above the diaphragm (approx. T6) is desirable over low catheterization (L3–L4) due to the greater

Table 2.3 Insertion depth of umbilical vein (UVC) and umbilical artery catheter (UAC)

Birth weight	UVC insertion depth from the umbilical ring (supra-diaphragmatic position, approx. T6–T8)	UAC insertion depth from the base of the cord (supra-diaphragmatic, approx. T6–T8)
≤1000 g	Approx. 6–7 cm	Approx. 12 cm
1000–1500 g	Approx. 7–8 cm	Approx. 13 cm
1500–2000 g	Approx. 8–9 cm	Approx. 14 cm
2000–3000 g	Approx. 9–10 cm	Approx. 15–17 cm
3000–4000 g	Approx. 11–12 cm	Approx. 17–19 cm

distance from the renal arteries[76]. However, some neonatologists believe low UA lines are safer.

- Infusion must run at a minimal rate of 0.5 ml/h (caution: volume overload in ELBW) Resistance may be encountered while inserting a UAC, especially after approximately 5 cm when entering the junction or confluence of the internal iliac artery. If the catheter cannot be advanced, this may be vasospasm of the artery.

If the resistance cannot be overcome by pressing gently, then remove the catheter and use the other umbilical artery. When there is no blood return, then the UAC may not have been advanced far enough, or it may have been sited incorrectly into a femoral artery. A catheter with no blood return is useless and thus must be removed!

Securing the catheter

Securing with sutures or tape:

- *Suturing*
    - Place a purse string suture around the stump of the cord
    - "Air knot" (e.g., place sterile forceps between skin and knot)
    - Tie a knot around the catheter
- *Fixation with tape*
    - Place two strips of tape vertically, using one on the right and one the left of the cord (Ω shaped), then fix the catheter horizontally, slightly above the stump to both Ω-shaped strips by using two short strips of tape
    - To protect the skin from the adhesive tape, skin-friendly tape may be placed underneath.

How long to use umbilical catheters after their initial sterile placement

- **UVC:** Due to the danger of infection and thrombosis, no longer than 14 days[77]. Many centers place a peripherally inserted central line (PICC) early when long-term central venous is indicated, and discontinue the UV line on day 1 or 2 of life
- **UAC:** Up to 7 days

! Complications from umbilical artery/vein catheters can be serious, therefore their need should be re-evaluated on a daily basis. Consider replacing UVC with PICC lines if long-term central access is anticipated.

! PICUs have started to use antibiotic-coated central venous catheters, however clinical data on their usefulness are preliminary.

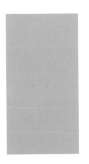

Central venous access (internal jugular vein)

Juan C. Ibla

Introduction

Central venous access is frequently necessary for the management of critical illness presenting in the neonatal period. Especial attention should be given to the anatomical landmarks and technique for safe and successful central venous cannulation and catheter placement. Here, basic indications and anatomy are reviewed. Then, a simple technique for internal jugular vein (IJV) cannulation and catheter placement is described that is useful in children of all ages but particularly in neonates. Sufficient experience is mandatory. Clinical judgment should be used to ensure the indication and safety of this procedure.

Indications

- Lack of peripheral intravenous access (PIV)
- Administration of multiple medications
- Need for inotropes/vasopressors not feasible for PIV access
- Tranfusions
- Blood sampling
- Central venous pressure (CVP) monitoring

Anatomy

The internal jugular vein (IJV; *vena jugularis interna*) drains blood from the brain, face, and neck. It originates from the jugular foramen at the base of the skull and travels down the side of the neck in a vertical direction towards the midline. Initially, the IJV runs lateral to the internal carotid artery, and then lateral to the common carotid, in contact with the posterior border of the sternocleidomastoid muscle (SCM), see Figures 2.30 and 2.31. At the root of the neck the IJV joins the subclavian vein to form the innominate vein (= brachiocephalic vein = vena anonyma) and enters the thoracic inlet to become the superior vena cava (SVC).

Materials

- Ultrasound system, e.g., TITAN TM®
- Pediatric Two-Lumen Central Venous Catheterization Kit®. Included: two-lumen indwelling polyurethane catheter (4 F × 5 cm × 22 G lumen), Tegaderm™ dressing
- 24 G ¾″ JELCO®
- 22 G 1″ JELCO®

Neonatal Emergencies: A Practical Guide for Resuscitation, Transport and Critical Care, ed. Georg Hansmann.
Published by Cambridge University Press. © Cambridge University Press 2009.

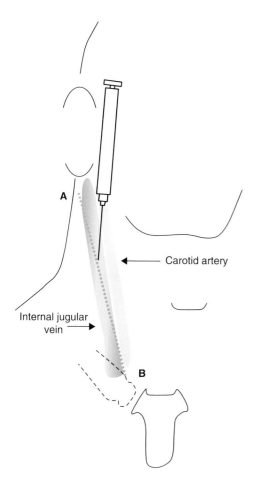

Figure 2.30 Anatomical relationship between the internal jugular vein (IJV) and carotid artery (CA). Note that the IJV travels lateral to the CA towards the midline between points A (=mastoid process of the temporal bone) and B (=jugular notch in the manubrium of the sternum). See color plate section for full color version.

Carotid artery

Internal jugular vein

A

B

- 25 G 5/8″ needle
- Spring-Wire Guide 0.18″ × 25 cm (see color plate section)

Anatomical and technical instructions for central venous catheter placement (IJV) are given below. Arrows refer to the appropriate solution in the "troubleshooting section" (pp. 115–16).

Technique

Various techniques for central venous access cannulation have been studied in infants and small children[78,79]. A modern approach to these techniques involves the use of ultrasound (U/S) for identification of patent veins and guidance of catheter placement[80–82]. We describe a modification of the Seldinger technique[83] which involves a combination of U/S interrogation of neck vascular anatomy and standard landmark based technique (→ **1**).

Goals for ultrasound examination
- Primary location of IJV
- Patency and size comparison between left- and right-sided veins
- Anatomical relationship between the IJV and carotid artery

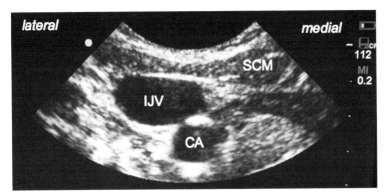

Figure 2.31 Ultrasound examination of the right neck. Note the internal jugular vein (IJV) is superficial and lateral to the carotid artery (CA) and in contact with the posterior border of the sternocleidomastoideus (SCM). Examine the anatomy with different degrees of head rotation, and observe their change in relation to each other.

Internal jugular vein location

For right-sided IJV cannulation, the patient is positioned supine with interscapular support (shoulder roll) and their head turned to the opposite side (left). Anatomical landmarks are determined by inspection and a straight line drawn from point A (mastoid process of the temporal bone) to point B (jugular notch in the manubrium of the sternum), see Figure 2.30. The C11/8–5 MHz transducer from the ultrasound system (2D Mode) is positioned perpendicular to the floor and a surveillance scan from points A to B is performed, see Figure 2.31. The IJV is identified and marked with respect to the line A–B (→ 2), see Figure 2.32a. Both IJVs are routinely examined and marked since occasionally the left IJV is larger in size (as in the case of L-SVC to coronary sinus anatomy). Additionally, various degrees of head rotation are inspected since, this can affect the relationship of the IJV with respect to the carotid artery (i.e., too much left-sided rotation of the head results in medial displacement of the IJV, placing the carotid artery directly underneath the IJV, increasing the incidence of carotid artery puncture or accidental cannulation).

Catheter placement (internal jugular vein)

Once the anatomy is identified, it is imperative not to change the patient's position. The usefulness of the Trendelenburg or head-down position in the neonate is not well established, but may be used it if increases the comfort of the operator.

- Skin and sterile field preparation
- Mount the 24 G ¾″ JELCO® (item b in Figure 2.33) on to the 1-ml syringe and prepare the Spring-Wire Guide 0.18″ × 25 cm (item d in Figure 2.33).
- Advance both JELCO® and the syringe as described in Figure 2.32b, taking care to minimize compression of the skin and the IJV directly underneath. In our experience, the IJV in the neonate is usually located no deeper than 1.25 cm from the point of entry at the skin. Occasionally the first attempt does not reveal evidence of venous puncture by the classic "back flush." Remove the needle from the catheter and withdraw the catheter slowly, no more than 1 mm at a time (→ 3). As soon as blood is noted in the catheter, the Spring-Wire Guide 0.18″ × 25 cm is advanced slowly (→ 4). We prefer to use this wire initially because of its shorter length, which makes it easier to manipulate through the 24 G ¾″ JELCO®. There should be no resistance

(a) (b)

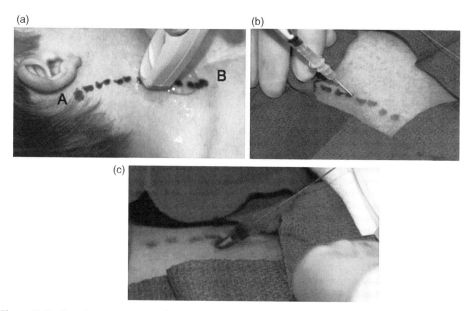

(c)

Figure 2.32 Central venous catheter placement. Once the anatomy is identified (a), the initial goal is to gain access to the internal jugular vein (IJV) with the Spring-Wire Guide 0.18″ × 25 cm minimizing tissue disruption by venous or arterial hematoma (b). The 24G ¾″ JELCO® is exchanged for the 22G 1″ JELCO® over the wire (c). This maneuver ensures secure access to the IJV, and allows advancement of the longer J tip 0.18″ × 45 cm PTFE-coated Spring-Wire Guide. Additionally, this catheter can be safely attached to a pressure transducer to rule out carotid artery cannulation. See color plate section for full color version.

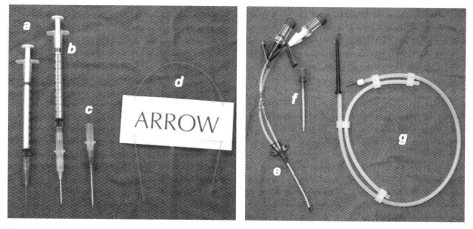

Figure 2.33 Materials required for internal jugular vein (IJV) cannulation. Items a, b, c and d are not included in the Central Venous Catheterization Kit and should be gathered separately. See color plate section for full color version.

to advancing the wire. If resistance is noted, start over (→ 5). If multiple attempts fail to identify the vein, we use the 25 G 5/8″ (item a on Figure 2.33) as a finder needle (→ 6)

- Once the wire has been advanced, the 24G ¾″ JELCO® is exchanged for a 22 G 1″ JELCO® (item c on Figure 2.33) over the Spring-Wire Guide 0.18″ × 25 cm as demonstrated in Figure 2.32c (→ 7)

115

- The 22 G 1″ JELCO® catheter can now accommodate the J tip 0.18″ × 45 cm PTFE-coated Spring-Wire Guide (item g on Figure 2.33) included in the Pediatric Two-Lumen Central Venous Catheterization Kit (→ 8). Observe the ECG for atrial or ventricular arrhythmia. If arrhythmia is noted, withdraw the wire slowly 0.5 cm

- Mount the short (2.5″, 6 cm, item f on Figure 2.33) tissue dilator on to the J tip 0.18″ × 45 cm PTFE-coated Spring-Wire Guide and make a skin incision with a sharp surgical blade. Advance the dilator half way (~2.5 cm or 1″) over the wire using a rotating motion. Usually there is no need to advance the tissue dilator the entire length since the platysma is relatively superficial and the only point of resistance for catheter advancement (→ 9).

- Remove the dilator and advance the two-lumen indwelling (4 F × 5 cm × 2 lumen) polyurethane catheter (item e on Figure 2.33) over the wire. No resistance should be encountered at this point. If resistance is found as the catheter is advanced, mount the dilator once more and repeat the previous step (→ 9)

- Secure the catheter (tape or suture) and apply sterile dressing (Tegaderm™)

Troubleshooting (see arrows/numbers in preceding text)

1. In premature and newborn patients we do not use the U/S real-time identification and cannulation of the internal jugular vein (IJV), since often, this requires a second sterile operator.

2. In our experience, the location of the IJV is inconsistently found precisely at the line A–B and is more frequently found medially and superficial to the carotid artery (CA).

3. In dehydrated patients, it is common not to observe a "back flush" due to low central venous pressure; often the 1-ml syringe is attached to the 24G ¾″ JELCO® after the introducer needle is removed and gentle aspiration is applied.

4. Apply gentle rotation pressure to the Spring-Wire Guide.

5. Ask a second operator to apply gentle sub-diaphragmatic pressure to increase central venous pressure. Consider giving a bolus of IV crystalloids 10–20 ml/kg.

6. Mount the 25 G 5/8″ needle on to a 1-ml syringe and identify the IJV by observing a "back flush." This technique minimizes the incidence of local hematoma formation even in the case of carotid artery puncture.

7. In premature and newborn patients with low systemic blood pressure and cyanosis we often attach a transducer to the 22 G 1″ JELCO®, if there is a question regarding possible carotid artery cannulation.

8. The 24 G ¾″ JELCO® can accommodate the 0.18″ wire guide of the 4 Fr Double-Lumen Venous Catheter Set produced by COOK® (Bloomington, IN, USA).

9. Particular attention should be paid not to bend or damage the J tip 0.18″ × 45 cm PTFE-coated Spring-Wire Guide.

Acknowledgment

This technique has been designed and modified by the Division of Cardiac Anesthesia, Department of Anesthesiology, Perioperative and Pain Medicine, Children's Hospital Boston and Harvard Medical School.

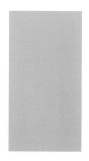

Intraosseous access

Andrea Zimmermann and Georg Hansmann

Indication

In emergency situations, when administering drugs, fluids, blood, and blood products, intraosseous (IO) access is indicated when attempts at obtaining peripheral or central venous access (e.g., UVC, femoral vein catheter) have failed (Figure 2.34). Intraosseous access has been successfully used during pediatric critical care transport[84], in intensive care units, and in emergency departments[85]. A recent retrospective study of pediatric critical care transport showed that IO access was performed in 2.6% of 1792 children with a first-attempt success rate of 78%[84]. However, in this study, only 23 patients were <1 year old. The first-attempt success rate in these infants was lower (74%)[84], indicating not only a need for further training but also an unjustified hesitation to place IO needles in infants and neonates.

- IO access can be established in all age groups (i.e., from newborns to adults).
- IO access can often be achieved in 30–60 seconds.
- The IO route of administration is preferred to the ET route.
- Any drug or fluid that is administered IV can be given IO (*PALS Manual*, 2006)[8].

Equipment

- Intraosseous (IO) needle (18 G, e.g., Cook™ "Standard Tip Design" or "Dieckmann modification model" with two sideholes at the tip of the IO needle). IO needles work by a careful-push-no-thread technique. You may use 16 G IO needles in newborns >3.5 kg body weight and older infants (no data). As an alternative to IO needles, you may use a disposable iliac bone marrow aspiration needle (18 G). Use 18 G IO needles in preterm babies.
- Skin disinfectant (e.g., povidone-iodine)
- Sterile drape with hole or sterile towels
- Sterile gloves, 4 × 4 sterile gauze pads, tape
- A 20- to 30-ml syringe attached to stopcock and tubing, filled with normal saline flush (20 ml)
- A 10-ml syringe for bone marrow aspiration (optional; not recommended by some experts)
- Local anesthetic (e.g., lidocaine 1%), 2- or 3-ml syringe, needle – optional
- **If no IO needle is available in an emergency situation**, a large butterfly needle (16–19 G) or a short 18–20 G lumbar puncture needle with a stylet may be used[85]

Neonatal Emergencies: A Practical Guide for Resuscitation, Transport and Critical Care, ed. Georg Hansmann.
Published by Cambridge University Press. © Cambridge University Press 2009.

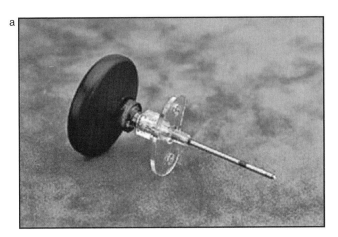

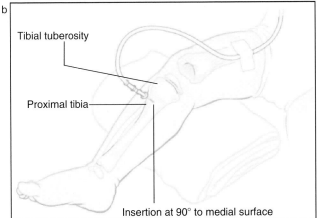

Tibial tuberosity

Proximal tibia

Insertion at 90° to medial surface

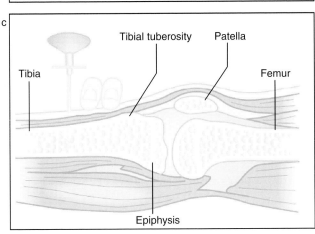

Tibial tuberosity   Patella

Tibia   Femur

Epiphysis

Figure 2.34 Intraosseous access. **a** Diekmann cannula. **b** Puncture technique: insertion site is the proximal tibia approx. 1–2 cm below the tibial tuberosity in the middle of the antero-medial aspect of the proximal tibia. Place a pillow or towel underneath the knee for support. Hold the calf/ankle with your left thumb, index, and middle finger. Work under sterile conditions. Look for puncture site and insert the needle perpendicular (approx. 90 degrees) to the bone using little pressure until loss of resistance is felt (if the needle has a thread, turn it counter clockwise); then remove the stylet and connect to tubing/syringe filled with normal saline. Local anesthesia is appropriate for a conscious patient. **c** Intraosseous needle placed in the proximal tibia – landmarks and vascular structures. Intraosseous cannulation provides access to a non-collapsible marrow venous complex, which serves as a rapid route for administration of drugs and fluids. The technique is based on the use of a rigid needle, preferably a specially designed intraosseous access needle (with stylet) or bone marrow puncture needle.

Technique (IO access, proximal tibia)[85]

- Place a towel, sandbag or IV bag behind the knee for support.
- Restrain the lower leg (assistant); sterile precautions if possible.
- Clean the area with povidone-iodine or an alternative disinfectant solution (drape optional)
- Hold the IO access device properly: grip the needle with the thumb and index finger approx. 1 cm proximal to the tip (1 cm is the approximate distance you have to advance the needle).
- Position the needle at the proximal tibia below the medial knee joint space, approx. 1–2 cm below the tibial tuberosity in the middle of the anteromedial surface of the tibia (or use the following rule of thumb: the distance from the medial joint space is approximately the width of the patient's hand).
- Insert the needle perpendicular (90°) to the bone, always away from the epiphyseal plate and joint cavity, perhaps with twisting motions (caution: some models have a thread and have to be advanced with a clockwise rotation motion).
- Carefully advance the needle (perhaps with twisting motions) by exerting moderate pressure along the axis of the needle with one's palm: usually no more than 1 cm is necessary.
- Moderate pressure along the axis of the needle is exerted by one's palm.
- A sudden decrease in "resistance" indicates entrance into the bone marrow space.
- Remove the stylet and connect to a syringe/tubing immediately.
- The needle should stand on its own if properly positioned, but should be fixed with tape to the skin and secured with supporting dressing (4 × 4 gauze, tape).
- If indicated and it is not an emergency situation: aspirate bone marrow at this point (culture, blood chemistry, blood gas, hemoglobin/hematocrit). Most experts argue that with bone marrow aspiration, IO needles (particularly 18 G and 20 G) tend to clot rapidly and therefore *aspiration of bone marrow should be avoided in any emergency situation.*
- Inject at least 20 ml normal saline slowly via the IO needle. You should not feel any resistance or observe any calf edema/local tissue swelling.
- Hypertonic or alkaline solutions (e.g., sodium bicarbonate) should be diluted 1:1 or 1:2 with normal saline.
- Use the IO needle for the shortest time possible: aim for <2 h and ≪24 h.
- Consider antibiotic coverage including *Staphylococcus aureus*, particularly if sterile precautions were limited/insufficient.

Alternative IO technique in preterm infants

A butterfly needle (18 G) was successfully used as tibial IO access in an edematous preterm infant of 25 weeks' gestation[86]. However, there are no safety data on the use of these lines in preterm infants.

Alternative sites of IO access

- Distal femur: approx. 1 cm above the patella in the midline
- Medial or lateral malleolus: approx. 1 cm superior to the malleolus in the midline. The medial malleolus is generally easier to penetrate than the lateral malleolus
- Iliac crest

Complications (IO access)

Overall, there is a low complication rate when used short term ($\ll 24\,h$; aim for $<2\,h$). The benefit in emergency situations outweighs the risks by far. Case reports/series describe:

- Fat or air embolism (always connect the IO needle immediately to NS prefilled tubing/syringe[87]
- Subperiosteal or soft tissue extravasation
- Compartment syndrome (high risk: incomplete penetration of the IO needle into cortex leading to fluid extravasation, IO infusion into a fractured limb or perforation of the bone with IO needle)
- Local cellulitis/abscess formation
- Osteomyelitis ($<1\%$, associated with hypertonic solutions, e.g., D50W or drug infusion)[85]
- Sepsis
- Abnormal bone growth (do X-ray to rule out fracture when patient is stable)
- Fractures (tibia) – extremely rare

Alternative access: ultrasound-guided peripheral venous access

For centers with sufficient expertise, this can be an alternative for emergency situations in which any access, but not necessarily central venous access, is needed (e.g., emergency rehydration).

Alternative access: central IV line (other than UVC or IO needle)

Ultrasound-guided central venous access (e.g., femoral vein, internal jugular vein, subclavian vein)[88,89]. More and more physicians apply this technique in pediatric emergency departments[90] and intensive care units[88,89]. It is especially useful in older neonates and young infants, when UVC is not feasible, or if long-term central venous access is required (see pp. 112–16).

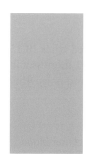

Cord clamping

Georg Hansmann

Cord clamping is part of the third stage of labor, i.e., the time between delivery of the infant and delivery of the placenta, and is usually achieved by applying two clamps. The cord is cut between the clamps thereby avoiding blood loss in either the infant or the mother through the placenta.

The optimal timing of cord clamping has been a controversial issue for decades; there are no formal practice guidelines. In developing countries, there is a trend toward delayed cord clamping (with a resulting increase in blood and iron received by the infant at birth) to counter the higher incidence of anemia during infancy in these countries. In the western hemisphere, the umbilical cord tends to be clamped soon after birth. There is huge variability between centers worldwide.

Before the clamps are applied, the infant can be placed on the mother's abdomen (above the level of the placenta), between the mother's thighs (at the level of the placenta) or held below the level of the placenta. Blood flow from the placenta to the infant will depend on which position is used, but there are no clear data suggesting an optimal position for infants in the first few minutes of life. Some birth attendants also "milk" the cord towards the infant before clamping, as it contains up to 20 ml of placental blood, although there is no consensus on whether this useful.

Technique of cord clamping

The most common way of cord clamping is a prophylactic disconnection with Péan clamps (umbilical cord length: 10–15 cm) and subsequent definitive clamping with a disposable plastic clamp approx. 3(−6) cm from the umbilicus. Cut with a sterile pair of scissors; while doing so, consider the possibility of taking a sterile umbilical smear (see pp. 129–30) and maybe also the necessity of placing an umbilical vessel catheter (then the stump should be at least 6 cm long).

The controversy in cord clamping

It has been estimated that, for a vaginally born full-term infant, delaying cord clamping by 2–3 min results in an increase in neonatal blood volume of approx. 20–30 ml/kg body weight (cesarean delivery has the same effect but to a lesser extent). This equals one-quarter to one-third of the newborn's intravascular volume! Delayed cord clamping may lead to neonatal hypertransfusion, a rise in hemoglobin from 16 g/dl (intrauterine) up to 24 g/dl (caution: polycythemia, p. 128), and subsequently to neonatal hyperviscosity, volume overload, tachypnea, and hyperbilirubinemia. A recent meta-analysis, however, advocates delaying cord clamping for a minimum of 2 minutes in (otherwise stable) full-term

Neonatal Emergencies: A Practical Guide for Resuscitation, Transport and Critical Care, ed. Georg Hansmann.
Published by Cambridge University Press. © Cambridge University Press 2009.

neonates[90]. This conclusion is based on the authors' analysis of 15 controlled trials (8/15 randomized) that showed a significantly lower incidence of anemia at age 2–3 months and an insignificant difference in the incidence of transient tachypnea, jaundice, and polycythemia in term infants with delayed cord clamping.

In cord clamping, placento–neonatal over-transfusion, as well as neonatal–placental blood loss can be prevented to a large extent if certain standards are followed (see below). Randomized controlled trials with sample sizes that are adequately powered for beneficial and potential adverse effects are needed before the practice of delayed clamping for term or preterm infants can be strongly endorsed.

Recommendations for cord clamping

- In the event of fetal distress, meconium-stained amniotic fluid, and/or neonatal depression, immediate resuscitation should take priority over placental transfusion; immediate clamping of the cord may be necessary so the infant can be resuscitated.
- After vaginal delivery of a vigorous term neonate (no hypoxia, first arterial pH and fetal scalp blood sampling pH >7.20), the baby should be laid on the mother and dried; cord clamping may be done approximately at the end of the pulsation of the cord, which is about 1 min after birth ("*moderate delay in cord clamping*") without previous "milking" of the cord. If the birth took place in a sitting or squatting position, the cord may be clamped earlier (30 s). However, others recommend longer delay in cord clamping (approx. 2 min, see below) and holding the baby approximately 20–30 cm below the introitus to allow gravity to aid the transfusion.
- Full-term, low-risk infants (no hypoxia, first arterial pH and fetal scalp blood sampling pH >7.20), especially those born in developing countries with limited postnatal follow-up (e.g., iron supplementation/sufficient nutrition), might benefit from delaying cord clamping for a minimum of 2 min[91]. The optimal position of the newborn remains unclear
- In preterm newborn infants (<37 weeks of gestation), delaying cord clamping by 30–120 seconds, rather than early clamping, seems to be associated with less need for transfusion and less intraventricular hemorrhage (Cochrane meta-analysis, 2004)[92].
- Cord clamping of a non-hypoxic neonate born by C-section should take place after milking the cord (exceptions below). Many obstetricians, however, do not milk the umbilical cord after C-sections as it is unclear whether the additional 20 ml of blood passes to the newborn.
- In chronic placental insufficiency (leading to intrauterine growth retardation and a small-for-gestational age infant), diabetic fetopathy or post term delivery (>42 weeks of gestation), the hematocrit is usually already elevated in utero, such that early cord clamping (without milking the cord after C-sections) is preferred.
- A fetal nuchal cord or an entangled cord should, if possible, be loosened immediately. Cord blood should then be re-transfused quickly by milking the cord if the baby does not need immediate resuscitation.
- If hypovolemia is suspected, e.g., loss of placental integrity/bleeding (abruption placentae, placenta previa, traumatic amniocentesis), twin – twin transfusion syndrome, the obstetrician may briefly milk but then clamp the cord immediately (early cord clamping) followed by neonatal resuscitation.

- After the birth of acidotic (e.g., FBS pH <7.2) or hypoxic babies (abnormal cardiotocogram (CTG)), cord clamping must be performed immediately after birth, so that the depressed newborn can be transferred to the resuscitation unit for treatment. These neonates – even if bleeding has not occurred – frequently have hypovolemia due to a volume shift towards the placenta (caused by vasoconstriction).

The management of neonatal polycythemia is described in the next chapter (p. 128).

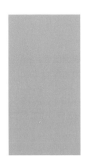

Management of high-risk infants in the delivery room

Georg Hansmann

Diagnostics in the delivery room

The pulse oximetry transducer (for S_aO_2 and HR monitoring) is secured with elastic tape by the second or third assistant, preferably on the neonate's right hand, after suctioning and drying (i.e., within first minute of life). Pulse oximetry is used for monitoring during neonatal resuscitation and transport (see pp. 131–2). S_pO_2 and blood pressure values obtained from the right arm and leg may provide information on right-to-left (ductal) shunting and outflow tract obstructions (e.g., coarctation of the aorta, interrupted aortic arch); the latter are rarely immediately evident in the delivery room since a large patent ductus arteriosus is common and may "bridge" outflow tract obstruction in these lesions. Capillary or venous blood gas analysis and blood glucose sticks (quick test with test strips) should be performed for all initially depressed neonates with metabolic acidosis (umbilical arterial pH <7.15), for preterm infants and for growth-restricted term infants. An arterial blood gas analysis is the gold standard for assessment of oxygenation and ventilation of the newborn. For the transport team (NETS), it is advisable to obtain and document these measurements (i.e., capillary or venous blood gas plus blood glucose), even in well-adapted neonates with a normal umbilical artery pH, approximately 30 min after birth or prior to transport (for legal reasons). If the newborn infant is depressed, blood gas sampling must be done earlier and should be repeated while the neonate's condition remains critical.

> *!* In extreme acrocyanosis (decreased peripheral perfusion), capillary blood gas analyses and pulse oximetry are unreliable. Venous (VBG) or arterial blood gas (AGB) sampling is required. An arterial blood gas analysis is the gold standard for assessment of oxygenation and ventilation of the newborn.

Differential diagnosis: delayed respiratory transition versus cyanotic heart disease

Transient tachypnea of the newborn (TTN; syn.: wet lung, retained fetal lung fluid) is a benign disease in term, near-term or large premature infants who have respiratory distress after delivery that usually resolves after 1–3 days. Delayed resorption of lung fluid and pulmonary immaturity are involved in the pathophysiology of TTN/delayed postnatal adaptation.

If a term/near-term or preterm newborn infant requires supplemental oxygen for more than 30 min after birth in order to maintain S_aO_2 levels ≥90% (pulse oximetry), hypoxemia is frequently due to delayed pulmonary adaptation (differential diagnosis (DDx): TTN, infection, primary surfactant deficiency due to immaturity) leading to respiratory distress

Neonatal Emergencies: A Practical Guide for Resuscitation, Transport and Critical Care, ed. Georg Hansmann.
Published by Cambridge University Press. © Cambridge University Press 2009.

(nasal flaring, rib retraction, tachypnea). However, if the S_aO_2 is reliably (i.e., good S_pO_2 tracing) lower than 85% in room air $\approx$30 min after delivery and does not increase by 5–10 percentage points despite oxygen supplementation (100%, 5–10 l/min), *cyanotic congenital heart disease* should be considered as an important DDx (DDx: *diffusion impairment in severe lung disease/sepsis* may also be associated with lack of a significant O_2 response).

> **!** Some experts recommend routine postductal S_pO_2 screening at 12–48 h of life (before discharge).
> Absence of a heart murmur does not exclude congenital heart disease

Central versus peripheral cyanosis

Obtain arterial PO_2 (P_aO_2) from the right half of the upper body, i.e., preductal P_aO_2 (e.g., right radial artery). In well-adapted term neonates, P_aO_2 should be $\geq$60 mmHg approx. 30 min after birth; if not, work up hypoxemia and *central cyanosis* (i.e., lips, tongue) (etiology: central nervous system, pulmonary, cardiac). *Peripheral cyanosis* (etiology: hypothermia, hypovolemia, shock) presents as bluish skin color in the limbs (acrocyanosis) with normal P_aO_2 ($>$60 mmHg) and S_aO_2 ($\approx S_pO_2$ $>$92%).

Cyanosis depends on the newborn's hemoglobin level

Cyanosis is clinically evident when 3–5 g/dl hemoglobin is desaturated (central cyanosis visible at oral soft tissue, e.g., tip of the tongue). This also means that neonates, who usually have a high hematocrit (Hct $>$55%; Hb $\geq$19 g/dl) and/or moderate peripheral hypoperfusion, may show signs of cyanosis in spite of an S_aO_2 of 90% (pulsoximetry is unreliable in significant peripheral hypoperfusion). On the other hand, anemic neonates (e.g., placental bleeding) or young infants with physiological anemia (Hb $\approx$11 g/dl at 3 months of age) may be pale rather than bluish (desaturated Hb $<$3 g/dl), even when cyanotic heart disease is the cause of hypoxemia (i.e., low P_aO_2).

Right-to-left shunts

So-called *differential cyanosis* is the result of significant right-to-left ductal shunting (pulmonary artery $\rightarrow$ descending aorta): the upper half of the body appears rosy while the lower part of the body is bluish. This may occur in persistent pulmonary hypertension of the newborn (PPHN with predominant right-to-left ductal shunting, or extreme left heart obstruction (aortic valve stenosis, coarctation of the aorta, interrupted aortic arch) with significant ductal right-to-left shunting. If a low P_aO_2 is obtained from the UAC or from the lower extremity, another sample from the upper body should be obtained and compared with a simultaneously drawn arterial sample from the lower part of the body to clarify the presence or absence of a right-to-left ductal shunt (perform Echo). Even when "differential cyanosis" is not present, a P_aO_2 difference of 10–15 mmHg between the upper-right (e.g., right radial artery) and lower body (e.g., UAC) is significant[16].

> **!** A preductal and postductal S_aO_2 or S_pO_2 of 90% does not completely rule out cyanotic heart disease, because the oxygen – hemoglobin dissociation curve is shifted to the left compared to that for adults. Hence, in newborns, an S_aO_2 of 90% can still be attained at a P_aO_2 of 45–55 mmHg, and an S_aO_2 of 50% is achieved with a P_aO_2 of 22 mmHg, the so-called P_{50}.[16]

> **!** Any significant S_pO_2 difference ($\approx$8–10 percentage points more than 30 min after birth), blood pressure or pulse difference between upper right and lower extremities, or between right arm (or right ear lobe if aberrant right subclavian artery present) and left arm evaluated by *urgent echocardiography* (e.g., coarctation of the aorta, interrupted aortic arch) must be further.

Hyperoxia test

Remarks

This test seems a bit outdated compared with modern-day imaging techniques (echocardiography), and carries underappreciated risks for the newborn infant, especially for those born preterm. However, if echocardiography is not readily available, and (gross) diagnosis of underlying congenital heart disease has an impact on further management and transport (e.g., admitting hospital), the hyperoxia test may still be useful (caution: oxygen toxicity, especially in preterm newborn infants).

Def.

If a 10- to 15-min exposure to supplemental oxygen (oxygen hood preferred: 100%, flow 5–10 l/min) leads to a rise in P_aO_2 by more than 10–30 mmHg *and* above 100–50 mmHg, then the cyanosis is most likely of respiratory (or central nervous) origin (caution: exceptions in heart disease with increased pulmonary blood flow or severe lung disease with large intrapulmonary right-to-left shunts; see box below).

If the oxygenation is abnormal in room air (approx. 30 min postnatally: S_pO_2 <85%; capillary PO_2 <40 mmHg, P_aO_2 <50 mmHg in term neonates), and does not improve with the hyperoxia test (i.e., pulse oximeter on the right hand $\rightarrow$ rise in S_aO_2 or S_aO_2 is less than 8 percentage points, or a rise in P_aO_2 obtained in the right temporal artery or radial artery is less than 10–30 mmHg) then *cyanotic heart disease* must be suspected – especially when the P_aO_2 is <35 mmHg during and after hyperoxia.

If duct-dependent (cyanotic or acyantotic) heart disease is suspected, *prostaglandin E$_1$ (PGE$_1$, alprostadil) infusion* should be initiated in the delivery room and continued throughout transport until the exact diagnosis is made by echocardiography (or additional imaging). If echocardiography is readily available ("in house"), then the hyperoxia test may be omitted, and a stable neonate may be started on PGE$_1$ infusion after the echocardiogram justifies this approach.

Unreliability of the hyperoxia test

Decreased peripheral perfusion and obtaining ABG samples from the left upper (occasionally postductal) or lower part of the body (left-to-right ductal shunt $\rightarrow$ low postductal P_aO_2) make the hyperoxia test unreliable. In all cases, echocardiography is far more accurate and superior to the hyperoxia test.

> **!** In cyanotic heart disease with increased pulmonary blood flow (e.g., TAC, TAPVR), P_aO_2 levels may exceed 60 mmHg (S_pO_2 then $\geq$90%) and increase with supplemental oxygen above 100 mmHg. In contrast, the hyperoxia test may not lead to a significant increase of P_aO_2 above 100 mmHg in severe lung disease with large intrapulmonary right-to-left shunts but normal cardiac anatomy[16].

Risks of the hyperoxia test

- Constriction of ductus arteriosus (caution in duct-dependent congenital heart disease)
- Pulmonary perfusion increases and systemic perfusion decreases (Qp:Qs $\gg$1) → **caution**: Shock possible, especially in defects with duct-dependent systemic perfusion, e.g., hypoplastic left heart
- For details about risks of default oxygen supplementation in preterm and term born infants; see p. 70, and chapter on critical cardiovascular disease (pp. 340–79)

More diagnostic criteria

The *hematocrit* (Hct) level is an important indicator of intravascular blood volume, especially when placental separation/bleeding is suspected, or when vacuum/forceps extraction has led to considerable cephalhematoma (determine Hct prior to volume bolus). Caution: acute bleeding initially may not affect Hct.

The *body temperature*, which is measured before the newborn leaves the delivery room (or earlier when delivery room care is prolonged), is an important criterion for the quality of resuscitation and the outcome for the neonate (avoid hyperthermia and hypopthermia). Adjust the temperature within the transport incubator to compensate for the current body temperature of the newborn (Figure 2.10). If the incubator has to be opened frequently, then set the temperature at the higher end of the recommended range.

> **!** If you don't take a temperature, you can't find a fever.[93]

Standard values for healthy, term newborn infants in the delivery room

- Body temperature: 36.5–37.5°C
- Heart rate: 110–170 bpm
- *Capillary blood gas approx. 30 min postnatal*:
  - PCO_2: 35–45 ($\pm$5) mmHg
  - PO_2: $\geq$40 mmHg
  - pH value: >7.30
- S_aO_2 measured by pulse oximetry (S_pO_2): 90%–96%
- Blood pressure: MAP (in mmHg) > GA (in weeks) (see Figure 5.3, appendix)
- Hct: 45%–60% ($\pm$10%)
- Hemoglobin: 14–20 g/dl
- Blood glucose (range not evidence-based)
  - 0–24 h after birth >40 mg/dl
  - More than 24 h after birth >45 mg/dl

Management of problems associated with abnormal laboratory values

> **!** A Hct of 70% is an indication for partial exchange transfusion/hemodilution.

Neonatal polycythemia

- Polycythemia (defined as Hct >65% by peripheral venous stick) occurs in 1%–4% of newborn infants, many of whom are asymptomatic.
- Polycythemia is rare in preterm infants <34 weeks of gestation, but very common in newborns of diabetic mothers (20%–30%) and SGA infants (placental insufficiency). Other causes of polycythemia are congenital adrenal hyperplasia (CAH), neonatal thyrotoxicosis, Beckwith–Wiedemann syndrome (EMG: exomphalos, macroglossia, gigantism), and chromosomal abnormalities (e.g., trisomy 13, 18, 21). Hct peaks at 2–3 h after birth. Late polycythemia (>48 h postnatally) may be a sign of dehydration.
- In blood obtained by heelstick, the Hct may be falsely elevated.
- Possible signs of neonatal polycythemia include respiratory distress/tachypnea, apnea, lethargy, irritability, jitteriness, seizures, hypoglycemia, poor feeding/vomiting, and cyanosis.
- Partial exchange transfusion/hemodilution is indicated in symptomatic newborns with central Hct >65%, and asymptomatic newborns with central Hct >70%. Whether treatment of this self-limiting problem justifies central venous catheter insertion underlies an ongoing debate (two large PIV, i.e. 22 G, may be sufficient for hemodilution). See also chapter on twin – twin transfusion syndrome, p. 240.

Partial exchange transfusion (hemodilution) in neonatal polycythemia in the NICU

Volume to be exchanged =
(patient's blood volume in ml) × [(Hct of patient – desired Hct) ÷ Hct of patient]
Blood volume is 80–85 ml/kg in term infants, and 90–100 ml/kg in preterm infants. Postnatal blood volume also depends on the delay in cord clamping. Desired Hct is usually 50%–55%.
Procedure: Sterile precautions. Use bubble-free, properly located UVC (exclude hepatic position by X-ray) or large 22 G PIV to remove blood in 10- to 20-ml aliquots from the circulation, and replace the same volume (1:1, i.e., 10 ml blood out, 10 ml NS in) with normal saline via a PIV.

Hypoglycemia (see also Hypoglycemia, p. 260)

! Most Dextrostix (D-stix) devices are not designed for neonatal use and are especially inaccurate for blood glucose levels below 45 mg/dl.

! Many portable dextrostix devices measure blood glucose at levels that are higher (by up to 15 mg/dl) than commonly used advanced glucose or combined blood gas-electrolyte-blood glucose apparatus.

! There is ongoing glycolysis in blood samples sent to the laboratory in serum and plasma tubes, causing falsely low glucose results. Therefore, always use appropriate tubes (e.g., sodium fluoride) instead.

Blood glucose <45 mg/dl prior to transport

For transport teams (NETS), the following procedure has been established for term/preterm infants with blood glucose levels <45 mg/dl (<50 mg/dl when >24 h of life) prior to transport (based on experience; no evidence-based data available):

- Give $D_{10}W$ 1–2 ml/kg slow push IV (if symptomatic $D_{10}W$ 3–5 ml/kg slow push IV).
- Check blood glucose once more; during transport give double the usual maintenance rate (i.e., start in this scenario $D_{10}W$ at 6 ml/kg/h IV = 10 mg/kg/min. IV).
- The latter approach (i.e., start off $D_{10}W$ at 6 ml/kg/h IV = 10 mg/kg/min. IV) is also valid for large-for-gestational-age (LGA) neonates s/p (gestational) maternal diabetes!.
- After arrival (or during long transport), titrate IV glucose to $D_{10}W$ 3–6 ml/kg/h IV to maintain blood glucose within the recommended range of 50–120 mg/dl (for older neonates and infants aim for 70–120 mg/dl).

Blood glucose borderline (40–50 mg/dl) and neonate asymptomatic

Dextrostix values in the low–normal/borderline range (40–50 mg/dl) should be confirmed with a separate dextrostix (there is often a different model in the nursery) or even a laboratory glucose measurement, in order to decide whether the neonate may remain in the birth clinic.

For low – normal blood glucose values in asymptomatic newborns without respiratory distress:

- Early feeding with formula. Check D-stix 30–60 min after feeding (goal >60 mg/dl). If the second glucose reading is 40 mg/dl or newborn is symptomatic, start $D_{10}W$ IV (bolus plus infusion), check glucose in the laboratory, and transport/admit patient
- Order dextrostix checks at 1, 3, 6, 12 and 24 hours after birth for all borderline glucose values, for infants of mothers with gestational diabetes, with type 1 or type 2 diabetes, and for all LGA infants
- If the second glucose reading is >40 mg/dl (goal >60 mg/dl) and the patient is asymptomatic, the newborn may stay with the mother in the birth clinic if early pediatric follow-up is available (see p. 260)

! Blood gas, blood glucose, body temperature, and total transport/treatment time must be well documented.

Suspect infection if premature rupture of the membranes (PROM) is evident (def.: ROM ≥18 h before delivery) and the following signs are present:

- Green–yellow, foul-smelling or even meconium-stained amniotic fluid,
- Maternal signs of infection (CRP >2 mg/dl, WBC >17 000/µl, temperature >38.0°C)
- Positive group B streptococci (GBS) smear
- Fetal tachycardia (>160 bpm), body weight below the 10th percentile or clinical signs of infection of the neonate (pale-grey-marbleized skin color, tachydyspnea, rash/petechiae)
  - If the neonate is stable, smears from the pharynx, ears, and nose or perhaps from the umbilical cord (immediately after birth) may be taken for bacterial or viral culture (many NICU no longer do this routinely)
  - Obtain aerobic blood culture under sterile conditions: blood can be withdrawn while placing a PIV catheter. Rather than using a 3-ml syringe with tubing (vein may collapse), let the blood drop into a 2- or 3-ml syringe (assistant removes the syringe's plunger and applies a sterile plug at the distal end of the syringe). Subsequently the blood should be transferred into a (prewarmed) blood culture bottle using a sterile needle

Afterwards, blood gas (VBG, capillary or arterial if indicated) and glucose samples as well as standard serum tubes (chemistry, CRP, IL-6/-8, perhaps HIV and hepatitis serology, electrolytes 6 hours afterwards, bilirubin, etc.) and one to two EDTA tubes (CBC, blood type and screen) are filled with blood. If the peripheral venous catheter has no blood return, then NETS may defer the blood draw to the admitting team, but obtain blood gas analysis and determine blood glucose concentration.

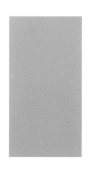

Monitoring in the delivery room and during neonatal transport

Georg Hansmann

> **!** Pulse oximetry (S_pO_2, HR) is part of standard monitoring in the delivery room and during transport.

Heart rate (HR)

Measurement of the HR (at the umbilical cord, by auscultation, by pulse oximetry or ECG) is the most objective indicator of: (1) the newborn's clinical condition, (2) the need for PPV (HR <100 bpm) or chest compressions (HR <60 bpm), and (3) a good response to one's resuscitation efforts (e.g., rise in HR after successful mask-PPV or endotracheal intubation plus PPV). The HR should correlate with the pulse palpated (brachial or femoral artery).

Pulse oximetry (S_pO_2, HR)

An analysis of six studies aimed at estimating the "normal S_pO_2 in newborn infants in the first minutes of life"[30] revealed that in term and near-term infants a (pre- or postductal) S_pO_2 of 90% was reached at about 5 minutes of life. The S_pO_2 at 1 min of life ranged from 40% to 70%. S_pO_2 was generally lower in preterm infants and in those delivered by cesarean section. Postductal S_pO_2 (feet) was 7–10 percentage points lower than preductal S_pO_2[30].

Heart rate and S_pO_2 tracings are more easily picked up when the transducer is placed at the hands rather than the feet (perfusion more often impaired in the feet). If the neonate shows no early signs of dyspnea (nasal flaring, retractions at about 5–15 min postnatally) and no longer needs supplemental oxygen, then the baby should be wrapped up warmly and laid on the mother's chest (if necessary, monitored with a pulse oximeter). The 10-min Apgar score and a 30-min postnatal blood glucose and blood gas analysis can be obtained thereafter.

> **!** Obviously, there is the future need for immediate and continuous monitoring of oxygen saturation and heart rate via pulse oximetry in the delivery room, and the need to vary inspired oxygen concentrations based on the individual status of newborn infants (i.e., tailored oxygen resuscitation)[4]. When providing additional oxygen, health care providers should keep in mind that oxygen saturation, if kept above 92%, is not reliable at detecting hyperoxia[36]. According to a worldwide survey from 2004, 20 of 40 centers still use 100% oxygen for the resuscitation of all babies at delivery, whereas the remaining centers have already changed their standards and use lower oxygen concentrations[41].

Neonatal Emergencies: A Practical Guide for Resuscitation, Transport and Critical Care, ed. Georg Hansmann.
Published by Cambridge University Press. © Cambridge University Press 2009.

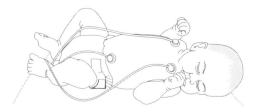

Figure 2.35 Attachment of ECG electrodes for ECG monitoring.

> ❗ We usually start neonatal resuscitation in the delivery room with room air (for exceptions[4,7] see *pp. 70–71*
>
> ❗ For S_pO_2 >85% in preterm and S_pO_2 >90% in term newborn infants, we usually *do not* recommend additional oxygen supplementation in the delivery room (i.e., use room air).

Blood pressure (BP)

When hemodynamic depression (capillary refill >2 s, pale-grayish skin color, weak or absent pulses, volume bolus required) or immaturity/dystrophy is present, *blood pressure* should be taken at regular intervals using a cuff (NIBP) of appropriate size (size 2–3; size 1 for infants <1000 g). Alternatively, the UA (or radial artery) catheter can be connected to a transducer and then calibrated to enable continuous arterial BP monitoring (frequently done in the NICU rather than the delivery room). If a pulse difference is observed between the upper and lower extremities (e.g., coarctation of the aorta/interrupted aortic arch), the blood pressure must be obtained from more than one extremity (right arm/leg; better: all four extremities). See also Figure 5.3, appendix.

Electrocardiogram (ECG)

Three standard leads (Figure 2.35). In VLBW preterm infant (<1500 g), ECG electrodes designed for preterm infants should be used (fragile, vulnerable skin). Continuous ECG monitoring is absolutely indicated in cases of prenatally diagnosed heart disease, pre- or postnatal cardiac arrhythmia, and during and after administration of drugs affecting the cardiovascular system (adenosine, epinephrine, atropine, calcium, or the like) and after resuscitation.

> ❗ Pulse oximeters (S_pO_2, HR), disposable colorimetric CO_2 detectors, cardiac monitors (BP, HR, ECG, RR), oxygen blenders, and pressure manometers (PIP and PEEP control) should be standard equipment in the delivery room[4]. These devices are valuable tools to assess the neonate's clinical condition, resuscitation efficiency, and the immediate need for IV drugs (epinephrine) or fluids (normal saline, packed red blood cells).
>
> ❗ Blood gas, glucose, and hematocrit analysis must be readily available in the delivery room.

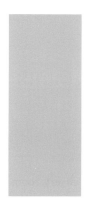

Hygiene in the delivery room and during neonatal transport (infection control)

Andrea Zimmermann

Resuscitation of neonates

- Wear gloves (not sterile) for your own protection
- Disinfect your hands thoroughly, in case neonates are held without gloves, e.g., to be transferred[94–96]
- Wear a mask (attending physician) in case of cold symptoms or Herpes simplex infection[97] (some NICU recommend staff not to work if these symptoms are present)
- It is recommended to wear a gown for your own protection. The gown does not have to be sterile[98]
- Before placing catheters and needles, the skin should be thoroughly disinfected with the proper disinfectant. For placing central lines, you should follow sterile precautions (head, mask, sterile gown, sterile gloves, sterile drape covering the field involved)
- Using alcohol-based solutions on the vulnerable skin of a very small preterm infant can lead to toxic dermatitis. Therefore, 2% 2-phenoxyethanol and 0.1% octenidine, a soft tissue disinfectant, can be used even though they are not approved for such use[12]. Be sure you give this soft tissue disinfectant at least 2 minutes of skin contact time before any further manipulation in the sterile field! Some institutions use chlorhexidine
- Keep everything sterile while connecting infusion tubing and injecting drugs, even if it is an emergency

Cleansing/disinfection

- Areas which have been close to or in contact with newborn patients, such as cables, tubes, and stethoscopes, as well as the transport incubator, must be cleansed with detergents after resuscitation and transport. The use of surface disinfectants is required if the patient is likely to have, or possibly has, an infection[99]
- The operating surfaces of the apparatus used on the transport incubator must be cleansed with detergents on a daily basis
- Bag-and-mask systems should be disinfected (thermally) after each use
- Blades should be sterilized or disinfected (thermally) after each use

> **!** Each hospital must establish its own infection control/standard precautions protocols.

Neonatal Emergencies: A Practical Guide for Resuscitation, Transport and Critical Care, ed. Georg Hansmann.
Published by Cambridge University Press. © Cambridge University Press 2009.

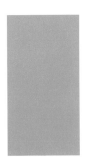

When to call a pediatrician to the delivery room

Georg Hansmann

The following is not an exclusive list of when to call a pediatrician to the delivery room. Consider additional antepartum and intrapartum risk factors (not listed here) associated with the need for neonatal resuscitation as indication for pediatric attendance at delivery[9].

Fetal emergencies and risk factors
- Meconium-stained amniotic fluid (MSAF)
- Cardiotocogram (CTG) shows:
  - Persistent late decelerations (Dip 2)
  - Severe variable decelerations
  - Persistent tachycardia or bradycardia
- Fetal scalp blood sampling with pH <7.20
- Umbilical cord hernia/prolapse
- Signs of placental separation/bleeding

Operative deliveries
- C-section
- Vacuum extraction
- Forceps delivery
- Vaginal breech presentation delivery

Premature delivery (<37 0/7 weeks of gestation)
- If <31 (+0 days) weeks of gestation: one to two pediatricians (or one pediatrician, one NICU nurse)

Multiple gestation or growth restriction
SGA/IUGR (<10th percentile according to ultrasound) or estimated weight <2500 g

Severe anomaly of the fetus, for example:
- Chromosomal anomalies according to amniocentesis
- Fetal hydrops
- Critical congenital heart disease
- Skeletal anomalies, gastrointestinal anomalies (e.g., gastroschisis), neural tube defects

Neonatal Emergencies: A Practical Guide for Resuscitation, Transport and Critical Care, ed. Georg Hansmann.
Published by Cambridge University Press. © Cambridge University Press 2009.

Maternal diseases and risk factors

- Signs of infection in the mother:
  - Temperature $>38.0°C$
  - WBC $>17,000/\mu l$
  - CRP >2 mg/dl
- Time between ROM and birth >18 h ($=$PROM) is associated with a greater risk of chorioamnionitis
- Severely compromised maternal health, for example:
  - Maternal systemic lupus erythematosus: 1%–5% of live births have congenital complete heart block (third-degree AV block), of which 50% require a pacemaker, and 15% die in the neonatal period[16]; risk of recurrence of complete heart block in subsequent pregnancies: 10%–15%
  - Insulin-dependent diabetes mellitus of the mother (leads to diabetic fetopathy)
- Gestational diabetes (controversial)
- Preeclampsia/arterial hypertension/HELLP syndrome (i.e., hemolysis, elevated liver enzymes, low platelet count)
- Medication and drug abuse by the mother: especially alcohol, heroin/methadone, ketamine, "sleeping tablets" including benzodiazepines, anticonvulsants, beta-blockers, warfarin, iodine, thyroid gland inhibitors (e.g., methimazole), sulfonamides, tetracycline, psychoactive drugs, tocolytics, cytostatic drugs
- Administration of drugs to the mother:
  - Morphine derivates (e.g., fentanyl, pethidine, tramadol) 0–4 h before delivery
- Placental insufficiency, placental presentation, separation of placenta
- Rhesus incompatibility: isoimmunization, positive Coombs test
- When obstetrician or midwife asks for attendance of a pediatrician

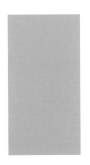

Checklist for the postnatal treatment of newborn infants

Georg Hansmann

Risk factors (pp. 134–5, 179–80)

- Fetal/neonatal: estimated birth weight, gestational age, abnormal growth (IUGR/SGA or LGA?), intrauterine status of the fetus (HR, decelerations?), prenatal diagnostic workup (titers, echocardiogram, aminiocentesis/chromosome analysis)?
- Maternal: fever/infection, medication/drugs, diabetes (gestational?, insulin-dependent?), hepatitis-B-antigen status (HBSAg), indication for operative delivery (vacuum extraction, forceps, C-section)?

Hygiene

- Gloves (always)
- Eye protection
- Mask for the physician if they have a cold or any (potential) Herpes simplex lesions

Stethoscope (size for infants)
Monitor

Connected to:

- Pulse oximeter transducer
- ECG electrodes (when <34 weeks' gestation, use "preterm" ECG electrodes)
- Blood pressure apparatus with adequate cuffs:
    - Size 1 fits neonates <1000 g
    - For birth weight >1000 g use size 2 (for large neonates and infants consider size 3)
- Temperature probe (preterm infants <35 weeks' gestation)

Suction catheters and suctioning device

- Term infants Ch 10 = 10 F
- Preterm/SGA infants Ch 8 (= 8 F) or Ch 6 (= 6 F)
- Check efficiency of suction device (–0.2 bar = –200 mbar = –200 cmH$_2$O; some NICUs use only 100 cmH$_2$O)
- "Meconium aspirator" (Figure 2.17) that is connectible to standard ET tubes
- Alternatively: have a rigid suction catheter at hand ("Yankauer's catheter")

Neonatal Emergencies: A Practical Guide for Resuscitation, Transport and Critical Care, ed. Georg Hansmann. Published by Cambridge University Press. © Cambridge University Press 2009.

> ! Do not place suction catheters under the radiant warmer (they melt!); instead keep the catheter attached to the suction tube device and put it on the side of the resuscitation table where there is less exposure to the radiant warmer.

Ventilatory support and O_2 supplementation

- Bag-and-mask ventilation, e.g., self-inflating bag with a closed reservoir (Figures 2.3, 2.5a–d):
  - PEEP valve +3 to +5 mbar (= cmH_2O)
  - O_2 flow 5 l/min (up to 10 l/min)
  - Adjust O_2 blender to 21% (certain exceptions, such as congenital diaphragmatic hernia, apply)
  - Test mask, seal ring and tubing (see below)
  - Place mask on your own palm. PIP should be sufficient to achieve adequate chest rise; for self-inflating 250-ml bags use thumb plus one finger per kilogram birth weight for adequate PIP (applies to 250-ml bags only)
  - Ventilation rate (applied plus spontaneous respiratory rate) 40–60 breaths/min
- Bag-and-mask ventilation, e.g., flow-inflating bag (Figure 2.4)
  - Flow-inflating bag systems need a higher flow rate (8–10 ml/min) and a better seal than those with self-inflating bags
- T-piece resuscitator, such as "Neopuff" or "Tom Thumb" (Figure 2.6):
  - Initial PIP (20−)25 mbar, PEEP +3 to +5 mbar, F_iO_2 21%, respiratory rate 40–50 breaths/min
  - $T_{in} : T_{exp} = 0.4$ s/0.9 s for term infants
  - Later, adjust parameters to the patient
- Simple "bubble CPAP" (Figure 2.7, CPAP with surge tank and water seal): a gas flow of 5 l/min generates, by tightly closing the mask, a PIP of approx. 20 mbar (cmH_2O). Adjust metal tube in the surge tank to achieve the target PEEP value of 5 cmH_2O
- Choose correct mask size:
  - Size 00 for preterm infants <1000 g
  - Sizes 00–0/1 for weights up to 2500 g
  - Size 0/1 for weights ≥2500 g

Complete intubation kit and additional intubation supplies

- Laryngoscope with straight blade:
  - Blade at sizes 00 (for infants <1000 g), 0 (for infants <2500 g) or 1 (for infants >2500 g)
  - Does the bulb work?
  - Extra set of batteries
- Correct tube size (if applicable, with surfactant application canal)
- Stylet for oral intubation (use as needed)
- Magill's forceps (two sizes)
- Equipment for ET tube fixation, e.g., 3 strips of tape (pre-cut), or special device for oral ET tube.

Radiant warmer

- Always set to maximum to start with
- *Adjust the radiant warmer to the gestational age and body temperature.* When the conditions in the delivery room are optimal, you may use the following guideline for the set surface temperature of the warmer to maintain a rectal temperature of 37.0°C in the newborn:
  - >30 weeks' gestation → 38.5°C/101.2°F
  - <30 weeks' gestation → 39.5°C/103°F
- Six to eight prewarmed cotton diapers/towels/mini-blankets
- Hat/bonnet for the infant's head (exception: therapeutic hypothermia in birk asphysia pp. 315–16)
- Plastic wrap/plastic bag for preterm infant <1500 g; commonly used in preterm infants <28 weeks of gestation

Timer

An Apgar timer should be available at the resuscitation unit.

Blood draw supplies

Blood gas capillaries, blood glucose measuring device (e.g., D-stix) with proper test strips (check expiration date). When indicated, prepare EDTA-coated and serum tubes (CBC, CRP, IL-6, etc.), and aerobic blood culture bottles (preferably prewarmed). Place them in the transport incubator when filled with blood (use plastic bag).

Prepare continuous infusion as needed

- Peripheral IV catheters (24 gauge or 26 gauge)
- Three strips of tape
- 30–50 ml $D_{10}W$ in 50-ml pump syringe with tubing; if neonate is expected to have hypovolemia prepare 50 ml of normal saline with tubing prewarmed to 37°C (98.6°C) (e.g., in incubator)
- 70% alcohol/soft tissue disinfectant and swabs for disinfection

Transport incubator

- Adequate temperature (at first, adjust to 37°C (98.6°F) and check using a thermometer, see Figure 2.10)
- Sufficient O_2 and compressed air
- Sterilized tubing (leak proof)
- Calibrated oxygen tension sensor

Umbilical catheter set (Figure 2.29)

- Umbilical catheter (3.5–5 Ch = 3.5–5 F)
- Two sets of sterile anatomical forceps and drapes (see pp. 106–10)

! A complete catheter set must always be available. Prepare UAC/UVC set prior to use: flush with normal saline (add heparin later, if necessary).

Drugs (Table 2.1, pp. 41–62)

- Check expiration date
- As needed, prepare epinephrine 1:10 000 (epinephrine 1:1000, which needs to be diluted 1:10 in normal saline; or use a pre-prepared 1:10 000 solution) and fill two 1-ml syringes
- As needed, surfactant ampules

Has the neonatal intensive care unit or nursery been informed about this admission?

! Pay attention to detail and prepare generously for the initial care/resuscitation of a newborn infant (even if you may not need all the supplies). It is very hard to find the proper equipment quickly during the resuscitation of a critically ill baby.

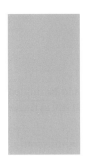

Assigning individual duties in the delivery room

Georg Hansmann

While the resuscitation unit is being prepared and checked, the emergency doctor (NETS-MD, pediatrician, anesthesiologist or obstetrician), nurse practitioner (NP), registered nurse (RN) or paramedic, and maybe a second or third physician, coordinate among themselves who is going to be in charge of which tasks, and in what order they should be achieved.

> ❗ One health care provider takes the leadership role early (i.e., prior to delivery), assigns duties and runs the initial care and neonatal resuscitation. The leader may be the one taking care of the airway (head position) or the leader may be an extra person – most often standing to the right of the head position – not involved in the resuscitation efforts.

Helper no. 1 (mostly the emergency doctor, pediatrician, anesthesiologist or obstetrician)

- Head position and leader. "Runs the code" if no extra help/supervising leader in the room
- Helper no. 1 stands directly in front of the resuscitation unit; the neonate is placed on the resuscitation unit with their forehead close to helper no. 1
- Helper no. 1 is responsible for:
  - Clinical assessment of the neonate and airway management:
    1. Suctioning (can also be performed by helper no. 2, after verbal agreement)
    2. Ventilation (bag-and-mask ventilation, CPAP, intubation)
- Fast and practical approach: wipe the neonate's wet face quickly with a cloth (right hand), and at the same time feel the pulse of the umbilical cord and determine the HR (bpm = umbilical cord pulse in 3 s × 20). These measurements should not take longer than 5 seconds. Drying the face makes bag-and-mask ventilation easier and counteracts hypothermia. Pulse amplitude and rate provide important information about the vitality of the neonate. Use a stethoscope to determine HR if you are unclear about the umbilical pulse/HR
- Next, helper no. 1 continues with suctioning: first mouth and pharynx, then nose (both nostrils). Deep suctioning (hypopharynx) during the first 5 minutes should not be performed except under unusual circumstances (e.g., meconium aspiration), because the vagal reflex can lead to significant bradycardia (→ then perform PPV, cardiopulmonary resuscitation)!

Neonatal Emergencies: A Practical Guide for Resuscitation, Transport and Critical Care, ed. Georg Hansmann. Published by Cambridge University Press. © Cambridge University Press 2009.

Helper no. 2 (mostly NP, RN, paramedic or midwife)
- Stands on the right-hand side of the head position at the right foot of the baby
- Responsible for:
  - Starting the Apgar timer
  - Suctioning (after agreement with helper no. 1)
  - Drying (torso, extremities), manual breathing stimulation (rub back, soles of the feet)
  - Preventing heat loss (e.g., ensuring that the door in the resuscitation room remains closed; cloth/blanket change when the child is stable after the first suctioning; for VLBW preterm infants use plastic wrap)
  - Oxygen supplemention (only if indicated) and continued respiratory stimulation
  - Attaching pulse oximeter ($\approx$ 1 min postnatally) and ECG electrodes
  - Handing over the supplies for ET intubation (including meconium aspirator adapter)
  - Administration of drugs, if indicated
  - Chest compressions (external cardiac massage), if HR <60 bpm (may be done by extra person)
  - May insert UA/UV or PIV catheters (may be done by extra person)
  - Obtaining capillary, venous blood or arterial blood gas and glucose samples, if indicated (obligatory for NETS)

Helper no. 3 (mostly, NP, RN, paramedic or midwife)
- "Relief person"
- Commonly stands on the left side of the baby
- Responsible for:
  - Handing over the instruments and the following supplies: peripheral IV catheters, tape strips; flushed tubing (short) connected to a three-way stopcock; smaller masks, etc., if indicated, an ETT/intubation kit (optimum: from the right side by helper no. 2)
  - Preparing and handing over the drugs
  - May perform chest compressions from the left side of the baby (two-thumb or two-finger techniques)

! When two physicians are present for the management of VLBW or ELBW preterms infants (<1500 g), the second physician should be positioned next to helper no. 2 at the right-hand side of helper no. 1 or at the baby's right foot. This way, they will be able to place a PIV or UV catheter quickly (i.e., while helpers no. 1 and no. 2 suction the airway and perform PPV). The second physician may change position with helper no. 2 in order to provide chest compressions 3:1 with PPV (performed by helper no. 1).

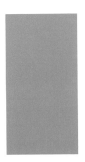

Clinical assessment of the newborn infant

Georg Hansmann

! The evaluation of neonates is based on three signs: *breathing, heart rate, and color*

! Evaluation → Decision → Action

! The one who waits for the umbilical artery pH to come back misses the train!

Breathing

Immediately after the initial postnatal chest excursions, the neonate should be able to breathe spontaneously during the next few seconds, and gradually turn rosy (beginning at the torso, then the extremities) and should maintain a heart rate >100 bpm.

Gasping, apnea and bradycardia (HR <100 bpm) are indications for initiating bag-and-mask ventilation/PPV (see below). Prolonged and severe hypoxia results in anaerobic glycolysis, hypoglycemia, lactic acidosis, peripheral vasoconstriction/shock, cardiac depression and subsequently cell death (CNS, myocardium, and other organs/tissues).

Heart rate

The heart rate (HR) is determined by quick palpation of the pulse at the base of the umbilical cord and/or cardiac auscultation. A HR >100 bpm and variation with breathing are normal.

If the HR is below 100 bpm in spite of 30 s of respiratory stimulation, apply (repeat) oropharyngeal suctioning quickly, then initiate mask-PPV and continue resuscitation according to the standard algorithm (Figure 2.38, p. 157).

Skin color

A well-adapted neonate has rosy mucous membranes without oxygen supplementation. Acrocyanosis (bluish extremities, rosy body) is usually normal for a neonate, but it may be a sign of low environmental temperature (peripheral vasoconstriction).

Signs of central cyanosis are seen on the face, torso and mucous membranes. Extreme pallor can indicate reduced cardiac output, severe anemia (in which case one does not see cyanosis), infection, hypovolemia, acidosis, and/or hypothermia.

Neonatal Emergencies: A Practical Guide for Resuscitation, Transport and Critical Care, ed. Georg Hansmann. Published by Cambridge University Press. © Cambridge University Press 2009.

It should be noted that a completely pink skin color (i.e., trunk and limbs, no acrocyanosis) in the first minutes of life is NOT mandatory, and – because of the risk of hyperoxia – should NOT be the goal of additional oxygen supplementation in the delivery room. For this reason, "pink skin color" as a criterion of excellent postnatal adaptation has been removed from the ILCOR 2005 algorithm on neonatal resuscitation. We generally do not recommend additional oxygen supplementation when a reliable preductal S_pO_2 of 85% (preterm) or 90% (term) is achieved within 5–10 min after birth (certain exceptions apply). The newborn's skin color, capillary refill and pulses, however, are good indicators of overall peripheral perfusion of the neonate. Measure postductal S_pO_2 simultaneously to detect ductal split.

Apgar score (see Table 2.4, p. 144)

The Apgar score (Dr. Virginia Apgar, 1909–1974, obstetric anesthesiologist, New York; http://www.neonatology.org/classics/apgar.html) is a well-established method for evaluating the general clinical condition of the neonate and to determine the baby's response to one's resuscitation efforts.

! Resuscitation must begin, if indicated, 30 s after birth, i.e., PRIOR to the assessment of the "1-min Apgar score."

! Apgar scores should not be used to dictate appropriate resuscitative actions, nor should interventions for depressed infants be delayed until the 1-min Apgar score has been taken.

The decision to perform resuscitation is primarily based on breathing, heart rate, and color (see above) and is – in cases of severe immaturity or malformations – also based on ethical grounds (see p. 184)[9].

Apgar scores are determined at 1, 5 and 10 min after delivery. When the 5-min score is less than 7, the baby's condition is critical, and additional scores should be assigned every 5 min for up to 20 min. Immaturity (reflex irritability, muscle tone, respiratory drive/chest are decreased), congenital malformations, and administered drugs can have a negative effect on the 5-min Apgar score.

- *The 5-min Apgar score* correlates with the survival rate better than the 1-min Apgar. However, the 5-min Apgar score is of limited value when diagnosing birth asphyxia or estimating the long-term outcome of birth asphyxia (for definition of birth asphyxia see p. 310 and Table 1.2 in which common abbreviations are listed).

A newborn infant with a 5-min Apgar score of 0–3 bears the highest neonatal mortality rate. For term neonates with such low Apgar scores (0–3 after 5 min), the neonatal mortality is 8-fold greater than that of term neonates with an umbilical arterial pH <7.00[99,100].

! *Interpretation of Apgar scores in term neonates*

- A 5-min Apgar score of 0–3 means "severe"; a score of 4–6, "moderate depression of the neonate".
- A 5-min Apgar score of 7–8 means "good"; a score of >8, "excellent condition of the neonate".
- A low 5-min Apgar score is a prognostic criterion with regard to the survival rate.

Table 2.4 Advanced documentation of Apgar score and neonatal resuscitation

APGAR SCORE

Sign	0	1	2	1 min	5 min	10 min	15 min	20 min
Breathing	Absent	Hypoventilation, gasp, weak cry	Regular, RR ≈ 40/min, Crying					
Heart rate	Absent	<100 bpm	>100 bpm					
Color	Blue or pale	Acrocyanosis	Completely pink, no acrocyanosis					
Muscle tone	Limp	Some flexion	Active motion					
Reflex irritability (e.g., on suctioning)	No response	Grimace	Cry, cough, or active withdrawal					
Total Apgar Score →								

Comments:

Initial neonatal care/ resuscitation

	1 min	5 min	10 min	15 min	20 min
Minutes after birth					
Oxygen (F_iO_2) (preductal S_pO_2, HR)					
PPV/N-CPAP (PIP und PEEP)					
ET tube: size/position (in cm from nostril/upper gum)					
Chest compressions					
Epinephrine (= adrenaline)					

Table 2.4 Advanced documentation of Apgar score and neonatal resuscitation. Apgar score (0–10) should be assigned at 1, 5 and 10 min after birth. When the 5-min score is less than 7, additional scores should be documented every 5 min for up to 20 min. These scores should not be used to dictate appropriate resuscitative actions, nor should interventions for depressed infants be delayed until the 1 min Apgar score is taken. Advanced resuscitative interventions (such as PPV, intubation) that might have to be initiated immediately after birth (i.e., prior to the 1-min Apgar score) should be documented in the appropriate fields and timepoints (see right lower fields "Initial neonatal care/ resuscitation"), and may include specific data (PIP, PEEP, F_iO_2, S_pO_2, HR). Complete documentation of the events taking place during a resuscitation must also include a narrative description of interventions performed (see left lower field "Comments"). If possible, the documentation should include important prenatal findings. The purpose of the Apgar score is to quantify the general clinical condition of the newborn infant, and to estimate the neonate's response to resuscitative interventions. If the 5-min Apgar score is less than 7, the neonate's condition is likely to be critical.

Note: A completely pink skin color (i.e., no acrocyanosis) in the first minutes of life is NOT mandatory, and – because of the risk of hyperoxia – should NOT be the goal of additional oxygen supplementation in the first minutes of life. For this reason, "pink skin color" as a measure of excellent postnatal adaptation has been removed from the ILCOR 2005 algorithm on neonatal resuscitation. PPV, positive pressure ventilation; N-CPAP, nasal continuous positive airway pressure; S_pO_2, pulsoximetric oxgen saturation; preduct, preductal.
Modified from: *The Apgar Score.* American Academy of Pediatrics, Committee on Fetus and Newborn, American College of Obstetricians and Gynecologists and Committee on Obstetric Practice. *Pediatrics* 2006; 117:1444–7.

- A 5-min Apgar score of 10 means "no acrocyanosis" and is rarely reached, and, because of the risk of hyperoxia, should NOT be the goal of additional oxygen supplementation in the delivery room

! Virginia Apgar created one "scoring system" for pediatricians, obstetricians, midwives, and anesthesiologists.

CRIB score

In high-risk neonates or term/preterm infants with a birth weight <1500 g, the CRIB score (Clinical Risk Index for Babies[102]) can be documented to estimate the risk-adjusted survival rate in the NICU. The CRIB score includes the birth weight, gestational age, base deficit, F_iO_2, and congenital deformities (Table 2.5).

Silverman–Andersen retraction score (Table 2.6)

The Silverman – Andersen retraction score is designed to provide a continuous evaluation of an infant's respiratory status (Table 2.6). An index of respiratory distress is determined by grading each of five criteria: chest lag, intercostal retraction, xiphoid retraction, nasal flaring, and expiratory grunt. The retraction score is computed by adding the values (0, 1, or 2) assigned to each factor that best describes the infant's condition at the time of a single observation. With 6 or more points, endotracheal intubation may be indicated. Respiratory rate and pattern, skin color (pallor, cyanosis?), and blood gases are evaluated as well.

Typical scenario: A grunting neonate in the nursery or "still" in the delivery room → Intubation prior to transport?

Umbilical artery pH value (UA pH)

Aside from the assessment of vital signs, the UA pH and arterial blood gases are other criteria used to evaluate the neonate. Of note, the correlation between UA pH and Apgar score is only weak (for postnatal arterial blood gas analysis see Table 2.7).

! An isolated UA acidosis without any symptoms or a single low 1-min Apgar score of 0–3 – increasing by 5 min postnatally – does not show any definite correlation with neurological sequelae[103].

A UA pH >7.20 is physiologic, whereas values between 7.10 and 7.20 indicate mild acidosis; values between 7.00 and 7.10, moderate acidosis; values below 7.00, severe acidosis.

! If the UA pH is below 7.15 a blood gas analysis should be performed approx. 30 min after birth (or earlier) – especially when vital signs (e.g., respiratory rate and pattern, S_pO_2) are not normal.

For legal reasons, the NETS team may consider repeating the blood gas analysis 30 min after the birth regardless of the UA pH value.

Table 2.5 CRIB Score (Clinical Risk Index for Babies)

Sample sheet

Newborn's name: ....

Date of birth:..

Weight: ....Weeks' of GA: ....Apgar:.................................

Diagnoses:...

CRIB score assessment at the age of:.. (usually at 12 h of life)...............................

By: ....

Factor	Score
Birth weight (g):	
>1350	0
851–1350	1
701–850	4
≤700	7
Weeks of GA:	
>24	0
≤24	1
Congenital malformations (without lethal malformations):	
None	0
Not acutely life threatening	1
Acutely life threatening[a]	3
Maximum base deficit during the first 12 hours (mmol/l):	
Positive up to −6.9	0
−7.0 to −9.9	1
−10.0 to −14.9	2
−15 or even more negative	3
Minimum F_iO_2 during the first 12 hours of life (P_aO_2 50–80 mmHg, S_aO_2 88%–95%):	
≤0.40	0
0.41–0.60	2
0.61–0.90	3
0.91–1.0	4
Maximum F_iO_2 during the first 12 h of life (P_aO_2 50–80 mmHg, S_aO_2 88%–95%):	
≤0.40	0
0.41–0.80	1
0.81–0.90	3
0.91–1.00	5
Sum (max. 23)	....

The CRIB score is applied to neonates with additional risk factors, and/or term/preterm infants with a birth weight less than 1500 g (VLBW, ELBW) in order to estimate the risk-adjusted survival rate in the NICU. The in-hospital mortality increases from <40% to >70% with a CRIB score of greater than 10. For accurate assessment of the CRIB score, lethal malformations, e.g., bilateral renal agenesis, Patau's syndrome (trisomy 13), Edward's syndrome (trisomy 18), Potter's sequence, or anencephaly are excluded.

[a]Namely, CoA, CHARGE, ornithine cycle (Krebs cycle) disorder, hydrops, hypoplasia of the lungs, omphalocele, polycystic renal degeneration, osteogenesis imperfecta, prune-belly syndrome, conjoined twins, tetralogy of fallot, VACTERL association.

Adapted from: Cockburn F, Cooke R, Gamsu H. The CRIB (Clinical Risk Index for Babies) score: a tool for assessing initial neonatal risk and comparing performance of neonatal intensive care units. The International Neonatal Network. *Lancet* 1993; 342(8865):193–8.

Table 2.6 **Silverman–Andersen retraction score**

	Score		
	0	**1**	**2**
Movements of upper chest	In synchrony with abdominal wall	Delayed (chest lag)	In opposite direction vs. abdominal wall
Intercostal retractions	None	Slight (intermittent)	Severe
Sternal retractions	None	Moderate (intermittent)	Severe
Nasal flaring	None	Subtle (intermittent)	Obvious
Expiratory groaning	None	Moderate (intermittent)	Severe

The Silverman–Andersen retraction score is a tool for assessing the clinical condition of term/preterm infants with a delayed respiratory adaptation during the first hours after birth. Six or more points indicate the need for endotracheal intubation. Respiratory rate and pattern, skin color (pallor, cyanosis?), and blood gas analysis are evaluated as well.

Table 2.7 **Perinatal arterial blood gas analysis in healthy term newborn infants**

	At birth (UA)	**After 10 min**	**After 60 min**
pH	7.24	7.21	7.33
P_aCO_2 (mmHg)	49	46	36
P_aO_2 (mmHg)	19	50	63
Base deficit (mmol/l, mEq/l)	−7	−10	−7
Sodium bicarbonate (mmol/l, mEq/l)	20	17	19

The difference between primary and secondary ("terminal") apnea (see Figure 2.36a, b; see pp. 150–1)

Hypoxia can occur for various reasons categorized as either intrauterine or intrapartum (during birth). The first vital sign that is affected and becomes abnormal is breathing (rate, amplitude, and pattern).

Primary apnea

After an initial period of fast breathing efforts (that usually begin in utero), the neonate shows periodic breathing/gasping or develops apnea. Heart rate begins to fall at about the same time the baby enters primary apnea[9]. After suctioning of the upper pharynx, respiratory stimulation (the back, the soles of the feet) is usually sufficient to restore adequate spontaneous breathing[4,9,35]. Oxygen supplementation is very rarely indicated in newborn infants with primary apnea[104].

Typical scenario for a term infant with primary apnea
- HR >80 bpm (usually >100 bpm within 30 s of effective stimulation of breathing), 1-min Apgar score 4–6, UA pH >7.00
- Immediate drying/stimulation of breathing is performed in room air

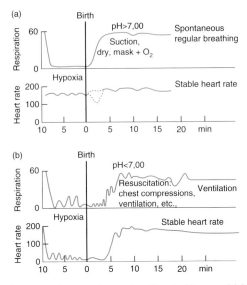

Figure 2.36 The difference between primary and secondary ("terminal") apnea. (a) Primary apnea. (b) Secondary ("terminal") apnea.

- Cerebral damage is very rare in neonates who respond well to these resuscitative measures
- However, primary apnea may be associated with bradycardia and progress to secondary ("terminal") apnea

> **!** A neonate who does not cry or breathe straight after delivery despite stimulation is most likely in a state of secondary (terminal) apnea and needs immediate ventilation (PPV) via bag-and-mask or T-piece device, pharyngeal tube or endotracheal intubation/PPV. Manual stimulation of breathing and oxygen supplementation will NOT solve the problem[9].

Secondary ("terminal") apnea

The time between the last gasp/breath and cardiac arrest is called the period of secondary or "terminal" apnea. There are *two ways* by which a newly born infant may enter a state of secondary (terminal) apnea:

1. *Either* by severe intrauterine/intrapartum hypoxia leading to the birth of a neonate with apnea and bradycardia/cardiac arrest
2. *Or* incessant primary apnea with irregular breathing pattern/gasping leading to secondary apnea

These neonates need immediate PPV (with prior oropharyngeal suctioning), by bag-and-mask ventilation, by pharyngeal-PPV or by (rapid) endotracheal intubation/PPV. The decision has to be made within the first 30 s after delivery – thus before the 1-min Apgar score is determined.

Table 2.8 **Petrussa index, a simple estimate of gestational age (≥30 weeks)**

Maturity signs	Points (+30 = gestational age in weeks)		
	0	**1**	**2**
Skin	Bright red, vulnerable thin and transparent	Rosy, more firm, more skin folds	Firm, fine peeling
Breasts	Mammary gland barely present	Mammary gland is palpable; areola is visible	Mammary gland and areola palpable; breast tissue above skin level
Ears	Almost no profile and no cartilage, soft	More profile, cartilage in tragus and anti-tragus	Thick and stiff cartilage
Soles of feet	Smooth, creases in the anterior third	Creases in the anterior and middle third	Creases over the entire sole
Genital organs	Inguinal testes, labia majora < labia minora	Testes partly descended, labia majora and labia minora equal in size	Testes fully descended, labia majora > labia minora

The Petrussa index serves as a simple estimate of gestational age. Somatic signs of maturity are assessed. GA in weeks post menstruation = 30 + attained points. Applicable for gestional ages ≥30 weeks. See also Dubowitz/Ballard assessment of gestational age. If the eyelids are fused, the infant is likely ≤27 weeks GA.

Typical scenario for a term infant with secondary (terminal) apnea

- HR <100 bpm (often <80 bpm), 1-min Apgar score mostly 0–3, UA pH frequently <7.00
- Rapid intubation and PPV performed, however no spontaneous breathing for several hours
- Cerebral edema and damage are common. Consider therapeutic hypothermia for an asphyxic newborn infant according to a published protocol[104]

> **!** It may be very difficult to distinguish between primary and secondary (terminal) apnea in the first seconds of life, and appropriate neonatal resuscitation should never be delayed just for the purpose of distinguishing between the two (see Standard algorithm, see Figure 2.38).

All newly born infants need to be evaluated immediately after birth according to the following five criteria (note that "pink color" has been removed from the ILCOR 2005 algorithm):

1. Are the amniotic fluid and the skin of the neonate free of meconium?
2. Is the initial heart rate >100 bpm?
3. Is the newborn breathing or crying?
4. Is the muscle tone good (active movement)?
5. Is the baby likely born at term? (For Petrussa index see Table 2.8)

If any of the five answers is NO, the newborn infant needs intensive (rather than routine) care (see standard algorithm, Figure 2.38).

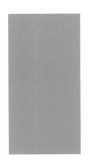

Cardiopulmonary resuscitation of newborn infants at birth

Georg Hansmann and Sam Richmond

Pathophysiology of perinatal hypoxia ("birth asphyxia")

If one does not understand the basic physiology of perinatal hypoxia ("birth asphyxia") then resuscitation of the newborn, however many algorithms you learn, becomes a series of ritual interventions that may be difficult to remember under stress. However, once this physiology is known, the process can be easily understood and the appropriate actions of the resuscitator seem to be logical, predictable, and essentially very simple.

Before delivery, the baby's respiration occurs via the placenta. Immediately following delivery the baby has to fill its lungs with air while disposing of the fluid currently filling them and massively increase the circulation to the lungs in order to establish independent respiration. While preparing for this change, the baby undergoing vaginal delivery must also cope with intermittent obstruction of placental gas exchange during each uterine contraction. These intermittent obstructions can each last for around 90 s and will occur maybe four times every 10 min for the 30–60 min of the second stage of labor (in this stage of delivery, the baby is at greatest risk for severe hypoxia).

Animal experiments performed in the 1950s provide very useful information on the response of fetal mammals to acute hypoxia[106]. The immediate fetal response to acute hypoxia is a rise in blood pressure, heart rate, and "breathing" movements. With continuing hypoxia the fetus becomes unconscious, breathing movements stop as higher breathing centers are disabled by hypoxia, and the heart rate rapidly falls as the fetus enters *early terminal apnea*. Cardiac output is initially maintained by anaerobic metabolism and peripheral vasoconstriction despite severe hypoxia. After a variable period primitive spinal centers, released from suppression by the higher breathing centers, stimulate the fetus to produce deep gasping movements at a rate of around 12 per minute. If hypoxia continues, the gasping movements gradually fade away and, though blood pressure is maintained for somewhat longer, this too is failing. Without external intervention (PPV, eventually chest compressions) the fetus will ultimately die. A baby subjected to severe hypoxia in utero may be delivered at any point during this process.

A baby born in *primary apnea* may be about to start gasping. If it does so with an open airway then air will enter the lungs and blood circulating through the lungs will carry this oxygen back to the heart, which will respond with a rapid increase in heart rate. As oxygen is further carried to the brain the baby will regain consciousness and start breathing again.

A just-delivered baby who experienced total asphyxia and a period of *terminal apnea in utero* is unconscious and severely acidotic, cardiac glycogen stores are virtually

Neonatal Emergencies: A Practical Guide for Resuscitation, Transport and Critical Care, ed. Georg Hansmann.
Published by Cambridge University Press. © Cambridge University Press 2009.

exhausted, and no more gasping/breathing efforts can be expected without external intervention. In this situation, the circulation is rapidly failing (heart rate ≪60 bpm or primary asystole). An attempt at lung inflation may have no effect on the heart rate, presumably because the circulation cannot return any oxygenated blood to the heart. However, having inflated the lungs, a brief period of chest compressions may successfully bring some oxygenated blood to the heart, which then responds (i.e., heart rate and blood pressure rise). As oxygen reaches the central nervous system, gasping, and then more normal breathing, returns (see Figure 2.36, p. 148).

Definition of "birth asphyxia"

It should be noted that neonatologists mean very different degrees of perinatal hypoxia when they talk about "birth asphyxia" (greek: pulselessness). Many use the old definition by Carter et al. (1993)[107], i.e., (1) extremely abnormal postnatal transition with cardiac arrest or severe bradycardia, apnea, cyanosis/pallor, and unconsciousness, i.e., 5-min Apgar score of 0–3, plus (2) severe UA acidosis: pH <7.00, plus (3) organ damage with a high risk of hypoxic ischemic encephalopathy (HIE), however there is no worldwide-accepted definition of "birth asphyxia."

Basic sequence of resuscitation (Figure 2.37)

Keep the baby warm – make sure the cord is securely clamped then dry the baby and wrap in warm, dry towels. With small preterm babies (<30 weeks of gestation) place the baby up to the neck in a food-grade plastic bag under a radiant heater (see below).

Assess the situation – while drying the baby you have time to assess the situation by checking the baby's *heart rate, breathing, tone, and color*. A healthy baby will be born blue, will be well flexed, with good tone, a heart rate of more than 100 bpm, and will cry within a few seconds of delivery. Most babies need very little intervention and healthy babies can take as long as 3 min to start breathing after delivery. A less well baby will have less good tone, a slower heart rate (<100 bpm) and may not have established adequate breathing by 90–120 s. A sick baby is likely to be pale rather than blue, floppy and has a slow, very slow or undetectable heart rate – such a baby would require rapid intervention but such intervention should follow exactly the same logical flow.

The heart rate is best checked using a stethoscope – a slowly pulsating umbilical cord may truly indicate a slow heart rate but it can also be found in the presence of a good heart rate.[108]

Having assessed the baby's tone, color, heart rate, and breathing at the start it is then necessary to repeat these observations at approximately 30-s intervals in order to note the effect of any interventions and to decide whether yet further intervention is needed. If intervention is required then the first sign of success will be a rapid increase in heart rate.

<u>Airway</u> – air cannot be drawn or pushed into the lungs unless the airway is clear – in floppy babies the commonest reason for a blocked airway is loss of pharyngeal tone. Place the baby on its back, support the head in the neutral position and, if the baby is floppy, provide jaw thrust (Esmarch's maneuver). In a very few babies lumps of blood, vernix or meconium can occasionally block the airway and may need removal with a large-bore suction catheter, preferably under direct vision.

Breathing – if the baby does not breathe, or is not breathing adequately, inflate the lungs using positive pressure ventilation (PPV) via a pressure-regulated mask and T-piece or a bag-valve-mask system. Air is probably perfectly adequate to start with and it can be supplemented with oxygen later if cyanosis persists. If the heart rate is slow one would expect a rapid increase in heart rate within a few seconds of successful lung inflation. If the baby's heart rate responds in this fashion you can safely assume that you have succeeded in aerating the lungs. Continue providing ventilation (~30–40 breaths per minute) sufficient to keep the heart rate above 100 bpm until the baby is breathing adequately.

If the baby's heart rate does not improve following lung inflation then either lung inflation has not been achieved (this is the most likely reason) or else the heart may be so affected by acidosis and hypoxia that it is unable to respond. Before moving on to chest compressions check that the chest is moving passively with each inflation – if it is not then consider the following:

- Is the baby's head in the neutral position?
- Do you need to provide jaw thrust?
- Would it help to use a longer inflation time or a higher inflation pressure?
- Do you need a second person's help with the airway (mask, endotracheal tube)?
- Could there be an obstruction in the oropharynx?
- Would an oropharyngeal airway (Guedel) help?

Circulation/chest compressions – if the heart rate remains below 60 bpm after the lungs have truly been inflated (i.e., if you can see passive chest movement in response to PPV) perform chest compressions. If sufficient skills are available then intubation is appropriate at this point (or earlier if no sufficient lung inflation is achievable). The currently recommended ratio for cardiopulmonary resuscitation (CPR) in this situation is three compressions to one breath performed at a rate of 120 "events" per minute (~90 compressions and 30 breaths per minute).

Drugs – very occasionally a newborn does not respond to lung inflation combined with chest compressions (Figure 2.37). Some of these babies will respond to drugs (epinephrine) but, if drugs are truly needed to achieve recovery, the babies so resuscitated have a poor prognosis.

This basic sequence of neonatal resuscitation (ABCD) not only tells you what to do but also tells you the order in which you should do it. Checking the baby's condition at delivery allows you to pause and judge whether any intervention at all is called for. It also allows you to assess the heart rate. From the physiology you know that the first response any baby will make to successful resuscitation efforts is an increase in the heart rate (see Figure 2.37). Furthermore, there is no point in trying to inflate the baby's chest without first ensuring that the airway is clear. There is also no point in providing chest compressions until you have placed some air in the lungs to allow oxygenation of any blood that you might succeed in pumping back to the heart.

Only 10% of all newly born babies require some kind of postnatal medical support. However, 1% need more extensive resuscitative measures (intubation, chest compressions, and/or medications) to survive[9]. In numbers, this means from an estimated 134 million births per year worldwide, 13.4 million require some kind of assistance (stimulation, CPAP, PPV) and 1.3 million require extensive intervention (PPV, intubation, chest compressions, and/or medications).

Basic sequence of neonatal resuscitation

A	Assess, Airways?	Amniotic fluid? Meconium? Blood? → Suctioning, jaw thrust (= Esmarch's maneuver) necessary?
B	Breathing?	Breathing excursions sufficient and the same on both sides?
		Respiratory frequency and pattern? → Supplemental oxygen needed?
		If HR <100 bpm → bag-and-mask or T-piece ventilation, LMA, pharyngeal PPV, or endotracheal intubation/PPV
C	Circulation?	Heart rate (auscultation, umbilical cord pulse) → may need to provide chest compressions after 30 s of effective ventilation (chest compressions : ventilation = 3 : 1)
		Umbilical cord, femoral or brachial artery pulse? → Subsequently check ABC! Arterial blood gas (ABG)

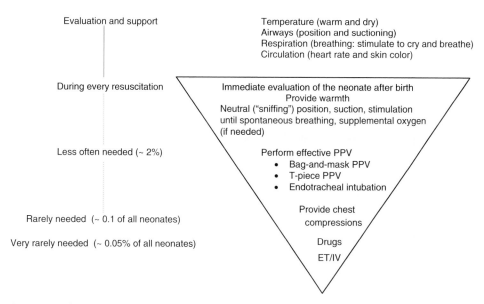

Figure 2.37 This inverted pyramid represents the frequency of applied ABCD procedures during the initial management of the newborn infant at birth in the absence of meconium-stained skin or fluid (no MSAF). Modified from: Kattwinkel J (2006) *Neonatal Resuscitation*, 5th edn. ELK Grove Village, IL: American Academy of Pediatrics and American Heart Association.

Epinephrine (adrenaline) and volume therapy
(See also Table 2.1.)

Epinephrine (Adrenaline) 1:10 000

- Either prepare 1 ml epinephrine 1:1000 + 9 ml normal saline or use 1:10 000 solution.
- Fill two 1- to 3-ml syringes with the 1:10 000 solution (0.1 ml = 0.01 mg).
- The preferred route is IV (PIV or UVC or IO).

- Initial dose 0.1 ml/kg/dose IV (= 0.01 mg/kg/dose) or 0.3–1 ml/kg/dose ET (= 0.03–0.1 mg/kg/dose ET).
- Repeat single dose, if needed. Give volume with second epinephrine dose.
- Increase single dose up to 0.3 ml/kg/dose IV (= 0.03 mg/kg/dose IV) or 1 ml/kg/dose ET (=0.1 mg/kg/dose ET). Higher IV doses are not evidence-based. No data on best ET dose.
- Maximum single dose is 0.03 mg/kg/dose IV; higher single doses are not more effective and are potentially harmful.
- Always flush with 5 ml normal saline IV.

Volume therapy

- Normal saline 10–20 ml/kg in 5–10 min IV. In VLBW infants, give 10 ml/kg in 30 min IV. May repeat volume bolus (goals: MAP $\geq$ gestational age in weeks, good pulses, capillary refill $\leq$2 s). Only crystalloid (normal saline) but not colloid solutions are recommended for the resuscitation of newborn infants[22].
- Consider packed red blood cells (PRBC) after significant feto-maternal blood loss, hemorrhagic shock or severe sepsis with capillary leak. Replace clotting factors as needed (e.g., fresh frozen plasma (FFP)).

For volume therapy and buffer solutions (sodium bicarbonate, THAM), see also separate Chapter, pp. 173–8.

> ! The ILCOR guidelines 2005[22] only recommend epinephrine (adrenaline) and volume therapy (normal saline, packed red blood cells) for the resuscitation of newborn infants in the delivery room.

Very rarely, sodium bicarbonate or vasopressors (others than epinephrine) may be useful during or after resuscitation.

Sodium bicarbonate 8.4% (1 M), i.e., 1 ml = 1 mmol = 1 mEq = 1 mval

- Sodium bicarbonate 4.2% (0.5 M) should be used as final concentration for IV application.
- After PPV, volume expansion and blood gas analysis, consider administering sodium bicarbonate 4.2% (0.5 M) safely through a large IV line.
- Required amount of sodium bicarbonate in mEq = mmol = (base deficit $\times$ kg body weight) $\div$ 3.
- Dilute sodium bicarbonate 8.4% 1 : 1 in sterile water (e.g., 10 ml + 10 ml, then 4.2% final concentration) and administer as continuous infusion in 30–60–120 min IV.
- Maximum speed: 0.1 mEq/kg/min = 6 mEq/kg/h (= 12 ml of the 1:1 solution/kg/h) IV.
- Only in an absolute emergency without the ability to determine the patient's pH/blood gas, e.g., 10 min ineffective resuscitation in the delivery room (external heart massage and IV epinephrine), you may "blindly" administer 1 mEq/kg/dose = 2 ml/kg of 4.2% sodium bicarbonate (0.5 M) per dose IV in 5–10 min. Consider THAM if repetitive buffer doses are indicated for severe metabolic or mixed acidosis.
- It should be noted that, especially in Europe, neonatologists are quite reluctant to use sodium bicarbonate or tris-hydroxymethyl aminomethane (THAM) in the delivery room, because of their adverse effects and insufficient evidence on their efficacy in neonatal resuscitation/post-resuscitation care. Neither sodium bicarbonate nor THAM is recommended any longer as first-line agent in neonatal resuscitation in the delivery room[22].

If hypernatremia is present, use THAM (very rarely indicated). Some use THAM for mixed acidosis when P_aCO_2 is high, although in this situation sufficient ventilation should have priority. THAM might bring some benefit for newborns with congenital diaphragmatic hernia (CDH) and persistent pulmonary hypertension of the newborn (PPHN); however, ILCOR does NOT recommend either sodium bicarbonate or THAM for the resuscitation of newly born infants in the delivery room.

THAM (tris-hydroxymethyl aminomethane) = Tris buffer (very rarely indicated)

- Required THAM (3 M) in ml = (base deficit × kg body weight) ÷ 10
- Required THAM (0.3 M) in ml = (base deficit × kg body weight)
- Caution (peripheral IV access):
  - If you have only the 3 M solution, dilute THAM (3 M) 1:10 with sterile water, to give a 0.3 M solution
- THAM 0.3 M solution is preferably diluted 1:1 in $D_{10}W$ (10 ml Tris 0.3 M + 10 ml $D_{10}W$)
- Then peripheral THAM infusion is possible
- Better: THAM up to 3 M diluted 1:1 in $D_{10}W$ via central venous line
- Replace half of the required THAM amount over 30 min (in asphyxia) to 60 (up to 120) min IV. Advantage of THAM over sodium bicarbonate is no increase of PCO_2 and sodium; adverse effects: hypertonic solution, hypoglycemia, apnea, liver cell necrosis, or the like; contraindications: uremia/anuria

For indications and contraindications of buffer solutions see pp. 176–8.

10% dextrose in water ($D_{10}W$, glucose 10%)

- Maintenance glucose infusion rate (GIR) 3 ml/kg/h = 5 mg/kg/min.
- In cases of hypoglycemia: 2–5 ml/kg/h IV bolus, give double the infusion rate (6 ml/kg/h).
- Never use dextrose solutions for volume replacement

Administer a maximum of 15% of dextrose in water by peripheral IV (if there is no emergency, maximum concentration is 12.5% dextrose continuously by peripheral IV). In highly normal or elevated blood glucose (e.g., after resuscitation/administering epinephrine) use 5% dextrose in water (D_5W) as maintenance IV infusion.

How to treat cerebral seizures of unknown etiology

- Administer 2 ml $D_{10}W$/kg per dose IV, or
- In confirmed hypocalcemia (ionized calcium): 10% calcium gluconate diluted 1:1 in $D_{10}W$: slowly inject 1 ml/kg of the solution through a secure IV, or
- In confirmed hypomagnesemia: 10% magnesium (1 ml = 0.315 mmol) 0.5 ml/kg over 5 min IV, or
- Phenobarbital 10(−20) mg/kg IV. (Caution: arterial hypotension, respiratory depression! Do not use phenobarbital primarily for sedation.). Flush with 3 ml normal saline IV. Alternative: *Lorazepam* 0.05–0.1 (−0.2) mg/kg per dose; *diazepam* 0.5–1 (−2) mg/kg IV; or (fos) phenytoin – if possible, under ECG monitoring in the NICU
- Evaluate for possible causes of cerebral seizures, including infection/meningitis, metabolic disorder, hypoxic-ischemic insult, anatomical CNS abnormalities, hemorrhage/bleeding disorder, hemorrhagic or thromboembolic stroke

Step-by-step guidelines for the resuscitation of a newborn infant at birth

> *!* Use all information and resources you have available.
>
> *!* Whatever you do, do it carefully but with determination.
>
> *!* The key to successful neonatal resuscitation is establishment of adequate ventilation.
>
> *!* Proper handling in the delivery room reduces postnatal morbidity (*"The Golden Hour After Birth"*).

Check ABCD (see above); see standard algorithm (Figure 2.38, p. 157):

- If meconium is present and newborn depressed: laryngoscopy and rapid tracheal suctioning (for meconium aspiration, see p. 269, Figure 3.5, *meconium algorithm*)
- Determine the heart rate (umbilical cord pulse and cardiac auscultation)
- Suctioning by helper no. 1 or 2 (oral/pharyngeal before nasal, avoid deep suctioning during the first few minutes, due to the vagal stimulation)
- Helper no. 2 dries and stimulates the neonate (exemption: thick, stained amniotic fluid, e.g., when meconium aspiration is suspected), supplement oxygen only if indicated, attach pulse oximeter and ECG electrodes, keep the neonate warm. Place the preterm infant in a plastic bag or cover with wrap (to prevent loss of heat and moisture)

Check after 30 s

In case of HR <100 bpm or apnea

- Either ventilate with bag-and-mask or T-piece system for at least 30 seconds (initially, a higher PIP is often necessary for lung expansion), or perform pharyngeal PPV (via LMA or tube)
- Or, immediate endotracheal intubation/PPV (see below); the decision must be made within the first 30 s after birth – thus before the 1-min Apgar score is determined

! Indication for bag-and-mask or T-piece mask ventilation

- Respiratory insufficiency (e.g., secondary apnea, RDS, s/p opioid exposure)
- If symptomatic: HR <100 bpm, severe cyanosis or pallor, muscular hypotonia plus dyspnea
- To support the infant until intubation is performed ("bridge")
- In between trials of intubation
- Tube obstruction in spite of tracheal suctioning (remove tube and begin bag-and-mask ventilation)

! **Contraindication for bag-and-mask or T-piece mask ventilation (mask-PPV)**

- (Suspected) diaphragmatic hernia
- (Suspected) aspiration of meconium, viscous mucus or blood
- Abdominal wall defects (omphalocele, gastroschisis)
- Esophageal atresia
- Strong suspicion of pneumothorax

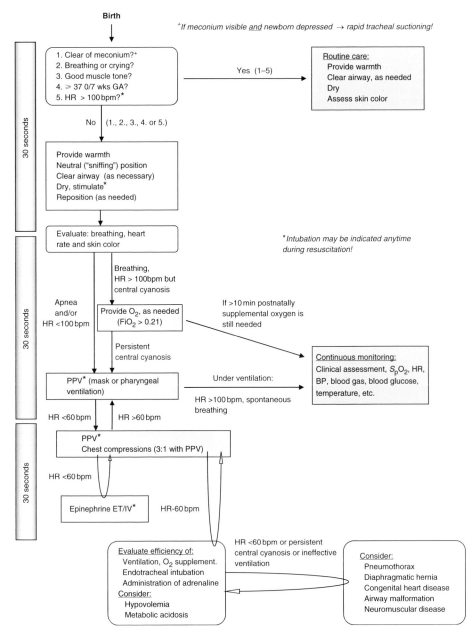

Figure 2.38 Standard algorithm for the initial management and resuscitation of the newborn infant. GA, gestational age. Modified from: ILCOR guidelines (2005) *Resuscitation* 2005; 67:293–303, and AHA/AAP guidelines (2005) *Circulation* 2005; 112:IV 188–195 and *Pediatrics* 2006; 117:e1029–1038; URL link http://pediatrics. aappublications.org/cgi/content/extract/117/5/e1029).

Check after 30 s of effective ventilation

HR < 60 bpm in spite of effective PPV (mask or endotracheal ventilation)

- Perform chest compressions coordinated with mask or endotracheal ventilation (compressions : PPV = 3:1)
- When chest compressions have been initiated, usually the next step is endotracheal intubation (if immediate intubation had not yet been performed)

> **!** Endotracheal intubation may be indicated at any time during neonatal resuscitation (see standard algorithm, Figure 2.38, p. 157)

! Indications for endotracheal intubation

- Immediate intubation (in the first minute after birth)
  - Severely depressed neonate ("birth asphyxia")
  - Depressed neonate with meconium aspiration and indication for endotracheal suctioning
  - Suspected congenital diaphragmatic hernia
  - Preterm infant <28 weeks' gestation *and* indication for prophylactic or early thera- peutic surfactant administration
- *Insufficient respiration and contraindication for bag-and-mask ventilation* (e.g., congenital diaphragmatic hernia, gastroschisis, omphalocele, esophageal atresia, meconium aspir- ation, strong suspicion of pneumothorax)
- When chest compressions are performed, i.e., HR <60 bpm (early rapid intubation preferred)
- When endotracheal administration of epinephrine is indicated (HR <60 bpm in spite of PPV/chest compressions over 30 s and no IV access)
- When there is *no response to bag-and-mask ventilation/pharyngeal-PPV* over at least 30 s – even though PPV had been correctly performed, i.e., HR <60 bpm, persistent cyanosis or pallor, and lack of sufficient chest rise, or when mask/pharyngeal-PPV is prolonged (e.g., recurring apnea when neonate is being weaned from PPV)
- *Persistently high inspiratory oxygen concentration:* in preterm infants >40%, in term infants >60% (for oxygen toxicity, see pp. 70–1).
- When instillation of surfactant is indicated (is stable transport without endotracheal intubation possible?)
- Respiratory exhaustion with a capillary or arterial PCO_2 >70 mmHg, pH value <7.25 and ineffective CPAP trial (blood gas analysis approx. 30 min after birth). A typical situation: dyspneic newborn in the delivery room/nursery before transport
- When transport out of the labor and delivery area does not seem to be safe without a stable airway (e.g., persistent stridor)
- Critically ill newborn prior to long transport (e.g., severe coarctation of the aorta on prostaglandin E_1 IV infusion)

When rapid intubation is performed, chest compression should be interrupted, whereas ventilation may be continued through the pharyngeal tube – depending on the experience of the resuscitators (Figure 2.42, p. 192). If mask ventilation is insufficient, rule out technical error and switch to pharyngeal-PPV (e.g., in ELBW) or immediate intubation (in the first minute of life).

Once the decision to intubate has been made (e.g., severe asphyxia/resuscitation), ventilation should be performed for the initial 30 s. If the heart rate does not exceed

60 bpm, then chest compressions in a 3:1 ratio with PPV for the next 30 s and subsequent administration of epinephrine IV/ET (0.01–0.03 mg/kg/dose IV, 0.03–0.1 mg/kg/dose ET) are indicated (see standard algorithm, Figure 2.38).

! Coordination of chest compression and intubation/PPV

- Chest compression and PPV are carried out in a 3:1 ratio with hardly any interrruptions
- During intubation and when PPV tidal volumes are applied, chest compression may be interrupted
- Theoretically, the goal is 120–150 compressions per minute (= 2 per second); however, since the PPV tidal volume ("squee-eeze" or "breath") is applied during the 3:1 pause, chest compressions actually amount to approximately 90 per minute (30 "PPV breaths" per minute; chest compressions plus "PPV breaths" = 120 events per minute)

Check after another 30 s

(See Table 2.9, Troubleshooting during neonatal resuscitation)
- Breathing, heart rate and skin color?

HR is still <60 bpm

- Administration of epinephrine
    - Initial single dose is epinephrine 0.01 mg/kg IV = 0.1 ml/kg of epinephrine 1:10 000 IV (in case helper no. 3 is able to place a peripheral IV or umbilical venous catheter in the meantime). If no IV/IO access available, give epinephrine 0.03–0.1 mg/kg ET = 0.3–1 ml/kg of epinephrine 1:10 000 ET
    - Obtain (second) peripheral venous access (PIV)
    - Place an umbilical venous catheter, if indicated/not done yet

Check after another 30 s

HR is still <60 bpm

- Give second epinephrine dose (0.01–0.03 mg/kg/dose IV)
- With second epinephrine dose give volume: normal saline 10–20 ml/kg IV
- If no improvement at this point, do trouble shooting (see Figure 2.38 and Table 2.9)
- Place a gastric tube (indicated after 2 min of PPV and always after intubation)
- D_5W or $D_{10}W$ dextrose infusion according to blood glucose level
- Eventually consider sodium bicarbonate or THAM according to blood gas analysis or course of resuscitation (e.g., if epinephrine has no effect)

Key points

⏐ Effective bag-and-mask or T-piece ventilation (PPV) for 30 s usually is sufficient to generate acceptable heart rate (HR >100 bpm) and cardiac output.

⏐ It seems reasonable to start resuscitation of newly born babies with room air[4,104], and increase F_iO_2 in 20% point increments if needed. 100% oxygen as back-up should be available at any time.

Table 2.9 Troubleshooting during neonatal resuscitation

Problem	Previous (preliminary) information/clinical signs	Decision and action
Mechanical airway obstruction		
• Blockage by meconium, blood or amniotic fluid/mucus (see Figures 2.17, 3.5; Algorithm MAS)	• Meconium-stained or otherwise stained and thick amniotic fluid, blood or mucus AND newborn infant depressed • Decreased chest rise	→ 1. Oral intubation and tracheal suctioning using a meconium aspirator (adapter connected to ETT) or → 2. Laryngoscopy and tracheal suctioning with rigid Yankauer suctioning catheter → Always (1 + 2) suction oropharynx and stomach → After (1) or (2). oral or nasal endotracheal intubation plus PPV plus gastric tube placement → Perhaps surfactant lavage (rarely indicated in the NICU; not in the delivery room, not evidence-based)
• Choanal atresia (see p. 432)	• Pink when crying, blue when quiet	→ Head in sniffing position, insert oral Guedel tube or LMA, oral endotracheal intubation and gastric tube placement
• Malformation of upper (pharyngeal) airways	• Persistent sternal and intercostal retractions, hardly any air movement/pulmonary air entry, or inspiratory stridor	→ Head in sniffing position, jaw thrust (Esmarch's grip), prone or lateral positioning may improve breathing. Oral Guedel tube, oro- or nasopharyngeal airway, pharyngeal CPAP/PPV, or LMA/PPV. May attempt endotracheal intubation. Gastric tube placement
Impaired lung function		
• Pneumothorax (see p. 410)	• High PIP was or is now needed • Breath sounds decreased or absent on the affected side, falling S_pO_2 • Possible circulatory decompensation/cardiac arrest (tension pneumothorax) • Distended abdomen	→ Transillumination and chest X-ray (AP view, cross-table lateral view, lateral decubitus view) only if vital signs stable (i.e., DO NOT DELAY pleural puncture in suspected tension pneumothorax) → Emergency pleural puncture with 21–24 G butterfly needle or angiocath (above the rib at 4th or 5th intercostal space in anterior axillary line, i.e., approx. 0.5 cm above the intermammillary line, or at 2nd or 3rd intercostal space in midclavicular line). Use stopcock and two 2-ml syringes for decompression. → Place chest tube and connect to water seal ± suction (−2 to −5 to max. −10 cmH$_2$O)
• Pleural effusions/ascites (see, p. 427; hydrops)	• Decreased breath sounds on affected side/decreased bowel sounds and distended abdomen • Persistent cyanosis, bradycardia • Oliguria in severe ascites • With additional pericardial effusion: distant or absent heart sounds, jugular vein distension, hepatomegaly, tachycardia	→ Pleural puncture and drainage (above the rib at 4th or 5th in middle or posterior axillary line and above the intermammillary line) → Drain ascites: for situs solitus in left lower quadrant, under ultrasound guidance. Do not remove more than 10 ml/kg at once. Consider volume replacement (if volume depletion likely, start IV replacement prior to drainage). Consider diuretics in NICU

- Congenital diaphragmatic hernia (CDH) (see, p. 404)

  • Asymmetrical breath sounds and chest rise
  • Decreased breath sounds ± bowel sounds on affected side
  • Sunken abdomen on affected side (cannot palpate spleen in left CDH)
  • Persistent bradycardia and/or cyanosis

  → Avoid bag-and-mask PPV
  → Immediate endotracheal intubation (first 30 s after birth), F_{O_2} 0.7–1.0 (PPHN), monitor pre- and postductal S_pO_2 and ABG, place gastric tube. In NICU, consider surfactant, HFOV, iNO (?), ECMO

- Pneumonia/sepsis (see, p. 280)

  • Often decreased bowel sounds, not always fine pulmonary crackles (amniotic fluid vs. infiltrate?), persistent pallor/cyanosis/bradycardia

  → Endotracheal intubation/PPV if indicated, then place gastric tube.
  → Volume IV (NS or Ringer's lactate, eventually PRBC)
  → CBC, CRP, IL-6, blood culture, ABG
  → 2–3 antibiotics IV

Impaired cardiovascular function

- Congenital heart disease (CHD) (see, p. 340)

  • Pallor or cyanosis
  • Capillary refill >2 s
  • Decreased or absent peripheral pulses
  • Symptoms most often observed outside the delivery room
  • The very young newborn who exhibits severe cyanosis (but has normal lung function) is likely to have one of the following: d-TGA, pulmonary atresia/IVS, or Ebstein's malformation[172]

  → Diagnostic work-up: BP and SpO2 at all 4 extremities, ECHO, ECG, chest X-ray,
  → When duct-dependent heart disease is suspected (and PPHN unlikely), start prostaglandin E1 (alprostadil) IV
  → Consider careful volume replacement IV; inotropic drugs are rarely needed
  → No oxygen supplementation in newborns with suspected duct-dependent systemic perfusion (e.g., HLHS) or d-TGA

- Fetal-maternal blood loss (see p. 304, algorithm for hemorrhage)

  • Severe pallor
  • No or weak response to resuscitation measures

  → ABCD measures
  → Repetitive volume replacement: NS or Ringer's lactate 10 ml/kg q 5–10 min IV
  → Give PRBC (O Rhesus negative) ASAP: in hemorrhagic shock, give 5 ml PRBC/kg in 10–15 min IV, then 5–10 ml PRBC/kg/h. If vital signs acceptable, give 3 ml PRBC/kg/h IV

- Cardiac arrhythmia (see, p. 325, algorithms)

  • Pallor (rarely cyanosis), tachypnea plus arrhythmia (see below)

  1. Sinus bradycardia

  → ABCD measures, ECG monitoring, 12-lead and right precordial ECG. Bradycardia often in the context of secondary (terminal) apnea or vagal stimulation (early deep suctioning)
  → ABCD measures, especially PPV, consider atropine 0.03 mg/kg/dose IV (minimum 0.1 mg IV)

  2. Second- or third degree heart block (AV block) with decreased cardiac function

  → ABCD measures, if epinephrine 0.01 mg/kg/dose ineffective → Atropine 0.03 mg/kg/dose IV (minimum 0.1 mg IV)

Table 2.9 (cont.)

Problem	Previous (preliminary) information/clinical signs	Decision and action
	3. Supraventricular tachycardia (SVT)	→ ABCD measures → Vagal stimulation (controversial, e.g., ice pad onto face), if ineffective → Adenosine (0.1 mg/kg/dose fast push IV, PIV right arm or central line; double dose and repeat if unsuccessful), if ineffective or unstable proceed to electric cardioversion (DCCV) → Cardioversion (0.5–1 J/kg/dose)
	4. Multiple ventricular ectopic beats (VEB), ventricular tachycardia (VTach) or flutter (VFlu) or ventricular fibrillation (VFib)	→ ABCD measures → For multiple VEB and VTach: amiodarone 5 mg/kg/loading dose in 30 min IV or lidocaine 1 mg/kg/loading dose IV → For VTach (or VFlu) with pulses and poor perfusion: cardioversion (0.5–1 J/kg/dose), if ineffective 2 J/kg/dose → For VFib or pulseless VTach: immediate defibrillation 2 J/kg/dose, if ineffective 4 J/kg/dose. Consider amiodarone or lidocaine loading dose after second shock with 4 J/kg/dose

! The key to successful neonatal resuscitation is establishment of adequate ventilation.

! Oxygen blenders, pulse oximeters, and pressure manometers are standard equipment in the delivery room.

New ILCOR recommendations on neonatal resuscitation at birth (2005)[22,103]

Ventilation strategies

The ILCOR consensus on science document concluded that *"When performed properly, positive pressure ventilation alone is effective for resuscitating almost all apneic or bradycardic newborn infants (level of evidence, LOE 5)[109]. The primary measure of adequate initial ventilation is prompt improvement in heart rate (LOE 6)[110,111,112]."* The resulting treatment recommendation was *"Establishing effective ventilation is the primary objective in the management of the apneic or bradycardic newborn infant in the delivery room. In the bradycardic infant, prompt improvement in heart rate is the primary measure of adequate initial ventilation; chest wall movement should be assessed if heart rate does not improve. Initial peak inflating pressures necessary to achieve an increase in heart rate or movement of the chest are variable and unpredictable and should be individualized with each breath. If pressure is being monitored, an initial inflation pressure of $20\,cmH_2O$ may be effective, but a pressure ≥ 30 to $40\,cmH_2O$ may be necessary in some term babies. If pressure is not being monitored, the minimal inflation required to achieve an increase in heart rate should be used. There is insufficient evidence to recommend optimal initial or subsequent inflation times."*

Air or oxygen for resuscitation at birth?

There is growing evidence that babies can be resuscitated as effectively at birth using air as with 100% oxygen. There are also increasing concerns that high concentrations of oxygen, even if only applied for a short time, can have detrimental effects[4,7,113]. The most recent ILCOR recommendation is as follows: *"There is currently insufficient evidence to specify the concentration of oxygen to be used at initiation of resuscitation. After initial steps at birth, if respiratory efforts are absent or inadequate, lung inflation/ventilation should be the priority. Once adequate ventilation is established, if the heart rate remains low, there is no evidence to support or refute a change in the oxygen concentration that was initiated. Rather the priority should be to support cardiac output with chest compressions and coordinated ventilations. Supplementary oxygen should be considered for babies with persistent central cyanosis."*

Peripartum management of meconium?

A multi-center randomized controlled trial published in 2000 showed that immediate intubation and suctioning of the airways of *vigorous* term infants born through meconium-stained fluid of any consistency did not reduce the incidence or meconium aspiration syndrome or other respiratory problems. A further multi-center randomized controlled trial published in 2004 has shown that, in the presence of meconium-stained fluid, attempts to clear the airway of the term baby before delivery of the shoulders, so-called intra-partum suctioning, did not reduce the incidence of meconium aspiration syndrome. The most recent ILCOR recommendation is as follows: *"Meconium-stained, depressed infants should receive tracheal suctioning immediately after birth and before stimulation, presuming the equipment and expertise is available. Tracheal suctioning is not necessary for babies with meconium-stained fluid who are vigorous."*

Confirmation of tracheal tube placement

Carbon dioxide detectors can be very useful to confirm correct placement of the tracheal tube, especially in babies who do not immediately respond to lung inflation via the tube with an increase in heart rate. With low or absent cardiac output, however, there might be little endtidal CO_2 despite successful endotracheal intubation.

Laryngeal mask airways (LMA)

These have been successfully used in resuscitation of term babies and in the stabilization of preterm babies at birth. However, there is insufficient evidence to recommend their use as a primary airway device in newborn resuscitation.

Epinephrine (adrenaline)

Despite the absence of evidence of the effectiveness of epinephrine in resuscitation of the human newborn, ILCOR still recommends the use of intravenous epinephrine should adequate lung inflation followed by adequate chest compressions fail to restore a normal heart rate at birth. The recommended intravenous dose is 10–30 µg/kg (0.01–0.03 mg/kg). Pediatric and animal studies suggest that higher doses intravenously are harmful.

Animal studies suggest that this dose given via the trachea is unlikely to be effective. For tracheal administration consider using a higher dose – up to 100 µg/kg (0.1 mg/kg). However, neither the safety nor the efficacy of these higher tracheal doses in babies have been studied.

Intravascular volume expansion

For reasons of cost and theoretical risks (infection, anaphylaxis), isotonic crystalloid rather than albumin should be used if volume expansion is considered urgent and suitable blood (PRBC) is not immediately available.

Naloxone

Naloxone should *not* be considered a resuscitation drug. In a sick baby the heart rate and oxygenation should be improved by supporting ventilation before naloxone is given.

Temperature control in preterm infants

When stabilizing the very small preterm baby at birth, covering the baby up to the neck in food-grade plastic whilst under a radiant heater is more effective at maintaining body temperature than more traditional methods.

Therapeutic hypothermia in asphyxiated term infants

A number of randomized studies of various means of cooling symptomatic asphyxiated term infants have suggested that the babies cooled by 3–4°C (i.e., to 33.5–34.0°C) for up to 72 h after a hypoxic-ischemic insult may have a better neurological outcome. However, ILCOR found that there are, as yet, insufficient data to recommend routine use of this approach and that further clinical trials are needed to confirm that cooling is beneficial, to identify infants who will benefit most, and to determine the most effective method and timing of cooling. However, we feel the current clinical data strongly indicate a consistent, robust beneficial effect of therapeutic hypothermia for neonatal post-resuscitation encephalopathy[104]. Thus we advocate for therapeutic hypothermia in clinical practice provided the practitioner follows the protocol of one of the published trials[114]. Many remaining questions on therapeutic hypothermia have to be answered in the coming years.

Withholding or discontinuing resuscitation

The ILCOR group statement is reproduced below. The authors of this book would like to draw attention to the fact that ILCOR felt it is important to state that these guidelines should be, "interpreted according to current regional outcomes and societal principles." In other words the gestation and birthweight "cut-offs" used as examples in this statement may reasonably be varied in accordance with varying survival and outcome in different countries.

"A consistent and coordinated approach to individual cases by obstetric and neonatal teams and parents is an important goal. Not starting resuscitation and discontinuation of life-sustaining treatment during or following resuscitation are ethically equivalent and clinicians should not be hesitant to withdraw support when functional survival is highly unlikely. **The following guidelines must be interpreted according to current regional outcomes and societal principles**.

- Where gestation, birth weight, and/or congenital anomalies are associated with almost certain early death, and an unacceptably high morbidity is likely among the rare survivors, resuscitation is not indicated. Examples from the published literature from developed countries include:
- Extreme prematurity (gestational age <23 weeks and/or birthweight <400 g)
- Anomalies such as anencephaly and confirmed Trisomy 13 or 18
- In conditions associated with a high rate of survival and acceptable morbidity, resuscitation is nearly always indicated
- In conditions associated with uncertain prognosis, where there is borderline survival and a relatively high rate of morbidity, and where the burden to the child is high, the parents' views on starting resuscitation should be supported"

If there are no signs of life after 10 minutes of *continuous and adequate resuscitation efforts*, it *may* be justifiable to stop resuscitation.

Special situations in the delivery room
(see Table 2.9.)

Meconium (see also p. 269)

A large randomized trial has shown that elective intubation of **vigorous** meconium-stained babies in an effort to remove meconium from the airways does not reduce the incidence of meconium aspiration syndrome (MAS)[24]. In a large randomized trial on newborns with meconium-stained amniotic fluid (MSAF) that was mainly conducted in Argentina, suctioning of the nose and mouth before delivery of the shoulders did not reduce the incidence of MAS and neonatal mortality among the enrolled babies[21]. Although the ILCOR (2005) no longer recommends intrapartum suctioning for babies with MSAF, it is questionable whether the findings of a single trial[21] should be applied to countries with more or different resources, or whether obstetricians should commence with intrapartum suctioning of meconium stained babies until further evidence becomes available[114]. This controversial point is open to debate.

It seems reasonable, however, to attempt to clear particulate meconium from the oropharynx of any meconium-stained baby who is not vigorous (i.e., depressed) at birth.

It seems equally reasonable to attempt to clear the trachea of such babies immediately after birth should appropriate skills and equipment be available.

Congenital malformations

(See also scenario chapters and Table 2.9.)

Congenital malformations are not a significant concern in relation to resuscitation at birth and the presence of a malformation usually does not increase the risk of hypoxic-ischemic stress in labor above that of any other baby. Many significant malformations are diagnosed before delivery allowing one to make appropriate plans for their management.

Malformations of the face and airways can cause problems within minutes of birth. Babies with bilateral choanal atresia or severe Pierre Robin syndrome are unlikely to have been diagnosed antenatally and may have difficulties maintaining an open airway – in either case placing an oro- or nasopharyngeal airway or LMA will help.

For congenital diaphragmatic hernia, congenital heart disease and hydrops, see Table 2.9 and separate scenario chapters.

Stabilizing the preterm baby

It is traditional to refer to the pediatric ministrations at the delivery of a significantly preterm baby as "resuscitation." However, this process should be more honestly referred to as "stabilization" given that one is much more likely to be providing careful handling ("minimal handling"), prophylaxis, and gentle support to an otherwise healthy but fragile baby, than undertaking life-saving interventions in a baby on the point of death (see p. 231).

The principles of management are exactly the same as for the more mature baby but with a few minor modifications as follows:

1. *Temperature*: In very small babies ($\leq$30 weeks' gestation) maintaining their body temperature is probably more effectively achieved by placing the baby up to the neck in a food-grade plastic bag under a radiant heater, than the more traditional approach of drying them and placing them under a radiant heater[116]. If the preterm is placed in a bag then drying is unnecessary.

2. *Avoid insufficient inflation and over-distension of the lungs*: The lungs of very preterm babies are more fragile and less compliant than at term. Repeated over-distension followed by collapse and re-expansion will damage lung tissue leading to inflammation, which may further progress to bronchopulmonary dysplasia. Consider initiating CPAP in the spontaneously breathing infant. If needed, gently inflate the lungs, perhaps starting with lower inflation pressures than used with term infants; avoid excessive chest wall excursions and use PEEP.

3. *Consider early administration of surfactant*: Administration of surfactant obviously requires intubation and there is some advantage in early administration. A degree of experience and skill is required to ensure that intubation does not cause additional trauma and hypoxia. Each neonatal unit should have its own policy as to exactly which babies should be routinely intubated at birth for this purpose, and by whom.

Babies who do not respond to resuscitation measures (see Table 2.9)

The most common reason for a baby's failing to respond to resuscitation at birth is failure to inflate the lungs due to inadequate management of the airway. If you are not achieving good lung inflation using a mask, and you are unable to intubate, then it is worth running through this checklist:

- Is the baby's head in the neutral position?
- Do you need to provide jaw thrust?
- Would it help to use a longer inflation time or a higher inflation pressure?
- Do you need a second person's help with the airway (mask, ET tube)?
- Could there be an obstruction in the oropharynx?
- Would an oropharyngeal airway (Guedel) help?

Blocked lower airway

If you are unable to inflate the lungs despite using high pressures via a well fitting tracheal tube then consider whether there might be impacted debris within the trachea, perhaps thick mucus, blood clot, vernix or meconium. If you apply suction to the tracheal tube while you remove it you may be able to remove the obstruction either by sucking it into the tracheal tube or by pulling it out of the trachea attached by suction to the end of the tube.

The baby who remains blue

If the baby remains blue despite adequate ventilation and with a normal heart rate then consider the possibility of persistent pulmonary hypertension of the newborn (PPHN). In this condition blood "bypasses" the lungs (via right-to-left atrial and/or ductal shunting exacerbated by V/Q mismatch) because of increased pulmonary vascular resistance, inadequate lung inflation, poor left ventricular function or a mixture of these causes. The remedy is adequate oxygenation and ventilation, inotropic support and, occasionally, pulmonary vasodilatation. Other less common possibilities include the various types of cyanotic congenital heart disease.

The baby who remains very pale

Very rarely the baby may have suffered an acute blood loss around the time of delivery. This can be caused by a number of rare situations such as ruptured vasa praevia, bleeding into the baby's own abdomen from damage to the liver or spleen, bleeding across the placenta into the maternal circulation, partial occlusion of the umbilical cord in such a way as to allow blood from the baby to continue to be pumped to the placenta but sufficient to obstruct the return flow into the baby via the umbilical vein. If the baby is severely hypovolemic then it may show persistent bradycardia – see p. 304. In less severe cases the baby will be likely to be pale and both tachypneic and tachycardic. Immediate volume replacement using normal saline should then be followed later by an appropriate blood transfusion. Of note, severe perinatal hypoxia without hemorrhage may lead to significant vasoconstriction, volume shift towards the placenta and hypovolemia in the newborn.

Pneumothorax

Spontaneous pneumothorax can occur but these are very seldom severe enough to cause problems in the delivery room. They normally reveal themselves later as a tachypneic baby with a significant oxygen requirement. Asymptomatic pneumothorax occurs in 1%–2% of neonates. The rate of pneumothoraces in preterm infants with respiratory distress syndrome ranges between 3% and 10%[117]. Upon PPV more than 10% of newborn infants may develop a pneumothorax (see also p. 410).

Baby affected by opiates administered to the mother

Opiates are often used for pain relief in labor. If maternal blood levels are sufficiently high the baby may have significant respiratory depression as a result. What usually happens is the baby responds normally and establishes breathing at delivery because of all the stimulation the baby is receiving at this moment, but the baby then becomes apneic when wrapped up warm and "secure" a few minutes later. In this situation the immediate response should be the standard ABC of resuscitation. Once appropriate skin color (pink trunk) and good heart rate are achieved by appropriate resuscitation, and the airway is secured (usually endotracheal intubation, or LMA), the baby should be transferred to the NICU (continuous monitoring). Only then is it the time to consider giving the competitive opioid receptor antagonist naloxone (rule out prepartal maternal IV or oral methadone use before administering naloxone). See also chapter on psychoactive substances p. 322. **Because of the risk of inducing neonatal opioid withdrawal by giving naloxone to a depressed baby s/p prenatal long-term opioid exposure, ILCOR 2005 states:**

> *"Naloxone is not recommended as part of the initial resuscitation of newborns with respiratory depression in the delivery room. . . . There is no evidence to support or refute the current dose of 0.1 mg/kg IV or IM."*

! To date, there is no evidence that **naloxone** reduces the indication for mechanical ventilation or intensive care in neonates. According to a Cochrane meta-analysis (2002), naloxone merely improves ventilation[118].

Postnatal presentations of newborn infants in the delivery room

Newly born infants, just seconds after birth, can be classified roughly into five groups[17].

1. The healthy, vigorous/active and well-perfused newborn infant

Clinical presentation

Good respiratory excursions/normal respiratory rate 40–50 breaths/min, heart rate >100 bpm, skin color mostly rosy (trunk), adequate muscle tone/moves all four extremities, 1-min Apgar score 7–10, usually umbilical arterial pH >7.2.

Management

- *Amniotic fluid is clear of meconium, skin is not stained with meconium, no meconium or blood/viscous mucus in the upper or lower respiratory tract*
  - No need for advanced treatment. Leave neonate mostly alone, i.e., suction only as indicated (if plenty of amniotic fluid in the oropharynx), dry/stimulate, keep warm, give baby to the mother, assess 10-min Apgar score, measure birth weight. Some centers pass a gastric tube prior to the first feeding. Vitamin K and hepatitis B vaccination on the first day of life (or prior to discharge depending on unit policy)
- *Meconium-stained amniotic fluid (MSAF) and/or newborn's skin stained with meconium and/or meconium or blood/viscous mucus found in the upper respiratory tract, however the neonate is vigorous and active with HR >100 bpm and making good respiratory efforts*
  - If the neonate is obviously vigorous and active, and if the upper respiratory tract is clear of meconium, then there is no indication for intubation/PPV, endotracheal suctioning or lavage[24]. Provide oropharyngeal suctioning, dry/stimulate, keep warm,

oxygen supplementation only if indicated, diagnostic work-up if necessary. Give the stable newborn to the mother, and consider continuous pulse oximetry and documenting S_pO_2 at intervals. Assess 10-min Apgar score, obtain weight. Some centers pass a gastric tube prior to the first feeding. Vitamin K and hepatitis B vaccination on the first day of life (or prior to discharge depending on unit policy).

2. The apneic or irregularly breathing newborn with good heart rate (likely primary apnea)

Clinical presentation
Apneic for 30 s to 2 min, then under stimulation, gasping/grunting, improving skin color, HR >80 bpm (with stimulation in first 30 s quickly >100 bpm), 1-min Apgar score approximately 4–6, umbilical arterial pH value >7.00.

Management
- *Term, eutrophic (appropriate for gestational age, AGA) neonate (37–42 weeks of gestation)*
  - Suction, dry, stimulate breathing. Supplement oxygen under S_pO_2 monitoring only if persistently cyanotic (aim for room air with certain heart defects). Keep warm, diagnostic work-up as needed. Give stable neonate with S_pO_2 monitoring to the mother, assess 10-min Apgar score, get weight. Some centers pass a gastric tube prior to the first feeding. Vitamin K and hepatitis B vaccination on the first day of life (or prior to discharge depending on unit policy)
- *Preterm infant (<37 weeks of gestation) or SGA (birth weight <10th percentile)*
  - Suction, dry, stimulate breathing. Supplement oxygen under S_pO_2 monitoring only if indicated, keep warm. Controversy exists over whether preterm infants of <30 weeks' gestation should be primarily intubated (followed by surfactant administration and extubation as soon as possible) or first ventilated by bag-and-mask PPV or pharyngeal-PPV followed by CPAP (if surfactant is indicated later on, proceed to intubation). Preterm infants <28 0/7 weeks of gestation benefit from early, so-called prophylactic endotracheal surfactant administration, i.e., 0–30 (–60) min after birth
  - Determine arterial (or capillary) blood gas and blood glucose approximately 30 min after birth (or earlier). If preterm infant is stable, transfer to high observation nursery (monitoring) or NICU. Some centers pass a gastric tube prior to the first feeding. Vitamin K and hepatitis B vaccination on the first day of life (or prior to discharge depending on unit policy)

3. The newborn with obviously delayed or insufficient cardiopulmonary adaptation (probably secondary = "terminal" apnea s/p severe perinatal hypoxia)

Incidence
- 0.2%–0.5% of all births

Clinical presentation
Apnea, bradycardia (HR <100 bpm, mostly <80 bpm and not rising), generalized cyanosis or more often pallor, 1-min Apgar score 0–3, usually umbilical arterial pH <7.00.

> **!** It's common that severely depressed ("asphyxic") newly born infants turn pink under bag-and-mask ventilation before spontaneous breathing occurs (unless they belong to the "problem group" of neonates described below), and that the severity of perinatal hypoxia (and postnatal prognosis) is indicated by the time lapsed until spontaneous breathing is observed under PPV[17].

Management

Quick but efficient suctioning (even endotracheal, if indicated), bag-and-mask ventilation or immediate intubation (aim for intubation 30–60 s after birth) followed by PPV via ET tube. If HR remains <60 bpm despite 30 s of efficient PPV, perform chest compression and PPV (3:1 ratio, 120 events per minute). Intubate at this point if you have not yet done so. Assistant inserts PIV or UV catheter (preferable) as soon as possible. If after 30 s of chest compressions/PPV the HR remains below 60 bpm, administer epinephrine (1:10 000) 0.1 ml/kg/dose IV (= 0.01 mg/kg/dose IV) via UV catheter or PIV, or give epinephrine (1:10 000) 0.3–1 ml/kg/dose ET (= 0.03–0.1 mg/kg/dose ET), and resume chest compressions/PPV. If indicated, repeat and increase single epinephrine dose (maximum 0.03 mg/kg/dose IV = 0.3 ml/kg/dose IV), give volume with the second epinephrine dose (normal saline 10 ml/kg/dose IV), and determine (preferably arterial) blood gas and blood glucose. Consider sodium bicarbonate IV or THAM in severe acidosis; when stable, transfer to NICU.

4. Stillbirth

Def.

Both *miscarriage* and *stillbirth* are terms describing pregnancy loss (fetal death), but they differ according to when the loss occurs. The distinction between both is arbitrary. The dividing line is variously set at 20 (USA) to 24 (UK) weeks of gestation in different countries (see Table 1.2 for abbreviations and definitions). Before that time it is a miscarriage (also called "spontaneous abortion"); after that time it is a stillbirth. If the gestational age is unknown or unclear, then countries register these fetal deaths as stillbirth if the birthweight is above 350 g (USA), 400 g (Australia) or 500 g (Canada).

Management

- *If the decision to resuscitate has been made*
  - Suctioning (even tracheal, if needed), immediate intubation (during the first minute postnatal). If a heart beat was recorded 10 min before birth, call for the second physician, start chest compressions and PPV (3:1) until HR >60 bpm. If after 30 s of chest compressions/PPV the HR remains below 60 bpm, administer epinephrine (1:10 000) 0.1 ml/kg/dose IV (= 0.01 mg/kg/dose IV) via PIV or UVC, or give epinephrine (1:10 000) 0.3–1 ml/kg/dose ET (= 0.03–0.1 mg/kg/dose ET), and resume chest compressions/PPV. If indicated, repeat and increase single epinephrine dose (maximum: 0.03 mg/kg/dose IV = 0.3 ml/kg/dose IV), give volume with second epinephrine dose (NS 10 ml/kg/dose IV), determine (preferably arterial) blood gas and blood glucose. Consider sodium bicarbonate IV or THAM in severe acidosis; when stable, transfer to NICU
- If a heart beat is not clearly recorded more than 10 min (ILCOR 2005) after birth, do not continue any further therapy (this interval may be extended to 30 min in certain

circumstances); see "Ethical aspects of neonatal resuscitation and postresuscitation care" below, see also p. 172 and "Ethics in neonatal intensive care," p. 184

- Withdraw or withhold therapy? See "Ethics in neonatal intensive care," p. 184
- Redirection of care? See also "Ethics in neonatal intensive care," p. 184
- Talk to the parents

5. "Problem group": newborn infants who do not adequately respond to PPV, chest compressions and/or epinephrine
See Standard algorithm, Figure 2.38, and Table 2.9.

Possible causes

- Technical errors (handling, equipment, esophageal intubation)
- *Severe perinatal asphyxia*, i.e., cyanosis, bradycardia, and unconsciousness even 5–10 min after birth (cause: e.g., severe intrauterine hypoxia, hemorrhagic shock)
- Critically ill neonate with underlying *severe lung disease* (hypoplasia/dysplasia, congenital diaphragmatic hernia, respiratory distress syndrome in ELBW preterm infants, meconium aspiration, congenital pneumonia/sepsis, etc.)
- *Pneumothorax* (see p. 410)
- Differential diagnosis (see Table 2.9, pp. 160–2)
  - Upper respiratory tract (choanal atresia, Pierre Robin's sequence, laryngotracheal malformations)
  - Lungs (hypoplasia, pleural effusions with/without hydrops, congenital malformation, pneumothorax, etc.)
  - Cardiovascular system (e.g., cyanotic heart disease – rarely symptomatic in the delivery room)
  - Other extrapulmonary causes (congenital diaphragmatic hernia, tumors, hepatosplenomegaly, ascites, etc.)
- The neonate is apneic due to *neuromuscular or central nervous disease* (seldom). Clinical presentation: persistent apnea and poor muscle tone with good heart rate (HR >100 bpm)
- Think of maternal narcotic drugs, especially when there are no signs of asphyxia, mother received opioids in the last 4 h before delivery, and newborn became apneic after initial breathing efforts. Caution: secure airway (intubation, LMA), transfer to NICU, get proper history (rule out maternal IV drug use, PO methadone, etc.), and then consider naloxone 0.1 mg/kg IV.

! The delivery room is not the place to get overly ambitious. Drugs – aside from oxygen – are rarely needed for the resuscitation of neonates at birth. The *quality* of neonatal resuscitation and transport comes first, "*speed*" comes second. Provide "minimal handling" whenever possible. However, the newly born infant is endangered especially by the **7 "H"**: hypothermia, hyperthermia, hypotension, hypoxia, hyperoxia, hypocarbia, and hypoglycemia. Fast and focused therapy in the delivery room lowers these 7 "H-risks" and shortens the time spent in the delivery room (*"The Golden Hour After Birth"*).

! When the baby is stable → rapid transport. No out-of hospital transfer without functional IV line ($D_{5-10}W$ infusion)

Performing excellent neonatal resuscitation in a stressful environment

The resuscitation of a newly born infant is often performed under very emotional circumstances and in a stressful environment. The parents had imagined the birth of their child as being completely different, and now find themselves with an emergency team they hardly know. Even the experienced health care provider (MD, NP, RN) in charge may not be free from stress. However, the outcome of resuscitated neonates is better than that of any other age group. Moreover, newly born infants can be resuscitated efficiently under unfavorable circumstances – with room air and, if necessary, with fluids and drugs that are available in every hospital (epinephrine, normal saline; consider sodium bicarbonate). Keep calm, foresee problems! Clearly say what you want to happen and what not. The motto should be: the worse the condition of the child, the more collegial the team work, and the more direct and uncomplicated the tone of the conversations!

Ethical aspects of neonatal resuscitation and post-resuscitation care

The question as to when and whether resuscitation should be initiated in the delivery room is a very complex matter and cannot be sufficiently discussed here (see p. 184). It is especially difficult when conflict arises and the parents' wishes differ from the neonatologist's or the emergency doctor's evaluation of the patient. We therefore dedicate a separate chapter to the ethical issues in neonatal resuscitation and post-resuscitation care (see p. 184).

Information obtained prior to or during neonatal resuscitation may not be reliable, e.g., a newborn infant may be "asystolic" for more than 10 min according to the obstetrician or "first responder," but actually, the very gentle heart beats (e.g., in pericardial effusion, situs inversus), were missed and the pulse not palpated. If in this situation PPV/chest compressions are performed sufficiently prior to arrival of the neonatology or NETS-teams, the outcome (neonatal mortality, long-term neurological outcome) is not necessarily poor. Resuscitation efforts should then be optimized and continued.

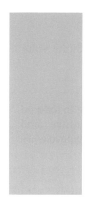

Volume therapy and sodium bicarbonate supplementation in preterm and term newborn infants

Georg Hansmann

There is hardly any other topic in the field of neonatal intensive care that bears such controversy.

- When (indication)? How much fluid (5, 10, 20 ml/kg IV)? Crystalloid or colloid solutions? How fast (bolus, in 10, 30, 60, 120 min?)
- When (indication)? How much sodium bicarbonate? How fast (bolus, in 10, 30, 60, 120 min)?

Pathophysiology[15]

Cardiac output principally is determined by all four of the following components: heart rate (main regulator in neonates), stroke volume, preload ($\approx$ end-diastolic volume of the ventricle; or simplified as $\approx$ intravascular volume) and afterload ($\approx$ combination of elastance of the great vessels, resistance of the small vessels, and ventricular wall stress).

In neonates, a low heart rate (HR <100 bpm) usually indicates respiratory failure and/or hemodynamic compromise. After birth, pulmonary vascular resistance (PVR) remains high whereas systemic arterial resistance (SVR) is low but starts rising when the umbilical cord is clamped.

The blood volume of a term neonate ranges between 80 and 85 ml/kg, in preterm infants between 90 and 100 ml/kg. Thus, administration of 50 ml volume IV given to a term newborn infant (body weight $\approx$ 3 kg) is equivalent to one-fifth of the intravascular volume (relative amount even higher in significant hypovolemia)! This will have notable impact on the hematocrit and hemoglobin value due to dilution effects (normal: 45%–60% and 14–20 g/dl, respectively). Oxygen delivery to the peripheral tissue and vital organs (brain, heart, kidneys) depends on perfusion pressure, total intravascular hemoglobin, and oxygenation (F_iO_2, lung function).

Shock with signs of peripheral hypoperfusion occurs, either because of significant intrauterine blood loss (e.g., placental abruption, placental anomaly, very large cephalohematoma, intracranial hemorrhage, twin – twin or feto – maternal transfusion syndrome) or severe perinatal hypoxia (e.g., nuchal cord, placental insufficiency, low cardiac output, e.g., third-degree AV block) or hypovolemia, with subsequent vasoconstriction and volume shift to the placenta (hypoxia $\rightarrow$ hypovolemia).

Goals of volume therapy

The aim of every volume therapy is to maintain adequate preload without accumulation of interstitial fluid (edema). Of note, the circulating blood volume may be low even in patients

Neonatal Emergencies: A Practical Guide for Resuscitation, Transport and Critical Care, ed. Georg Hansmann.
Published by Cambridge University Press. © Cambridge University Press 2009.

with peripheral or pulmonary edema, therefore edema per se does not indicate volume overload.

> **!** In an emergency, it is extremely difficult to distinguish low cardiac output due to reduced myocardial contractility associated with high end-diastolic ventricular pressure (and volume) from low cardiac output because of insufficient preload (primary hypovolemia; Frank–Starling curve shifted to the left)[15].

Therefore, in a severely depressed newborn infant, volume therapy (normal saline, packed red blood cells) as well as positive inotropic drugs (initially epinephrine, then for example dopamine ± milrinone) will be applied.

> **!** In a state of poor peripheral perfusion and shock (tissue malperfusion, hypoxia → suspicion of lactic acidosis), adequate volume therapy is often sufficient to restore proper circulation and will improve acidosis, so that buffer therapy may be omitted.

Crystalloid solutions
Normal saline
Crystalloids, such as normal saline, remain in the intravascular space for a short period before diffusing into the interstitial space (25% intravascular for 1–2 h; intravascular half-life approx. 30 min). Crystalloids only have a short-lived effect on the systemic perfusion, however they provide other advantages: electrolytes are substituted, there is no risk of anaphylaxis and infection, and costs are low. The benefit of Ringer's lactate solution is that it contains less sodium than normal saline. Hypo-osmolar solutions, such as D_5W and $D_{10}W$, remain intravascular for a short time and are not appropriate for volume expansion since they can cause dangerous intracerebral volume shifts.

Colloid solutions
Human albumin (5%)
Colloid solutions, such as human albumin 5% remain in the intravascular space for hours and therefore rapidly support the systemic blood pressure; however, they may also lead to peripheral/pulmonary edema in the long run, due to late diffusion into the interstitium where they increase oncotic pressure. This should be taken into account, especially with respect to the lungs (interstitial pulmonary edema), when endothelial dysfunction and increased vascular permeability is likely (e.g., sepsis → capillary leak). Further adverse effects of human albumin solutions are hypocalcemia, coagulation disorders and platelet dysfunction, as well as a higher risk for anaphylaxis and infections when compared to crystalloid solutions.

The risk of platelet dysfunction and a relative high risk for anaphylaxis excludes HAES (6% hydroxyethyl starch (HES 200/0.5) in isotonic sodium chloride solution) and dextran solutions from their use in the first month (first year?) of life (limited data available).

> ⚠ The ILCOR guidelines 2005[22] recommend only epinephrine (adrenaline) and volume therapy (normal saline, packed red blood cells) for the resuscitation of newborn infants. Colloid solutions that contain albumin (serum protein solutions or 5% human albumin) are not recommended for the resuscitation of newly born infants (infection risk, eventually higher mortality).

Procedures

If the neonate has poor peripheral perfusion (capillary refill >2 s with cyanotic or pale-grayish skin color, weak or absent pulse, MAP <40 mmHg), but is otherwise vigorous with S_aO_2 $>70\%$ and HR >100 bpm, then proceed as follows:

- Normal saline solution:
  - 10 ml/kg over 30–60 min IV (may give over 60–120 min in preterm infants)
  - Repeat volume as needed

> ⚠ Be sure not to use colloid solutions (serum protein solution, human albumin) – particularly when infection/sepsis is suspected (caution: capillary leakage/"third spacing").

During the resuscitation of a neonate (e.g., shock/bradycardia, no pulse, MAP <25 mmHg in a term neonate), status post feto-maternal *bleeding* (abruptio placentae), proceed as follows:

- 10–20 ml/kg in 5–10 min IV
- In preterm infants (especially with body weight <1500 g) cautiously start with 10 ml/kg in 10–30 min IV
- Repeat volume, as indicated, after 5–10 min
- Give packed red blood cells (O Rhesus negative) early if hemorrhagic shock is likely (see the following section)

Blood transfusion (packed red blood cells)

> ⚠ After an episode of significant bleeding and an initial hematocrit (Hct) of $<35\%$ ($<40\%$ in a patient with cyanotic heart disease; always determine Hct prior to volume therapy), blood transfusion is indicated. Packed red blood cell (PRBC) transfusion is sometimes required in the delivery room, e.g., in life-threatening hemorrhagic shock (ensure availability of type-O, Rhesus-negative, lysine-free PRBC at adequate temperature). Caution: An acute bleeding episode may initially be accompanied by a normal Hct value.

Packed red blood cell transfusion

PRBC volume to be transfused in ml =
[(desired Hct – actual Hct) ÷ Hct of PRBC bag] × blood volume (ml) of the infant
  PRBC bag Hct: approx. 55%–60%
  Blood volume: for term neonates 80–85 ml/kg, for preterm infants 90–100 ml/kg

Calculation of PRBC volume useful in non-acute anemia (for hemorrhagic shock, see below and p. 304)

Remember: 1 ml PRBC/kg raises the Hct by approx. 1%, whereas 3 ml PRBC/kg raises the Hgb by approx. 1 g/dl. Before any blood transfusion, draw blood for blood typing of the infant.

PRBC transfusion rate

- In hemorrhagic shock 10 ml PRBC/kg in 10 min IV, followed by 5–10 ml/kg/h IV (caution: hyperkalemia, intracerebral hemorrhage, heart failure with rapid transfusion)
- Otherwise 3 ml PRBC/kg/h IV (no life-threatening emergency)

The indication for transfusion of preterm neonates is dependent on vital signs, age, and PPV/F_iO_2 requirements. If a coagulation disorder (±signs of active bleeding) is present, the transfusion of fresh frozen plasma (FFP) and platelets may be necessary.

Buffer solutions

The use of buffer solutions, such as 4.2% sodium bicarbonate (dilute 8.4% 1:1 with sterile water), is very restrictive, but indicated when resuscitation efforts are ineffective (severe acidosis reduces the effect of inotropes) and/or severe metabolic acidosis (e.g., sepsis, asphyxia, hypoplastic left heart syndrome), as well as heart disease (especially) with duct-dependent lung perfusion.

> ! Usually sodium bicarbonate should only be given when the pH is <7.20 and the base deficit is at least −10 mmol/l, and only when effective ventilation/oxygenation and volume therapy have not led to rapid improvement of arterial blood gases[17,120].

"Blind" use of buffer solutions is only legitimate when resuscitation is prolonged (>10 min ineffective administration of chest compressions/epinephrine) and a blood gas apparatus is not available. The correction of metabolic acidosis also improves the myocardial contractility and the effect of epinephrine, systemic and lung perfusion, movement of the diaphragm and surfactant synthesis, and reduces the work of breathing.

Hyperosmolarity (sodium) and volume expansion with risks of intraventricular hemorrhage (especially in preterm infants) and cerebral edema, intracellular acidosis, hypercarbia, poorer oxygenation of tissues, a decrease in PVR (may be deleterious in single ventricle and left ventricular outflow tract obstruction, e.g., hypoplastic left heart syndrome), tissue necrosis due to extravasations, hypokalemia, and hypocalcemia are disadvantages of IV use of sodium bicarbonate solutions[17,120,121].

8.4% Sodium bicarbonate (1 M)

(1 ml = 1 mmol = 1 mEq, 2000 mosm/l)

Indication

Consider buffer therapy with: pH <7.15 (<7.20), low standard bicarbonate, a base deficit of −10 mmol/l (or more negative) *and* $PaCO_2$ <60 mmHg (first blood gas usually is approx. 30 min postnatal; earlier during resuscitation).

> ❗ Under continuous buffer therapy, monitoring the status of pH, PCO_2, bicarbonate and base deficit should be performed regularly via blood gas sampling.

Administration of sodium bicarbonate infusion by syringe pump should be considered *after* effective ventilation, volume expansion, and blood gas sampling.

Sodium bicarbonate 8.4% (1 M), i.e., 1 ml = 1 mmol = 1 mEq = 1 mval

- Sodium bicarbonate 4.2% (0.5 M) should be used as the final concentration for IV application
- After PPV, volume expansion and blood gas analysis, consider administering sodium bicarbonate 4.2% (0.5 M) safely through a large IV line
- Required amount of sodium bicarbonate in mmol = (base deficit × kg body weight) ÷ 3 = mEq sodium bicarbonate required
- Dilute sodium bicarbonate 8.4% 1 : 1 in sterile water (e.g., 10 ml + 10 ml, then 4.2% final concentration) or use pre-prepared 4.2% solution, and administer as continuous infusion in 30–60–120 min IV
- Maximum IV infusion rate: 0.1 mmol/kg/min = 6 mmol/kg/h (= 12 ml/kg/h of the 4.2% solution) IV = 6 mEq/kg/h
- Only in an absolute emergency without the ability to determine the patient's pH/blood gas, e.g., 10 min of ineffective resuscitation in the delivery room (chest compressions and IV epinephrine) you may "blindly" administer 1 mEq/kg/dose = 2 ml/kg of 4.2% sodium bicarbonate (0.5M) per dose in (5–)10 min IV. Consider THAM if repetitive buffer doses are indicated for severe metabolic or mixed acidosis

Continuous infusion rate for sodium bicarbonate

The maximum IV infusion rate for neonates is 0.1 mmol/kg/min = 6 mmol/kg/h = 6 mEq/kg/h of the 4.2% solution. We DO NOT recommend rapid sodium bicarbonate IV administration at a rate of 0.5 mmol/kg/min (=0.5 mEq/kg/min) or even up to 1 mmol/kg/min (=1 mEq/kg/min), as suggested by other authors, even if birth asphyxia is obvious (→ cerebral hemorrhage).

In the case of hypernatremia use Tris buffer (= THAM). THAM, administered in the delivery room may have some benefit for newborns with congenital diaphragmatic hernia and persistent pulmonary hypertension of the newborn; however, ILCOR 2005 does NOT mention THAM for the resuscitation of newly born infants[22].

Do not buffer in the delivery room. . .

- When acidosis is mainly respiratory ($PCO_2 > 60$ mmHg and base deficit ≤ -9; exceptions such as congenital diaphragmatic hernia may apply)
- In metabolic acidosis plus hypoventilation (especially with deficient spontaneous breathing)
- When only brief cardiopulmonary resuscitation has to be performed
- When IV access is not definitely intravascular
- In hypernatremia, then use Tris buffer (THAM 3 M, 1 ml = 3 mmol, 3000 mosmol/l, use in appropriate dilution)

> ❗ Sodium bicarbonate should be given rarely and slowly, with good ventilation into a large vein.

Rare indications for sodium bicarbonate

- Hyperkalemia
- Hypermagnesemia
- Intoxication with tricyclic antidepressant

THAM (Tris-hydroxymethyl-aminomethane) = Tris buffer (very rarely indicated)

- Required THAM (3 M) in ml = (base deficit × kg body weight) ÷ 10
- Required THAM (0.3 M) in ml = (base deficit × kg body weight)
- Caution (peripheral IV access):
  - If you have only the 3 M solution, dilute THAM (3 M) 1:10 with sterile water, to give a 0.3 M solution
- THAM 0.3 M solution is preferably diluted 1:1 in $D_{10}W$ (10 ml Tris 0.3 M + 10 ml $D_{10}W$)
- Then peripheral THAM infusion is possible
- Better: THAM up to 3 M diluted 1:1 in $D_{10}W$ via central venous line
- Replace half of the required amount over 30 min (in asphyxia) to 60 (up to 120) min IV. (Advantage of THAM over sodium bicarbonate → no increase of PCO_2 and sodium; adverse effects: hypertonic solution, hypoglycemia, apnea, liver cell necrosis, or the like; contraindications: uremia/anuria)

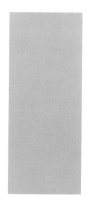

Absolute and relative indications for neonatal transport and NICU admission

Georg Hansmann

Indications for neonatal transport and NICU admission depend on the availability of a pediatrician with sufficient experience in neonatology (i.e., clinical follow up in birth hospital). Recommendations may vary based on local protocols, settings, and staffing. Newborns who are stable but transferred for further work-up and short-term treatment should return to the mother as soon as possible. Alternatively, the mother may be transported to the hospital where the newborn receives advanced care. Separation of the mother from her newborn child should be limited to a minimum period. The following section lists the most common, but not all, indications for neonatal transport.

Absolute indications for neonatal transport

- Immaturity (<35 0/7 weeks of gestation)
- Intrauterine growth retardation (IUGR) with birth weight <3rd percentile
- Respiratory disorder
- Persistent cyanosis
- UA–pH <7.0
- Obvious or suspected congenital malformations, to be transferred for further work–up
- Symptomatic or potentially harmful cardiac arrhythmias
- Confirmed or suspected metabolic or endocrinological disorders, including:
  - Hypoglycemia
    - Blood glucose <40 mg/dl (<2.3 mmol/l) in the first 24 h of life
    - Blood glucose <45 mg/dl (<2.5 mmol/l) after the first 24 h of life
  - Diabetic fetopathy (in babies born to a diabetic mother) and its complications (e.g., respiratory distress syndrome)
  - Rhesus hemolytic disease (*Morbus haemolyticus neonatorum*, isoimmune haemolytic anemia)
  - Polycythemia (symptomatic and/or Hct >70%)
  - Anemia (Hct <35%) in the first week of life
  - Hyperbilirubinemia (see www.bilitool.com and p. 516)
    - Visible jaundice (icterus) in the first 24 h of life
    - Total bilirubin >20 mg/dl despite phototherapy in an otherwise healthy term newborn infant

Neonatal Emergencies: A Practical Guide for Resuscitation, Transport and Critical Care, ed. Georg Hansmann.
Published by Cambridge University Press. © Cambridge University Press 2009.

- Total bilirubin >17 mg/dl despite phototherapy in a term newborn infant with additional risk factors
- Immune thrombocytopenia
- Confirmed or suspected intracranial (most often subependymal or intraventricular) hemorrhage
- Confirmed or suspected infection/sepsis
- Newborn infant of a (IV) drug-using or methadone–substituted mother

Relative indications for neonatal transport
If an experienced pediatrician and/or sufficient equipment is not available around the clock:
- 35 0/7 weeks ≤ GA <37 0/7 weeks (for GA <35 0/7 weeks decide on a case-by-case basis whether to transport)
- IUGR with birth weight between the 3rd and 10th percentile
- Newborn infants born to a insulin–dependent diabetic mother
- Hyperbilirubinemia for further diagnostics and treatment
- Polycythemia (asymptomatic with Hct >65%)
- Abnormal neurological findings on examination which do not require immediate treatment
- Suspected infection by history and normal examination, until sepsis is ruled out
- Minor or non-urgent congenital malformations
- Non-urgent cardiac arrhythmias
- Non-urgent problems with PO feeding/nutrition

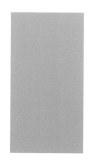

Communication with mother and father

Georg Hansmann

The team that attends the delivery and performs the initial newborn care and eventually neonatal resuscitation should introduce themselves to the mother and father – given that the resuscitation unit is prepared and there is enough time prior to delivery. The same applies to the non-emergent inter-hospital transport of neonates. If postnatal transport is warranted, parents should be informed about the main reason for the transport team's arrival (e.g., postnatal tachypnea). Later, the need for the newborn's transfer to a tertiary NICU should be explained and at the same time the parents should be reasonably reassured.

A well-adapted newborn infant should not be transferred, but dried and warmly wrapped up and placed on the mother's chest – if there is any doubt, early assessment by a pediatrician and strict observation, which may include pulse oximetry, are required.

If basic measures have to be performed on the resuscitation unit (suctioning, stimulation, oxygen supplementation; e.g., after C–section), the father may be brought to the baby when spontaneous breathing/crying is established, and the newborn appears to be adapting well and appears stable. Let the father know what you are doing and how his child's transition into the ex utero world is going (i.e., in most cases, give reassurance).

Conversations with the parents may be difficult and demanding when the condition of the baby is critical. The physician performing the resuscitation/intensive care should mention and emphasize the critical condition of the newborn with sensitivity, empathy, and honesty. It is important to underline that the intensive care will be continued by the admitting NICU team, which is specialized in taking care of critically ill babies. In extreme cases, a newborn infant may have undergone advanced resuscitation s/p severe asphyxia, be suffering from hypoxic ischemic encephalopathy (HIE) and is transported to a level III NICU for evaluation, continuation of intensive care or redirection of care.

- Talk to the parents before or after, but not during, neonatal resuscitation (unless you are not directly involved in its performance). However, it is important that a health care provider updates the parents during the resuscitation/intensive care of their newborn child.
- Before any neonatal transport, show the infant to the mother – even when the baby is already in the incubator. The parents need to be informed about the reasons for transfer and the clinical condition of the newborn infant.

Neonatal Emergencies: A Practical Guide for Resuscitation, Transport and Critical Care, ed. Georg Hansmann.
Published by Cambridge University Press. © Cambridge University Press 2009.

Coordinating neonatal transport and patient sign-out to the NICU team

Georg Hansmann

When deciding on the level of care a sick newborn infant should receive (nursery, high observation unit vs. NICU level I–III), evaluate not only the patient's clinical condition but also other factors, such as the distance between the birth hospital and the parents' home, staffing as well as personal experiences gained from previous deliveries and neonatal transfers.

The transport physician (NETS-MD) calls the neonatology department and lets the doctor in charge know that an admission to the NICU (with or without mechanical ventilation) is needed. If the physician is still performing resuscitation, a midwife or RN should be assigned to make the call. As soon as the NETS-team leaves, the midwife or RN must confirm to the admitting unit that the NETS-team – with the patient – is on its way. Just to make sure, the NETS-MD should also announce their own arrival, for instance by mobile phone, shortly before the ambulance or aircraft reaches the children's hospital.

The initial sign-out to the admitting neonatologist should contain information that is most up-to-date and most important to the patient's current clinical condition.

- Actual problems, such as "suspected pneumothorax" must be underlined and mentioned first (chest X-ray and drain are more important than the gestational age), followed by the ventilatory setting for an intubated/assisted patient, ET tube size and inserted length, infusion rates for the most important infusions (prostaglandin, volume, buffer, inotropic agents, dextrose, etc.)
- Then continue with a *chronological presentation*:
  - Maternal risk factors (time of rupture of membranes, signs of infection, preeclampsia, etc.)
  - Prenatal drugs/medications (steroids, antibiotic therapy) and lab results (maternal CRP, WBC)
  - Time and place of birth, spontaneous vs. operative (forceps, vacuum extraction, C-section)
  - Birth weight, gestational age in weeks
  - Postnatal course and adaptation (including Apgar score)
  - Procedures during the resuscitation, including blood glucose, blood gas analysis, temperature, and Hct, as well as diagnostic tests (CBC, CRP, blood culture), complications, notable findings on physical examination
- Finally, provide additional information on the *mother and child*: maternal age, previous pregnancies/births/miscarriages/abortions, drug abuse, medications during pregnancy, maternal HBsAg status, as well as mother's blood type. Clarify whether a direct Coombs test was performed, and whether vitamin K and hepatitis B vaccination were given.

Neonatal Emergencies: A Practical Guide for Resuscitation, Transport and Critical Care, ed. Georg Hansmann.
Published by Cambridge University Press. © Cambridge University Press 2009.

Documentation and feedback after neonatal emergency transport

Georg Hansmann

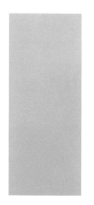

Neonatal resuscitation and transfers are always documented in written form, and obstetricians, nursery/NICU and NETS are provided with a copy of the transport chart. Aside from the hand-written form, a detailed report may be faxed to the admitting team (nursery, NICU) after completion of the transport and verbal sign-out of the patient. Usually, all specifications mentioned in chronological order on p. 182 belong to documentation of both the standard initial care/resuscitation in the delivery room and NETS (resuscitation, stabilization, transport). In particular, the Apgar score, initial UA pH value and at least one blood gas analysis and one blood glucose value (D-stix), together with total transport time, must be documented in a transport protocol (legal backup). The original, labeled blood gas analysis printout should be stapled to the protocol. Further mandatory information should be documented: maternal HBsAg status, HIV status and blood type, perinatal drugs/medication/antibiotic prophylaxis/maternal signs of infection, and, if performed, hepatitis B vaccination and vitamin K administration. The admitting team also needs full prenatal laboratory test results, which can be faxed by the birth hospital, but is better provided as a photocopy. The complete physical examination after birth should also be documented, as should additional data such as the time of the emergency call, time of arrival at the delivery site, and time of arrival at the admitting children's hospital/NICU. Also, the most important vital signs obtained in the delivery room, during the transport and those obtained upon arrival in the NICU (HR, MAP, S_aO_2, blood gas, blood glucose, core temperature; see pp. 131–2) must be documented.

Special remarks on complications or complaints about the equipment (e.g., "local blood gas analyzer not functional") should be documented in an extra field.

> **!** Blood gas analysis, blood glucose, body temperature, and total transport time must be documented by the neonatal emergency transport (NETS) team.

After initial care/resuscitation, or after transport, the neonatal emergency doctor and paramedics/NP/RN should summarize and discuss the prior transport case, in order to explain the pathophysiological background, and to highlight areas for future improvement and extraordinary performance.

Neonatal Emergencies: A Practical Guide for Resuscitation, Transport and Critical Care, ed. Georg Hansmann.
Published by Cambridge University Press. © Cambridge University Press 2009.

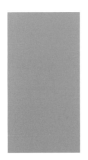

Ethics in neonatal intensive care

Christoph Bührer

Neonatal resuscitation and intensive care may need certain restrictions and limits if it is to be in the best interests of the newborn infant. There are circumstances in which treatments that merely sustain "life" neither restore health nor confer other benefit and hence are no longer in the child's best interest. Imposing resuscitation or advanced critical care medicine on an infant requires a greater justification than mere survival. There must be a rationale on which doctors decide the infant may face not merely pain and suffering, but rather a realistic chance of long-term survival without devastating sequelae[122]. Survivability is not the only issue at stake. Both suffering inflicted by medical procedures and severe long-term morbidity might be considered an even greater tragedy than death. This issue poses problems across multiple medical specialties, not just neonatology, and the ethical principles regarding resuscitation and advanced critical care of newborns are not different from those applicable to older children and adults. However, as the body of a newborn, particularly that of an extremely preterm infant, is still developing, both vulnerability and the potential for adaptive recovery exceed those of older children or adults.

Opinions and beliefs

The very nature of medicine implies inherent interference with the natural course of a disease. Doctors have powerful means, the use of which must be wisely considered. However, withholding or withdrawing medical care from patients with a poor prognosis raises challenging ethical, moral, legal, and emotional dilemmas. At first glance, an easy opt-out of such difficult decisions is the *vitalistic "sanctity-of-life" view* that considers all human lives, irrespective of their quality or kind, equally valuable and inviolable, and that life is always preferable to death. The 2004 Texas Supreme Court decision justifying the resuscitation of a preterm baby girl of 23 weeks' gestational age and 615 g birth weight against the explicit wishes of her parents[123] is based on this view. The baby went on to have intracranial hemorrhage and survived severely handicapped. The vitalistic position permits doctors to err on the side of the preservation of life and mandates them to resuscitate a neonate no matter how premature, how unlikely to survive, how likely to incur severe disabilities, or how strongly the parents object. Several proponents of the vitalistic position come from a rather rigid monotheistic background, sometimes welcoming human suffering as God's will – even in cases when it is actually rather the result of human action.

The appeal of the vitalistic view is that it is straightforward and provides a clear-cut answer to a difficult question. It also puts up a firm stance against attempts to deliberately eliminate handicapped people, who inflict huge medical and financial expenditures. However, resuscitation at all costs is neither tenable nor realistic. The percentage of infants dying in hospitals as a result of a professional end-of-life decision has been rising steadily

Neonatal Emergencies: A Practical Guide for Resuscitation, Transport and Critical Care, ed. Georg Hansmann.
Published by Cambridge University Press. © Cambridge University Press 2009.

alongside the advances in neonatal intensive care[124,125]. In former decades, however, decisions on withdrawing or withholding treatment in severely ill neonates were "quiet decisions," made by the physician in charge. Awareness on the subject matter steadily increased in the medical community after the extent of this practice and its ethical dilemma were made public in 1973[124].

In a survey of neonatologists across Europe, most doctors reported having been involved at least once in setting limits to intensive care because of incurable conditions (61%–96%), while slightly smaller proportions reported such involvement because of a baby's poor neurological prognosis (46%–90%)[126]. Practices such as continuation of current treatment without intensification and withholding any emergency maneuvers were widespread, whereas withdrawal of mechanical ventilation was reported by variable proportions (28%–90%). Only in France (73%) and the Netherlands (47%) was the administration of drugs with the aim of ending life reported with substantial frequency. Age, length of professional experience, and the importance of religion in the physician's life affected the likelihood of reporting non-treatment decisions, but the country of where the physicians were practising remained the most important predictor of physicians' opinions and practices. In the Flemish-speaking part of Belgium, 79% of neonatologists surveyed found that the physicians' duties sometimes included the prevention of unnecessary suffering by hastening death[127]. The expected quality of life and the parents' wishes should have a role in decision-making according, respectively, to 88% and 93% of the surveyed neonatologists.

Thus, most neonatologists now recognize that decisions in borderline cases should no longer be solely based on presumed sanctity of human life. In the anglo-american literature, *the four principles – autonomy, non-maleficence, beneficence and justice –* are often invoked as the cornerstones of ethical considerations and decisions. However, applying the principle of autonomy is difficult in newborn infants, as decisions are always made by proxy. French neonatologists, who perceive themselves as moderately *paternalistic*[126], base their decisions on three principles: the best interests of the infant, the actual and expected quality of life, and sound procedures applied to end-of-life decisions[128]. In the optional intensive care borderline zone, conflict between such principles is inevitable, and decisions cannot be made without some violation of principles and loss of value.

Ethical guidelines for neonatal resuscitation

The American Academy of Pediatrics (AAP) and the American Heart Association (AHA) have jointly issued guidelines for withholding and discontinuing resuscitation of newborn infants[129], encouraging doctors to withdraw support when gestation, birth weight, or congenital anomalies are associated with almost certain early death and when unacceptably high morbidity is likely among the rare survivors. Examples cited are extreme prematurity (gestational age <23 weeks or birth weight <400 g), anencephaly, and chromosomal abnormalities incompatible with life, such as trisomy 13.

The AAP/AHA guidelines further recommend supporting parental desires concerning initiation of resuscitation in conditions associated with uncertain prognosis in which survival is borderline, the morbidity rate is relatively high, and the anticipated burden to the child is high.

Most congenital malformations and gestational age ≥25 weeks (unless there is evidence of fetal compromise such as intrauterine infection or hypoxia-ischemia) are considered conditions in which resuscitation is nearly always indicated, as the rates of survival are high, and morbidity is perceived as acceptable. These guidelines from the AAP/AHA specify a borderline zone, exemplified by a 2-week gestational age window between 23 0/7 and 24 6/7 weeks, where decisions as to what course of treatment is appropriate should be based on the individual circumstances of each baby and the wishes of the parents of that particular baby[129].

Meanwhile, nearly all published national or local recommendations now recognize that there is a borderline zone, spanning about 2 weeks of gestational age, when it comes to the issue of extreme prematurity. In this borderline zone, an individualized prognostic strategy appears to be more appropriate than a dogmatic policy of not treating patients born at less than a certain gestational age, or treating all live-born infants regardless of gestational age. While such a gray zone of uncertainty (i.e., questionable appropriateness of neonatal intensive care) is widely recognized, it is its precise determination in gestational weeks that is fiercely debated[130,131]. In countries with maximum medical resources, this borderline zone in which advanced treatment may be initiated or not ranges from 22 0/7 to 23 6/7 weeks in guidelines from Austria and Germany[132] (available at www.docs4you.at/Content. Node/Spezialbereiche/Neonatologie/Erstversorgung_von_Fruehgeborenen.pdf, accessed 13 November 2008), to 23 0/7 to 25 0/7 weeks in the United Kingdom (Nuffield Council on Bioethics[133]; available at http://www.nuffieldbioethics.org/fileLibrary/pdf/Conclusions_an-d_recommendations.pdf, accessed 13 November 2008), to 24 0/7 to 25 6/7 weeks in those from Switzerland[134] (available at http://www.neonet.ch/assets/doc/Infants_born_at_the_li-mit_of_viability_-_english_final.pdf, accessed 13 November 2008) or the St. Vincent Medical Center in Portland, Oregon[135], despite similar long-term outcomes. Although most statistics show that chances for intact survival are much better for preterm girls as compared to boys[136,137], the issue of sex is not addressed in any of the guidelines published. The personal views of doctors drafting these guidelines obviously play a large role when the provision of intensive care is optional.

Opinions among neonatal health care providers (often between RN, nurse practitioners and doctors of the same neonatal intensive care unit) vary widely regarding the benefits and disadvantages of aggressive therapies in newborns at the limits of viability. However, determining whether or not the risks and benefits warrant the use of aggressive technology is a value judgment, not a medical assessment. As such, it properly belongs to those who, along with the infant, will bear the burden of a decision to resuscitate: the parents.

End-of-life decisions
Preparing an end-of-life decision

Time permitting, end-of-life decisions constitute a two-step process that begins with a thorough determination of diagnosis and estimation of prognosis, assessing potential futility of treatment and quality-of-life issues based on gestational age and conditions of the baby, as well as published and local outcome data. Obtaining the most reliable data sources available constitutes part of the professional duty of the doctors involved. Morbidity and mortality for newborns vary according to region and availability of resources. Outcome data require constant updating, and doctors need to remain informed of changing statistics and new trials.

Decisions to be made are best elaborated in a continuing dialogue between all parties involved. Because decisions frequently have to be made within a short period of time, it is helpful that the members of the perinatal team have previously discussed and agreed upon a standard approach in such situations[138]. A structured decision-making process that attempts to integrate the best interests of the infants and their parents, the possibilities of high-tech neonatal intensive care interventions, and the perspective of the nurses and doctors has been shown to shorten futile intensive care and thereby decrease suffering for infants, parents, and possibly caregivers[139].

Caregivers need to be vigilant to their own biases. Apprehension has been voiced by the pioneer neonatologist William A. Silverman (1917–2004)[140,141]. He stressed that neonatologists become self-appointed guardians of the rights of barely viable (i.e., borderline) neonates and that this decision-making power is trumping the competing rights of families and society[130]. To ensure an unbiased discussion, it is important that those who make decisions regularly receive input from external sources. Whenever possible, end-of-life decisions should be made by a team, not by sole individuals. Disagreement voiced during consensus-finding is inherent to this process and indicative of its quality.

Involving the parents

After the caregiving team has prepared an end-of-life decision, professionals must then counsel the parents and provide them with the most reliable outcome data available. Through a process of communication and value exploration between the well-meaning parents and well-intentioned doctors, the goal is to reach a consensus decision that respects parental authority and promotes physician beneficence, with the best interests of the infant placed in the center of the analysis. It is impossible to avoid quality-of-life judgments since there is a close link between the patient's quality of life on the one hand, and her/his best interests on the other. Another important goal is that parents are at peace and will stay at peace with a decision to initiate, to continue, to withhold or to withdraw life support.

Results from studies assessing parents' perceptions of counseling and decision-making[142,143] suggest that most parents desire a larger role in decisions to initiate resuscitation and continue life support of severely compromised newborns. Parents apparently favor a model of shared decision-making, playing an active but not autonomous role in decisions made for their infants. To be involved in the decision-making process, parents feel they need information and recommendations from physicians, but also encouragement and hope. At certain gestational ages, doctors feel parents are the decision-makers, but doctors may become very directive at other gestational ages. Counseling may heighten parents' anxiety during and after their infant's hospitalization, but that does not diminish their recalled satisfaction with counseling and the decision-making process. Prenatal counseling, e.g., on a threatening delivery of an extremely immature infant, should be conducted by a limited number of health care providers so that information and assessments provided to the parents are clear and not conflicting. Parents, however, should feel free to ask for a second opinion.

Doctors should strive to provide parents with the medical information critical for informed decision-making, and foster parental involvement in life-support decisions to the extent appropriate to them and local cultural norms. However, implementing this recommendation is heavily influenced by the parents' values and the doctor's conception of parental autonomy[144]. When the parents' values are well-defined, fixed and known to themselves, the doctor may assume the role of a competent technical expert and just provide relevant factual information and later on implement the selected intervention (*informative style*). However, if the parents' values are inchoate and conflicting, the doctor's role will also somehow involve elucidating these values in addition to providing factual information (*interpretive style*). In cases where parents are open to development and revision through discussion, the doctor may articulate his or her own values separately from informing the parents (*deliberative style*). In contrast to scenarios whereby directivity is kept to a minimum, doctors may also see themselves primarily as the infant's guardian and promote the neonate's best interests, as perceived by them, independently of the parents (*paternalistic style*).

The parents' views may be determinative unless they conflict seriously with the interpretation of the child's best interests by those who are providing care[145]. It is best if parents and staff can agree on the need for intensive treatment of the infant. When there is an irresolvable disagreement, parents – while having the legal right to consent to treatment for their children – do not have an absolute right either to refuse treatment judged to be in the best interests of the child or to demand treatment to sustain the life of their child[146].

A helpful framework for decision-making in cases with uncertain diagnoses and some kind of disagreement between parents and doctors[147,148] is based on the prospects for the individual infant. *Treatment decisions for newborns may be divided into four categories: mandatory, optional, investigational, and unreasonable.* They are explained as follows.

- Mandatory: if the parents ask the physician to withhold or withdraw medical support that has a very high likelihood of benefiting a child, the treating physician's independent obligation to foster the best interest of the patient prohibits them from following the parents' request. An example would be parents who ask the physician to remove ventilation from a full-term newborn unless the physician can guarantee that their child will be "normal," or parents of an infant with trisomy 21 who request ending all medical treatment[145]

- Optional: when the risks are very high and the benefits are at best uncertain or extremely low, the parents have the option of accepting or rejecting the proposed resuscitation. In this "gray zone" the parents' decision to either accept or reject support should be followed

- Investigational: when outcome data are such that the best we can tell parents is that the intervention is so new or its effects on this category of patients so unproven that it is basically an experimental procedure. Such procedures necessarily require informed patient or proxy consent

- Unreasonable: if the parents are demanding attempts at resuscitation, when in the physician's best judgment there is no expectation of efficacy. Indeed, an attempt to initiate resuscitation or any other medical treatment when there is no possible benefit to the patient would constitute an assault or battery. When it does not provide a benefit, intensive treatment can be ethically and legally withdrawn, even if the parents disagree[146]

Dying on a neonatal intensive care unit

When intensive care is withheld or withdrawn, palliative comfort care enters the foreground of the stage. Care is given to the same patient but with a different goal in mind, i.e., care continues but is redirected to a maximum of comfort. The humane and compassionate care provided to the infant includes diligent handling, maintaining a neutral thermal environment, and gentle monitoring of vital signs.

In addition to comfort care for the dying infant, support of the parents becomes a second important focus of the health care team. The family should be treated with dignity and compassion, and the parents' ethnic background, beliefs and religion should be respected and accommodated whenever possible. The support of the parents should include the acknowledgment of the birth of the infant[149]. When medical support is discontinued or death is inevitable, time should be allowed for the parents and other family members to hold, touch, and interact with the infant if they desire to do so, both before and after the infant has died. Naming the infant, obtaining a photograph and a tuft of hair may be very important to the parents, and a crib card and name band should be provided to the family, as well as birth weight and other measurements. Clergy and members of the extended family should be allowed access to the infant in a setting that maintains the dignity of both the family and infant. Many hospitals now have palliative care suites and well-trained staff to address these needs.

Support should be provided to the family by physicians, nurses, and other staff prior and beyond the time of the infant's death. Perinatal loss support groups, intermittent contact by telephone, and a later conference with the family to review the medical events surrounding the infant's death and to evaluate the grieving response of the parents may be considered.

Provisional and end-of-life care for neonates

While end-of-life decisions require intensive deliberations, they also sometimes need to be done in due time because of apparent futility or dismal prospects. Varying proportions of neonatologists prefer to resuscitate the baby and start provisional intensive care, provided that intensive care can later be withdrawn if the baby's prognosis appears poor[150]. An evaluation at a later point in time may provide a more solid basis for a decision to continue or abort intensive care measures (*redirection of care*). However, procrastinating a decision could also run the risk of creating a situation where withholding treatment is no longer apt to stop suffering but is rather the beginning of it. The American Academy of Pediatrics vindicates discontinuation of treatment in infants without signs of life (no heart beat and no respiratory effort) after 10 minutes of continuous and adequate resuscitative efforts, because these infants show either a high mortality or severe neurodevelopmental disability[129]. Continuing resuscitation may save the infant's life but not its brain. The parents may end up with an infant who is able to breathe on its own but without any prospects for development. This infant will not fulfil brain death criteria, so treatment cannot be stopped legally.

In 2001, the Ethics Working Group of the Confederation of European Specialists in Paediatrics clearly rejected every form of intentional killing of such infants[151]. Euthanasia in severely ill newborns is illegal and subject to criminal prosecution in all countries in the world, including the Netherlands[152]. However, the Dutch Medical Association and the Dutch Pediatric Association have issued reports on the legitimacy of end-of-life decisions in very severely affected newborns[153]. They argue that in these infants, it is not the life-ending decisions but the life-prolonging decisions that must be legitimized. In their opinion, the physician should initiate treatment if there is a chance of a favorable outcome or to win time to establish a diagnosis. If the child survives but the condition of the child is such that it could have been foreseen at the beginning and the treatment should not have been started, the doctor must be prepared to take the responsibility to discontinue the treatment. Discontinuation of treatment is indicated if the quality of life, as judged by the child's expected ultimate level of communication, suffering, dependency on others, autonomy, and personal development, is viewed to be so miserable as not to be worth living. Both reports declare that if after discontinuation of treatment a situation of severe suffering occurs, euthanasia can be an acceptable choice.

The Groningen protocol

In the Netherlands, as in all other countries, ending someone's life, except in extreme conditions, is considered murder. A life of suffering that cannot be alleviated by any means might be considered one of these extreme conditions. A framework, known as the

Groningen protocol, has been developed to actively end the life of a newborn to alleviate the infant's suffering after extensive discussions with the parents and various physicians, including at least one not directly involved in the care of the infant[154]. An external legal body determines after the infant's death whether the decision was justified and all necessary procedures have been carefully followed. It has been applied solely to infants with the most serious forms of spina bifida who are not dependent on intensive medical treatment but for whom a very poor quality of life, associated with sustained suffering and without hope of improvement, is predicted.

While there is a shift towards ethics that does not ask or seek to preserve human life as such but only a life that is worth living, the Groningen protocol has evoked public outcries in various countries. Of note, one of its main authors had been involved only a few years earlier in the draft of the Ethics Working Group of the Confederation of European Specialists in Paediatrics that clearly rejected every form of intentional killing[151]. All infants killed according to the Groningen protocol so far suffered from severe spina bifida, which most likely would have been easily recognized early during pregnancy by prenatal ultrasound. What strikes many as hypocritical is the fact that the Groningen protocol is being practised in a country that has mostly abandoned publicly funded prenatal ultrasound screening. In addition, society shies away from directly taking legal responsibility for the decision to kill the infant but instead places the legal burden on the doctor. *In summary, while the Groningen protocol has opened the door to many important discussions, it is not helpful for neonatologists caring for infants at the limits of viability and has not been adopted anywhere outside the Netherlands.*

Permissibility of infanticide relies crucially on a particular concept of personhood that excludes a theological dimension. The dispute between the proponents of infanticide and their religious opponents is difficult to resolve because one side's perspective on the infant is shaped by a metaphysics that is emphatically rejected by the other. It is reminiscent of the debate on abortion ravaging Western countries for several decades. For the near future, the lack of any consensus on the issue of infanticide keeps the pressure up on doctors involved in neonatal intensive care to make end-of-life decisions not only wisely but also timely.

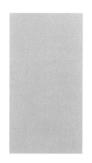

Perinatal images of preterm and term infants

Georg Hansmann and Andrea Zimmermann

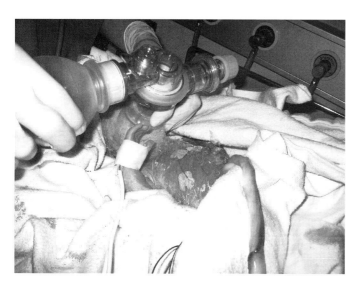

Figure 2.39 Bag-and-mask ventilation in a preterm infant with insufficient spontaneous breathing, muscular hypotonia, central cyanosis, and heart rate 70–90 bpm. The chest is covered with plastic wrap to prevent heat loss. Three small ECG leads are placed and connected. A pulse oximeter probe is attached to the right hand. See color plate section for full color version.

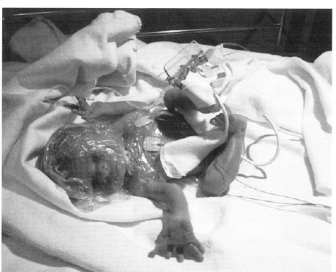

Figure 2.40 Preterm infant (32 3/7 weeks' gestation) with appropriate postnatal adaptation approx. 15 min after birth. Head and body are covered with plastic wrap (alternative: plastic bag). A peripheral venous catheter has been placed in the dorsal left hand. Monitoring via small ECG leads and pulse oximeter. See color plate section for full color version.

Neonatal Emergencies: A Practical Guide for Resuscitation, Transport and Critical Care, ed. Georg Hansmann.
Published by Cambridge University Press. © Cambridge University Press 2009.

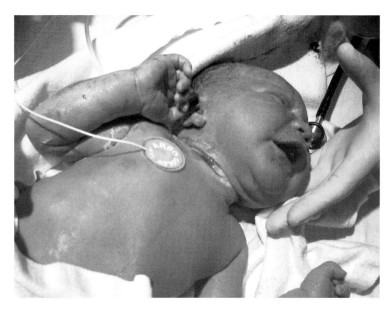

Figure 2.41 Term neonate with d-transposition of the great arteries without VSD ("simple, TGA"). Central cyanosis in the delivery room; 6 h after birth a balloon atrioseptostomy (ballon atrial sepostomy = Rashkind procedure) was performed because of significant blood flow restriction through the PFO/ASD (left-to-right shunt). See color plate section for full color version.

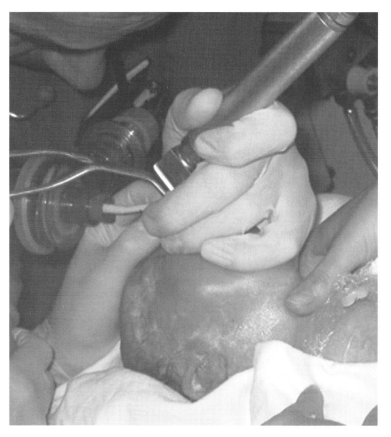

Figure 2.42 Nasotracheal intubation of a term neonate under continuous nasopharyngeal ventilation by an experienced team: assistant no. 1 secures the tube and ventilates, assistant no. 2 gently applies external pressure on the larynx. See color plate section for full color version.

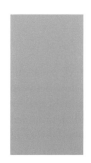

Mechanical ventilation of the neonate

Juan C. Ibla and John H. Arnold

Advances in the understanding of pulmonary pathophysiology and experience with the various ventilatory modalities have improved early and late outcomes in patients with respiratory failure and have reduced overall complications. In this chapter we discuss generally accepted strategies for mechanical ventilation and methods for optimizing the delivery of oxygen in frequently encountered pediatric clinical situations. We present general guidelines for ventilatory therapy intended to aid in the care of complex patients. The reader should realize that individual differences between patients exist and therapy should be modified to meet specific patient requirements.

Conventional mechanical ventilation (CMV)

The following topics will be discussed:

- Volume ventilation (VV)
- Pressure ventilation (PV)
- Indications for mechanical ventilation
- Modes of mechanical ventilation
  - BabyLog 8000
  - Siemens Servo 300
- General principles of CMV

Volume ventilation (VV)

Initially designed by the US Army, volume-cycled ventilation was commercially introduced in 1970 (Hamilton Standard PAD). Time-cycled, volume-limited ventilators were used in the early stages of ICU development in pediatric and mostly adult settings. Volume ventilation has not been a popular mode of ventilation historically in NICUs due to difficulty in achieving accurate delivery of small tidal volume (V_T) in neonates or premature infants. Volume ventilation assures adequate minute ventilation by delivering a preset V_T and rate independent of lung compliance. V_T is maintained at the expense of mean airway pressure ($\bar{P}_{aw}$) and peak inspiratory pressure (PIP), increasing the risk of barotrauma. Additionally, a large leak around the endotracheal tube poses significant disadvantages since V_T cannot be easily achieved. Modern modes of VV (Siemens Servo 300) have circumvented most of the disadvantages of this ventilation mode in neonates.

Neonatal Emergencies: A Practical Guide for Resuscitation, Transport and Critical Care, ed. Georg Hansmann.
Published by Cambridge University Press. © Cambridge University Press 2009.

Pressure ventilation (PV)

Pressure ventilation is the most frequently used mode of ventilation in the NICU; constant-flow, time-cycled, pressure-limited devices provide a constant inspiratory gas flow between breaths, improving ventilation and oxygenation by supporting functional residual capacity (FRC). The pressure-limited feature allows a preset PIP to be reached and maintained during the inspiratory cycle despite changes in compliance. Time cycling allows delivery of mandatory breaths at fixed intervals. Modern ventilators can sense inspiratory efforts and synchronize a mandatory cycle. Pressure ventilation in general also allows spontaneous breaths that may or may not trigger a mandatory breath; this feature makes this mode appealing for weaning from high ventilatory settings. Relative safety exists if using PV as sudden decreases in compliance (coughing, migration of ET tube) do not increase PIP. On the other hand, if compliance worsens so does V_t. If compliance increases (e.g., following surfactant therapy), there is a potential risk for overdistention.

Indications for mechanical ventilation

- Respiratory failure (tachypnea, cyanosis) at any gestational age
- Extreme prematurity ($\leq$26 0/7 weeks gestational age) (individual physiological factors may affect this indication)
- Selected clinical conditions (meconium aspiration syndrome, congenital diaphragmatic hernia (CDH), respiratory distress syndrome, congenital heart disease)

Modes of mechanical ventilation (see Table 2.10)

Dräger Babylog 8000 Ventilator

The Babylog 8000 is an electrically and pneumatically powered, electronically controlled mechanical ventilator. This device is one of the most popular ventilators used in neonatal intensive care due to its versatility and reliability. It is designed for use in infants up to 10 kg. The Babylog 8000 has been used in nearly all modes of ventilation (CMV/IMV, SIMV, A/C, PSV/NPS, and CPAP), and is preferred due to its high sensing accuracy and achievement of respiratory synchrony. During conventional ventilation, synchronization has been shown to decrease the work of breathing in preterm[155] and neonates recovering from cardiac surgery[156]. In addition to triggered modes, the Babylog 8000 is used for volume guaranteed ventilation (pressure-regulated volume control (PRVC) and pressure support volume guarantee (PSVG)), proven to be helpful to establishing weaning protocols. The Babylog 8000 *plus* is now available with a leak adapted synchronization feature that automatically adjusts inspiratory time to individual patient's needs. The inspiratory hold has been eliminated from this model, reducing the chance of active expiration against positive pressure. The Babylog 8000 is also capable of delivering high-frequency ventilation (5–20 Hz) (www.draeger-medical.com). See Table 2.10 for description of the different modes of ventilation.

Leak test
- Turn ventilator on
- Ventilator will ask to calibrate flow sensor; press confirm
- Set mode to CPAP
- Set peak inspiratory pressure to 80
- Set inspiratory flow to 2
- Press confirm
- Keep manual inspiratory pressed; bar graph pressure displays pressure of $80 \pm 2\,cmH_2O$

Table 2.10 Modes of mechanical* ventilation

Mode	Description
Intermittent mandatory ventilation (IMV)	Time cycled, volume/pressure-limited mandatory breaths are delivered at a fixed rate. This mode is generally reserved for small premature infants with minimal inspiratory effort or for patients who have received muscle relaxants. This is a standard feature on most ventilators, rarely used in "vigorous" neonates, since the lack of synchronization usually impairs ventilation and oxygenation
Synchronous intermittent mandatory ventilation (SIMV)	SIMV is considered the first line of therapy for pediatric patients with respiratory failure of different etiologies[174]. With the institution of SIMV, positive airway pressure and spontaneous inspiratory effort occur simultaneously. Synchronicity of these two components results in adequate gas exchanges with lower peak airway pressures reducing the risk of barotrauma. SIMV can be achieved in patients with an intact respiratory drive and is a common mode of ventilation used to wean patients off high ventilatory settings[175]. Most effective at lower rates since high rates reduced the expiratory time and may lead to air trapping
Assist control (AC)	This is a synchronized mode of ventilation that requires a mandatory minimum preset rate. In AC all breaths (triggered or mandatory) are fully assisted (pressure/volume limited). With AC the patient controls its own MV by triggering spontaneous/assisted respiratory cycles above a minimum preset value. Is not designed for weaning from the ventilator since the minimum rate is fixed, only PIP or tidal volume can be modified
SIMV-PS (pressure support, PS)	This modality exists in both pressure and volume control modes. As in SIMV a minimum MV target is selected allowing spontaneous breaths to be augmented by positive pressure (i.e., $+5$ to $+10\,cmH_2O$). Ideal for weaning since the minimum MV can be maintained entirely by patient-triggered assisted breaths. The degree of PS can also be adjusted to the minimum to overcome the resistance of the respiratory circuit before extubation
Pressure-regulated volume control (PRVC)	In this mode the minimum inspiratory pressure will be used to achieve a preset tidal volume V_T. If the minimum inspiratory pressure (i.e., $+10\,cmH_2O$) fails to achieve the preset V_T on the first breath, it will make small breath-to-breath adjustments until the pre-set V_T is achieved.
Pressure support volume guarantee (PSVG)	This mode is used almost exclusively used for weaning. PSVG is a pressure-limited mode with a preset V_T. If compliance improves the PIP needed to achieve the V_T will decrease. If the patient requires increased support another mode should be selected

Initial settings (see Figure 2.43)
- Calibrate flow sensor
- Set mode to CMV
- Set inspiratory pressure to $20\,cmH_2O$ (Figure 2.43A)
- Set inspiratory flow to 10; bar graph will display $20 \pm 4\,cmH_2O$ (Figure 2.43B)
- Set T_{in} to 0.4 and T_{exp} to 0.6 (Figure 2.43C)
- Set PEEP/CPAP to $0\,cmH_2O$, then set PEEP/CPAP to $10\,cmH_2O$ (Figure 2.43D)

Calibration of O_2 sensor
- Performed automatically every 24 h
- Must be performed manually after replacing a used O_2 sensor
- Can be performed manually at any time

195

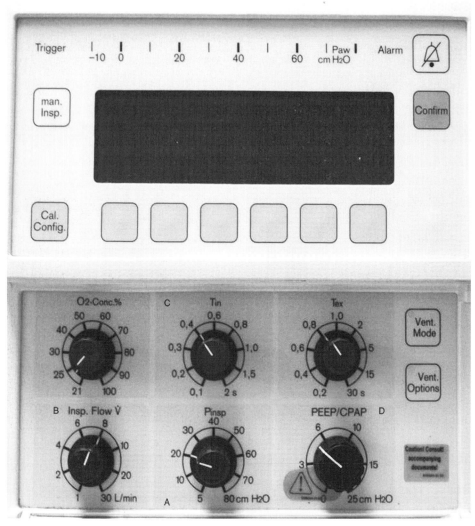

Figure 2.43 BabyLog 8000 plus control panel. Individual control of inspiratory time and pressure allows for the use of multiple ventilatory modes. See color plate section for full color version.

To calibrate
- Press Cal config
- Press O₂ cal
- After 5 min O₂ cal disappears from the screen, cal is complete

Calibration of flow sensor
- Required each time the vent is switched on
- After exchanging a flow sensor

To calibrate
- Press Cal config
- Press Vcal, disconnect from patient and seal the other end of the sensor

Table 2.11 Initial settings for the Siemens Servo 300. See Figure 2.44

Parameter	Neonatal	Pediatric
Preset tidal volume (ml)	2–39	10–399
Max. flow rate (l/min)	13	33
Bias flow rate (l/min)	0.5	1.0
Flow trigger (l/min)	0.17–0.5	0.3–1.0
Apnea alarm interval (s)	10	15
Auto mode apnea interval (s)	5	8

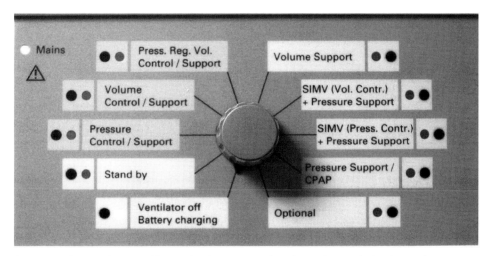

Figure 2.44 Siemens Servo 300. This ventilator's programmed modes can be switched with a single control button. See color plate section for full color version.

- Press start, Flow sensor calibrated will appear on vent
- Reconnect to endotracheal tube

Siemens Servo 300

These ventilators are capable of a wide variety of ventilatory modes (Figure 2.44; Table 2.11) but differ from constant-flow ventilators in that there is no gas flow from the ventilator between breaths in the adult and pediatric settings (the ventilator automatically adjusts flow in the circuit to maintain the set level of PEEP or CPAP despite patient's spontaneous breathing; hence, the flow is "servo-controlled"). In the neonatal mode there is low (0.5 l/min) continuous flow of gas through the circuit. SERVO ventilation relates to the feedback that the ventilator obtains from the patient's respiratory mechanics. This feature is exemplified by the PRVC mode available in this particular device. It can be used for both volume and pressure ventilation, but is known for its accuracy in the preset V_T delivered in all volume guarantee modes. It is widely used for volume ventilation of small infants; mode of ventilation assist control (AC) and CPAP (www.somatechnology.com). See Table 2.10 for general guidelines of initial ventilatory settings.

Initial settings (select PEDIATRIC range and PRESSURE CONTROL mode)
- Upper pressure limit to $60\,cmH_2O$
- Pressure control level $0\,cmH_2O$
- Pressure support level $0\,cmH_2O$
- PEEP $40\,cmH_2O$
- Trigger sensitivity $-17\,cmH_2O$
- CMV frequency 20 breaths/min
- Inspiratory time 25%
- Pause time 10%
- Inspiratory rise time 5%
- SIMV frequency 16 breaths/min
- Upper alarm limit 60 l/min
- Lower alarm limit 0 l/min
- O_2 concentration 21%

Tightness test
- Verify that PEEP level displayed in the end expiratory window is $40\,cmH_2O$
- Turn the PAUSE HOLD control to *EXP*. And hold for 30 s
- Verify that displayed PEEP drop is $<5\,cmH_2O$ at the end of 30 s

Special functions
- Oxygen breaths: deliver 100% O_2 for 1 min or 20 breaths
- Start breath: manually triggers a mandatory breath, typically used to initiate PRVC
- Expiratory hold: "freezes" expiratory phase for a maximum of 30 s, typically used to measure $PEEP_{auto}$
- Inspiratory hold: "freezes" inspiratory phase for a maximum of 5 s, typically used to measure plateau pressure
- Automode: option that provides automatic switching between a control mode and a support mode. Can be set to switch between volume controlled (VC), PRVC and pressure controlled (PC) and pressure support (PS). Switches from control mode to support mode with two consecutive patient-triggered breaths. If apnea is detected, switches from support mode to control mode

General principles of conventional ventilation
Ventilation
- Minute ventilation = frequency (rate, breaths/min) $\times$ tidal volume (ml)
- Parameters affecting frequency: inspiration time (T_{in}), expiration time (T_{exp}) and I:E ratio
- Parameters affecting tidal volume: driving pressure (PIP – PEEP) and tissue time constant (airway resistance), lung compliance (ΔVolume/Δpressure).
- *To increase ventilation: $\uparrow$ frequency, $\uparrow$ T_{in}, and $\uparrow$ PIP*

Oxygenation
- Oxygenation = mean airway pressure $\bar{P}_{aw} \times F_iO_2$
- $\bar{P}_{aw} = (T_{exp} \times PIP) + (T_{exp} \times PEEP)/T_{in} + T_{exp}$

Table 2.12 General ventilatory indications for high-frequency oscillatory ventilation (HFOV)

Parameter	Consider HFOV	Start HFOV
MAP	8	9
PIP	18–22	>22
F_iO_2	30–40	>40
Rate	20–30	>30
Lung disease		Air leak, early intervention

*Consider HFOV if the oxygenation index (O.I.) is >13 in two consecutive arterial blood gas samples in a period of 6 h. O.I. = $F_iO_2 \times \bar{P}_aw \times 100 / P_aO_2$.
$\bar{P}_{aw}$, mean airway pressure; PIP, peak inspiratory pressure.

> **!** To increase oxygenation: ↑ F_iO_2 or ↑ mean airway pressure by increasing PIP or PEEP

High-frequency oscillatory ventilation (HFOV)

The following topics will be discussed:

- Definition of HFOV
- General indications and strategies for HFOV
- Parameters for HFOV
- Initial settings for HFOV SensorMedics 3100A

Definition of HFOV

High-frequency ventilation was developed in the early 1980s based on the concept that HFOV is superior to CMV in its ability to provide adequate ventilation and oxygenation using lower mean airway pressures, thus reducing barotrauma. Initial results in HFOV[54,157] failed to demonstrate a significant difference in the rate of chronic lung disease and mortality in neonates with respiratory failure. Despite initial disappointing results HFOV has proven to lead to significant improvement in oxygenation in VLBW infants as well as in patients with severe respiratory failure[158]. A recent Cochrane analysis concluded that the use of HFOV in preterm populations results in a modest reduction in chronic lung disease[159]. HFOV is used to recruit and maintain optimal lung volumes in pediatric patients with diffuse alveolar disease and air leak syndromes. HFOV is indicated in patients with respiratory failure not responding to conventional ventilation[160]. See Table 2.12 for general ventilatory indications of HFOV.

General indications and strategies for HFOV

- Alveolar disease of diverse etiology ($\bar{P}_{aw} \geq 10$)
- Early intervention. Traditionally HFOV ventilation has been reserved as a rescue therapy for hypoxemic respiratory failure when CMV has failed in later stages of treatment. Although not widely studied in humans, early intervention is defined as the use of HFOV in the first 24 h of mechanical ventilation in preterm neonates
- For VLBW neonates. The care of VLBW (<1000 g or <28 weeks' gestation) with HFOV has been suggested to be beneficial; however, additional studies are needed to definitely recommend its use for this purpose. Our ventilator strategy in VLBW

neonates is of permissive hypercapnia with a target pH of 7.25–7.33, P_aCO_2 of 50–60 mmHg and S_pO_2 between 87% and 94%

- Air leak syndrome. Pneumothorax is a commonly encountered complication of mechanical ventilation of preterm and term infants. The use of HFOV as a lung-protective ventilatory strategy allows adequate ventilation minimizing air leak at low $\bar{P}_{aw}$.

Exclusion criteria
- Elevated intracranial pressure
- Significant cardiovascular instability
- Passive pulmonary blood flow (e.g., Fontan physiology) with normal compliance

General considerations
- Establish arterial line for mean arterial pressure (MAP) and ABG monitoring
- Consider CVP monitoring to maintain a minimum of 8 mmHg
- Transcutaneous CO_2 monitoring at 38–40°C for initiation and follow trend information
- Pulse oximetry.

Ventilation strategies (HFOV)
- High volume strategy. Uses high $\bar{P}_{aw}$ to recruit alveoli in infants with respiratory failure and low lung volumes and is also used in the early intervention strategy
- Low volume strategy: uses low $\bar{P}_{aw}$ to maximize oxygenation in patients with significant air leaks and when ventilating VLBW infants. Careful assessment of patient's general conditions should be done before initiating any of these strategies

F_iO_2 can be weaned in increments (i.e., 5%–10 %) to 0.60 and then $\bar{P}_{aw}$ should be weaned. $\bar{P}_{aw}$ should not be weaned more that 1–2 cmH$_2$O each *time*. If lung disease improves and $F_iO_2 \leq 0.60$ consider alternating weaning $\bar{P}_{aw}$ and F_iO_2.

See Table 2.13 and Figure 2.45 for parameters of HFOV; the alarms and alerts of HFOV are shown in Table 2.14 and Figure 2.46.

Table 2.13 Parameters of HFOV. See Figure 2.45

Controls	Function	Range
Power ON switch	Turn the oscillator on. Green LED indicates power	
Mean airway pressure/ adjust (Figure 2.45A)	Adjust $\bar{P}_{aw}$ by valve restriction. Partial occlusion of the valve prevents exit of bias flow from the patient circuit. Changes in bias flow, I$_T$, Hz, power, piston location can affect $\bar{P}_{aw}$	3100A = 3–45 cmH$_2$O 3100B = 3–55 cmH$_2$O
Power control (ΔP or amplitude) (Figure 2.45B)	Amount of driving power moves piston back and forth. Effect is to change the % displacement of the oscillator piston. An increase improves ventilation	0–10
% Inspiration time (Figure 2.45C)	Percentage of cycle time that the piston is moving forward and remains at full inspiratory pattern. Changing the % T_{in} has an effect on the % displacement of the piston. An increase results in increased tidal volume	33%–50%
Frequency (Hz) (Figure 2.45D)	Sets the frequency in breaths per minute (1 Hz = 60 breaths/min)	3–15 (180–900 breaths/min)
Bias flow (Figure 2.45E)	Sets flow of continuous gas that moves past the patient airway. Adjust to "fine tune" $\bar{P}_{aw}$. Increasing bias flow will increase $\bar{P}_{aw}$	0–60 l/min (5 l/min increments). Internally limited to 40 l/min

Alarms and Alerts	Function	Range
Limit (3100A only)	Limits the proximal $\bar{P}_{aw}$ within the patient circuit	10–45 cmH$_2$O (standard = 45 cmH$_2$O)
Set Max. $\bar{P}_{aw}$ (Figure 2.46, A)	Set maximum $\bar{P}_{aw}$ with thumbwheel switch. Activation is indicated by audible and visual alarm. Does NOT limit $\bar{P}_{aw}$. Dump valve will open if $\bar{P}_{aw}$ >50 cmH$_2$O or <20% of set max. $\bar{P}_{aw}$	0–49 cmH$_2$O (standard = >5 cmH$_2$O)
Set min. $\bar{P}_{aw}$ (Figure 2.46, B)	Sets minimum $\bar{P}_{aw}$ with thumbwheel switch. Audible and visual alarm. Auto-reset after correction	0–49 cmH$_2$O (standard = >5 cmH$_2$O)
Power failure (Figure 2.46, C)	Red LED indicates loss of power. Audible alarm. Reset by pressing reset button even if condition corrected	
Start/stop	Manual toggle between on/off. Green LED = ON if the LED is not lit, the oscillator is disabled	
Reset (Figure 2.46, D)	Button reset all alarms. Depressed together with the START/STOP enabled until the dumb valve closes and airway pressure builds to >20% set max. MAP	
Piston centering (3100A only)	Determines the center position of the oscillator piston by adjusting the mean pressure on the back side of the piston. Acts in opposition to the $\bar{P}_{aw}$ on the front side of the piston, resulting in a centering effect. Clockwise rotation shifts the piston center closer to max. inspiratory limit. Counterclockwise rotation shifts the center toward the max expiratory limit	Allowing the piston to strike the mechanical stop for an extended period may reduce the life of the mechanism
Source gas low (Figure 2.46, E)	LED indicates gas pressure or air-cooling pressure <30 PSIG. Yellow LED resets after correction	
Oscillator overheated (Figure 2.46, F)	Oscillator coil is overheated; may be due to low gas pressure, loose gas source connection or filter blockage. Yellow LED resets after correction	
Oscillator stopped (Figure 2.46, G)	Indicates that the oscillator is enabled but ΔP <5–7 cmH$_2$O. Audible and red LED	

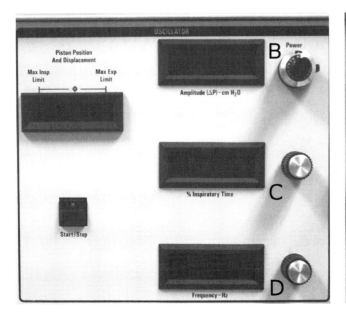
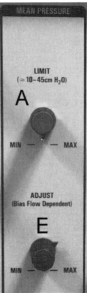

Figure 2.45 SensorMedics 3100A. Location of the principal control functions of HFOV.

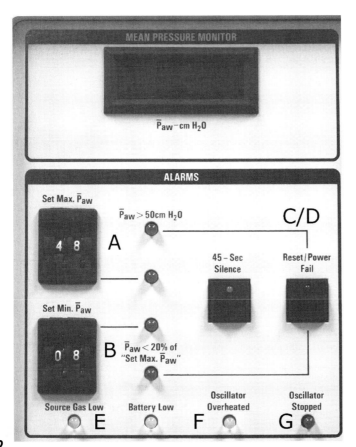

Figure 2.46 SensorMedics 3100A. Location of the alarm system.

Pre HFOV

Monitoring	Obtain baseline vital signs, S_pO_2/P_aO_2 and $P_aCO_2/tcPCO_2$
Cardiovascular	Verify adequate intravascular volume/cardiac output
Respiratory	Verify adequate position of ETT radiographically. Suction ETT
Neurological	Verify if sedation and muscle relaxation are required
Lung volume recruitment	Optimize lung volume with hand ventilation and inspiratory hold maneuvers as tolerated hemodynamically. Use caution in air leak syndrome

Neonatal HFOV settings.

$\bar{P}_{aw}$	High volume strategy: 3–5 cmH$_2$O > $\bar{P}_{aw}$ on CMV
	Air leak strategy: 2–3 cmH$_2$O > $\bar{P}_{aw}$ on CMV
	Early intervention: 10–14 cmH$_2$O
	For all: if S_pO_2 falls rapidly and below 90%, ↑ $\bar{P}_{aw}$ incrementally
ΔP	Full term: 25 cmH$_2$O or greater
	Pre term: 16 cmH$_2$O or greater
Frequency (Hz)	Full term: 12–15 Hz
	Pre term: 15 Hz
Bias flow	8–15 l/min
Inspiratory time	33%
F_iO_2	0.3–1.0 (use the lowest concentration required for adequate oxygenation)

Management of HFOV

Oxygenation^a	High volume strategy: increase $\bar{P}_{aw}$ by 1–2 cmH$_2$O and decrease F_iO_2 until ≤0.6 with acceptable P_aO_2/S_pO_2
	Air leak strategy: tolerate F_iO_2 0.8–1.0 (especially for the first 24 h to minimize $\bar{P}_{aw}$ while achieving acceptable P_aO_2/S_pO_2)
	Early intervention: adjust $\bar{P}_{aw}$ to maintain $F_iO_2 = 0.3$, S_pO_2 88%–92%
Ventilation^b	Adjust ΔP: 2–5 cmH$_2$O to achieve P_aCO_2 change of 3–5 mmHg
	Adjust ΔP: >5 cmH$_2$O to achieve P_aCO_2 change of 5–10 mmHg
	Hz: decrease only if P_aCO_2 is refractory to changes in ΔP
Chest X-ray	Obtain 1–2 h post-initiation, as often as every 6–8 h until stable. Thereafter every 24 h and repeat only after significant ventilatory changes
Suctioning ETT	Use closed suctioning system (e.g., Trach Care), but limit as much as possible, especially during the initial 24 h. Consider for acute or progressive increase in P_aCO_2. Perform manual recruitment maneuvers as tolerated

^{a}Hypoxemia may be treated by increasing F_iO_2 if <1.0 or by increasing $\bar{P}_{aw}$ until S_pO_2 ≥90%.
^{b}If adequate ventilation cannot be achieved by increasing ΔP with the maximum power, frequency may be decreased. The lower frequency will allow a longer inspiratory time by providing a longer equilibration time between the proximal airway and the alveolus, thus increasing tidal volume.

Weaning off HFOV

ΔP	↓ incrementally while maintaining adequate P_aO_2/S_pO_2 and $P_aCO_2/tcPCO_2$
$\bar{P}_{aw}$	↓ by 1–2 cmH$_2$O, in full-term and preterm transition to CMV when = to 10–12 cmH$_2$O
	↓ by 1–2 cmH$_2$O, in VLBW transition to CMV when <10 cmH$_2$O Consider CPAP in absence of apnea or bradycardia

SensorMedics 3100A

This high-frequency oscillatory ventilator utilizes a linear motor, which displaces a diaphragm-seated piston. In essence the patient's circuit constitutes a high-flow CPAP system in which oscillations of adjustable degrees are superimposed by an electrically driven diaphragm. It is the only HFOV ventilator approved for use in infants and pediatric patients <35 kg. It is the most frequently used ventilator in VLBW infants and patients selected for early intervention[161]. For patients >35 kg, the Sensormedics 3100B is the device of choice (www.sensormedics.com).

Inhaled nitric oxide (iNO) therapy

The following topics will be discussed:
- Definition of iNO therapy
- Indications for iNO therapy
- Patient optimization during iNO therapy
- iNO protocol

Definition of iNO therapy

Nitric oxide (NO) has been used in clinical practice since 1991 – shortly after its discovery by Ignarro and Moncada in 1987. iNO was only approved by the FDA for its use in hypoxic newborns in the year 2000. Despite its widespread use, PPHN was the only approved indication of iNO. The selectivity of a pulmonary specific vasodilator has proven of significant benefit to preterm neonates with lung disease and patients with pulmonary hypertension[162]. Recent trials have addressed the role of iNO therapy suggesting potential benefit for premature infants at risk for bronchopulmonary dysplasia[162,163,164], and additional studies in this area are needed to definitely recommend its use for this purpose.

Indications for iNO therapy

Prematurity	Infants >34 weeks started on mechanical ventilation
Respiratory failure	O.I. >25 in two ABG 30 min apart
Primary pulmonary hypertension	Obtain echocardiogram to rule out congenital heart disease
Aspiration syndrome	Meconium, blood, amniotic fluid

Patient optimization during iNO therapy

- Ensure adequate oxygenation/ventilation: adequate $\bar{P}_{aw}$ and oxygenation generally via HFOV
- Ensure adequate lung volume: order chest X-ray before iNO
- Ensure adequate oxygenation: P_aO_2 >80 mmHg, PCO_2 <40 mmHg and pH $\geq$7.45
- Ensure adequate hemodynamic parameters: BP >45–50 mmHg, use volume expansion or pressors
- Ensure adequate sedation and consider muscle relaxation before iNO

iNO protocol

Intervention	Result
Start iNO at 20 ppm	A 20% improvement in P_aO_2 with S_pO_2 >90% should occur within 15–30 min. S_pO_2 should be stabilized within 15–30 min.
	Rarely a dose of 40 ppm is needed if no improvement in O.I. is seen at 20 ppm
Decrease iNO to 10 ppm	If P_aO_2 ≥60 mmHg on F_iO_2 ≤0.60 and S_pO_2 >90%
	If S_pO_2 ↓ by >5% and <90%, return to 20 ppm
Decrease iNO in 10–15 min intervals from 10 to 5 to 1 ppm	If P_aO_2 ≥60 mmHg on F_iO_2 ≤0.60 and S_pO_2 >90%.
	If S_pO_2 ↓ by >5% and <90%, stop weaning and maintain at previous iNO dose
Discontinue iNO	If P_aO_2 ≥60 mmHg on F_iO_2 ≤0.40 and S_pO_2 >90%; ↑F_iO_2 to 0.60
	Wean F_iO_2 to ≤0.40 over 60 min
Re-start iNO at 1 ppm	If F_iO_2 >0.60, S_pO_2 is labile and/or ventilator settings ↑ after 60 min off iNO
Attempt to discontinue iNO	4–8 h after initiating iNO
Obtain MetHb 24 h after initiating iNO	If MetHb 1%–5% follow values daily. If MetHb <1% no need for further evaluation. If MetHb >5%, treat with Methylene Blue
	(Urolene Blue), 1 mg/kg IV over 5 min and decrease iNO dose

Extracorporeal membrane oxygenation (ECMO)

The following topics will be discussed:
- Definition of ECMO
- Indications for ECMO

Definition of ECMO

The concept of extracorporeal circulation was developed in the 1950s by Lillehei and has provided the fundamental basis for the development of ECMO. The first clinical use was reported in 1972 and since then has evolved with controversy to be an acceptable therapy for various neonatal respiratory and cardiac diseases[165]. The main goal of ECMO is to stabilize acute and reversible cardiorespiratory conditions and either: (1) provide support that allows cardiac or pulmonary recovery, or (2) provide a bridge to definitive therapy.

Indications for ECMO

Hypoxia, for longer than 4 h:
- If O.I. >40 in two or more ABG
- If alveolar–arterial oxygen difference [(A–a)DO$_2$] > 400 mmHg
- If P_aO_2 <40 mmHg
- Despite maximized ventilatory therapy (CMV, HFOV, iNO)

Acidosis
- If pH <7.0 despite maximum medical therapy (alkalinization therapy, hyperventilation, NaHCO$_3$ infusion)
- Acute heart failure in the absence of major congenital heart disease despite maximum hemodynamic support

Surgical
- Inability to separate from cardiopulmonary bypass or postoperative complications of cardiac surgery

Selection criteria
- Reversible disease
- Gestational age $\geq$34 weeks
- Weight $\geq$1.8 kg
- Mechanical ventilation for $\leq$14 days
- Predicted mortality $\geq$80% by historical criteria

Exclusion criteria
- Overwhelming sepsis
- Severe coagulopathy
- Gestational age <34 weeks
- Weight <1.8 kg
- Intraventricular hemorrhage >Grade 1
- Evidence of brain/kidney/liver damage
- Lung disease not reversible in 14 days
- Parental refusal

Non-invasive assessment of lung volume

Measurement of lung volume is a difficult and critical aspect of the care for mechanically ventilated patients. In the past, multiple techniques involving sophisticated imaging systems have been reported[166,167], however these are expensive and usually require physical transport of the patient outside the ICU. Bedside reproducible techniques have emerged as acceptable alternatives allowing the clinician to optimize lung recruitment and minimize overdistention. Here we will discuss two methods of lung volume assessment (respiratory inductance plethysmography, electrical impedance tomography) with potential use in routine clinical practice.

Respiratory inductance plethysmography (RIP)

RIP quantifies changes in cross-sectional area of the chest and abdomen by attaching two elastic bands containing Teflon-coated wires. These wires produce independent signals and the summation of these signals is calibrated against a known gas volume. Gothberg et al.[167] have shown that RIP-derived measurements correlate closely with injected gas volumes ($r^2 = 0.98$–0.99). Brazelton et al.[169] reported that RIP is capable of tracking volume changes during HFOV in animal models of acute respiratory distress syndrome.

Advantages
- Correlates closely with lung volumes
- Can create pressure–volume curves during HFOV[168]
- Real-time continuous data (i.e., comparing before and after ET tube suctioning)
- Portable
- Bedside technique

Limitations

- Peak-to-trough pressure changes (amplitude) during HFOV cannot be quantified
- Does not provide information about the regional distribution of lung volume/collapse

Electrical impedance tomography (EIT)

EIT hardware injects small amounts of electrical current sequentially, using electrodes applied circumferentially to the patient's chest. The receiving electrodes calculate the voltage differential and determine the impedance change (see Figure 2.47a). A cross-sectional image of the lung composed of 1024 data points (32×32 array) creates a topographic representation depicting the distribution of tissue electrical properties in a cross-sectional fashion.

Advantages

- Accurate (lung volume measurements correlate with CT images, Figure 2.47b)
- Portable
- Bedside measurements
- Scanning rate between 13 and 44 scans per second (44 cross-sectional images per second)

(a)

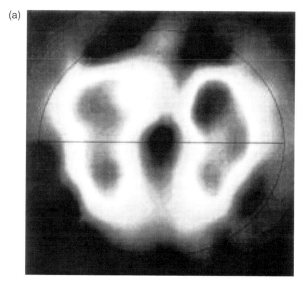

Figure 2.47
(a) Electrical impedance tomography (EIT). Representative data analysis depicting the heterogeneous distribution of lung volume in a mechanically ventilated patient. (b) Electrical impedance tomography (EIT). Data in contrast with CT images in a mechanically ventilated patient.

(b)

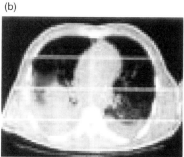 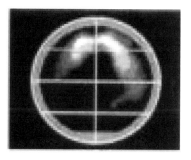

- Impedance measurements up to 30 min in length
- Quantifies regional and global changes in lung volume[169]
- Can record simultaneous ventilatory pressures (correlate impedance changes with airway pressures)
- Capable of tracking lung volume changes during HFOV

Limitations

- Requires experience in data interpretation (different tissues in the thorax can cause changes in lung tissue impedance)
- Cardiopulmonary interactions during mechanical ventilation affect EIT signal
- Electrical interference is produced by 50 mA currents generated by patient monitoring devices[170]
- Decreased resolution with small tidal volumes

Ventilatory considerations in selected clinical conditions (see Table 2.15)

Table 2.15 General ventilatory considerations in selected clinical conditions

Condition	CMV	HFOV	iNO	ECMO
RDS	Volume targeted ventilation is superior to PV in VLBW <1000 g for some clinical outcomes*[176,177] When using IMV in 700–1000 g neonates adding PS is beneficial[177]	No effect on overall morbidity.[179] Significant improvement in oxygenation in severe respiratory failure[160,179]. May decrease the incidence of CLD[181]	Effective in reducing the risk of brain injury associated with MV[164]. May be associated with improving the risk of CLD[182]	Not indicated in neonates <1800 g or <34 weeks Less indicated as alternative new modalities have emerged
MA	In mild to moderate cases effective when combined with exogenous surfactant replacement and bronchoalveolar lavage[183]. Controversy whether inhaled or IV steroids improves outcome[184,185]	Effective alternative in patients who fail CMV Effective if combined with exogenous surfactant replacement and bronchoalveolar lavage[183]	May improve oxygenation in combination with CMV or HFOV.[186] No outcome data available in humans	Indicated in infants with severe respiratory failure[165]
CDH	SIMV-PS with permissive hypercapnia is the first line of therapy[187]	Effective as initial therapy[188]. Unclear whether superior to CMV	Improves outcomes and decreases the need for ECMO if in combination with either CMV or HFOV[189]	Not indicated as initial therapy. Reserved for severe respiratory failure[190]

CDH, congenital diaphragmatic hernia; CLD, chronic lung disease; CMV, convention mechanical ventilation; ECMO, extracorporeal membrane oxygenation; HFOV, high-frequency oscillatory ventilation; IMV, intermittent mandatory ventilation; MA, meconium aspiration; RDS, respiratory distress syndrome.
*Duration of ventilation, pneumothorax, intraventricular hemorrhage, and incidence of bronchopulmonary dysplasia.

Respiratory distress syndrome (RDS; see "Management of very preterm newborn infants (VLBW, ELBW)," p. 231)

RDS the most common respiratory disorder in preterm neonates. An immature lung parenchyma with various degrees of surfactant deficiency is common to all etiologic forms of RDS[171,172]. Patients with RDS are usually the product of preterm labor requiring endotracheal intubation and mechanical ventilation at birth. Significant advances have been made in management of this disease, including antenatal steroids and exogenous surfactant replacement; however mechanical ventilation is needed in the vast majority of these patients.

Meconium aspiration (see "Meconium spiration," p. 269)

This is a common respiratory complication of often otherwise healthy neonates. Meconium aspiration syndrome is usually induced by fetal distress during labor. Mechanical obstruction of the airways and diffusion impairment by meconium induce various degrees of respiratory failure. Depending on the severity of the hypoxemia, neonates may require intensive support ranging from from conventional mechanical ventilation to ECMO.

Congenital diaphragmatic hernia (see "Congenital diaphragmatic hernia," p. 404)

CDH is a common congenital malformation of the diaphragm, which allows the migration of abdominal organs to occupy the thoracic cavity during the early stages of lung development. As as a result, pulmonary hypoplasia and pulmonary vascular hypertension generally mandate immediate ventilatory support at birth. Ventilatory management of neonates with this disease has evolved alongside the different ventilatory modalites, reflecting in part the evolution to more modern therapy[190].

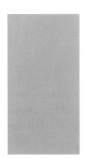

Questions for review (basics)

1. Especially for obstetricians and midwives:
   When is a pediatrician needed in the delivery room? See p. 134.
2. Review the checklist for neonatal resuscitation (preparation). Then look up p. 136.
3. How are the different helper roles assigned prior to an upcoming neonatal resuscitation? See p. 140.
4. Procedures: what are the most important primary measures during the resuscitation of a (slightly to severely) depressed newly born infant? What should you keep in mind and avoid while performing neonatal resuscitation? See pp. 66–123, pp. 150–72.
5. Clinical assessment of the newborn infant in the delivery room: the initial evaluation of the neonate is dependent on which three signs? What is the main difference between "primary" and "secondary (terminal) apnea"? What Five questions need to be answered by the person who performs the initial care/resuscitation? When after birth do you have to decide whether more extensive resuscitative measures have to be initiated (PPV, etc.)? To what extent do the 1-min and 5-min Apgar scores allow a statement on the general condition and prognosis of a newborn? See pp. 142–9, pp. 191–2.
6. Taking all signs and symptoms together (vital signs, 1-min Apgar score, initial umbilical artery pH value), newborns at birth can be roughly divided into five groups, including a "problem group (non-responders)." How are each of these neonates managed? See pp. 168–71.
7. What are the 7 "H"s that endanger the newly born term and preterm infant? See p. 171.
8. Cardiopulmonary resuscitation of the newborn infant. Recapitulate in your mind and then look up the following: ABCD measures, standard algorithm of neonatal resuscitation, and techniques/procedures (e.g., bag-and-mask ventilation, endotracheal intubation? When to perform PPV? When to do chest compressions? When to intubate?), including the dosage of the most important drugs (epinephrine). See pp. 150–72, Fig. 2.37, Fig. 2.38.
9. Does the International Liaision Committee on Neonatal Resuscitation (ILCOR 2005) recommend a specific oxygen concentration to be used in the delivery room? See p. 163.
10. Why is it reasonable to start neonatal resuscitation with room air and have up to 100% oxygen available as a back-up (certain exceptions apply)? See pp. 70–1, p. 312.
11. What do you have to keep in mind when administering volume and buffer solutions (sodium bicarbonate, THAM) to a term newborn – and especially to a preterm infant? See pp. 176–8.

Neonatal Emergencies: A Practical Guide for Resuscitation, Transport and Critical Care, ed. Georg Hansmann.
Published by Cambridge University Press. © Cambridge University Press 2009.

12. Review absolute and relative indications for transfer of a newborn infant! See pp. 179–80.

13. Mechanical ventilation: what variables can be manipulated during mechanical ventilation to improve oxygenation and ventilation in the neonate. See pp. 198–9.

14. Mechanical ventilation: name commonly accepted indications for establishing high-frequency oscillatory ventilation (HFOV) in the neonate. See pp. 199–200.

15. Mechanical ventilation. List indications for nitric oxide therapy in the neonate. See p. 204.

16. Mechanical ventilation. List exclusion criteria for extracorporeal membrane oxygenation (ECMO). See p. 206.

17. Mechanical ventilation. What ventilatory interventions have been proven to be of clinical benefit in patients with meconium aspiration syndrome? See p. 208, Table 2.15.

References (Section 2)

1. O'Donnell C, Davis P, Morley C. Positive end-expiratory pressure for resuscitation of newborn infants at birth. *Cochrane Database Syst Rev* 2004(4):CD004341.

2. Stenson BJ, Boyle DW, Szyld EG. Initial ventilation strategies during newborn resuscitation. *Clin Perinatol* 2006;**33**(1): 65–82, vi–vii.

3. Leone TA, Rich W, Finer NN. A survey of delivery room resuscitation practices in the United States. *Pediatrics* 2006;**117**(2):e164–75.

4. Hansmann G. Neonatal resuscitation on air: it is time to turn down the oxygen tanks [corrected]. *Lancet* 2004;**364**(9442):1293–4.

5. Davis PG, Tan A, O'Donnell CP, Schulze A. Resuscitation of newborn infants with 100 % oxygen or air: a systematic review and meta-analysis. *Lancet* 2004;**364**(9442):1329–33.

6. Saugstad OD, Ramji S, Vento M. Resuscitation of depressed newborn infants with ambient air or pure oxygen: a meta-analysis. *Biol Neonate* 2005;**87**(1):27–34.

7. Vento M, Sastre J, Asensi MA, Vina J. Room-air resuscitation causes less damage to heart and kidney than 100 % oxygen. *Am J Respir Crit Care Med* 2005;**172**(11):1393–8.

8. Ralston M, Hazinski MF, Zaritsky AL, Schexnayder SM, Kleinman ME. *PALS Provider Manual.* Dallas: American Heart Association and American Academy of Pediatrics, 2006.

9. Kattwinkel J. *Neonatal Resuscitation*, 5th edn. Elk Grove Village: American Academy of Pediatrics and American Heart Association, 2006.

10. O'Donnell CP, Davis PG, Lau R, Dargaville PA, Doyle LW, Morley CJ. Neonatal resuscitation 2: an evaluation of manual ventilation devices and face masks. *Arch Dis Child Fetal Neonatal Ed* 2005;**90**(5):F392–6.

11. Leone TA, Lange A, Rich W, Finer NN. Disposable colorimetric carbon dioxide detector use as an indicator of a patent airway during noninvasive mask ventilation. *Pediatrics* 2006;**118**(1):e202–4.

12. Bührer C, Bahr S, Siebert J, Wettstein R, Geffers C, Obladen M. Use of 2 % 2-phenoxyethanol and 0.1 % octenidine as antiseptic in premature newborn infants of 23–26 weeks gestation. *J Hosp Infect* 2002; **51**(4):305–7.

13. Young TE, Mangum B. *Neofax 2007*, 20th edn. London: Thomson PDR, 2007.

14. Allen HD, Driscoll DJ, Shaddy RE, Feltes TF. *Moss and Adams' Heart Disease in Infants, Children, and Adolescents: Including the Fetus and Young Adult*, 7th edn. Philadelphia: Lippincott Williams and Wilkins, 2008.

15. Nichols DG, Ungerleider RM, Spevak PJ, et al. *Critical Heart Disease in Infants and Children*, 2nd edn. Philadelphia: Mosby, 2006.

16. Park MK. *Pediatric Cardiology for Practitioners*, 5th edn. St. Louis: Mosby, 2008.

17. Rennie JM, Robertson NRC. *Robertson's Textbook of Neonatology*, 4th edn. Edinburgh: Churchill Livingstone, 2005.

18. Kliegman R. Fetal and neonatal medicine. In: Behrman R, Kliegman R, eds. *Nelson Essentials of Pediatrics*, 4th edn. Philadelphia: W. R. Saunders Company, 2002: 179–249.

19. Roth P, Harris M, Vega-Rich C, Marro P. Neonatology. In: Polin RA, Ditmar MF eds. *Pediatric Secrets*. Philadelphia: Hanley & Belfus, 2001: 409–65.

20. Cordero L, Jr., Hon EH. Neonatal bradycardia following nasopharyngeal stimulation. *J Pediatr* 1971;**78**(3):441–7.

21. Vain NE, Szyld EG, Prudent LM, Wiswell TE, Aguilar AM, Vivas NI. Oropharyngeal and nasopharyngeal suctioning of meconium-stained neonates before delivery of their shoulders: multicentre, randomised controlled trial. *Lancet* 2004;**364**(9434):597–602.

22. International Liaison Committee on Resuscitation. 2005 International Consensus on Cardiopulmonary Resuscitation and Emergency Cardiovascular Care Science with Treatment Recommendations. Part 7: Neonatal resuscitation. *Resuscitation* 2005;**67**(2–3):293–303.

23. Halliday HL. Endotracheal intubation at birth for preventing morbidity and mortality in vigorous, meconium-stained infants born at term. *Cochrane Database Syst Rev* 2001 (1):CD000500.

24. Wiswell TE, Gannon CM, Jacob J, et al. Delivery room management of the apparently vigorous meconium-stained neonate: results of the multicenter international collaborative trial. *Pediatrics* 2000;**105**(1):1–7.

25. Niermeyer S, Kattwinkel J, Van Reempts P, et al. International Guidelines for Neonatal Resuscitation: an excerpt from the Guidelines 2000 for Cardiopulmonary Resuscitation and Emergency Cardiovascular Care: International Consensus on Science. Contributors and Reviewers for the Neonatal Resuscitation Guidelines. *Pediatrics* 2000;**106**(3):E29 (http://pediatrics.aappublications.org/cgi/reprint/106/3/e29).

26. Wiswell TE, Knight GR, Finer NN, et al. A multicenter, randomized, controlled trial comparing Surfaxin (Lucinactant) lavage with standard care for treatment of meconium aspiration syndrome. *Pediatrics* 2002;**109**(6):1081–7.

27. Kattwinkel J. Surfactant lavage for meconium aspiration: a word of caution. *Pediatrics* 2002;**109**(6):1167–8.

28. Lundstrom KE, Pryds O, Greisen G. Oxygen at birth and prolonged cerebral vasoconstriction in preterm infants. *Arch Dis Child Fetal Neonatal Ed* 1995;**73**(2):F81–6.

29. Beasley R, McNaughton A, Robinson G. New look at the oxyhaemoglobin dissociation curve. *Lancet* 2006;**367**(9517):1124–6.

30. Saugstad OD. Oxygen saturations immediately after birth. *J Pediatr* 2006;**148**(5): 569–70.

31. Collins MP, Lorenz JM, Jetton JR, Paneth N. Hypocapnia and other ventilation-related risk factors for cerebral palsy in low birth weight infants. *Pediatr Res* 2001;**50**(6):712–19.

32. Fabres J, Carlo WA, Phillips V, Howard G, Ambalavanan N. Both extremes of arterial carbon dioxide pressure and the magnitude of fluctuations in arterial carbon dioxide pressure are associated with severe intraventricular hemorrhage in preterm infants. *Pediatrics* 2007;**119**(2):299–305.

33. Askie LM, Henderson-Smart DJ, Irwig L, Simpson JM. Oxygen-saturation targets and outcomes in extremely preterm infants. *N Engl J Med* 2003;**349**(10):959–67.

34. Tin W, Milligan DW, Pennefather P, Hey E. Pulse oximetry, severe retinopathy, and outcome at one year in babies of less than 28 weeks gestation. *Arch Dis Child Fetal Neonatal Ed* 2001;**84**(2):F106–10.

35. Finer NN, Rich WD. Neonatal resuscitation: raising the bar. *Curr Opin Pediatr* 2004;**16**(2):157–62.

36. Tin W, Walker S, Lacamp C. Oxygen monitoring in preterm babies: too high, too low? *Paediatr Respir Rev* 2003;**4**(1):9–14.

37. Saugstad OD, Rootwelt T, Aalen O. Resuscitation of asphyxiated newborn infants with room air or oxygen: an international controlled trial: the Resair 2 study. *Pediatrics* 1998;**102**(1):e1 (http://pediatrics.aappublications.org/cgi/content/full/102/1/e1).

38. Vento M, Asensi M, Sastre J, Garcia-Sala F, Pallardo FV, Vina J. Resuscitation with room air instead of 100 % oxygen prevents oxidative stress in moderately asphyxiated term neonates. *Pediatrics* 2001;**107**(4):642–7.

39. Vento M, Asensi M, Sastre J, Lloret A, Garcia-Sala F, Vina J. Oxidative stress in asphyxiated term infants resuscitated with 100 % oxygen. *J Pediatr* 2003;**142**(3):240–6.

40. Niermeyer S, Vento M. Is 100 % oxygen necessary for the resuscitation of newborn infants? *J Matern Fetal Neonatal Med* 2004;**15**(2):75–84.

41. O'Donnell CP, Davis PG, Morley CJ. Positive pressure ventilation at neonatal resuscitation: review of equipment and international survey of practice. *Acta Paediatr* 2004;**93**(5):583–8.

42. Jobe AH, Bancalari E. Bronchopulmonary dysplasia. *Am J Respir Crit Care Med* 2001;**163**(7):1723–9.

43. Jobe AH, Kramer BW, Moss TJ, Newnham JP, Ikegami M. Decreased indicators of lung injury with continuous positive expiratory pressure in preterm lambs. *Pediatr Res* 2002;**52**(3):387–92.

44. Naik AS, Kallapur SG, Bachurski CJ, et al. Effects of ventilation with different positive end-expiratory pressures on cytokine expression in the preterm lamb lung. *Am J Respir Crit Care Med* 2001;**164**(3):494–8.

45. Vanpee M, Walfridsson-Schultz U, Katz-Salamon M, Zupancic JA, Pursley D, Jonsson B. Resuscitation and ventilation strategies for extremely preterm infants: a comparison study between two neonatal centers in Boston and Stockholm. *Acta Paediatr* 2007;**96**(1):10–16; discussion 8–9.

46. Lindner W, Pohlandt F. Oxygenation and ventilation in spontaneously breathing very preterm infants with nasopharyngeal CPAP in the delivery room. *Acta Paediatr* 2007;**96**(1):17–22.

47. Halamek LP, Morley C. Continuous positive airway pressure during neonatal resuscitation. *Clin Perinatol* 2006;**33**(1):83–98, vii.

48. Courtney SE, Barrington KJ. Continuous positive airway pressure and noninvasive ventilation. *Clin Perinatol* 2007;**34**(1): 73–92, vi.

49. Van Marter LJ, Allred EN, Pagano M, et al. Do clinical markers of barotrauma and oxygen toxicity explain interhospital variation in rates of chronic lung disease? The Neonatology Committee for the Developmental Network. *Pediatrics* 2000;**105**(6):1194–201.

50. Blennow M, Jonsson B, Dahlstrom A, Sarman I, Bohlin K, Robertson B. [Lung function in premature infants can be improved. Surfactant therapy and CPAP reduce the need of respiratory support.] *Lakartidningen* 1999;**96**(13):1571–6.

51. Stevens TP, Blennow M, Soll RF. Early surfactant administration with brief ventilation vs selective surfactant and continued mechanical ventilation for preterm infants with or at risk for respiratory distress syndrome. *Cochrane Database Syst Rev* 2004(3):CD003063.

52. Kribs A. Is it safer to intubate premature infants in the delivery room? *Pediatrics* 2006;**117**(5):1858–9; author reply 1859.

53. Kribs A, Pillekamp F, Hunseler C, Vierzig A, Roth B. Early administration of surfactant in spontaneous breathing with nCPAP: feasibility and outcome in extremely premature infants (postmenstrual age ≤27 weeks). *Paediatr Anaesth* 2007;**17**(4):364–9.

54. Clark RH, Gerstmann DR, Jobe AH, Moffitt ST, Slutsky AS, Yoder BA. Lung injury in neonates: causes, strategies for prevention, and long-term consequences. *J Pediatr* 2001;**139**(4):478–86.

55. Auten RL, Vozzelli M, Clark RH. Volutrauma. What is it, and how do we avoid it? *Clin Perinatol* 2001;**28**(3):505–15.

56. Carlton DP, Cummings JJ, Scheerer RG, Poulain FR, Bland RD. Lung overexpansion increases pulmonary microvascular protein permeability in young lambs. *J Appl Physiol* 1990;**69**(2):577–83.

57. Carlton DP, Cho SC, Davis P, Bland RD. Inflation pressure and lung vascular injury in preterm lambs. *Chest* 1994;**105**(3 Suppl):115S–116S.

58. Bittigau P, Sifringer M, Genz K, et al. Antiepileptic drugs and apoptotic neurodegeneration in the developing brain. *Proc Nat Acad Sci USA* 2002;**99**(23):15089–94.

59. Roberts KD, Leone TA, Edwards WH, Rich WD, Finer NN. Premedication for nonemergent neonatal intubations: a randomized, controlled trial comparing atropine and fentanyl to atropine, fentanyl, and mivacurium. *Pediatrics* 2006;**118**(4):1583–91.

60. Barrington KJ, Byrne PJ. Premedication for neonatal intubation. *Am J Perinatol* 1998;**15**(4):213–16.

61. Dempsey EM, Al Hazzani F, Faucher D, Barrington KJ. Facilitation of neonatal endotracheal intubation with mivacurium and fentanyl in the neonatal intensive care unit. *Arch Dis Child Fetal Neonatal Ed* 2006;**91**(4):F279–82.

62. Saarenmaa E, Huttunen P, Leppaluoto J, Meretoja O, Fellman V. Advantages of fentanyl over morphine in analgesia for ventilated newborn infants after birth: a randomized trial. *J Pediatr* 1999;**134**(2):144–50.

63. Hall RW, Kronsberg SS, Barton BA, Kaiser JR, Anand KJ. Morphine, hypotension, and adverse outcomes among preterm neonates: who's to blame? Secondary results from the NEOPAIN trial. *Pediatrics* 2005;**115**(5):1351–9.

64. van Straaten HL, Rademaker CM, de Vries LS. Comparison of the effect of midazolam or vecuronium on blood pressure and cerebral blood flow velocity in the premature newborn. *Dev Pharmacol Ther* 1992;**19**(4):191–5.

65. Ghanta S, Abdel-Latif ME, Lui K, Ravindranathan H, Awad J, Oei J. Propofol compared with the morphine, atropine, and suxamethonium regimen as induction agents for neonatal endotracheal intubation: a randomized, controlled trial. *Pediatrics* 2007;**119**(6):e1248–55.

66. Mellon RD, Simone AF, Rappaport BA. Use of anesthetic agents in neonates and young children. *Anesth Analg* 2007;**104**(3):509–20.

67. O'Donnell CP, Kamlin CO, Davis PG, Morley CJ. Endotracheal intubation attempts during neonatal resuscitation: success rates, duration, and adverse effects. *Pediatrics* 2006;**117**(1):e16–21.

68. Falck AJ, Escobedo MB, Baillargeon JG, Villard LG, Gunkel JH. Proficiency of pediatric residents in performing neonatal endotracheal intubation. *Pediatrics* 2003; **112**(6 Pt 1):1242–7.

69. Grein AJ, Weiner GM. Laryngeal mask airway versus bag-mask ventilation or endotracheal intubation for neonatal resuscitation. *Cochrane Database Syst Rev* 2005(2):CD003314.

70. Micaglio M, Trevisanuto D, Doglioni N, Zanette G, Zanardo V, Ori C. The size 1 LMA-ProSeal: comparison with the LMA-Classic during pressure controlled ventilation in a neonatal intubation manikin. *Resuscitation* 2007;**72**(1):124–7.

71. Goldmann K, Roettger C, Wulf H. The size 1(1/2) ProSeal laryngeal mask airway in infants: a randomized, crossover investigation with the Classic laryngeal mask airway. *Anesth Analg* 2006;**102**(2):405–10.

72. Shem S. *House of God*. New York: Dell Publishing, 1978.

73. Kabra NS, Kumar M, Shah SS. Multiple versus single lumen umbilical venous catheters for newborn infants. *Cochrane Database Syst Rev* 2005(3):CD004498.

74. Anderson J, Leonard D, Braner DA, Lai S, Tegtmeyer K. Videos in clinical medicine. Umbilical vascular catheter isahon. *N Eng 1 J Med* 2008;**359**(15):e18.

75. Barrington KJ. Umbilical artery catheters in the newborn: effects of catheter design (end vs side hole). *Cochrane Database Syst Rev* 2000(2):CD000508.

76. Barrington KJ. Umbilical artery catheters in the newborn: effects of position of the catheter tip. *Cochrane Database Syst Rev* 2000(2):CD000505.

77. O'Grady NP, Alexander M, Dellinger EP, et al. Guidelines for the prevention of intravascular catheter-related infections. The Hospital Infection Control Practices Advisory Committee, Center for Disease Control and Prevention, US. *Pediatrics* 2002;**110**(5):e51.

78. Cetta F, Graham LC, Eidem BW. Gaining vascular access in pediatric patients: use of the P.D. access Doppler needle. *Catheter Cardiovasc Interv* 2000;**51**(1):61–4.

79. Latto IP, Rosen M. *Percutaneous Central Venous and Arterial Catheterisation*, 3rd edn. London: Saunders, 2000.

80. Alderson PJ, Burrows FA, Stemp LI, Holtby HM. Use of ultrasound to evaluate internal jugular vein anatomy and to facilitate central venous cannulation in paediatric patients. *Br J Anaesth* 1993; **70**(2):145–8.

81. Verghese ST, McGill WA, Patel RI, Sell JE, Midgley FM, Ruttimann UE. Ultrasound-guided internal jugular venous cannulation in infants: a prospective comparison with the traditional palpation method. *Anesthesiology* 1999;**91**(1):71–7.

82. Arai T, Yamashita M. Central venous catheterization in infants and children – small caliber audio-Doppler probe versus ultrasound scanner. *Paediatr Anaesth* 2005;**15**(10):858–61.

83. Higgs ZC, Macafee DA, Braithwaite BD, Maxwell-Armstrong CA. The Seldinger technique: 50 years on. *Lancet* 2005; **366**(9494):1407–9.

84. Fiorito BA, Mirza F, Doran TM, et al. Intraosseous access in the setting of pediatric critical care transport. *Pediatr Crit Care Med* 2005;**6**(1):50–3.

85. Engle WA. Intraosseous access for administration of medications in neonates. *Clin Perinatol* 2006;**33**(1):161–8, ix.

86. Lake W, Emmerson AJ. Use of a butterfly as an intraosseous needle in an oedematous preterm infant. *Arch Dis Child Fetal Neonatal Ed* 2003;**88**(5):F409.

87. Hillewig E, Aghayev E, Jackowski C, Christe A, Plattner T, Thali MJ. Gas embolism following intraosseous medication application proven by post-mortem multislice computed tomography and autopsy. *Resuscitation* 2007;**72**(1):149–53.

88. Haas NA, Haas SA. Central venous catheter techniques in infants and children. *Curr Opin Anaesthesiol* 2003;**16**(3):291–303.

89. Haas NA. Clinical review: vascular access for fluid infusion in children. *Crit Care* 2004;**8**(6):478–84.

90. Skippen P, Kissoon N. Ultrasound guidance for central vascular access in the pediatric emergency department. *Pediatr Emerg Care* 2007;**23**(3):203–7.

91. Hutton EK, Hassan ES. Late vs early clamping of the umbilical cord in full-term neonates: systematic review and meta-analysis of controlled trials. *J Am Med Assoc* 2007;**297**(11):1241–52.

92. Rabe H, Reynolds G, Diaz-Rossello J. Early versus delayed umbilical cord clamping in preterm infants. *Cochrane Database Syst Rev* 2004(4):CD003248.

93. Sham S. *House of God.* New York: Dell Publishing, 1978.

94. Brady MT. Health care-associated infections in the neonatal intensive care unit. *Am J Infect Control* 2005;**33**(5):268–75.

95. Lam BC, Lee J, Lau YL. Hand hygiene practices in a neonatal intensive care unit: a multimodal intervention and impact on nosocomial infection. *Pediatrics* 2004;**114**(5):e565–71.

96. Brunetti L, Santoro E, De Caro F, et al. Surveillance of nosocomial infections: a preliminary study on hand hygiene compliance of healthcare workers. *J Prev Med Hyg* 2006;**47**(2):64–8.

97. CDC. Recommendations and Reports. *MMWR Morb Mortal Wkly Rep* 2002;51.

98. Webster J, Pritchard MA. Gowning by attendants and visitors in newborn nurseries for prevention of neonatal morbidity and mortality. *Cochrane Database Syst Rev* 2003(3):CD003670.

99. Dettenkofer M, Wenzler S, Amthor S, Antes G, Motschall E, Daschner FD. Does disinfection of environmental surfaces influence nosocomial infection rates? A systematic review. *Am J Infect Control* 2004;**32**(2):84–9.

100. Casey BM, McIntire DD, Leveno KJ. The continuing value of the Apgar score for the assessment of newborn infants. *N Engl J Med* 2001;**344**(7):467–71.

101. Papile LA. The Apgar score in the 21st century. *N Engl J Med* 2001;**344**(7):519–20.

102. Cockburn F, Cooke R, Gamsu H. The CRIB (Clinical Risk Index for Babies) score: a tool for assessing initial neonatal risk and comparing performance of neonatal intensive care units. The International Neonatal Network. *Lancet* 1993;**342** (8865):193–8.

103. Nelson KB, Emery ES, 3rd. Birth asphyxia and the neonatal brain: what do we know and when do we know it? *Clin Perinatol* 1993;**20**(2):327–44.

104. Richmond S. ILCOR and neonatal resuscitation 2005. *Arch Dis Child Fetal Neonatal Ed* 2007;**92**(3):F163–5.

105. Gunn AJ, Hoehn T, Hansmann G, et al. Hypothermia, an evolving treatment for neonatal hypoxic ischemic encephalopathy. *Pediatrics* 2008;**121**:648–49.

106. Dawes GS. Birth asphyxia, resuscitation, and brain damage. In: *Foetal and Neonatal Physiology.* Chicago: Year Book Publisher, 1968:141–59.

107. Carter BS, Haverkamp AD, Merenstein GB. The definition of acute perinatal asphyxia. *Clin Perinatol* 1993;**20**(2):287–304.

108. Owen CJ, Wyllie JP. Determination of heart rate in babies at birth. *Resuscitation* 2004;**60**:213–17.

109. Perlman JM, Risser R. Cardiopulmonary resuscitation in the delivery room – associated clinical events. *Arch Pediatr Adolesc Med* 1995;**149**:20–5.

110. Adamsons K, Jr., Behrman R, Dawes GS, James LS, Koford C. Resuscitation by positive pressure ventilation and Tris-hydroxymethylaminomethane of Rhesus monkeys asphyxiated at birth. *J Pediatr* 1964;**65**:807–18.

111. Campbell AG, Cockburn F, Dawes GS, Milligan JE. Pulmonary blood flow and cross-circulation between twin foetal lambs. *J Physiol (Lond)* 1966;**186**(2): 96P–97P.

112. Dawes GS. Circulatory adjustments in the newborn. *Heart Bull* 1963;**12**:17–19.

113. Richmond S, Goldsmith J. Air or 100 % oxygen in neonatal resuscitation? *Clin Perinatol* 2006;**33**(1):11–27.

114. Hoehn T, Hansmann G, Bührer C, et al. Therapeutic hypothermia in neonates. Review of current clinical data, ILCOR recommendations and suggestions for implementation in neonatal intensive care units. *Resuscitation* 2008;**78**(1):7–12.

115. Hansmann G, Humpl T, Zimmermann A, et al. [ILCOR's new resuscitation guidelines in preterm and term infants: critical discussion and suggestions for implementation.] *Klin Padiatr* 2007;**219**(2):50–7.

116. Vohra S, Roberts RS, Zhang B, Janes M, Schmidt B. Heat loss prevention (HeLP) in the delivery room: a randomized controlled trial of polyethylene occlusive skin wrapping in very preterm infants. *J Pediatr* 2004;**145**:750–3.

117. Cotten CM, Goldberg RU. Air leak syndromes. In: Spitzer A (ed.) *Intensive*

Care of the Fetus and Neonate, 2nd edn. Philadelphia: Elsevier Mosby, 2005; pp. 715–18.

118. McGuire W, Fowlie PW. Naloxone for narcotic-exposed newborn infants. *Cochrane Database Syst Rev* 2002(4): CD003483.

119. Rennie J, Chorley G, Boylan G, Pressler R, Nguyen Y, Hopper, R. Non-expert use of the cerebral function monitor for neonatal seizure detection. *Arch Dis Child Fetal Neonatal Ed* 2004;**89**(1):F37–40.

120. Ammari AN, Schulze KF. Uses and abuses of sodium bicarbonate in the neonatal intensive care unit. *Curr Opin Pediatr* 2002;**14**(2):151–6.

121. Dixon H, Hawkins K, Stephenson T. Comparison of albumin versus bicarbonate treatment for neonatal metabolic acidosis. *Eur J Pediatr* 1999; **158**(5):414–15.

122. Moore FD. The desperate case: CARE (costs, applicability, research, ethics). *J Am Med Assoc* 1989;**261**(10):1483–4.

123. Annas GJ. Extremely preterm birth and parental authority to refuse treatment – the case of Sidney Miller. *N Engl J Med* 2004;**351**(20):2118–23.

124. Duff RS, Campbell AG. Moral and ethical dilemmas in the special-care nursery. *N Engl J Med* 1973;**289**(17):890–4.

125. Ryan CA, Byrne P, Kuhn S, Tyebkhan J. No resuscitation and withdrawal of therapy in a neonatal and a pediatric intensive care unit in Canada. *J Pediatr* 1993; **123**(4):534–8.

126. Cuttini M, Kaminski M, Garel M, Lenoir S, Saracci R. End-of-life decisions in neonatal intensive care. *Lancet* 2000;**356** (9248):2190–1.

127. Provoost V, Cools F, Mortier F, et al. Medical end-of-life decisions in neonates and infants in Flanders. *Lancet* 2005; **365**(9467):1315–20.

128. Gold F. Exigence et refus de soins en néonatologie: le point de vue d'un pédiatre néonatologiste. [When parents require or refuse neonatal intensive care: one French neonatologist's opinion.] *Arch Pediatr* 2006;**13**(7):1005–8.

129. 2005 American Heart Association (AHA) guidelines for cardiopulmonary resuscitation (CPR) and emergency cardiovascular care (ECC) of pediatric and neonatal patients: neonatal resuscitation guidelines. Pediatrics 2006;117(5):e1029–38.

130. Silverman WA. Compassion or opportunism? *Pediatrics* 2004;**113**(2):402–3.

131. Janvier A, Barrington KJ. Advocating for the very preterm infant. *Pediatrics* 2006; **118**(1):429–30; author reply 430–2.

132. Österreichische Gesellschaft für Kinder- und Jugendheilkunde. Erstversorgung von Frühgeborenen an der Grenze zur Lebensfähigkeit. *Monatsschrift Kinderheilkunde* 2005;**153**:711–15.

133. Nuffield Council on Bioethics. *Critical Care Decisions in Fetal and Neonatal Medicine: Ethical Issues – Conclusions and Recommendations*. London: The Nuffield Council on Bioethics, 2006.

134. Berger TM, Büttiker V, Fauchère JC, et al. Empfehlungen zur Betreuung von Frühgeborenen an der Grenze der Lebensfähigkeit (Gestationsalter 22–26 SSW). *Schweizerische Aerztezeitung* 2002;**83**:1589–95.

135. Kaempf JW, Tomlinson M, Arduza C, et al. Medical staff guidelines for periviability pregnancy counseling and medical treatment of extremely premature infants. *Pediatrics* 2006;**117**(1):22–9.

136. Wood NS, Marlow N, Costeloe K, Gibson AT, Wilkinson AR. Neurologic and developmental disability after extremely preterm birth. EPICure Study Group. *N Engl J Med* 2000;**343**(6):378–84.

137. Marlow N, Wolke D, Bracewell MA, Samara M. Neurologic and developmental disability at six years of age after extremely preterm birth. *N Engl J Med* 2005;**352**(1):9–19.

138. Hentschel R, Lindner K, Krueger M, Reiter-Theil S. Restriction of ongoing intensive care in neonates: a prospective study. *Pediatrics* 2006;**118**(2):563–9.

139. Baumann-Hölzle R, Maffezzoni M, Bucher HU. A framework for ethical decision making in neonatal intensive care. *Acta Paediatr* 2005;**94**(12):1777–83.

140. Oransky I. William Silverman. *Lancet* 2005;**365**(9454):116.

141. Raju TN. William Sealy Gosset and William A. Silverman: two "students" of science. *Pediatrics* 2005;**116**(3): 732–5.

142. Kavanaugh K, Savage T, Kilpatrick S, Kimura R, Hershberger P. Life support decisions for extremely premature infants: report of a pilot study. *J Pediatr Nurs* 2005;**20**(5):347–59.

143. Partridge JC, Martinez AM, Nishida H, et al. International comparison of care for very low birth weight infants: parents' perceptions of counseling and decision-making. *Pediatrics* 2005;**116**(2):e263–71.

144. Emanuel EJ, Emanuel LL. Four models of the physician–patient relationship. *J Am Med Assoc* 1992;**267**(16):2221–6.

145. van der Heide A, van der Maas PJ, van der Wal G, Kollee LA, de Leeuw R, Holl RA. The role of parents in end-of-life decisions in neonatology: physicians' views and practices. *Pediatrics* 1998;**101**(3 Pt 1): 413–18.

146. Isaacs D, Kilham H, Gordon A, et al. Withdrawal of neonatal mechanical ventilation against the parents' wishes. *J Paediatr Child Health* 2006;**42**(5):311–15.

147. Tyson JE, Broyles RS. Progress in assessing the long-term outcome of extremely low-birth-weight infants. *J Am Med Assoc* 1996;**276**(6):492–3.

148. Tyson JE, Younes N, Verter J, Wright LL. Viability, morbidity, and resource use among newborns of 501-g to 800-g birth weight.National Institute of Child Health and Human Development Neonatal Research Network. *J Am Med Assoc* 1996;**276**(20):1645–51.

149. Perinatal care at the threshold of viability. American Academy of Pediatrics Committee on Fetus and Newborn. American College of Obstetricians and Gynecologists Committee on Obstetric Practice. [No authors listed.] Pediatrics 1995;96(5 Pt 1):974–6.

150. De Leeuw R, Cuttini M, Nadai M, et al. Treatment choices for extremely preterm infants: an international perspective. *J Pediatr* 2000;**137**(5):608–16.

151. Sauer PJ. Ethical dilemmas in neonatology: recommendations of the Ethics Working Group of the CESP (Confederation of European Specialists in Paediatrics). *Eur J Pediatr* 2001;**160**(6):364–8.

152. McHaffie HE, Cuttini M, Brolz-Voit G, et al. Withholding/withdrawing treatment from neonates: legislation and official guidelines across Europe. *J Med Ethics* 1999;**25**(6):440–6.

153. Verhagen E, Sauer PJ. The Groningen protocol – euthanasia in severely ill newborns. *N Engl J Med* 2005;**352**(10):959–62.

154. Verhagen AA, Sauer PJ, Verhagen E, Sauer PJ. End-of-life decisions in newborns: an approach from The Netherlands. The Groningen protocol – euthanasia in severely ill newborns. *Pediatrics* 2005; **116**(3):736–9.

155. Polimeni V, Claure N, D'Ugard C, Bancalari E. Effects of volume-targeted synchronized intermittent mandatory ventilation on spontaneous episodes of hypoxemia in preterm infants. *Biol Neonate* 2006;**89**(1):50–5.

156. Imanaka H, Nishimura M, Miyano H, Uemura H, Yagihara T. Effect of synchronized intermittent mandatory ventilation on respiratory workload in infants after cardiac surgery. *Anesthesiology* 2001;**95**(4):881–8.

157. High-frequency oscillatory ventilation compared with conventional mechanical ventilation in the treatment of respiratory failure in preterm infants. The HIFI Study Group. [No authors listed.] N Engl J Med 1989;320(2):88–93.

158. Courtney SE, Durand DJ, Asselin JM, Hudak ML, Aschner JL, Shoemaker CT. High-frequency oscillatory ventilation versus conventional mechanical ventilation for very-low-birth-weight infants. *N Engl J Med* 2002;**347**(9):643–52.

159. Henderson-Smart DJ, Bhuta T, Cools F, Offringa M. Elective high frequency oscillatory ventilation versus conventional ventilation for acute pulmonary dysfunction in preterm infants. *Cochrane Database Syst Rev* 2003(4):CD000104.

160. Arnold JH, Hanson JH, Toro-Figuero LO, Gutierrez J, Berens RJ, Anglin DL. Prospective, randomized comparison of high-frequency oscillatory ventilation and conventional mechanical ventilation in pediatric respiratory failure. *Crit Care Med* 1994;**22**(10):1530–9.

161. Calvert S. Prophylactic high-frequency oscillatory ventilation in preterm infants. *Acta Paediatr Suppl* 2002;**91**(437):16–18.

162. Day RW, Lynch JM, White KS, Ward RM. Acute response to inhaled nitric oxide in

newborns with respiratory failure and pulmonary hypertension. *Pediatrics* 1996;**98**(4 Pt 1):698–705.

163. Ballard RA, Truog WE, Cnaan A, et al. Inhaled nitric oxide in preterm infants undergoing mechanical ventilation. *N Engl J Med* 2006;**355**(4):343–53.

164. Kinsella JP, Cutter GR, Walsh WF, et al. Early inhaled nitric oxide therapy in premature newborns with respiratory failure. *N Engl J Med* 2006;**355**(4):354–64.

165. Kugelman A, Gangitano E, Taschuk R, et al. Extracorporeal membrane oxygenation in infants with meconium aspiration syndrome: a decade of experience with venovenous ECMO. *J Pediatr Surg* 2005; **40**(7):1082–9.

166. Simon BA. Non-invasive imaging of regional lung function using X-ray computed tomography. *J Clin Monit Comput* 2000;**16**(5–6):433–42.

167. Weber T, Tschernich H, Sitzwohl C, et al. Tromethamine buffer modifies the depressant effect of permissive hypercapnia on myocardial contractility in patients with acute respiratory distress syndrome. *Am J Respir Crit Care Med* 2000;**162** (4 Pt 1):1361–5.

168. Gothberg S, Parker TA, Griebel J, Abman SH, Kinsella JP. Lung volume recruitment in lambs during high-frequency oscillatory ventilation using respiratory inductive plethysmography. *Pediatr Res* 2001; **49**(1):38–44.

169. Brazelton TB, 3rd, Watson KF, Murphy M, Al-Khadra E, Thompson JE, Arnold JH. Identification of optimal lung volume during high-frequency oscillatory ventilation using respiratory inductive plethysmography. *Crit Care Med* 2001; **29**(12):2349–59.

170. Wolf GK, Arnold JH. Noninvasive assessment of lung volume: respiratory inductance plethysmography and electrical impedance tomography. *Crit Care Med* 2005;**33**(3 Suppl):S163–9.

171. Greenough A. Expanded use of surfactant replacement therapy. *Eur J Pediatr* 2000;**159**(9):635–40.

172. Finer NN. Surfactant use for neonatal lung injury: beyond respiratory distress syndrome. *Paediatr Respir Rev* 2004;**5** (Suppl A):S289–97.

173. Silberbach M, Hannon D. Presentation of congenital heart disease in the neonate and young infant. *Pediatr Rev* 2007;**28**(4):123–31.

174. Greenough A, Milner AD, Dimitriou G. Synchronized mechanical ventilation for respiratory support in newborn infants. *Cochrane Database Syst Rev* 2004(4): CD000456.

175. Mizuno K, Takeuchi T, Itabashi K, Okuyama K. Efficacy of synchronized IMV on weaning neonates from the ventilator. *Acta Paediatr Jpn* 1994;**36**(2):162–6.

176. McCallion N, Davis PG, Morley CJ. Volume-targeted versus pressure-limited ventilation in the neonate. *Cochrane Database Syst Rev* 2005(3):CD003666.

177. Singh J, Sinha SK, Clarke P, Byrne S, Donn SM. Mechanical ventilation of very low birth weight infants: is volume or pressure a better target variable? *J Pediatr* 2006; **149**(3):308–13.

178. Reyes C, Chang LK, Waffarn F, Mir H, Warden MJ, Sills J. Delayed repair of congenital diaphragmatic hernia with early high-frequency oscillatory ventilation during preoperative stabilization. *J Pediatr Surg* 1998;**33**(7):1010–14; discussion 1014–16.

179. Marlow N, Greenough A, Peacock JL, et al. Randomised trial of high frequency oscillatory ventilation or conventional ventilation in babies of gestational age 28 weeks or less: respiratory and neurological outcomes at 2 years. *Arch Dis Child Fetal Neonatal Ed* 2006;**91**(5):F320–6.

180. De Jaegere A, van Veenendaal MB, Michiels A, van Kaam AH. Lung recruitment using oxygenation during open lung high-frequency ventilation in preterm infants. *Am J Respir Crit Care Med* 2006;**174**(6):639–45.

181. Bhuta T, Henderson-Smart DJ. Elective high-frequency oscillatory ventilation versus conventional ventilation in preterm infants with pulmonary dysfunction: systematic review and meta-analyses. *Pediatrics* 1997;**100**(5):E6.

182. Hoehn T, Krause MF, Buhrer C. Meta-analysis of inhaled nitric oxide in premature infants: an update. *Klin Padiatr* 2006;**218**(2):57–61.

183. Lin HC, Su BH, Lin TW, Tsai CH, Yeh TF. System-based strategy for the management

of meconium aspiration syndrome: 198 consecutive cases observations. *Acta Paediatr Taiwan* 2005;**46**(2):67–71.

184. Sinn JK, Ward MC, Henderson-Smart DJ. Developmental outcome of preterm infants after surfactant therapy: systematic review of randomized controlled trials. *J Paediatr Child Health* 2002;**38**(6):597–600.

185. Ward M, Sinn J. Steroid therapy for meconium aspiration syndrome in newborn infants. *Cochrane Database Syst Rev* 2003(4):CD003485.

186. Huang QW, Sun B, Gao F, et al. Effects of inhaled nitric oxide and high-frequency ventilation in rabbits with meconium aspiration. *Biol Neonate* 1999;**76**(6): 374–82.

187. Boloker J, Bateman DA, Wung JT, Stolar CJ. Congenital diaphragmatic hernia in 120 infants treated consecutively with permissive hypercapnea/spontaneous respiration/elective repair. *J Pediatr Surg* 2002;**37**(3):357–66.

188. Cacciari A, Ruggeri G, Mordenti M, et al. High-frequency oscillatory ventilation versus conventional mechanical ventilation in congenital diaphragmatic hernia. *Eur J Pediatr Surg* 2001;**11**(1):3–7.

189. Okuyama H, Kubota A, Oue T, et al. Inhaled nitric oxide with early surgery improves the outcome of antenatally diagnosed congenital diaphragmatic hernia. *J Pediatr Surg* 2002;**37**(8):1188–90.

190. Lally KP, Lally PA, Van Meurs KP, et al. Treatment evolution in high-risk congenital diaphragmatic hernia: ten years' experience with diaphragmatic agenesis. *Ann Surg* 2006;**244**(4):505–13.

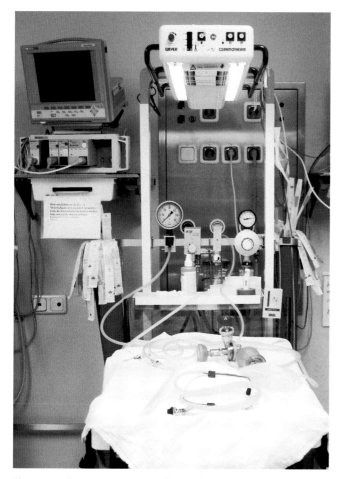

Figure 2.1 Resuscitation unit: a well-secured resuscitation table with side guards (down in the picture), covered with soft cotton blankets, with radiant warmer (here on stand-by), stethoscope, bag-mask-ventilation system (here self-inflating bag manufactured by Laerdal, model "infant," 250ml) with PEEP-valve, pressure gauge (manomometer for PIP monitoring), oxygen blender and flowmeter (both regulate inspiratory gas), mechanical suction with manometer (measured here in bar), suction catheters in various sizes (5–14 F, 5–18 Ch), Apgar timer, thermometer, sterile gauze, disinfectant solution, cardiopulmonary monitor (SpO_2, respiratory rate, heart rate, BP-NIBP or BP-arterial, CVP, ECG), oxygen and compressed-air wall supply.

Not shown: heating pad (K-pad), drawers with additional face masks, bulb syringe, meconium aspirator (ET tube adapter), intubation kit (laryngoscope, straight blades nos. 0 and 1, Magill forceps), endotracheal tubes (2.0–4.0), stylet (optional), laryngeal mask airway (optional), tape, scissors, extra bulb and battery for laryngoscope, oropharyngeal airways (Guedel sizes: 0, 00, 000 or 20-, 40-, and 50-mm lengths), CO_2 detector (colorimetric) or capnograph, umbilical vein/artery catheter equipment, alcohol sponges/swabs, angiocaths (24G, 26G) plus utensils for peripheral venous access, butterfly (22G, 24G), plastic wrap or reclosable, food-grade plastic bag (1-gallon size for preterms babies or abdominal wall defects), emergency drugs, normal saline, sodium bicarbonate 4.2% (5mEq/10ml = 5mmol/10ml), dextrose 10%, utensils for blood draw (blood gases, blood glucose and other labs, blood culture) and smears. Transport incubator to maintain baby's temperature on transport to the nursery. CVP, central venous pressure; ET, endotracheal tube; LMA, laryngeal mask airway; NIBP, non-invasive blood pressure; PEEP, positive end-expiratory pressure; PIP, peak inspiratory pressure.

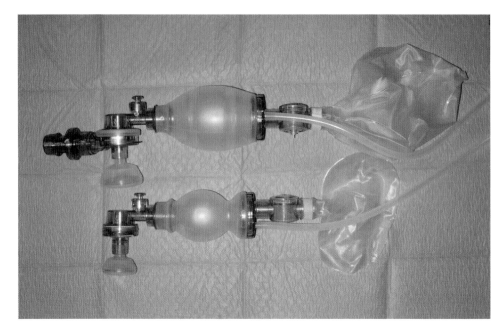

Figure 2.3 Two self-inflating bag-and-mask systems (Laerdal): upper device = model "child" (500ml, with PEEP valve); and lower device model: "infant" (250ml, here suboptimally without a PEEP valve). Safety pop-off valves make overinflation less likely. Refills even if not attached to compressed air source, but also refills if there is not a good seal between the mask and the patient's face. Can deliver PEEP if PEEP valve is added.

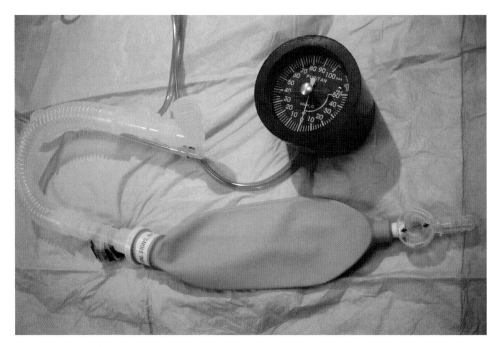

Figure 2.4 Flow-inflating bag-and-mask system (floppy "anesthesia bag"), 400ml. Can deliver CPAP and PEEP (regulate PEEP with flow-control valve). Disadvantages: requires a compressed air source. Requires a tight seal between the mask and the patient's face to remain inflated. Usually does not have a safety pop-off valve and therefore carries the risk of overinflation (check the connected pressure gauge frequently!). Note: flow-inflating bag systems need higher flow (8–10ml/min) and better seal than those with self-inflating bags. CPAP, continuous positive airway pressure; PEEP, peak end-expiratory pressure.

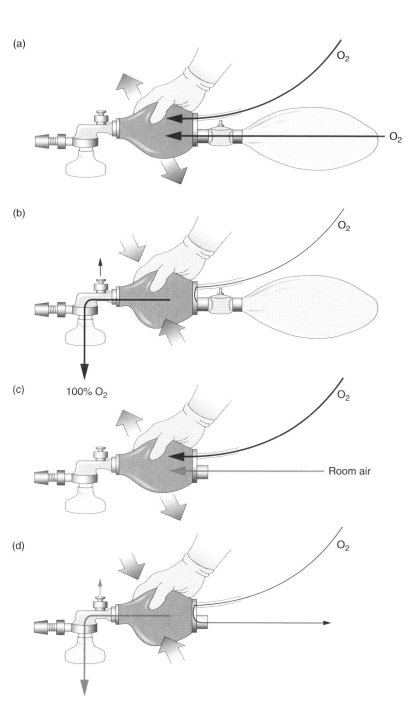

Figure 2.5a–d (a) Self-inflating bag-and-mask system with oxygen tubing, pop-off valve and PEEP valve. The gas mixture exhaled by the patient ends up in the atmosphere (a, c). (a) Bag re-expansion: O_2 flows from the source and the reservoir to the ventilation bag (ca. 100% O_2). (b) Bag compression: with a reservoir, almost 100% O_2 is delivered to the patient. (c) Re-expansion of the bag without a reservoir: with 5 l pure O_2/min flow → approx. 40%–50% O_2 in the bag. (d) Compression of bag without a reservoir: with a flow of 5 l pure O_2/min flow → ca. 40% O_2 will reach the patient. Modified from Ralston et al. (2006). *PALS Provider Manual.* American Heart Association and American Academy of Pediatrics.

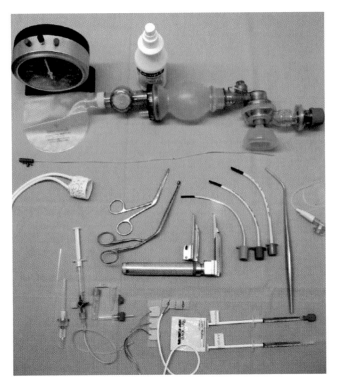

Figure 2.8 Ready-to-use equipment for initial care and resuscitation of neonates: timer, suction catheters, Yankauer suction catheter (not shown: meconium aspirator = tube adapter, Figure 2.16), bag-and-mask-system with inflatable reservoir and PEEP valve, intubation set [laryngoscope, straight blades (nos. 0 and 1), ET tubes (ETT shown here by Vygon) and Magill's forceps for nasal intubation (here two sizes: nasal intubation frequently performed in Europe), stylets for oral intubation (not shown; stylet optional; caution especially in preterm infants]. Oral intubation is standard technique in North America), two 1-ml syringes with epinephrine 1:10 000 (0.1 ml = 0.01 mg), gastric tube, utensils for blood workup: arterial blood gases, blood sugar, and chemistry (optional: blood cultures, smears), sphygmomanometer, ECG electrodes (here for preterm infants).

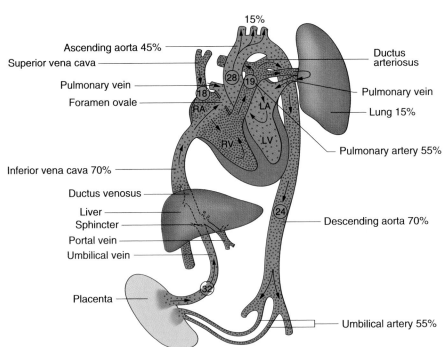

Figure 2.15 Fetal circulation with the four shunts: placenta, ductus venosus, foramen ovale, ductus arteriosus. The density of the dots is inversely proportional to the oxygen saturation: the less dense, the higher the oxygen partial pressure (PO₂). The numbers marked in the heart chambers and vessels correspond with the PO₂ in mmHg (circles). The percentages outside the cardiovascular structures stand for the relative flow in the main in-flow and outflow tracts of both heart chambers. The output of both ventricles adds up to 100%. VCI = V. cava inferior, LA = left atrium, LV = left ventricle, RA = right atrium, RV = right ventricle, VCS = V. cava superior. Modified from: Guntheroth WG et al. (1983) Physiology of the circulation: fetus, neonate and child. In: Kelly VC (ed.) Practice of Pediatrics, Vol. 8. Philadelphia: Harper & Row.

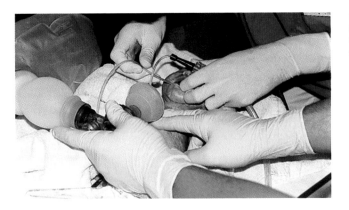

Figure 2.16 Oropharyngeal suctioning of amniotic fluid (here with simultaneous oxygen supplementation).

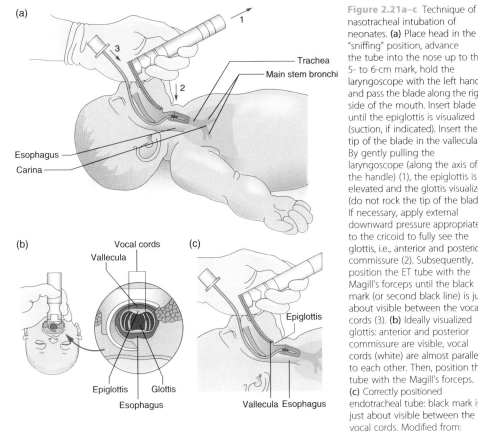

(a)

1

3

2

Trachea

Main stem bronchi

Esophagus

Carina

(b)

Vocal cords

Vallecula

(c)

Epiglottis

Epiglottis Glottis

Esophagus

Vallecula Esophagus

Figure 2.21a–c Technique of nasotracheal intubation of neonates. **(a)** Place head in the "sniffing" position, advance the tube into the nose up to the 5- to 6-cm mark, hold the laryngoscope with the left hand and pass the blade along the right side of the mouth. Insert blade until the epiglottis is visualized (suction, if indicated). Insert the tip of the blade in the vallecula. By gently pulling the laryngoscope (along the axis of the handle) (1), the epiglottis is elevated and the glottis visualized (do not rock the tip of the blade). If necessary, apply external downward pressure appropriately to the cricoid to fully see the glottis, i.e., anterior and posterior commissure (2). Subsequently, position the ET tube with the Magill's forceps until the black mark (or second black line) is just about visible between the vocal cords (3). **(b)** Ideally visualized glottis: anterior and posterior commissure are visible, vocal cords (white) are almost parallel to each other. Then, position the tube with the Magill's forceps. **(c)** Correctly positioned endotracheal tube: black mark is just about visible between the vocal cords. Modified from: Kattwinkel J, 2006. *Neonatal Resuscitation*, 5th edn. Elk Grove Village, IL: American Academy of Pediatrics and American Heart Association.

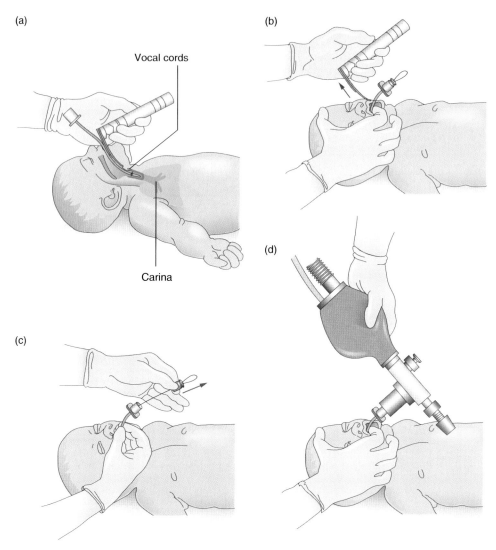

Figure 2.22a–d Technique of orotracheal intubation of neonates. **(a)** Place head in "sniffing" position, hold the laryngoscope with the left hand and pass the blade along the right side of the mouth. Insert blade until epiglottis is visualized (suction, if indicated). Insert the tip of the blade in the vallecula. By gently pulling the laryngoscope (along the axis of the handle) (step 1), the epiglottis is elevated and the glottis visualized (do not rock the tip of the blade). If necessary, apply external downward pressure appropriately to the cricoid to fully see the glottis, i.e., anterior and posterior commissure (step 2). Subsequently, advance the ET tube through the glottis until the black mark (or second black line) is just about visible between the vocal cords (step 3). **(b)** Hold the tube firmly with the right index finger against the maxillary ridge, then remove the laryngoscope. **(c)** Still holding the tube tightly with the right index finger, carefully remove the stylet from the tube. **(d)** PPV through the endotracheal tube (which is not yet taped) and always confirm correct ET tube position. (Are the chest movements sufficient and symmetrical? Are lungs equally ventilated? Is skin color more rosy? Rise of HR and SaO_2?). Then tape tube securely. Modified from: Kattwinkel J (2006) *Neonatal Resuscitation.* 5th edn. Elk Grove Village, IL: American Academy of Pediatrics and American Heart Association.

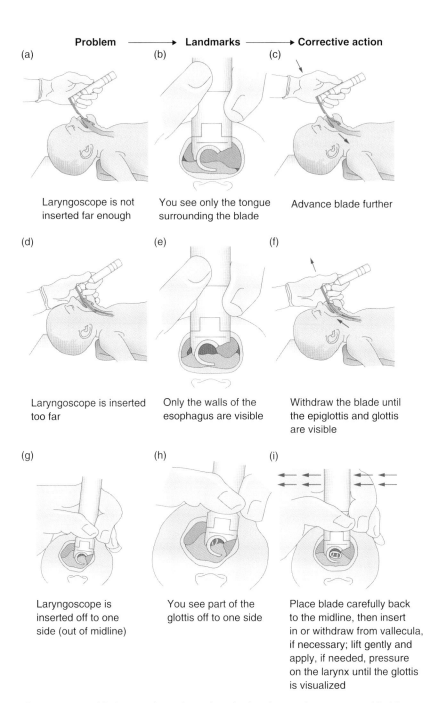

Problem →	Landmarks →	Corrective action

(a)

(b)

(c)

Laryngoscope is not inserted far enough

You see only the tongue surrounding the blade

Advance blade further

(d)

(e)

(f)

Laryngoscope is inserted too far

Only the walls of the esophagus are visible

Withdraw the blade until the epiglottis and glottis are visible

(g)

(h)

(i)

Laryngoscope is inserted off to one side (out of midline)

You see part of the glottis off to one side

Place blade carefully back to the midline, then insert in or withdraw from vallecula, if necessary; lift gently and apply, if needed, pressure on the larynx until the glottis is visualized

Figure 2.23 Troubleshooting during the endotracheal intubation of a neonate. Modified from: Kattwinkel J (2006) *Neonatal Resuscitation*, 5th edn. Elk Grove Village, IL: American Academy of Pediatrics and American Heart Association.

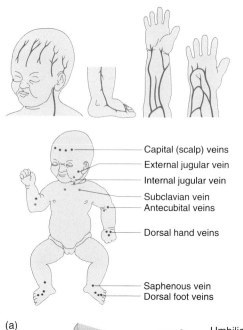

Capital (scalp) veins
External jugular vein
Internal jugular vein
Subclavian vein
Antecubital veins

Dorsal hand veins

Saphenous vein
Dorsal foot veins

Figure 2.28 Venous access. Possible venous insertion sites in neonates and infants. Central venous access (green), peripheral venous access (red).

(a)

(b)

(c)

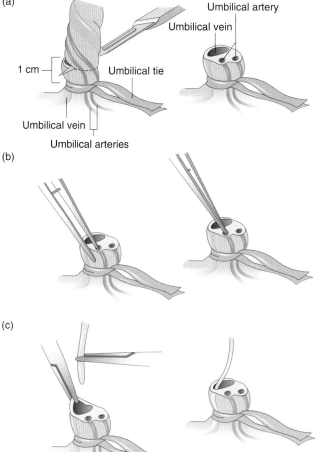

Umbilical artery
Umbilical vein

1 cm
Umbilical tie

Umbilical vein
Umbilical arteries

Figure 2.29 a–c Umbilical artery and umbilical vein catheterization (UAC, UVC). **(a)** Cutting the umbilical cord. **(b)** UAC placement: one helper gently dilates the umbilical artery with forceps. Then insert the UAC to a depth according to a depth as indicated in Table 2.3
(c) UVC placement: the helper or physician identifies the umbilical vein. Next insert the UVC to a depth as indicated in Table 2.3. In an emergency (full resuscitation including chest compressions) with no possibility of immediate radiographic control, insert the UVC tip only 3–5 cm until blood can be aspirated.[74]

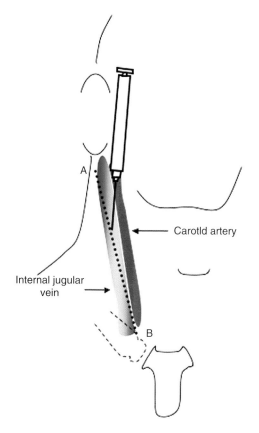

Figure 2.30 Anatomical relationship between the internal jugular vein (IJV) and carotid artery (CA). Note that the IJV travels lateral to the CA towards the midline between points A (= mastoid process of the temporal bone) and B (= jugular notch in the manubrium of the sternum).

Carotld artery

Internal jugular vein

Figure 2.32 Central venous catheter placement. Once the anatomy is identified (a), the initial goal is to gain access to the internal jugular vein (IJV) with the Spring-Wire Guide 0.18″ × 25cm minimizing tissue disruption by venous or arterial hematoma (b). The 24G ¾″ JELCO® is exchanged for the 22G 1″ JELCO® over the wire (c). This maneuver ensures secure access to the IJV, and allows advancement of the longer J tip 0.18″ × 45cm PTFE-coated Spring-Wire Guide. Additionally, this catheter can be safely attached to a pressure transducer to rule out carotid artery cannulation.

(a)

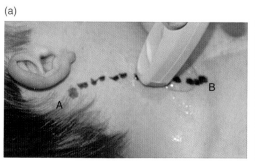

(b)

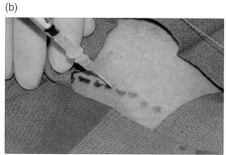

(c)

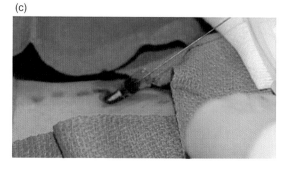

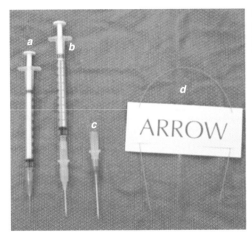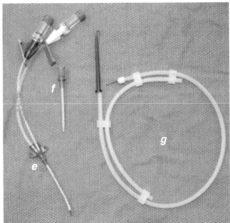

Figure 2.33 Materials required for internal jugular vein (IJV) cannulation. Items a, b, c and d are not included in the Central Venous Catheterization Kit and should be gathered separately.

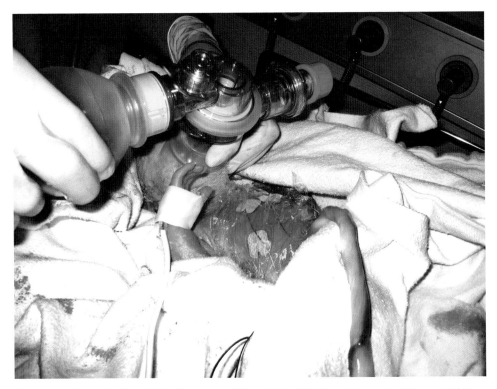

Figure 2.39 Bag-and-mask ventilation in a preterm infant with insufficient spontaneous breathing, muscular hypotonia, central cyanosis, and heart rate 70–90 bpm. The chest is covered with plastic wrap to prevent heat loss. Three small ECG leads are placed and connected. A pulse oximeter probe is attached to the right hand.

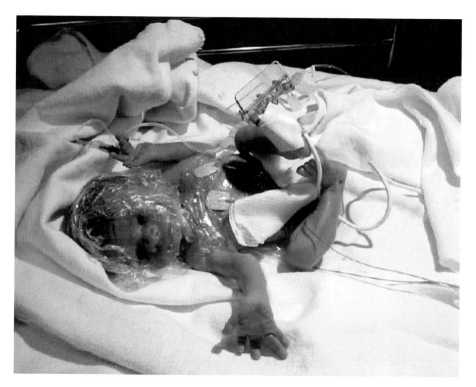

Figure 2.40 Preterm infant (32 3/7 weeks' gestation) with appropriate postnatal adaptation approx. 15 min after birth. Head and body are covered with plastic wrap (alternative: plastic bag). A peripheral venous catheter has been placed in the dorsal left hand. Monitoring via small ECG leads and pulse oximeter.

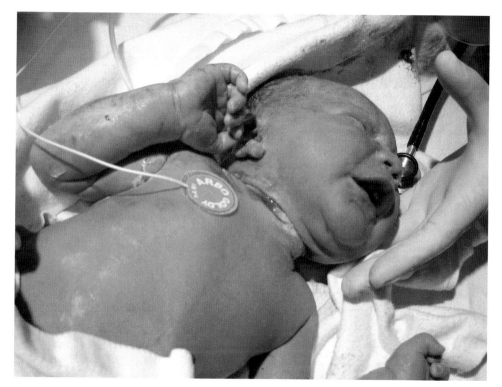

Figure 2.41 Term neonate with d-transposition of the great arteries without VSD ("simple, TGA"). Central cyanosis in the delivery room; 6 h after birth a balloon atrioseptostomy (ballon atrial sepostomy = Rashkind procedure) wase performed because of significant blood flow restriction through the PFO/ASD (left-to-right shunt).

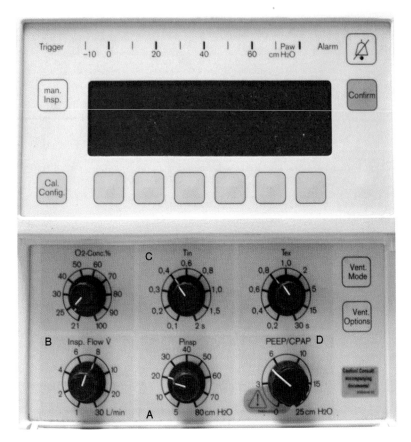

Figure 2.43 BabyLog 8000 plus control panel. Individual control of inspiratory time and pressure allows for the use of multiple ventilatory modes.

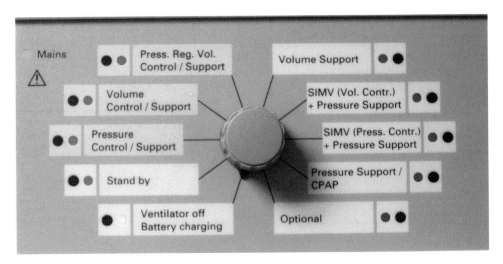

Figure 2.44 Siemens Servo 300. This ventilator's programmed modes can be switched with a single control button.

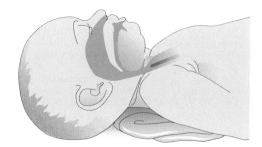

Figure 2.18 So called sniffing position of the head for bag-and-mask ventilation, pharyngeal tube ventilation and intubation. Note that the tip of the nose is the highest point in the lateral view. Modified from Ralston *et al.* (2006). *PALS Provider Manual*. American Heart Association and American Academy of Pediatrics.

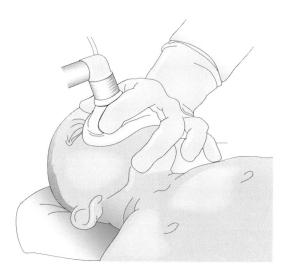

Figure 2.19 C-grip: left thumb and index finger hold the mask in a "figure of C" and the mask is cautiously, but tightly, placed over the mouth and nose ("sealed"); left middle and ring finger lift the chin and the prominent mandible (without the soft tissue) and hold it forward/up (moderate extension of head). Modified from: Hansmann G (2004) *Neugeborenen-Notfälle*. Thieme, Stuttgart, New York.

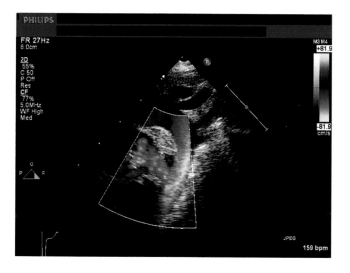

Figure 3.18 Patent ductus arteriosus (PDA) with right-to-left shunting (pulmonary artery → ductus → aorta) in a patient with coarctation of the aorta (CoA).

(a)

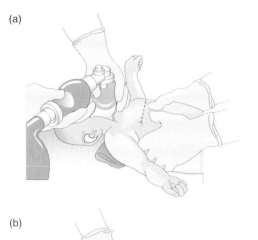

Figure 2.26 Chest compressions. **(a)** Two-thumb (encircling hands) technique for chest compressions. This technique is the method of choice (may have the advantage of producing greater peak systolic and coronary perfusion pressure). For small preterm infants (<1500g): consider superimposing the thumbs (one over the other) or using the two-finger technique. **(b)** Two-finger technique for chest compressions. Method of second choice: it has advantages for very small preterm infants (<1000g) and during umbilical vein catheterization. Modified from: Ralston M *et al*. (2006) *PALS. Provider Manual.* Dallas, TX: American Heart Association and American Academy of Pediatrics.

(b)

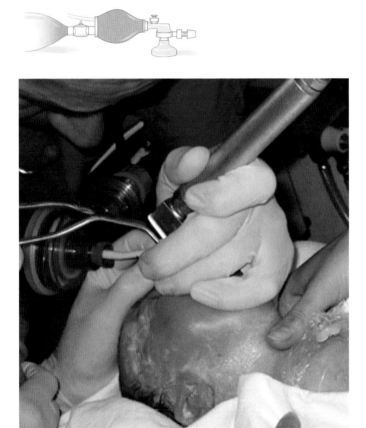

Figure 2.42 Nasotracheal intubation of a term neonate under continuous nasopharyngeal ventilation by an experienced team: assistant no. 1 secures the tube and ventilates, assistant no. 2 gently applies external pressure on the larynx.

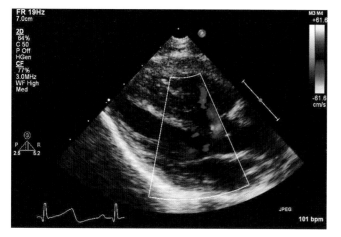

Figure 3.26 Tetralogy of Fallot (ToF). Echocardiography, long axis view. Key features of ToF include: (1) perimembranous ventricular septal defect (VSD), (2) the aorta overriding the VSD (aorta normally overrides the intact septum to some extent), (3) valvular and subvalvular (infundibular) pulmonary stenosis (PS; not shown in this view), (4) significant right ventricular hypertrophy (RVH).

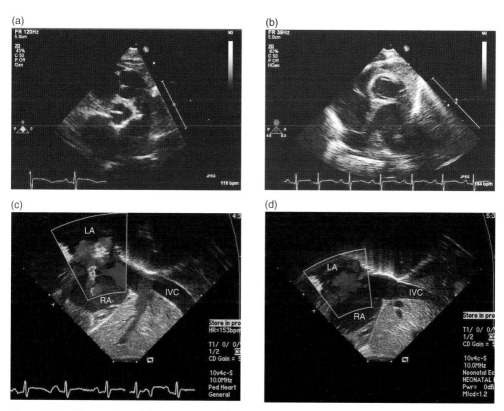

Figure 3.29 d-Transposition of the great arteries (d-TGA) without VSD. Echocardiography, atrial communication, subcostal view. Left atrium (LA), shunt through atrial septum, right atrium (RA, closest to the transducer) and inferior vena cava (IVC) are shown. (a) *Normal anatomy, short axis view*: central aorta with pulmonary artery (PA) crossing anteriorly, so-called circle (aorta) and sausage (PA). (b) *d-TGA, short axis view*: transversal views of both aorta and PA, with aorta right and anterior of the PA, so-called double circle image typical for d-TGA. (c) *Small, restrictive ASD/PFO, little left-to-right atrial shunting, systemic arterial desaturation* (severe cyanosis; SO$_2$ in the aorta approx. 30%–50%.). (d) *Unrestrictive ASD after balloon atrioseptostomy* (BAS = Rashkind procedure), SO$_2$ in the aorta ≈80%.

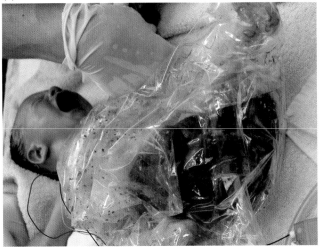

(a)

(b)

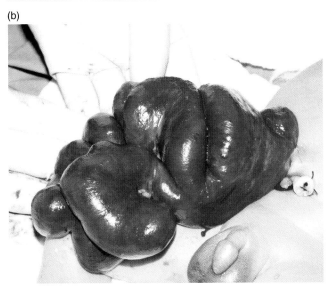

(c)

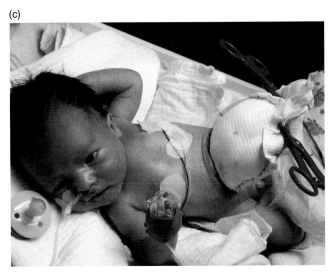

Figure 3.35a–c Gastroschisis. **(a)** Initial care of a preterm infant (35 + 5 weeks of gestation) with large gastroschisis after primary cesarean section. Umbilical artery pH 7.30, Apgar 9/10/10. Lower extremities and trunk have already been placed in a sterile plastic bag, no bag-and-mask ventilation, no nasal continuous positive airways pressure (CPAP). Later management included elective nasotracheal intubation 10min postnatally, volume IV for arterial hypotension, surgery during the first hours of life. **(b)** Gastroschisis, surgical field right before surgery: abdominal hernia with eventration of the whole small bowel and large bowel including parts of the sigma. The bowel wall is massively swollen and partly fibrinous. Intestinal non-rotation. **(c)** Status post abdominal surgery with two GoreTex® patches (Schuster's plastic).

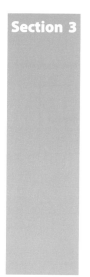

Classic and rare scenarios in the neonatal period

Management of healthy, term newborn infants (vaginal delivery, cesarean section, vacuum extraction, forceps delivery)

Georg Hansmann

Figure 3.1 shows the standard algorithm for the initial management and resuscitation of a newborn infant.

Clinical presentation

Vigorous newly born infant (Figure 3.1), i.e.:

- Apparent, equal chest movements, no distress, respiratory rate 40–50 breaths/min
- HR >100 bpm, trunk gradually turns rosy
- Newborn has adequate muscle tone (limbs flexed) and moves all four extremities
- Usually, 1-min Apgar score >6, initial umbilical artery pH >7.20

Meconium visible?

Yes (less common)

- *Meconium-stained amniotic fluid (MSAF) and/or meconium-stained skin and/or meconium or blood/viscous secretions in the upper respiratory tract, however, neonate is vigorous:*
  - Management
    - O_2 supplementation only as needed, no initial bag-and-mask ventilation
    - Laryngoscopy: if the neonate is vigorous and inspection shows the upper airways to be clear of meconium, there is no indication for intubation/endotracheal suctioning/PPV. If the baby is already vigorously crying/breathing and the vital signs are reassuring, then laryngoscopy can be omitted. If the status is unclear or there is possible vital depression, perform laryngoscopy, intubation/endotracheal suctioning, and optionally PPV
    - Oropharyngeal suctioning
    - Dry, stimulate, keep warm
    - Diagnostic tests, as indicated

Neonatal Emergencies: A Practical Guide for Resuscitation, Transport and Critical Care, ed. Georg Hansmann.
Published by Cambridge University Press. © Cambridge University Press 2009.

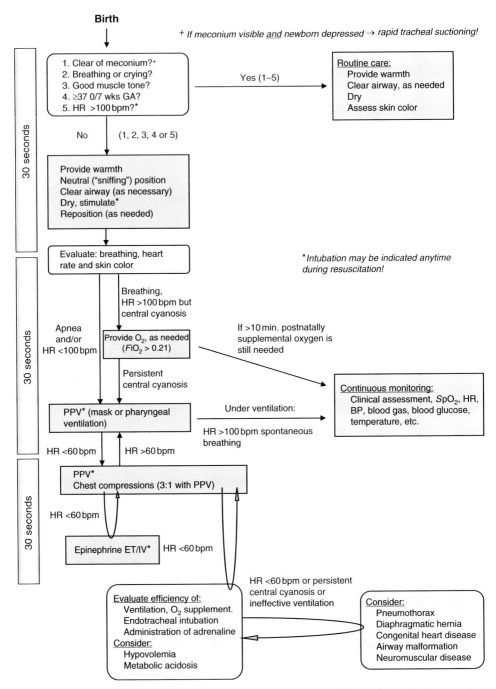

Figure 3.1 Standard algorithm for the initial management and resuscitation of the newborn infant. GA, gestational age. Modified from: ILCOR guidelines (2005), *Resuscitation* 2005; 67:293–303, and AHA/AAP guidelines (2005) *Circulation* 2005; 112:IV 188–195 and *Pediatrics* 2006; 117:e1029–1038; http://pediatrics.aappublications.org/cgi/content/full/117/5/e978, accessed 17 November 2008.

- Give baby to the mother when stable for early skin-to-skin contact (SSC), monitor with pulse oximeter (HR, S_aO_2) as indicated since late neonatal respiratory arrests are possible
- Determine 10-min Apgar score
- Consider inserting a gastric tube prior to the first feeding (some providers perform this only when choanal or esophageal atresia is suspected)
- Weigh the baby
- Vitamin K on the first day of life. Hepatitis B vaccine

No (regular case)
- *Amniotic fluid is clear and free of meconium, skin is clear of meconium, no meconium or blood/viscous secretions in the upper respiratory tract, neonate is vigorous:*
  - Management
    - Minimal handling
    - Suction only if there is a lot of fluid in the oropharynx
    - Dry, provide warmth, stimulate
    - O_2 supplementation only if indicated
    - Give stable neonate to the mother, determine 10-min Apgar score (often omitted in the USA)
    - Consider inserting a gastric tube prior to the first feeding (optional)
    - Weigh the baby
    - Vitamin K on the first day of life. Hepatitis B vaccine

General principles
For time and technique of cord clamping see pp. 121–3.

A vigorous newly born infant, who starts crying within the first 5–10 s and whose amniotic fluid is clear, does not need to be suctioned. Unnecessary *suctioning* irritates the neonate, can lead to lesions of the soft tissue and may cause both reactive bradycardia and apnea[1].

Indications for suctioning of the upper respiratory tract (e.g., much or green amniotic fluid, preterm infant, apnea) are given on pp. 66–9.

The *Apgar scores* can be determined while the infant, still lying warmly wrapped up on the mother's chest, turns rosy and is clinically stable. Encourage early skin-to-skin contact (SSC). If indicated, monitor with pulse oximeter (HR, S_aO_2), since late neonatal respiratory arrests are described (30 min to hours after birth).

You may attempt to insert a feeding tube through both nostrils and via the esophagus into the stomach to rule out choanal and esophageal atresia (many centers do this only in the presence of clinical signs or on the basis of a prenatal ultrasound). This procedure and the first physical examination of the newborn should be performed underneath a radiant heater on a well thermoregulated examination table (e.g., resuscitation unit).

Bag-and-mask ventilation and lung expansion (via CPAP) are not "standard initial care in the delivery room," however both may be indicated e.g., after a cesarean section and unsatisfactory lung expansion or prolonged grunting of the neonate.

Blood gas and blood glucose should be obtained – regardless of the initial umbilical arterial (UA) pH value – approximately 30 min after the birth as a routine if the UA pH is <7.15, or as routine prior to neonatal transport. If the clinical condition of the neonate is critical, blood gas analysis should be performed earlier and more frequently.

The *hematocrit value* (venous, arterial) gives important information about intravascular blood volume, for instance after a vacuum extraction (VE) with subsequent severe cephalohematoma or a premature separation of the placenta/bleeding.

The *body temperature* taken before leaving the delivery room is an important criterion for both the quality of the initial care/neonatal resuscitation and the outcome of the neonate[2].

Normal values and parameters in the first hours of life for healthy neonates born at term

- *Weight*: if birth weight >10th percentile and/or between 2800 g and 4000 g, weight-related problems are rare
- *Temperature*: 36.5–37.5°C (97.7–99.5°F)
- *Breathing*:
  - Respiratory rate (RR) 30–60 breaths/min
  - Regular, symmetrical breathing/intermittent crying
  - Equal breath sounds with satisfactory lung expansion, often with some fine basal crackles
- *Heart*:
  - HR 100–160 bpm
  - Mild respiratory arrhythmia possible
- *Pulse*: all palpable, no pulse difference between the extremities
- *Blood pressure: numerical value of* MAP (mmHg) ≥ gestational age in weeks p.m. (Figure 5.3),
- *Skin*:
  - Trunk with rosy skin color (i.e., not gray, not pale, no mottled appearance)
  - Sometimes mild peripheral cyanosis (acrocyanosis)
  - Warm
  - Capillary refill <2 s
- *Muscle tone*:
  - Limbs flexed with good muscle tone
  - Equal spontaneous movements (clavicular fracture? Moro reflex asymmetrical?)
- *Reflexes*: sucking reflex present, palmar and plantar reflex present
- *Capillary blood gas: heelstick, with good perfusion (no acrocyanosis, prewarm heel), approximately 30 min after birth:*
  - PCO_2: 35–45 (±5) mmHg
  - PO_2: ≥40 mmHg
  - pH value: >7.30 (±0.05)
  - Standard bicarbonate : ≥19 mmol/l
  - base excess or deficit: −9 to +3 mmol/l
- S_aO_2: 90%–96% by pulse oximetry (S_pO_2)
- CBC:
  - Hct: 45%–60%
  - Hemoglobin: 16–20 g/dl
  - WBC (leucocytes): 8000–30 000/µl (bands: day 1, 15%; day 2, 10%; day 3, 5%; I:T ratio on day 2 of life <0.2 (i.e., immature neutrophils:absolute neutrophils)
  - Platelets (thrombocytes): (125 000)–150 000–400 000/µl

- *Bilirubin*
  - Total: <7 mg/dl (<120 µmol/l) during the first 24 h of life, then <15 mg/dl (<256 µmol/l). See also http://www.bilitool.com
  - Conjugated (= direct): <1.5 mg/dl (−26 µmol/l) and less than 20% of total bilirubin. In biliary atresia (pale stools, dark urine), the direct bilirubin peak occurs between 3 and 5 weeks of life (caution especially in breastfed neonates with somewhat improving jaundice)
- *Clotting (0–72 h after birth)[3]:*
  - PTT: approx. 35–65 s
  - Activated PTT (ratio) approx. 1.29–1.96
  - INR approx. 1.0–1.46
  - Fibrinogen, factor I: approx. 160–300 (–375 mg/dl) mg/dl
  - AT III: approx. 38%–62%
  - D-dimers: <100 ng/ml (normal values for term/preterm neonates?)

Coagulation laboratories must develop age-related reference ranges specific to their own assays.

> **!** If Hct is >55%, the greater citrate dilution of the plasma can lead to false laboratory results.

- *Lactate:* <2 mmol/l (<18 mg/dl)
- *Blood glucose range for term and preterm neonates (not evidence-based, see Chapter "Hypoglycemia", p. 260):*
  - In the first 24 h after birth: minimum 40 mg/dl (>2.2 mmol/l)
  - After the first 24 h: minimum 45 mg/dl (>2.5 mmol/l)
  - Acceptable blood glucose values up to 150 mg/dl (8.2 mmol/l). The dextrostix only gives estimated values: particularly in the low blood glucose range (<60 mg/dl), the values are not accurate and often too high!

> In the neonatal emergency transport service, the following approach has been established for neonates/preterm infants with blood glucose levels <50 (or <45) mg/dl facing neonatal transfer: 2–5 ml $D_{10}W$/kg slow IV push (if necessary, use $D_{12.5}W$ IV solution via PIV). Caution: rebound hypoglycemia after IV glucose bolus is common. Check blood glucose once more and double the usual glucose infusion rate (GIR) during neonatal transport, i.e., give 6 ml $D_{10}W$/kg/h IV = GIR of 10 mg/kg/min for neonates at high risk for (recurrent) hypoglycemia.

- *Electrolytes:*
  - Sodium: 135–145 mmol/l
  - Potassium: 4.0–5.5 mmol/l
  - Calcium (total): 2.3–2.6 mmol/l
  - Phosphate (inorganic): 1.6–3.1 mmol/l (4.8–9.5 mg/dl)
  - Magnesium: 0.67–0.97 (−1.5) mmol/l

- *Renal function:*
  - Creatinine: up to 1.2 mg/dl ($= 106 \, \mu mol/l$), preterm $>$ term, down to normal adult values by approx. 3 weeks of life
  - Blood urea nitrogen (BUN): up to 7.1 mmol/l ($= 20$ mg/dl)
- *Protein:*
  - Total protein: 4.6–6.8 g/dl
  - Albumin: 3.2–4.5 g/dl
- *Urine output (UOP):*
  - 1st and 2nd day: 0.3–0.5 ml/kg/h
  - Starting the 2nd day: 1–3 ml/kg/h
  - Specific gravity: up to 1.015 g/ml
- *Inflammation/infection* (see p. 296):
  - See CBC
  - IL-6 $<$ 30 pg/ml (caution: short half-life, peaks at 6 h)
  - IL-8 $<$ 25 pg/ml
  - CRP $<$ 1 mg/dl

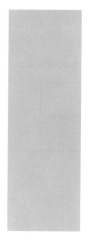

Management of preterm and moderately depressed term newborn infants with a birth weight $\geq$ 1500 g

Georg Hansmann

Figure 3.2 shows the standard algorithm for the initial management and resuscitation of newborn infants, including preterm infants >1500 g.

Clinical presentation

Apneic or inadequately breathing newly born infant with initial HR >80–100 bpm, probably with primary apnea (Figure 3.2):

- Skin pale or blue (cyanotic)
- Initial umbilical arterial pH >7.00
- 1-min Apgar score 4–6

Course

- 1–2 min of apnea or insufficient breathing
- Under stimulation $\pm$ O_2 supplementation $\rightarrow$ spontaneous breathing
- HR increases above 100 bpm
- Trunk gradually turns pink

Meconium visible?

Yes

- Meconium-stained amniotic fluid and/or meconium-stained skin and/or meconium or blood/mucus in the upper respiratory tract, however neonate is vigorous:
  - Management, see pp. 221–6, pp. 269–79
- Meconium present and newborn depressed (apneic, floppy, HR <100 bpm):
  - Management, see pp. 269–79 "Meconium aspiration" and/or see pp. 66–9 "Suctioning"

No

Estimated gestational age?
- *Term neonate (37–42 weeks of gestation p.m.)*
  - Management:
    - Suctioning

Neonatal Emergencies: A Practical Guide for Resuscitation, Transport and Critical Care, ed. Georg Hansmann.
Published by Cambridge University Press. © Cambridge University Press 2009.

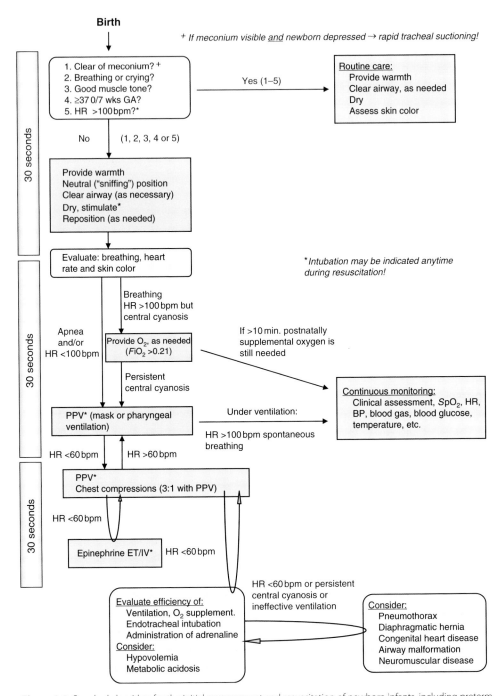

Figure 3.2 Standard algorithm for the initial management and resuscitation of newborn infants, including preterm infants ≥1500 g and the moderately depressed, term newborn infant. GA, gestational age. Modified from: ILCOR guidelines (2005), *Resuscitation* 2005; 67:293–303, and AHA/AAP guidelines (2005) *Circulation* 2005; 112:IV 188–195 and *Pediatrics* 2006; 117:e1029–1038; http://pediatrics.aappublications.org/cgi/content/full/117/5/e978.

- Dry, stimulate, keep warm
- O_2 supplement and CPAP depending on the S_pO_2 and breathing pattern
- Depending on general condition, body weight, blood glucose: indication for neonatal transport to higher level NICU and peripheral venous access
- Diagnostics, if indicated: blood gas, blood glucose, Hct/CBC, blood culture, CRP/IL-6, smears ($\rightarrow$ NICU)
- Give *stable* neonate to mother under continuous S_pO_2 monitoring (pulse oximeter)
- Determine 10-min (15-min, 20-min) Apgar scores, reassess frequently
- Blood gas and glucose approx. 30 min after birth (if needed earlier; always for NETS)
- Insert gastric tube before the first feeding (optional)
- Weigh the baby
- Vitamin K on the first day of life; hepatitis B vaccine
- If a transfer is indicated (see pp. 179–80) and the initially depressed neonate is now stable for transport: show the baby to the mother, explain the reason for transfer, provide D_5W or $D_{10}W$ continuous IV infusion at 3 ml/kg/h IV (double rate if at risk for hypoglycemia), transfer to NICU or high observation nursery with sufficient monitoring

> ! Only capillary or arterial blood gas analysis is adequate for assessing ventilation and oxygenation (PO_2, PCO_2). Arterial samples are considered the "gold standard".

- *Preterm infant (<37 0/7 weeks of gestation p.m.)*
  - Management:
    - Suctioning
    - Dry, stimulate, keep warm
    - O_2 supplement and CPAP depending on S_pO_2 and breathing pattern
    - If needed, ECG electrodes for preterm infants and plastic wrap (for BW <2000 g)
    - For preterm infants <32 weeks' gestation ($\approx$ VLBW), see pp. 231–9 (indications for bag-and-mask ventilation and endotracheal intubation, see pp. 156–8 and below)
    - All preterm infants <35 + 0 weeks' gestation or <2000 g, should receive intravenous fluids (first: $D_{10}W$ 3 ml/kg/h; in case of hypoglycemia: dextrose bolus, then $D_{10}W$ 6 ml/kg/h; for high–normal or elevated blood glucose levels: use D_5W)
    - If necessary, initiate diagnostics with PIV access: blood gas and glucose CBC/blood culture, CRP, blood culture, smears ($\rightarrow$ NICU)
    - Give well-adapted preterm infant with pulse oximeter monitoring to the mother
    - Determine 10-min Apgar score
    - Insert gastric tube before the first feeding
    - Obtain blood gas and blood glucose approx. 30 min after birth (if necessary, earlier; obligatory for Neonatal Emergency Transport Service = NETS)

- If neonatal transfer is indicated (see pp. 179–80) and the initially depressed preterm infant is now in stable condition for transport: show preterm infant to the mother, explain the reason for transfer to the parents, give D_5W or $D_{10}W$ 3 ml/kg/h IV, transfer with monitoring to NICU or high observation nursery with proper monitoring
- On the NICU/ high observation nursery: initiate further diagnostic work-up if indicated (laboratory tests, chest X-ray, etc.) and therapy

The newborn is still depressed 30 s after birth

Clinical presentation

- Apnea, HR <100 bpm
  - Bag-and-mask ventilation (technique: see pp. 70–80; for indications see pp. 156–8)

Check 15–30 s after start of bag-and-mask ventilation

No response under bag-and-mask ventilation

- Technical error? check technique, see pp. 70–80
- Ventilation with pharyngeal tube easier (e.g., in ELBW)? For technique, see pp. 79–80
- Intubation and tracheal ventilation indicated? For indications, see p. 158
- After stabilization of the newborn: is transfer to the NICU indicated?

Good response to bag-and-mask ventilation and oxygen supplementation (HR >100 bpm), but still pale and tachypneic

- Start with nasal (pharyngeal) CPAP or mask-CPAP in the delivery room
- O_2 only when needed (check S_pO_2 continuously, use room air when S_pO_2 >85%–90%)
- Attach electrodes and connect to monitor, obtain blood gas, glucose (dextrostix, glucometer) and temperature
- If the preterm infant is stable: move baby to incubator
- If necessary, adjust humidity (depending on the gestational age)
- If a pediatrician remains at the bedsite (no transport):
  - Start documentation using a standard protocol and delegate continuous observation
- If no pediatrician can stay with the patient:
  - Rapidly transport the patient with NETS to NICU
- If the condition of the child is borderline or unstable:
  - Reassess indication for intubation prior to transport
  - Immediate and rapid transfer to NICU

> ! For the differential diagnosis "delayed pulmonary adaptation (transition)" versus "cyanotic heart disease," see pp. 124–6.

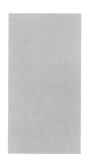

Management of very preterm newborn infants (VLBW, ELBW)

Christoph Bührer and Andrea Zimmermann

Definition

- Very low birth weight (VLBW) infants (birth weight <1500 g) and extremely low birth weight (ELBW) infants (birth weight <1000 g) constitute approximately 1.2% and 0.4% of all newborn babies in industrialized countries, respectively
- Induction of fetal lung maturation by betamethasone and prenatal transfer to a perinatal level III center prior to delivery of any such tiny infant is of paramount importance. This way, the most experienced doctors and nurses available perform or supervise the initial care of very immature infants. If prenatal transport is not possible due to rapid birth progression, call the Neonatal Emergency Transport Service (NETS) at the earliest available opportunity.
- Many details of the initial care of very preterm infants are controversial. Health care providers, while striving for the best evidence available, may follow locally established guidelines to benefit from the experience in a particular environment and to ensure a team approach

Questions prior to delivery

- Prenatal transfer allows the health care team to discuss treatment options with expectant parents before delivery in cases of borderline viability (see Chapter "Ethics in neonatal intensive care," pp. 184–90).
- Is there a reliable estimate of gestational age?
- What is the estimated birth weight?
- Has fetal lung maturation been induced (e.g., betamethasone: how many doses and how many hours prior to delivery)?
- Are there signs of fetal distress? for example, fetal tachycardia or bradycardia
- Are there signs of perinatal infection (maternal fever, CRP, GBS status, etc.)?

Preparations in the delivery room
Temperature

- Increase room temperature to 25–30°C if possible
- Turn on radiant heaters
- Keep doors closed
- Have prewarmed cotton towels or food-grade, heat-resistant plastic wrapping or bags ready

Neonatal Emergencies: A Practical Guide for Resuscitation, Transport and Critical Care, ed. Georg Hansmann.
Published by Cambridge University Press. © Cambridge University Press 2009.

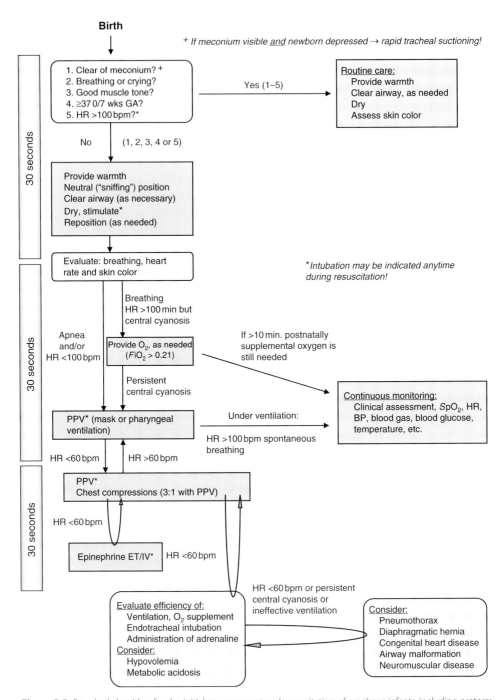

Birth

+ *If meconium visible and newborn depressed → rapid tracheal suctioning!*

30 seconds

1. Clear of meconium? +
2. Breathing or crying?
3. Good muscle tone?
4. ≥37 0/7 wks GA?
5. HR >100 bpm?*

Yes (1–5) →

Routine care:
 Provide warmth
 Clear airway, as needed
 Dry
 Assess skin color

No (1, 2, 3, 4 or 5)

Provide warmth
Neutral ("sniffing") position
Clear airway (as necessary)
Dry, stimulate*
Reposition (as needed)

Evaluate: breathing, heart rate and skin color

Intubation may be indicated anytime during resuscitation!

Breathing
HR >100 min but
central cyanosis

Apnea
and/or
HR <100 bpm

Provide O_2, as needed (FiO_2 > 0.21)

If >10 min. postnatally
supplemental oxygen is
still needed

Persistent
central cyanosis

PPV* (mask or pharyngeal ventilation)

Under ventilation:

HR >100 bpm spontaneous breathing

Continuous monitoring:
 Clinical assessment, SpO_2, HR,
 BP, blood gas, blood glucose,
 temperature, etc.

HR <60 bpm   HR >60 bpm

30 seconds

PPV*
Chest compressions (3:1 with PPV)

HR <60 bpm

30 seconds

Epinephrine ET/IV*   HR <60 bpm

HR <60 bpm or persistent
central cyanosis or
ineffective ventilation

Evaluate efficiency of:
 Ventilation, O_2 supplement
 Endotracheal intubation
 Administration of adrenaline
Consider:
 Hypovolemia
 Metabolic acidosis

Consider:
 Pneumothorax
 Diaphragmatic hernia
 Congenital heart disease
 Airway malformation
 Neuromuscular disease

Figure 3.3 Standard algorithm for the initial management and resuscitation of newborn infants, including preterm infants <1500 g. GA, gestational age. Modified from: ILCOR guidelines (2005), *Resuscitation* 2005; 67:293–303, and AHA/AAP guidelines (2005) *Circulation* 2005; 112:IV 188–195 and *Pediatrics* 2006; 117:e1029–1038; http://pediatrics. aappublications.org/cgi/content/full/117/5/e978.

Airway
- Turn on suctioning (-0.2 bar $= -200$ mbar $= -150$ mmHg), 8 F suction catheters

Breathing
- Turn on gas supply for self-inflating bag or T-piece resuscitator (Neopuff™, Perivent™, Neovent™, Tom Thumb™), with PEEP set at 4–5 mbar, PIP at 18 mbar ($= 18$ cmH$_2$O). Oxygen blender set at 21%
- Small round silicone mask (size 0 or 00)
- 2.0 and 2.5 (and 3.0) mm ET tube (soft for nasotracheal intubation, e.g., Vygon®; stiff for orotracheal intubation, e.g., Portex®, Mallinckrodt®)
- Check laryngoscope light, small blade (e.g., Miller, size 00, 0 or 1)
- Small Magill's forceps for nasotracheal intubation
- Strips of tape to secure ET tube or ET tube holder (for oral ET tube)
- Surfactant (minimum of two vials)

Circulation
- Plastic cord clamp, sterile scissors and gauze pads
- Umbilical venous catheter (3.5 G or 5 G) and umbilical arterial catheter (2.5 G or 3.5 G), to be filled with saline and fitted with three-way stop cock in sterile fashion. Alternatively, peripheral 24 G or 26 G venous access for preterm infants who may not require central venous access (>27 weeks' gestation). Flush tubing with saline. Have tape ready
- May use octenidine (0.1%) phenoxyethanol (2%) solution for local disinfection.[4] This soft tissue disinfectant needs 2 min of topical incubation time. Alcohol-based disinfectants will harm the immature skin
- Dry, sterile swabs
- Check source of O Rhesus-negative packed red blood cells (in case of perinatal hemorrhage)

Drugs
- Epinephrine (adrenaline) 1:10 000 – have it readily available
- D$_{10}$W solution IV (10% glucose)
- Normal saline (NaCl 0.9%)

Procedure/therapy in the delivery room
Be gentle ("minimal handling")
- Overzealous resuscitative efforts will get you and the baby in trouble – a determined but careful approach is most appropriate
- Start Apgar timer at birth
- Place infant in supine position, head facing towards the MD/NP responsible for the airway
- Avoid cold stress (thermal control)
- Initiate care in a small, prewarmed room (conductive heat loss)
- Close curtains of windows (the best resuscitation rooms have no windows)
- Turn on radiant heater

- Keep doors closed to avoid convective heat loss
- Dry infant in prewarmed cotton towels, exchange wet towels for dry ones
- Or, cover infant in food-grade, heat-resistant plastic wrapping or bag (convective, radiant and evaporative heat loss)

Airway management
- Gently and briefly suction anterior parts of mouth and nose. Avoid touching hypopharyngeal vagal trigger zones, which may induce bradycardia/apnea

Breathing
- While drying the infant with prewarmed towels and rubbing their back, gently stimulate breathing
- Spontaneous breaths are superior to those administered by PPV. If infant remains apneic, begin PPV via bag-and-mask or T-piece resuscitator. Continue stimulation to support respiratory efforts
- Do not be overzealous as long as heart rate is >100 bpm. Institute CPAP (PEEP 3–6 cmH$_2$O) by face mask, nasal prongs or pharyngeal tube (2.5-mm-diameter tube, advance tube just past the choanae, equivalent to 3–5 cm behind the tip of nose)
- Use supplemental oxygen in a very restricted fashion to prevent oxygen toxicity (see pp. 70–1, p. 312)
- Institute early preductal pulse oximetry (right upper extremity) and aim at preductal oxygen saturations of 85%–92%
- Consider early endotracheal intubation (2.5-mm-ID tube) if infant is below 27 weeks of gestation (i.e., fused eyelids) to administer exogenous surfactant (see pp. 85–93)
- For nasal ET tubes: depth of insertion (cm) = 5.5 + 1.5 × (kg body weight); for oral ET tubes: depth of insertion (cm) = 4.5 + 1.5 × (kg body weight). See also Table 2.2.
- Exogenous surfactant is usually given if a preterm infant requires supplemental oxygen exceeding a F_iO_2 of 0.4 for more than approx. 15–30 min to achieve a preductal oxygen saturation of 90%. Moreover, preterm infants <27–28 weeks, gestation who are intubated in the delivery room for respiratory insufficiency benefit from early surfactant administration – probably regardless of the initial F_iO_2 needed (see surfactant replacement therapy below). However, very early nasal CPAP instituted in the delivery often obviates the need for ET intubation and subsequent surfactant administration also in very preterm infants, especially in those who have received a complete course of fetal lung maturation by betamethasone (see pp. 79–80)
- Surfactant is administered through a side port of the tube or via a sterile feeding tube (must have the same length as the ET tube). Both fractionated and bolus administration appear to work well
- Before administering surfactant, check that the ET tube is not advanced too far into the trachea, as inadvertent intubation of the right main bronchus and uneven surfactant administration may occur. Is insertion depth commensurate with the value in Table 2.2, p. 85? Use your eyes (symmetrical chest rise?), stethoscope (for auscultation of equal breath sounds on both sides), and laryngoscope (for visual inspection of the tube at the laryngeal entrance). In the NICU, a chest X-ray should be obtained in order to confirm the position of the ET tube (tube tip seen at the level of second or third thoracic vertebra), to rule out pneumothorax, and to radiographically determine the degree of respiratory distress syndrome

- Do not administer surfactant to infants with a pneumothorax unless the pneumothorax has been efficiently drained (chest tube), as uneven distribution of surfactant may aggravate the pneumothorax
- Infants may respond to exogenous surfactant administration with a rapid and persistent rise in P_aO_2. Be prepared to turn the oxygen blender from 100% to 21% in less than a minute! After surfactant administration, lung compliance may initially decrease, but shortly thereafter usually improves quickly. Always monitor adequate chest rise and adjust ventilation. If possible (i.e., with mechanical ventilator) monitor and adjust tidal volumes (V_T) by reducing PIP for a V_T goal of 4–6 ml/kg

Circulation

- Chest compressions are rarely indicated (persistent bradycardia: HR <60 bpm despite adequate ventilation), as is administration of epinephrine (0.01 mg/kg/dose IV). Epinephrine by the intratracheal route does not work once the infant is in shock (IV route always preferred)
- If HR <60 bpm despite endotracheal PPV, perform chest compressions for 30 s and reassess HR. If HR remains below 60 bpm, administer epinephrine (0.01 mg/kg/dose IV), and continue chest compressions. If, after an additional 30 s of chest compression/PPV, HR remains below 60 bpm, give second dose of epinephrine (0.01 mg/kg/dose IV) and volume (NaCl 0.9%, 10 ml/kg/bolus IV)
- Rapid venous access (UVC, PIV) is required for rapid drug administration and in hypovolemic shock (pale skin, HR >180 bpm). Pre- or perinatal acute blood loss may not be in the perinatal history. Insert umbilical cord venous catheter and slowly administer prewarmed NaCl 0.9% 10–20 ml/kg per bolus (may be repeated). Heart rate will decrease once cardiac preload is optimized
- Getting hold of type-O Rhesus-negative packed red blood cells rapidly and transfusing slowly (in aliquots, up to 60 ml/kg total) may be live-saving in hypovolemic or septic shock
- If skin is very immature, avoid taping, and secure umbilical lines with sutures instead

Drugs

- Use of epinephrine (adrenaline) is rarely indicated in very preterm infants – remember the infant's heart has been pumping blood through the infant's body as well as through the placenta just recently at arterial oxygen tensions of less than 30 mmHg (see Figure 2.15)
- Start administering glucose intravenously (glucose infusion rate, GIR = 5 mg/kg/min IV, equivalent to $D_{10}W$ solution at 3 ml/kg/h IV) within 30 min of birth
- There is no point in masking metabolic acidosis (due to lactate accumulation) by administering sodium bicarbonate[5] or THAM. The use of sodium bicarbonate has been associated with intraventricular hemorrhage[6]
- Give vitamin K 0.5 mg slowly IV or IM
- Administer empiric antibiotics if infection is suspected after obtaining a blood culture. Surface swabs from the ear and gastric fluid are also helpful for identifying the bacteria causing chorioamnionitis and subsequent pneumonia/sepsis, and determine their antimicrobial susceptibility. Surfactant: 100–200 mg/kg/dose (see below) – natural surfactant preparation preferred

Areas of uncertainty in clinical practice (VLBW, ELBW)
Plastic wrap/bag

- While preventing heat loss by plastic barriers (wrap, bag) has been found to be effective in randomized controlled trials[7], other techniques (e.g., transwarmer mattresses, radiant heaters) to maintain temperature during stabilization of the VLBW infant in the delivery room are being used successfully as well[8]. They have not been evaluated in controlled trials, or compared with the plastic-wrap technique. Both hypothermia and hyperthermia are associated with poorer outcome in VLBW infants

Surfactant replacement therapy (SRT)[9]

- *Prophylactic surfactant administration* decreases the risk of air leak (pneumothorax, pulmonary interstitial emphysema) and may decrease mortality. However, even brief endotracheal intubation in the delivery room may increase the risk for prolonged oxygen requirement[10] and associated diseases (e.g., retinopathy of prematurity, BPD/CLD). At present, it remains unclear which criteria should be used to stratify at-risk infants who would benefit from prophylactic surfactant administration[11]. Gestational age-based limits for prophylactic surfactant use range from 25 to 28 weeks. A substantial proportion of very preterm infants with completed betamethasone-induced fetal lung maturation may actually be successfully managed by early CPAP alone[12,13]. At a gestational age of 25 weeks[10] or a birth weight around 750 g[14], about 50% of infants can be successfully managed with early nasal CPAP started in the delivery room, without the need for subsequent endotracheal intubation or surfactant administration. The success of early nasal CPAP appears to improve not only with increased gestational age but also with staff experience over time
- *Early selective surfactant administration* given to infants with respiratory distress syndrome (RDS) requiring assisted ventilation decreases the risk of acute lung injury (decreased risk of pneumothorax and pulmonary interstitial emphysema), chronic lung disease and neonatal mortality when compared to delaying treatment of such infants until they develop established RDS[15]. An oxygen requirement of 40% or more is commonly used as a threshold for surfactant administration
- To avoid the risks of mechanical ventilation altogether, surfactant may be administered either via ET tube by INSURE (i.e., short **in**tubation, **sur**factant administration, **ex**tubation)[12,16,17] or in spontaneously breathing infants via a thin gastric tube inserted into the trachea[18,19]

Limits of viability

- The AAP recommends to defer from resuscitating extremely preterm infants with a gestational age <23 weeks or a birth weight <400 g, and advocates support of parental wishes in the zone of uncertainty when it comes to infants with a gestational age between 23 0/7 and 24 6/7 weeks[20]. While all published guidelines recognize such gray zones of uncertainty, their precise implementation is fiercely debated (see Chapter, "Ethics in neonatal intensive care," p. 184

Endotracheal intubation of very preterm infants
(Indications: p. 158)

Special anatomical features of very preterm infants <1500 g

The *larynx* of VLBW infants is located (in relation to the cervical spine) considerably *higher* than in older infants *and tilted anteriorly*. Hold the blade parallel to the tongue and pull the laryngoscope in the direction of the handle. Do not pry open! We discourage the use of a style for the endotracheal intubation of very preterm infants <1500 g.

The opening of the larynx is small, while the entrance to the esophagus is bigger and not surrounded by the epiglottis. In very small infants, the glottis may not be visualized.

With **nasal** intubation, you may either:

1. First advance the tube blindly (no stylet!) to the calculated depth – it will end up in the esophagus. The open hole above the tube is the entrance to the trachea. Retract the tube, advance it anteriorly (e.g., by Magill forceps), and insert again, this time into the trachea.
2. Advance the nasal tube just past the choanae (3–5 cm from nostril), advance the blade of the laryngoscope carefully into the esophagus and, while pulling back, visualize the glottis (use left small finger to apply cricoid pressure). See Chapter, "Endotracheal intubation and gastric tube placement," p. 81).

Ventilation and oxygenation goals for very preterm infants (VLBW, ELBW)

* S_pO_2 85%–92%
* P_aO_2 and/or transcutaneous PO_2 (tcPO_2) 45–65 mmHg (may use calibrated, reliable transcutaneous PO_2)
* P_aCO_2 and/or tcPCO$_2$ 40–55 mmHg (may use calibrated, reliable transcutaneous PCO_2)
*   pH approx. (7.25–) 7.30–7.45
*   If indicated, permissive hypercarbia (i.e., allow higher P_aCO_2 in order to decrease barotrauma and volutrauma

---

! Trouble/shooting when heart rate remains below 60 bpm

Rule out esophageal intubation:
*   Laryngoscopy
    *   If necessary, retract the tube carefully and do pharyngeal PPV or remove tube and perform PPV via bag-and-mask or T-piece resuscitator
*   Next, try endotracheal intubation once more
*   If the tube is in the trachea but there is no increase in HR after 15–30 s of efficient PPV (see chest movements)
    *   Give epinephrine (1:10 000) 0.3 (–1) ml/kg/dose ET (= 0.03–0.1 mg/kg/dose), even before securing the tube, or 0.01 mg/kg/dose IV (preferred, if IV access available)
    *   As long as HR <60 bpm, perform chest compression 3:1 with PPV
*   Differential diagnosis: consider pneumothorax if patient is unstable but correctly intubated. When suspicion is high, perform emergent pleural puncture/chest tube (see algorithm Figures 3.3, and 3.34)

Assess the very preterm infant before transport (NETS)

- HR >100 bpm?
- Chest movements: sufficient and symmetrical?
- Pulse oximeter: S_pO_2 constantly >85%?
- Infant begins to move?
- Capillary refill <2 s?
- Body temperature acceptable? (36.5–36.9°C)
- Acceptable blood gas analysis and blood glucose?
- IV access functional? $D_{10}W$ 3 ml/kg/h IV running?

Brain damage in preterm infants

Epidemiology

- Intraventricular hemorrhage (IVH) grades I/II and III/IV affect about 20% and 5% of VBLW infants, respectively, while rates of cystic periventricular leukomalacia (PVL) have dropped to less than 5% in VLBW infants in recent years[21–23]. IVH, but not PVL, is more common in boys and in multiple births
- Immaturity constitutes the most important clinical risk factor for IVH – rates of IVH steeply increase with decreasing gestational age[21,22,24]. In contrast, PVL rates do not vary with gestational age in VLBW infants
- IVH in a term infant should prompt searching for an underlying cause (e.g., coagulation profile, platelet function, cerebral venous sinus thrombosis, trauma)

Etiology/pathophysiology

- IVH
  - Subependymal vessels of the germinal matrix are exquisitely fragile between 16 and 36 weeks of gestation. Fragility of these vessels is partly mediated by locally produced prostaglandins[25]
  - Antenatal fetal lung maturation, avoidance of postnatal transport, and late cord clamping are protective[6,24,26]
  - Progression to severe IVH (grade III/IV) is associated with use of vasopressors, buffering, and extreme PCO_2 (high and low)[6,27,28,29], while indomethacin given during the first 6 h of life is protective[30,31], especially in boys[31]
- PVL
  - Risk factors for PVL are quite different from those for IVH[22], only infection[32] and hypocapnia[33,34] are consistently associated with PVL[35]
  - Infants who go on to develop IVH or PVL have rather increased blood pressure[35,36]

Diagnosis in the NICU

- Transcranial ultrasonography on days 7–10 of life and at 36 weeks' gestational age[37]. In high-risk infants, schedule additional sonography at day 3 and day 28 of life
- While over 90% of IVH happen during the first 5 days of life[38], PVL usually does not become apparent until 10–14 days of age
- Any sudden clinical deterioration during the first 5 days of life may herald severe IVH
- PVL is clinically silent until several months of age

Prognosis

Major IVH and cystic PLV constitute the strongest risk factors for cerebral palsy in VLBW infants[39]. While cystic PVL is almost inadvertently an antecedent of cerebral palsy (mostly spastic diplegia), the burden of disease associated with IVH varies greatly with the extent of IVH[23]. Unilateral grade IV hemorrhage is associated with hemiplegia and posthemorrhagic hydrocephalus after grade II or III hemorrhage may require shunt placement or some other drainage 2–6 weeks after birth. About 50% of VLBW infants with grade III/IV hemorrhage die (or are allowed to die), and 90% of the survivors show some neurological deficit[23]. Hemorrhage grade I and II, formerly considered innocuous, is also associated with gray matter loss[40] and neurodevelopmental impairment[41].

! **General recommendations for preventing IVH and PVL**

- Antenatal transfer to a tertiary perinatal center (i.e., level III NICU)
- Late cord clamping (controvesial)[26,42]
- Avoid P_aCO_2 <40 mmHg in ventilated infants
- Avoid rapid rise in P_aCO_2 (such as with pneumothorax)
- Avoid buffering (treat the baby, not the blood gas analysis)
- Avoid vasopressors (treat the baby, not the mean arterial pressure)
- Prevent nosocomial infections
- Consider indomethacin within the first 3–6 h of life in high-risk infants (e.g., male multiples <26 weeks' gestational age; see Chapter, "Patent ductus arteriosus of the preterm infant," p. 380

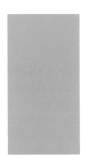

Twin–twin (feto–fetal) transfusion syndrome

Andrea Zimmermann

Definition/epidemiology

- *Twin gestation:*
    - Dichorionic-diamniotic twin gestation (approx. 70%): two placentas and two amniotic cavities, dizygotic or monozygotic fetuses
    - Monochorionic-diamniotic twin gestation (approx. 29%): one shared placenta, two amniotic cavities, monozygotic fetuses
    - Monochorionic-monoamniotic twin gestation (approx. 1%): shared placenta and amniotic cavities, monozygotic fetuses
    - Monochorionic-monoamniotic-monozygotic: conjoined twins/fused twins (high mortality)
- *Twin–twin (syn. feto–fetal) transfusions syndrome (TTTS, FFTS):* intrauterine transfusion between two fetuses via vascular anastomoses in monochorionic twin pregnancies
    - TTTS (syn. FFTS) occurs in up to 15% of monochorionic twin gestations[43]

Prenatal diagnosis

Sonography during the first trimester is most sensitive. In a monochorionic pregnancy with evidence of polyhydramnios and a gastric bubble in one twin, a diagnosis of TTTS should be considered.

Pathophysiology

- *Complications associated with twins:*
    - Increased perinatal morbidity and mortality: intrauterine fetal death[44], preterm labor, IUGR, discordant growth in up to 20% of all twin gestations[45], malformations[46], developmental dysplasia of the hip (DDH; formerly called congenital dysplasia of the hip)[47], premature placental abruption, and hypertensive disorders[48]
- *Monochorionic twin gestation and TTTS:*
    - TTTS is caused predominantly by arterio–arterial anastomoses in monochorionic-monoamniotic twin gestations, and by veno–arterial anastomoses in monochorionic-diamniotic twin gestations[49]
    - The result is an unbalanced circulation with net blood flow from the donor to the recipient and transfusion of corpuscular blood cells and plasma proteins
    - *Risk for the recipient:* polyhydramnios, edema progressing to fetal hydrops, cardiomegaly, intrauterine death, dilatation of the urinary bladder, polycythemia/hyperviscosity with impaired microcirculation and increased risk of thrombosis[43]

Neonatal Emergencies: A Practical Guide for Resuscitation, Transport and Critical Care, ed. Georg Hansmann.
Published by Cambridge University Press. © Cambridge University Press 2009.

- *Risk for the donor:* oligohydramnios, varying degrees of acute or chronic hypovolemia, IUGR, intrauterine death, hypoglycemia, anemia, hypoproteinemia, impaired cerebral perfusion and its sequelae[43]

Prenatal therapy

- Amnioreduction or laser coagulation of the placental anastomoses before 26 weeks' gestation[50–52]

> **!** If there is strong suspicion of TTTS, the pregnant woman must be transferred urgently to a perinatal center, as long as there is no indication for emergent delivery.

Clinical presentation/diagnosis/procedure/therapy in the delivery room (See Table 3.1.)

Diagnosis in the NICU

- Sonography of head, abdomen, heart
- Chest X-ray
- CBC, spun Hct $\times$ 2

Procedure/therapy in the NICU

- Treatment of side-effects or complications
- Depending on Hct and clinical presentation: transfusion and partial exchange transfusion

Table 3.1 Twin–twin (feto–fetal) transfusion syndrome

	Recipient	Donor
Clinical presentation	• Plethoric or cyanotic skin color • Hypoglycemia, hypocalcemia • *In advanced stages*: generalized edema, fetal hydrops, respiratory failure, apnea, seizures, irritability, lethargy, tachycardia or bradycardia, cardiac failure	• Pallor, anemia • Low birth weight • Hypoglycemia • Tachycardia • *In advanced stages*: tachycardia or bradycardia, hypotension, muscular hypotonia, apnea/respiratory failure
Monitoring	• Heart rate • Respiration • Oxygen saturation • Blood pressure	• Heart rate • Respiration • Oxygen saturation • Blood pressure
DDx	• Cyanosis and edema due to congenital heart defect • Hydrops of other origin • Congenital infection • Materno–fetal transfusion	• Premature abruptio placentae • Placenta praevia bleeding • Feto–maternal transfusion • Congenital infection • Placental insufficiency
Diagnosis in the delivery room	• ABG, blood glucose • Complete blood count (polycythemia?) • Draw a sufficient blood sample and store for future testing	• ABG, blood glucose • Complete blood count (anemia?) • Draw blood from the umbilical cord and store for future testing

Table 3.1 (*cont.*)

	Recipient	Donor

Therapy in the delivery room	Symptomatic treatment according to clinical presentation:
	• Checking vital signs
	• Intubation if indicated
	• Venous access and blood draw, PIV, usually place UVC, determine CVP
	• Immediate determination of Hct and blood sugar
	• Maintenance $D_{10}W$ 3 ml/kg/h IV
	In case of:
	• Hypoglycemia: $D_{10}W$ 2 ml/kg/dose IV, then increase $D_{10}W$ infusion
	• Polycythemia: If Hct > 65%: hemodilution with crystalloid solution, e.g., NS 10 ml/kg/ bolus (slowly)
	• If Hct >70% without neurological symptoms: hemodilution. No evidence for benefit of partial exchange transfusion[362]
	• Hct >70% and neurological symptoms: partial exchange transfusion with normal saline in the delivery room may be indicated[363]
	• Partial exchange volume is calculated according to the following formula (estimating the blood volume of the neonate to be ≈80 ml/kg): blood volume × body weight × [(observed Hct – desired Hct) ÷ observed Hct] = volume to be exchanged exchange in ml
	• For partial exchange transfusion draw blood by peripheral venous (if no central line available), by arterial or by central venous access and substitute continuously with equal volume of crystalloid solution (isovolumetric exchange, preferably through a central venous line, e.g., UVC)[362]
	• It may be sufficient to only withdraw 25% to 50% of the calculated exchange volume in the delivery room substituting it continuously with crystalloid solution
	• Check Hct 1, 4, and 24 h after partial exchange transfusion
	• For hydrops, see p. 427
	• Alert the admitting NICU, arrange for immediate transfer
		Symptomatic treatment according to clinical presentation:
		• Checking vital signs
		• Intubation if indicated
		• Venous access and blood draw,
		• PIV, may place UVC and determine CVP
		• Immediate determination of Hct and blood glucose
		• Maintenance $D_{10}W$ 3 ml/kg/h IV
		In case of:
		• Hypoglycemia: $D_{10}W$ 2 ml/kg/dose IV, then increase $D_{10}W$ infusion
		• Chronic hypovolemia and sufficient BP: intravenous crystalloid 10 ml/kg/24 h
		• Hypovolemic shock:
		  • Volume expansion with crystalloid solution, e.g., NS 10 ml/kg/bolus IV for 10–30 min (may repeat)
		  • Transfuse PRBC 5–10–20 ml/kg, O Rhesus-negative, lysine-free (preferably cross-matched with mother's plasma, if not an emergency), after having drawn a sample for the baby's blood type and cross
		• Inadequate blood pressure, i.e., MAP << 40 mmHg (or <GA in weeks) despite sufficient volume expansion?
		  1 Placement of UVC and administration of dopamine 4 – 20 µg/kg/min IV, titrated to maintain MAP above acceptable limit. In the emergency situation, dopamine may be given via peripheral venous access
		  2 Second choice: dobutamine via peripheral or central venous access (caution: may cause peripheral vasodilatation and tachycardia)
		• Alert the admitting NICU and arrange immediate transfer

Complications	Hyperviscosity carries risks of thrombosis and respiratory, neurological, renal, gastrointestinal, and cardiac problems[44,364]	Impending hypoxic-ischemic perfusion disorder of brain (HIE) and other organs[44,364]

ABG, arterial blood gas; CUP, central venous pressure; DDX, differential diagnosis; GA, gestational age; Hct, hematocrit; HIE, hypoxic ischemic encephalopathy; MAP, mean arterial pressure; NICU, neonatal intensive care unit; PIV, peripheral intravenous access; PRBC, packed red blood cells; UVC, umbilical vein catheter.

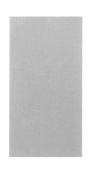

An apparently trivial call from the term baby nursery

Andrea Zimmermann

Measures after the arrival of the NETS/pediatrician in the delivery room

- Physical examination (see Table 3.2)
- Monitoring:
  - Pulse oximetry (S_pO_2, HR)
  - Blood pressure (right arm/left arm/leg; or right ear lobe and leg)
  - Core temperature
  - ECG
- Check vital signs. Achive and maintain stable vital signs by ABCD measures:
  - Oxygen supplementation if S_aO_2 <85% and adequate spontaneous breathing (be careful with supplemental oxygen when suspecting duct-dependent congenital heart disease with left heart obstruction, e.g., hypoplastic left heart syndrome (HLHS), coarctation of the aorta (CoA), interrupted aortic arch (IAA)! see pp. 340–79).
  - Bag-and-mask ventilation or nasal CPAP if required; intubation in cases of severe bradycardia, apnea or insufficient breathing (indications: see p. 158)
  - Venous access (PIV, IVC, IO) and blood sampling for blood gas analysis (normalization of neonatal pH within $\approx$1 h after birth), blood glucose, complete CBC, electrolytes, additional laboratory tests, CRP/IL-6, and blood culture if sepsis is suspected. If S_aO_2 <85%, a capillary or arterial (preferred) blood gas analysis is indicated for evaluation of oxygenation and ventilation (choose radial artery or UAC; consider placing a radial arterial line)
  - During transport to the NICU: give $D_{10}W$ 3 ml/kg/h IV (=5 µg/kg/min) as maintenance infusion. For hypoglycemia, give glucose bolus and double infusion rate to 6 ml/kg/h. Use D_5W or reduce rate of $D_{10}W$ infusion for preterm/term infants with elevated blood glucose levels (>180–200 mg/dl)

! Neonates with abdominal signs/symptoms should be transferred to a level III NICU with an adjacent department of pediatric surgey (tertiary center) well experienced in neonatal abdominal surgery.

! If congenital cardiovascular disease is suspected, transfer the patient to a NICU/pediatric cardiac ICU associated with an experienced pediatric cardiology and pediatric cardiothoracic surgery service (i.e., pediatric heart center).

Neonatal Emergencies: A Practical Guide for Resuscitation, Transport and Critical Care, ed. Georg Hansmann.
Published by Cambridge University Press. © Cambridge University Press 2009.

Table 3.2 Manifestation of critical neonatal disease in the first days of life: common differential diagnoses and initial clinical management

Symptoms	History and clinical findings	Suspected diagnosis	Initial management
Pallor	Tachypnea since birth? Grunting expiration, costal retractions, nasal flaring? Poor general condition? Cyanosis? Fever or hypothermia? Tachycardia?	Transient tachypnea of the newborn (TTN = wet lung), hypothermia, shock, SVT	• Venous access • Blood gas analysis, blood glucose, CBC, electrolytes, CRP/IL-6, blood culture, blood group • Oxygen supplement, nasal CPAP or intubation/PPV, as indicated[366]
	Poor general condition, whimpering, grunting, tachypnea, retractions? Poor peripheral perfusion? Tachycardia? Fever or hypothermia? Prenatal history: signs of maternal peripartal infection? Positive GBS smears?	Infection: pneumonia, sepsis (see p. 280), shock	• Venous access • Blood gas analysis, blood glucose, CBC, electrolytes, CRP/IL-6, lactate, blood culture, blood type and screen/cross • Blood, stool, CSF for enterovirus (see pp. 285–7) PCR and culture, CSF analysis and bacterial culture • Empiric antibiotics IV • Oxygen supplementation, nasal CPAP or intubation/PPV as indicated[366] • Volume (normal saline, PRBC) IV, as indicated • Rapid transfer to NICU
	Acute or chronic blood loss before or during delivery? Vaginal-operative delivery? Twin-twin (=feto–fetal) (see p. 240) or feto–maternal transfusion syndrome? Postpartal blood loss, e.g., bloody stools, progressive cephalohematoma/subdural hematoma? Has vitamin K been given? Rhesus or ABO incompatibility? Jaundice?	Anemia due to peripartal blood loss, vitamin K deficiency, intracerebral hemorrhage, hemolytic disease (p. 423)	• Venous access • Blood gas analysis, blood glucose, CBC and reticulocyte count, blood smear/RBC morphology, bilirubin (direct/indirect), direct Coombs test • Blood culture, blood type and screen/cross • Administer vitamin K IV/IM if not done yet • Volume (normal saline, PRBC) IV, as needed • Oxygen supplementation, nasal CPAP or intubation as indicated[366] • Head ultrasound
	Poor general condition? Vomiting?	Inborn errors of metabolism, gastrointestinal stenosis/atresia, sepsis, shock	• Venous access • Blood gas analysis, blood glucose, lactate, ammonia (later advanced metabolic work-up), CBC, electrolytes, bilirubin (direct/indirect), CRP, blood culture, blood type and screen/cross

Sign	Findings / questions	Diagnosis	Management
Pale or grayish (dusky) skin color, ± cyanosis	Increasing respiratory rate? Heart murmur absent or present? Decreased systemic perfusion (capillary refill >2 s, weak peripheral pulses, oliguria)? Blood gas analysis: metabolic acidosis? Lactate elevated?	Heart disease with left heart obstruction (=duct-dependent systemic perfusion) (see p. 340), e.g., hypoplastic left heart[367] (HLH, also CoA, IAA; see p. 340), sepsis, shock	• Volume (normal saline) IV • $D_{10}W$ 3–6 ml/kg/h (1× to 2× maintenance) IV, depending on blood glucose level • Venous access • Blood gas analysis, blood glucose, lactate, CBC, electrolytes, bilirubin, CRP, blood culture, blood type and screen/cross • Careful with oxygen supplementation (with final diagnosis pending, aim for max. S_pO_2 of 85%), nasal CPAP or intubation as indicated[366] • ECHO, as soon as possible • PGE_1 infusion (start with 50–100 ng/kg/min IV) • Pre- and postductal S_aO_2 • Blood pressure on all 4 extremities
Pallor or cyanosis	Intrapartal meconium-stained amniotic fluid (look at nail bed, stump of umbilical cord)? Increasing respiratory rate with dyspnea (retractions)?	Transient tachypnea (TTN=wet lung), (meconium) aspiration (p. 269), infection pneumonia/sepsis[366] ± PPHN[368] , shock	• Clear and secure airways • Oxygen • Supplementation, nasal CPAP or intubation as indicated[366] • Venous access • Blood gas analysis, blood glucose, CBC, electrolytes, bilirubin, CRP, blood culture, blood type and screen
Cyanosis	Increasing respiratory rate with dyspnea? Cyanosis? Poor general condition	Transient tachypnea (TTN=wet lung), pneumonia, beginning or manifest PPHN[368] (see p. 392), air leak (pneumothorax, pneumomediastinum) (see p. 410), diaphragmatic hernia (CDH; see p. 404), CCAML (see p. 417), congestive heart failure (see pp. 348–50)	• Clear and secure airways • Supplemental oxygen, nasal CPAP or intubation, as indicated[366] • Venous access • Blood gas analysis, blood glucose, lactate, CBC, electrolytes, CRP, blood culture, blood type and screen
Peripheral (± central) cyanosis?	Peripheral (± central) cyanosis? Poor peripheral perfusion (capillary refill ≫2 s)? History: Maternal diabetes? Suspected twin–twin (feto–fetal) or materno – fetal transfusion syndrome?	Polycythemia (see p. 128)	• Venous access • Blood gas analysis, blood glucose, CBC, electrolytes, blood culture, blood group • Volume (normal saline) IV • Consider partial blood exchange if symptomatic and Hct >70%

Table 3.2 (cont.)

Symptoms	History and clinical findings	Suspected diagnosis	Initial management
	Cyanosis? Adequate general condition? Heart murmur? Heart defect prenatally known/ suspected?	Cyanotic heart disease (see p. 340), e.g., congenital heart disease with right heart obstruction (=duct-dependent pulmonary perfusion (see p. 340)), PPHN (see p. 392)	• Venous access • Blood gas analysis, blood glucose, CBC, electrolytes, blood culture, blood type and screen/cross • Clear and secure airways • Supplemental oxygen, nasal CPAP or intubation, as indicated[366] • ECHO, as indicated • If PPHN is ruled out or unlikely: PGE infusion (start with 50–100 ng/mg/min IV) • Pre- and postductal S_pO_2 • Blood pressure on all 4 extremities
Jaundice	Child is remarkably sleepy; poor feeding? Dehydration? Ethnicity? Maternal blood group? Excessive bruising? Family history?	Severe jaundice? Rhesus immunization, Rhesus or ABO incompatibility, sepsis, dehydration, inborn errors of metabolism	• Venous access • Blood gas analysis, blood glucose, lactate, ammonia (later more advanced metabolic work-up), CBC, electrolytes, bilirubin, CRP, blood culture, blood type and screen, direct Coombs test • Volume expansion IV
Muscular hypotonia	General condition affected? Abnormal face or signs of dysmorphism? Skin color? Floppy infant?	Infection/sepsis, jaundice, seizures, intracerebral hemorrhage, neuromuscular or metabolic disorder[369]	• Venous access • Blood gas analysis, blood glucose, CBC, CRP, electrolytes, bilirubin • Blood pressure, volume expansion, as indicated • Neurological work-up[370] • Head ultrasound
Muscular hypertonia	General condition affected? Abnormal face or signs of dysmorphism? Skin color? Abnormal eye movement (e.g., deviation of eyes)? Newborn is drowsy/ apathetic? Change of skin color?	Pain, seizures, neuromuscular or metabolic disorder, intracerebral hemorrhage, metabolic disorder	• Venous access • Blood gas analysis, blood glucose, lactate, ammonia (later more advanced metabolic work-up), CBC, CRP, electrolytes, bilirubin • Neurological work-up[370]

Jitteriness	Poor feeding? Vomiting? Maternal diabetes mellitus or gestational diabetes? Immaturity? Maternal drug abuse?	Hypoglycemia, hypocalcemia, hypomagnesemia, hypophosphatemia, neonatal opioid withdrawal	• Venous access • Blood gas analysis, blood glucose, CBC, CRP, electrolytes including Ionized calcium, magnesium, phosphorus, bilirubin • Toxicology screen (mother and baby) • Neurological work-up[370]
Abdominal distension, bilious vomiting	General status and vital signs stable? Pallor? Poor feeding? Unusual abdominal finding? Unusual respiratory finding?	Nausea, bilious vomiting, suspected intestinal obstruction: intestinal stenosis/atresia, ileus (mechanical, paralytic), NEC, volvulus (see pp. 437–49)	• Venous access • Blood gas analysis, blood • Glucose, CBC, CRP electrolytes, lactate, bilirubin • Volume expansion IV • Nasogastric tube, no oral feeding, D_{10}W-based maintenance IV fluids • Abdominal ultrasonography[371] • Abdominal X-ray (KUB) • Consult pediatric surgery
Bloody stools	Stool considerably or slightly blood-stained? Guaiac positive? General condition and vital signs stable? Poor peripheral perfusion? Poor feeding? Unusual abdominal finding, distension? Anal fissure? Oliguria?	Intestinal infection, NEC, volvulus, intestinal duplication, anal fissure (see pp. 437–449), enterovirus infection (pp. 285–7), coagulation disorder, vitamin K deficiency, formula intolerance	• Venous access • Blood gas analysis, blood glucose, CBC, CRP, electrolytes, coagulation studies, bilirubin • Bacterial and viral stool culture, send stool for rotavirus antigen, Clostridium difficile diagnostics, enterovirus PCR • Volume expansion IV • No oral feeding and D_{10}W maintenace infusion • Abdominal X-ray (KUB) • Abdominal ultrasonography[371]
Diarrhea	Stool considerably or slightly blood-stained? Guaiac positive? (see under Bloody stools) General condition and vital signs stable? Poor peripheral perfusion? Poor feeding? Unusual abdominal finding, distension? Anal fissure? Oliguria?	Intestinal infection, enterovirus infection (pp. 285–287), (see also under Bloody stools)	• Venous access • Blood gas analysis, blood glucose, CBC, CRP, electrolytes, coagulation studies, bilirubin • Bacterial and viral stool culture, send stool for rotavirus antigen, C. difficile diagnostics, enterovirus culture and PCR • Volume expansion IV • No oral feeding and D_{10}W maintenace infusion

Table 3.2 (cont.)

Symptoms	History and clinical findings	Suspected diagnosis	Initial management
No meconium within 48 h after birth	Meconium passed during labor? General condition affected? Unusual abdominal finding? Inadequate tissue perfusion? Bilious vomiting? Distended abdomen? Bowel sounds are present, weak, or absent? Prenatal diagnostic clues?	Intestinal stenosis/atresia, NEC, volvulus, meconium plug	• Abdominal X-ray (KUB) • Abdominal ultrasonography[371] • Venous access • Blood gas analysis, blood glucose, CBC, electrolytes • Abdominal X-ray (KUB) • Abdominal ultrasonography[371]
No urine for more than 24 h after birth	Urine output absent or reduced? General condition affected? Prenatal diagnostic clues for kidney disease? Dehydration?	*Prerenal failure:* Hypovolemia (insufficient feeding?), medications *Renal failure:* agenesis, shock, infection, renal vein thrombosis *Postrenal failure:* urethral stricture[372]	• Venous access • Blood gas analysis, blood glucose, CBC, CRP, electrolytes, creatinine, nitrogen, coagulation, bilirubin, (urinanalysis) • Initiate or increase IV fluids ($D_{10}W \pm NS$) • Abdominal ultrasonography

CBC, complete blood count; CCAML, congenital cystic adenomatoid malformation of the lung; CoA, coarctation of the aorta; CPAP, continuous positive airways pressure; CRP, C-reactive protein; CSF, cerebrospinal fluid; ECHO, echocardiography; IAA, interrupted aortic arch; IL-6, interleukin-6; IM, intramuscularly; IV, intravenously; NEC, necrotizing enterocolitis; PGE, prostaglandin; PPHN, persistent pulmonary hypertension of the newborn; PRBC, packed red blood cells; PCR, polymerase chain reaction; SVT, supraventricular tachycardia.

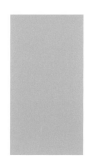

Out of hospital birth

Tilman Humpl

The term "out of hospital birth" was coined in the twentieth century. Before 1900 it was the exception rather than the rule to give birth at a hospital. At this time fewer than 5% of all births took place at a hospital, increasing to almost 50% in 1940, and 99% in the 1970s. Several studies have demonstrated that planned home birth attended by appropriately qualified caregivers is safe. However, for this to be true, there should be no significant difference in morbidity and mortality when compared to standard hospital delivery. A healthy woman without contraindications (see below) has a low risk, both for herself and for the newborn infant[53]. Midwives and/or obstetricians should discuss the advantages and possible risks of home birth with the expecting parents.

Outcome: the perinatal mortality of "intended home birth" in the USA, Canada, UK and Australia (studies from 1969 to 1996) ranges between 0.9/1000 and 5.1/1000[54-58].

Important factors influencing the mortality rate of the newborn

- Underestimation of the risks associated with post-term birth
- Twin pregnancy
- Breech presentation
- Lack of response to fetal distress

> **!** It is important to differentiate a *"planned home birth"* (with the presence of a skilled attendant, e.g., midwife) from an *"unplanned home birth,"* which can rapidly turn into an emergency situation.

Normal spontaneous delivery

Definition

Spontaneous in onset, low risk at the start of labor and remaining so throughout labor and delivery. The infant is born spontaneously in the vertex position between 37 and 42 completed weeks of pregnancy (normal spontaneous vaginal delivery, NSVD). Mother and infant are in good condition following delivery.

Focused assessment of the pregnant woman

- Subjective and objective condition of the pregnant woman (and of the fetus – if possible)
- Check records/history of the pregnant women

Neonatal Emergencies: A Practical Guide for Resuscitation, Transport and Critical Care, ed. Georg Hansmann.
Published by Cambridge University Press. © Cambridge University Press 2009.

- Calculate gestational age
- Prenatal exams
- Prenatal ultrasound reports
- Estimated birth weight
- Clarify fetal position
- Expected date of delivery
- History of bleeding
- Fetal movement
- Previous deliveries
- Blood group
- HBsAg
- Antibody titers
- GBS status
- Allergies
- Use of medication
- Time, amount, and content of last oral intake
- Other risk factors

Clinical examination

- Contractions
  - Beginning when?
  - How often?
  - How strong?
- Temperature
- Listen to fetal heart rate for a full minute (best audible along the side between the umbilicus and symphysis). If there are fetal heart rate abnormalities (<100 or >180 bpm), suspect fetal distress
- Even with normal heart rates, always check again after a contraction
- If bradycardia is present
  - Provide oxygen
  - Guide towards deep inspirations
  - Suggest change in position (lateral positioning – avoid supine position to prevent compression of the vena cava and supine hypotensive syndrome)
  - More invasive measures of intrauterine resuscitation: IV crystalloid solution (1000 ml), nitroglycerin spray (400 µg s.c., 2–4 puffs), albuterol HFA (90–100 µg, 2–4 puffs), terbutaline (250 µg, subcutaneously)
  - Results of previous vaginal examination (available?) If not: ask the pregnant woman if she has the urge to push or to defecate (if present: the second stage of labor may have started)

! In the absence of any abnormalities, the fetal heart rate should be checked immediately after a contraction or at least every 30 min and then every 15 min during the second stage.

Pelvic examination
- Inspection
  - Rupture of membranes?
- Palpation of the cervix
  - Dilatation
  - Effacement
- Palpation of the presenting part
  - Identification of the presenting part
- Check fetal position

Orientation of the presenting part within the maternal pelvis

Cephalic		Any position of the baby in which the head presents first (syn.: vertex, crown presentation). Most common is the occiput anterior presentation (easiest to deliver: head is sharply flexed, the chin is in contact with the thorax). Abnormal cephalic presentations include brow, face, and posterior occiput presentations at the time of delivery
Occiput	96%	Occiput anterior presentation: the upper back part of the fetal head is the presenting part. Occiput posterior presentation (5% of occiput presentations): back of the baby's head is facing the mother's spine (abnormal cephalic presentation leads to prolonged labor and complications)
Breech	3%	Buttocks or legs enter the birth canal before the head (leads to complications)
Shoulder	0.3%	Transverse lie. The baby's back is usually anterior (leads to complications)
Face	0.5%	Fetal head and neck are hyperextended (abnormal cephalic presentation leads to complications)
Brow	0.01%	Fetal head is midway between full flexion (vertex) and hyperextension (face) along a longitudinal axis. Fetal brow palpable on vaginal examination (abnormal cephalic presentation leads to complications)
Compound	0.1%	One or more limbs lie alongside and present with the head (leads to complications)

Observation of birth process
The following timelines are useful as guidelines.

The duration of the **first stage of labor** in the primipara ranges over 6–18 hours, while it is 2–10 hours in multipara. The rate of cervical dilatation during the active phase is about 1 cm per hour in the first pregnancy and approximately 1.5 cm per hour in subsequent pregnancies. The duration of the **second stage of labor** in the primipara ranges from 30 minutes to 3 hours, and 5 minutes to 30 minutes in multipara. The **third stage of labor** takes up to 30 minutes.

Identification of labor

True labor
- Contractions occur at regular intervals
- Interval between contractions steadily shortens
- Intensity of contractions steadily increases
- Discomfort predominantly in the back and abdomen

- Dilatation of the cervix
- Discomfort does not improve with sedation

False labor
- Contractions occur at irregular intervals
- Intervals between contractions are long
- Intensity of contractions is unchanged
- Discomfort is predominantly in the lower abdomen
- No cervix dilatation
- Relieve of discomfort with sedation

First stage of labor (stage of dilatation)
Definition
From the onset of contractions to the complete opening of the cervix (10 cm).
Duration of delivery depends on many factors that also contribute to the length of delivery, such as:

- Size relation of pelvis/child
- Previous birth
- Socio-economic status
- Psyche of mother
- Environment
  Duration of the dilatation period is highly variable:
- Primiparae: approx. 4–10 h (other data: 12 + 4 h)
- Multiparae: approx. 2–4 h (other data: 7 + 4 h)
  The stage of dilatation ends when the cervix is completely dilated (10 cm).

> ! As long as the cervix can be felt, i.e., as long as the cervix is *not yet 10 cm dilated*, the pregnant woman should *not push.*

Rupture of membranes (ROM)
Definition
- "Timely": at the end of the dilatation period
- Premature: rupture of membranes before labor begins
- Early: rupture of membranes before the cervix is fully dilated, i.e., <10 cm (additional definition: ROM before a cervix diameter of 6 cm is reached)

> ! If the membranes are ruptured and the head of the fetus is not yet engaged in the pelvis, the expectant mother should only be transported in a lying position (with the pelvis in an elevated position).

Procedure/therapy
Evaluation of the further course of the delivery: if frequency of contractions is less than two every 5 min and dilatation of cervix is not complete, consider transport to a hospital in primapara.

The second stage of labor

Definition

Period between the complete dilatation of the cervix and delivery of the newborn. Strong contractions occur every 2–3 min and last approximately 60 seconds.

Length of the second stage of labor:

- Primiparae: approximately 30–60 min (around 20 pushes)
- Multiparae: approximately 5–30 min (a few pushes)

Procedure/therapy

- Check position of the child's head: if the head has reached the mother's pelvis (the head is now seen in the vagina), birth will most likely begin within the next few minutes
- The woman should be guided to breathe during pauses of contractions. If possible, provide oxygen and allow slow and deep breaths (optimize the child's oxygenation)

! The second stage of labor is the most sensitive stage with the highest risk for hypoxia for the infant

---

Further course of delivery:

- The presenting part of the fetus is the posterior fontanel, i.e., usually the anterior occiput when the head passes the pelvis by flexion and rotation
- No pushing while the head is being born
- Protection of the perineum: controlled gradual delivery of the head and avoidance of fast pushes (the midwife supports the back of the head with the left hand and leads the head from the perineum with the right hand)
- Birth of the shoulders by lowering the head, then leading the body over the symphysis to the mother's abdomen. Do not pull the child straight!
- If the umbilical cord is wrapped around the neck, try to loosen and thrust back the umbilical cord before delivering the child

Clamping of the cord. The newborn may be placed at or below the level of the vaginal introitus for 1–2 minutes to shift blood from the placenta to the neonate. The umbilical cord is usually cut between two clamps placed 4–5 cm from the abdomen of the neonate. Subsequently, a plastic umbilical cord clamp is applied 2–3 cm from the abdomen of the neonate.

! The naked abdomen of the mother is the warmest place for the child. Determining the Apgar score and monitoring can also be done there; cover the child well, especially the head (e.g., with pre-warmed towel, cap).

Episiotomy

Available data do not support liberal or routine use of episiotomy. Nonetheless, there is a place for episiotomy for maternal or fetal indications, such as avoiding severe maternal lacerations or facilitating or expediting difficult deliveries[59].

> **!** *Episiotomy:* Restricted rather than routine use.
> Median episiotomy is associated with higher rates of injury to the anal sphincter and rectum than is mediolateral episiotomy.
> Routine episiotomy does not prevent pelvic floor damage (leading to incontinence).

Third stage of labor

Definition
The period between the birth of the child and when the uterus expels the placenta.
- Duration: about 10–30 minutes
- Physiological blood loss: around 200–400 ml

Procedure/therapy
- Observe the separation and birth of the placenta (do not pull on the cord without control: danger of ripping)
- Examine the placenta (complete?)
- Continue observation for bleeding and of the height of the uterus (level of navel)
- If heavy bleeding persists, administer oxytocin or methylergonovine and compress the uterus with the thumb and forefinger (Credé maneuver; contraindications apply)
- Observe maternal condition

Intended home birth
The course of the planned birth at home depends on many factors:
- Good prenatal care and examination (ruling out multiple gestations, malposition, malformations, growth retardation, etc.)
- Competence of obstetrics (mostly the midwife)
- Preparation for emergencies (depending on the local facilities: telephone number of NETS (neonatal emergency transport service) or children's hospital, paramedics, emergency physician, hospital)
- The exact estimation of gestational age: home birth can take place in the 37th–42nd weeks of gestation

Contraindications to intended home births

Maternal contraindications
- Contractions before completing 37 weeks or after the 42nd week of gestation
- Uterus malformations
- Polyhydramnios
- Oligohydramnios
- Chronic and acute diseases of the mother, such as:
  - Hypertension (e.g. preeclampsia, HELLP syndrome)
  - Diabetes mellitus (also gestational diabetes)
  - Extreme obesity
  - Pre-existing renal insufficiency
  - Neurological–psychiatric illnesses
  - Infections (e.g., fever, urinary tract infection, venereal diseases, HSV, VZV, HBV, HIV)

- Positive GBS smear (vaginal and/or cervical)
- Placental anomalies (e.g., placenta previa)
- Complications in previous deliveries:
  - Previous still birth
  - Previous preterm deliveries
  - Previous operative deliveries
- Earlier complications in the period of afterbirth

Fetal contraindications
- Abnormal positions
- Macrosomia
- SGA
- Malformations
- Placental anomalies
- Prematurity ($<37 + 0$ weeks' gestation)
- Postterm pregnancy ($>42 + 0$ weeks' gestation)
- Other fetal conditions that raise suspicion of a compromised newborn after birth

Indication for intrauterine transfer of the mother and fetus
- Impending premature delivery <35 weeks' gestation
- Oligo- or polyhydramnios
- Suspected malformation in the prenatal ultrasound

Complications already present during the early phase of contractions
- Unusual position
- Relative disproportion
- Persistent change of the fetal heart rate (<120 bpm or >160 bpm, late decelerations, variable decelerations)
- Suspected chorioamnionitis
- Abnormal amniotic fluid (foul smelling, meconium stained)
- Bleeding (more than smears, stronger than menstrual bleeding)
- Uterine tetany
- Uncoordinated contractions
- Stagnation of labor
- Unstable hemodynamics of the expectant woman

Initial care of the newborn after home birth
See Algorithm (Figure 3.1). Avoid drastic environmental changes in ambient light, noise, and temperature.

Equipment for intended home birth
- Cord clamping (p. 121)
  - Sterile cord clamps
  - Sterile scissors
  - Sterile gauze pads (packed)

- Tools for the initial care of the newborn after intended home birth (p. 25)
  - Clean, warm and bright surroundings
  - Radiant heater
  - Prewarmed, dry and absorbent towels (cotton diapers are better than terry cloth)
  - Firm surface (for potential resuscitation of the newborn)
  - Stethoscope
  - Bag-and-mask system with a closed reservoir, pop-off and PEEP valves
  - Oxygen tank with intact tubing
  - Portable suctioning device (–200 mbar)
  - Suction catheters in various sizes (Ch 6–12)
  - Blood glucose measuring device (e.g., glucometer) with test strips (air protected; check expiration date!)
  - Standard equipment for newborn resuscitation including adrenaline, normal saline, dextrose, intubation equipment, and endotracheal tubes in different sizes

Quick assessment of respiration, heart rate and skin color immediately after birth (see p. 142)

- Palpate the umbilical cord or auscultate the heart to assess HR: is HR > 100 bpm?
- Is meconium present? (If yes: see Chapter "Meconium aspiration," p. 269)?
- Chest movements/crying?
- Is the newborn already pink?
- Clear airway, as needed (p. 66)
- Always dry and keep warm
- If pallor/cyanosis/inadequate respiration is present:
  - Stimulation (with four fingers on the back while drying at the same time, then the soles or sternum)
  - O_2 supply (F_iO_2 0.5–1.0; flow 5 l/min)

Check 30 seconds after birth
- Chest movements sufficient and symmetric? crying?
- HR >100 bpm?
- Is the skin color turning rosy?

If there is persistent pallor, cyanosis, insufficient breathing, and/or HR <100 bpm
- Clear airways (suction pharynx, nose)
- Bag-and-mask ventilation (for indications and contraindications, see pp. 156–8)
- Provide warm environment
- Call NETS/pediatrician/paramedics

In a stable neonate (normal respiratory efforts, trunk rosy, HR >100 bpm)
- Place the neonate on the mother's belly
- Clamp the cord (if not done yet)
- Determine Apgar score
- Administer vitamin K on the first day of life

Further procedures after the adaptation of the newborn

A physical examination of the newborn should be performed immediately after birth.

- Detection of life-threatening conditions and apparent injuries
- If necessary emergency procedures may be initiated
- Data on pregnancy, delivery, Apgar score, measurements (weight, head circumference, length), maturity, and malformations must be recorded

---

Essential components of newborn care:
- Use sterile techniques at the time of delivery
- Ensure spontaneous, sufficient breathing and heart rate of the baby
- Ensure maintenance of warmth for the baby
- Identify at-risk neonates

Instructing the mother/parents in the care of the newborn (support may also be provided by a midwife)

- Monitor for sufficient food intake and weight gain
- Monitor for urine and stool (the neonate should pass urine and stool during the first 24 hours of life)
- Monitor for increasing jaundice during the first 24 hours of life or later
- Monitor other skin changes (cyanosis, pallor, hematomas, petechie)
- Monitor abnormal behavior (lethargy, jitteriness, continuous crying, irritability, etc.)

! If abnormal clinical symptoms are present, refer the newborn to a pediatrician or to a children's hospital without delay.

The second physical examination (early discharge examination)

Between the 3rd and 10th days of life, the baby should be examined by a physician with substantial experience in neonatology. The weight is checked, jaundice ruled out, and heel stick sampling performed (and documented) to screen for inborn metabolic disorders. If the parents opt for PO vitamin K prophylaxis (IM prophylaxis recommended in the USA), the second PO vitamin K dose is given at this time point. Some experts recommend postductal S_pO_2 screening in all newborns (12–48 hours after birth).

Outcome of home births

Planned home birth for low-risk women under supervision of certified professional midwives is associated with relatively low rates of medical interventions and similar intrapartum and neonatal mortality when compared to low-risk in-hospital births in developed countries. Post partal transport of the newborn (especially due to delayed respiratory adaptation, suspected infection or to examine malformations) is necessary in about 1.2% of cases.

When does a pediatrician need to be called immediately?

Examples:

- Meconium-stained amniotic fluid (MSAF)
- Primary asystole or severe bradycardia

- A 1-min Apgar score <5
- A 5- or 10-min Apgar score <7
- Respiratory rate >60 breaths/min with nasal flaring, grunting, retractions (30–60 min after birth)
- HR <80 bpm or >160 bpm (when quiet)
- Arrhythmia
- Neurological abnormalities (e.g., suspected seizures)
- Suspected infection of the newborn
- Intermittent apnea
- Central cyanosis
- Distended abdomen
- Gestational age (calculated or clinically) <37 + 0 weeks or signs of postmaturity
- Arterial Hypotension
- Projectile vomiting
- Vomiting of blood
- Birth weight <2300–2500 g (e.g., SGA) or >4500 g (undetected gestational diabetes?)
- Traumatic birth
  (These recommendations are well established, but do not claim to be complete.)

Unintended out of hospital birth
Definition
Midwives, emergency doctors and/or neonatal emergency doctors are called because of:
- A pregnant woman with incessant contractions
- A pregnant woman who is in labor
- A home birth, which has just taken place

Possible scenarios at the site
- No or only minimal information on the course of the pregnancy
- Hemodynamic instability of the mother (e.g., bleeding)
- Preeclampsia/eclampsia/HELLP syndrome
- Preterm or SGA delivery
- Birth asphyxia
- Postnatal asphyxia
- Meconium aspiration
- Chorioamnionitis/sepsis
- Respiratory distress syndrome (RDS)
- Malformations
- Twins

Disadvantages of an unintended out of hospital birth
- No midwife present
- Anxious, overburdened expectant woman
- Small, relatively cold rooms

- Absence of an adequate area for newborn resuscitation
- Stressed family members

Procedure/therapy

Assigning tasks (especially if multiple health care professionals are present):

- Who takes care of the mother? Usually the emergency physician (or the midwife)
- Who takes care of the newborn? Usually the neonatal team (or the midwife)
- Keep calm or ask other health care professionals to help with reassuring measures
- Provide the expectant mother with a safe and secure environment
- Prepare area for initial care/resuscitation of the newborn

> **❗ *Provide warmth to neonate***
> Suction and dry the neonate, and cover well (e.g., with warm towel, cap), especially the head. If a warm place is not available for the infant, the best place is the naked abdomen of the mother; additional covering with towels may be necessary.

- Meticulous physical examination of the newborn
- Exact documentation:
  - Time of arrival?
  - Condition of the neonate?
  - Age of the neonate?
  - Which measures were initiated by other health care professionals: midwife, NETS, emergency physician?
- The threshold to transfer the newborn to a children's hospital should be low!
- Preferably, the mother and the neonate are transferred to the same hospital
- Contact both the neonatal pediatric and the obstetric departments
  See also standard algorithm for the resuscitation of newborn infants, Figure 3.1.

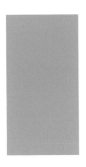

Hypoglycemia

Tilman Humpl

Definition

Hypoglycemia in neonates is a relatively common, heterogenous and potentially serious problem. A consistent definition of hypoglycemia does not exist in the literature or in clinical practice[60,61].

Epidemiology

- Hypoglycemia is a frequent concern in neonatology
- For the majority of healthy term infants, low glucose levels reflect metabolic adaptation to extrauterine life
- If the first feeding is delayed by 3–6 h, 10% of healthy neonates are not able to maintain their blood glucose level above 30 mg/dl (1.7 mmol/l). After 12 h of life (and feeding) the risk for symptomatic hypoglycemia declines, but still exists for the term infant with low birth weight (<2500 g; SGA), with high birth weight (LGA), and postasphyxic newborns[62].

Diagnosis

The diagnosis of hypoglycemia may be made in the symptomatic neonate with a low blood glucose concentration and resolving symptoms after normalization of the blood glucose concentration. Transient hypoglycemia in the first few hours after birth is relatively frequent. Hypoglycemia that is persistent requires further investigation.

WHO guidelines – hypoglycemia of the newborn[63] (continued on p. 262)

- Healthy term newborns who are breastfeeding on demand do not need to have their blood glucose routinely checked and need no supplementary foods or fluids
- Healthy term newborns do not develop "symptomatic" hypoglycemia as a result of simple underfeeding. If an infant develops signs suggesting hypoglycemia, look for an underlying cause. This usually means drawing a blood sample (serum tube, better: sodium fluoride tube) at the time of hypoglycemia prior to treatment. Detection of the cause is as important as immediate correction of the blood glucose level
- Thermal protection (the maintenance of normal body temperature) in addition to breast-feeding is necessary to prevent hypoglycemia
- Newborns at risk for hypoglycemia include those who are preterm and/or SGA, those who suffered intrapartum asphyxia or who are sick, and those born to diabetic mothers

---

Neonatal Emergencies: A Practical Guide for Resuscitation, Transport and Critical Care, ed. Georg Hansmann.
Published by Cambridge University Press. © Cambridge University Press 2009.

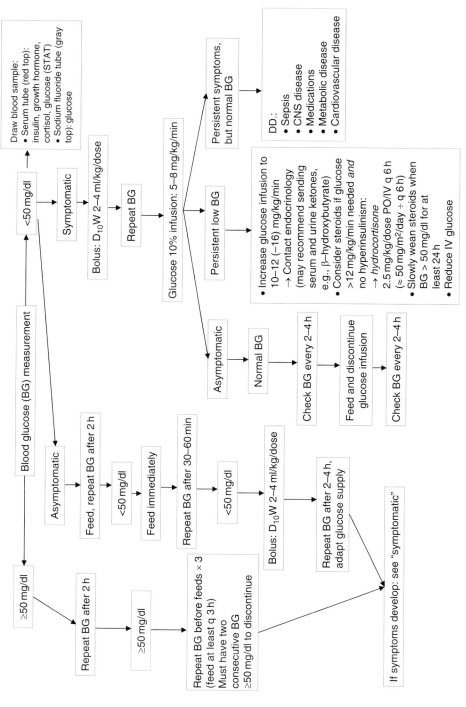

Figure 3.4 Algorithm for the initial management of neonatal hypoglycaemia. BG, blood glucose concentration.

- In newborns at risk, hypoglycemia is likely to occur in the first 24 h of life, as the infant adapts to extrauterine life. Hypoglycemia which presents after the first day of life, or which persists or recurs, does not necessarily indicate inadequate feeding. It may indicate underlying disease such as infection, or a wide range of metabolic conditions.
- For newborns at risk, breast milk is the safest and nutritionally most appropriate food. However, it may need to be supplemented with specific nutrients for some very low birth weight infants.
- For newborns at risk, the blood glucose concentration should be measured at around 4–6 h after birth, before a feed, if reliable laboratory measurements are available. Measurements using glucose-oxidase-based reagent paper strips have poor sensitivity and specificity in newborns, and should not be relied upon as an alternative.
- For newborns at risk *who do not show abnormal clinical signs* ("asymptomatic"), the blood glucose concentration should preferably be maintained at or above 47 mg/dl (2.6 mmol/l).
- If reliable laboratory measurements of blood glucose are not available (e.g., out-of-hospital birth, developing country), newborns at risk should be kept warm and breastfed. If breastfeeding is not possible they should be given supplements of expressed breast milk (PUMP) or an appropriate breastmilk substitute by bottle or gavage at least every 3 h. In the absence of hypoglycemia, supplemental nursing systems (SNS) (special bottle hung around the mother's neck, with two tubes taped to her breasts so that the ends reach her nipples) is well suited to providing babies with breast milk or formula supplement at the breast, e.g., for premature babies, babies with sucking difficulties, adopted babies, children with deft lip/palate or for stimulating milk production in a natural way after a break in breast feeding.

Practical (but not evidence-based) blood glucose levels for term neonates

- 0–24 h after birth: blood glucose minimum 40 mg/dl (2.2 mmol/l)
- >24 h after birth: blood glucose minimum 45 mg/dl (2.5 mmol/l)
- Aim for blood glucose 60–100 mg/dl (3.3–5.6 mmol/l)
- Blood glucose levels up to 150 mg/dl (8.3 mmol/l) are tolerable (some accept levels up to 180 mg/dl = 10 mmol/l)
- The use of rapid bedside measurement devices (D-stix) is not recommended for neonates, as values below 60 mg/dl (3.3 mmol/l) are inaccurate (often too high), but they may allow immediate recognition and initiation of therapy
- Low–normal blood glucose levels between 40 and 50 mg/dl (2.2–2.8 mmol/l), and those below 40 mg/dl (2.2 mmol/l), measured with rapid bedside analyzers (glucometer; D-stix), must be verified with the core laboratory immediately
- Of note, if the blood was collected in regular plasma (USA: green top) or serum tubes (USA: red top) instead of those with sodium fluoride (USA: gray top), there is ongoing glycolysis resulting in falsely low blood glucose levels (a reduction of 2 mg/dl per hour), especially when the samples are not processed immediately (color code may vary between countries and institutions)
- A neonate with low–normal blood glucose levels (40–50 mg/dl = 2.2–2.8 mmol/l in the first 24 h of life) should be fed early with 10% glucose solutions or formula. Check glucose level after 1, 3, 6, 12, and 24 h. If the blood glucose levels remain >50 mg/dl (2.8 mmol/l), there is usually no need to transfer the baby for further metabolic work-up

! The following approach is recommended for term/preterm infants with blood glucose levels <50 mg/dl (2.8 mmol/l) before or during transport (see Figure 3.4):
- In the absence of common risk factors for hypoglycemia (see below, e.g., prematurity, IUGR, SGA and LGA infants, maternal diabetes including gestational diabetes, birth asphyxia), in late (>48 h of life) or severe hypoglycemia <30 mg/dl (1.65 mmol/l), we strongly recommend drawing blood samples for advanced diagnostic testing at the time of hypoglycemia (serum tube (USA: red top): insulin, growth hormone, cortisol, glucose (STAT); sodium fluoride tube (USA: gray top): glucose), e.g., at the time of PIV placement, then 2–5 ml $D_{10}W$/kg/bolus IV.
- The blood glucose level should be checked once more before departure and double the amount of the usual maintenance glucose should be given during transport (i.e., 6 ml $D_{10}W$/kg/h IV = 10 mg/kg/min), anticipating rebound hyperinsulinemia/hypoglycemia s/p $D_{10}W$ bolus.
- High glucose maintenance infusion (approx. 10 mg/kg/min) may also be given to macrosomic neonates if there is a high suspicion of undiagnosed or poorly controlled (gestational) diabetes mellitus.

Etiology/pathophysiology

Hypoglycemia may be related to:
- Decreased glucose production
- Inadequate glucose supply and/or increased glucose utilization
- *Inadequate production or substrate deficit:*
  - Insufficient or delayed feeding
  - Insufficient or delayed parenteral supply
  - Abnormal hormone regulation of glucose and lipid metabolism
  - Transient immaturity in glucoregulatory mechanisms, leading to a reduction of endogenous glucose production (gluconeogenesis)
  - Decreased cerebral glucose transport (e.g., perinatal hypoxia/ischemia)
  - Suppression of gluconeogenesis and glycogenolysis
  - Fatty acid oxygenation disorders
  - Inborn errors of amino acid metabolism (e.g., propionic and methylmalonic acidemia)
- *Increased utilization:*
  - Hyperinsulinism
  - Increased calorie requirement (e.g., thermoregulation in LBW and SGA infants)
  - Increased calorie requirement in increased muscle activity (e.g., increased respiratory exertion)
  - Hemodynamic or respiratory shift from aerobic to anaerobic metabolism (e.g., hypoxemia, hypoventilation, septic shock)
  - Relative dominance of glucose-dependent organs (high parenchyma quotient in SGA)
  - Inborn errors in metabolism
  - Acute CNS damage (e.g., meningitis, encephalitis, hemorrhage)

! A single blood glucose sample does not give any information about the duration of hypoglycemia[64].

Neonates at high risk for hypoglycemia

- Preterm infant with very low body weight ($<1500\,g$)
- IUGR, SGA (birth weight below the 10th percentile)
- Smaller of discordant twins (weight difference $>25\%$)
- Very low birth weight infants ($<1250\,g$)
- LGA neonates (birth weight over the 90th percentile)
- Persistent imbalance in maternal glucose regulation/gestational diabetes
- Insulin-dependent diabetes mellitus of the mother
- Massive obesity of the mother
- High parenteral glucose supply to the mother during the birth
- Fast parenteral glucose supply to the mother before the birth
- Perinatal distress, e.g., 5-min Apgar score <5
- Fatty acid oxidation disorder of the newborn
- Inborn errors of amino acid metabolism
- Hypoxemia (e.g., heart or lung diseases)
- Hypoperfusion/shock
- Severe anemia
- Congenital genetic disorders associated with hypoglycemia
- Microcephalic neonates
- Neonates with midline defects
- Persistent hyperbilirubinemia
- Isolated hepatomegaly
- Neonates with Beckwith-Wiedemann syndrome (omphalocele-macroglossia-gigantism syndrome)
- Positive family history for neonates with hypoglycemia or sudden infant death syndrome (SIDS)

Clinical presentation

- *No symptoms*
- Irritability
- Jitteriness
- Tremor
- Hypotonia
- Seizures
- Apnea, irregular respiration, tachypnea
- Lethargy
- Poor feeding (which may improve with initial feeding and rise in blood glucose)
- High-pitched cry
- Temperature instability

Differential diagnosis

- Related to symptoms:
  - Other metabolic disorders
  - Sepsis
  - Primary neurological disorder (e.g., bleeding, malformation)
- A comprehensive list of differential diagnoses is given below

Differential diagnosis of transient, recurring or persistent hypoglycemia[65,66]

If high glucose supply (GIR >6–7 mg/kg/min) is required to maintain normoglycemia, it is not transient hypoglycemia, and further investigation is warranted.

Hyperinsulinemic hypoglycemia

Transient hypoglycemia

- Days: infant of mother with diabetes mellitus
- Weeks: birth asphyxia or other perinatal insult, or SGA neonate

Persistent hypoglycemia

- ATP-sensitive potassium (K_{ATP}) channel defects
- Glucokinase-activating mutations
- Glutamate dehydrogenase-activating mutation
- Undefined
  - Autosomal dominant
  - Autosomal recessive
- Congenital disorders of glycosylation (CDGs)
  - CDG-Ia
  - CDG-Ib (phosphomannose isomerase deficiency)
  - CDG-Id
- Short-chain L-3-hydroxyacyl-CoA dehydrogenase mutation
  - β-cell adenoma: multiple endocrine neoplasia type I
  - Beckwith–Wiedemann syndrome
  - Insulin administration (Münchausen by proxy)
  - Oral sulfonylurea drugs

Hormone deficit

Congenital hypopituitarism

- Aplasia of the anterior pituitary

Primary hormone deficiency

- Isolated growth hormone deficiency
- Cortisol deficiency adrenocorticotropin hormone (ACTH) unresponsiveness
- Glucagon deficiency
- Congenital adrenal hyperplasia
- Adrenal hemorrhage

Congenital disorders of carbohydrate metabolism
- Glycogen storage diseases (glucose-6-phosphatase deficiency)
- Fructose intolerance
- Glycogen synthase deficiency
- Fructose-1,6-diphosphatase deficiency

Congenital disorders of amino acid metabolism
- Maple syrup disease
- Type I tyrosinemia
- Propionic acidemia
- Methylmalonic acidemia
- 3-Hydroxy-3-methylglutarate CoA lyase deficiency

Congenital disorders of fatty acid metabolism
- Acyl-CoA-dehydrogenase deficiency for medium-chain (MCT) and long-chain fatty acids
- Mitochondrial β-oxidation deficiency

Diagnosis/monitoring (see Figure 3.4)

> **!** Rapid bedside analyzers can only estimate blood glucose levels, so have at least one value tested by the core laboratory in the appropriate tube and within a reasonable time frame (30 min).

- Screening and monitoring of all neonates at risk (see WHO guidelines on pp. 260–2)
- Confirmation of low glucose levels with appropriate technique (i.e., testing in the core laboratory)
- Observation and documentation
- Draw critical sample
- Serum tube, red top: insulin, growth hormone, cortisol, glucose (STAT)
- Sodium fluoride tube, gray top: glucose
- Consult endocrinology early for evaluation and need for additional diagnostic testing
- Advanced diagnostics: serum amino acid analysis, serum long-chain fatty acids, urine organic acids, serum and urine ketones, e.g. β-hydroxybutyrate

Therapy in the delivery room/in the nursery/in the NICU (see Figure 3.4)
- In the symptomatic neonate do not wait for the laboratory results, but treat with IV infusion (see Table 3.3).
- Consider IV glucose bolus if indicated (see below)
- Proven hypoglycemia in neonates, i.e., blood glucose <40 mg/dl (2.2 mmol/l): give 2–5 ml/kg 10% glucose IV. During transport, double the maintenance dose, i.e., $D_{10}W$ 6 ml/kg/h ($= 10$ mg/kg/min IV)

Table 3.3 Infusion table for dextrose (D) continuous intravenous infusion

mg/kg/min	4		5		6		7		8	
g/kg/day	5.8		7.2		8.8		10		11.5	
Weight (kg)	D_5W (ml/h)	$D_{10}W$ (ml/h)	D_5W (ml/h)	$D_{10}W$ (ml/h)	D_5W (ml/h)	$D_{10}W$ (ml/h)	D_5W (ml/h)	$D_{10}W$ (ml/h)	D_5W (ml/h)	$D_{10}W$ (ml/h)
1	4.8	2.4	6	3	7.2	3.6	8.4	4.2	9.6	4.8
2	9.6	4.8	12	6	14.4	7.2	16.8	8.4	19.2	9.6
3	14.4	7.2	18	9	21.6	10.8	25.2	12.6	28.8	14.4
4	19.2	9.6	24	12	28.8	14.4	33.6	16.8	38.4	19.2

mg/kg/min	8		9				10			
g/kg/day	11.5		13				14.5			
Weight (kg)	$D_{20}W$ (ml/h)	$D_{40}W$ (ml/h)	D_5W (ml/h)	$D_{10}W$ (ml/h)	$D_{20}W$ (ml/h)	$D_{40}W$ (ml/h)	D_5W (ml/h)	$D_{10}W$ (ml/h)	$D_{20}W$ (ml/h)	$D_{40}W$ (ml/h)
1	2.4	1.2	10.8	5.4	2.7	1.4	12	6	3	1.5
2	4.8	2.4	21.6	10.8	5.4	2.7	24	12	6	3
3	7.2	3.6	32.4	16.2	8.1	4.1	36	18	9	4.5
4	9.6	4.8	43.2	21.6	10.8	5.4	48	24	12	6

Supply per kg and minute (mg/kg/min; GIR = glucose infusion rate) and day (g/kg/day; for calorie count). Dextrose concentration in percent (%; mg/dl). D_5W, dextrose 5%; $D_{10}W$, dextrose 10%; $D_{20}W$, dextrose 20%; $D_{40}W$ dextrose 40%. Rate of continuous infusion according to weight (kg birthweight), provided in ml/h.

- In the NICU: continuous infusion according to the flow sheet/infusion table (see Figure 3.4 and Table 3.3). Consider hydrocortisone 2.5 mg/kg/dose PO/IV q 6 h ($\approx$50 mg/m$_2$/day $\div$ q 6 h) if glucose >12 mg/kg/min needed *and* no hyperinsulinism
- Further *medical treatment for infants with hyperinsulinism* is usually initiated at a specialized center (pediatric endocrinology). Main drugs include:
  - *glucacon* (acts by releasing hepatic glycogen stores; emergency drug),
  - *diazoxide* (opens potassium channels in the beta cells and prevents both depolarization and subsequent insulin release): mainly used in congenital hyperinsulinemic hypoglycemia = persistent hyperinsulinemic hypoglycemia of infancy), 8–10 mg/kg/day PO divided q8 h initially; titrate to effect, or
  - *octreotide* (inhibits calcium channels in the beta cells and inhibits insulin release)[67]

! The maximum concentration of IV dextrose that can be administered peripherally is 12.5%.

Outcome
The effect of neonatal hypoglycemia on neurodevelopmental outcomes remains unclear[68]. Low glucose levels for more than 24 h or multiple episodes over a period of days are more likely to be associated with poor outcome.

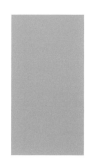

Meconium aspiration

Georg Hansmann

> **!** The ABCD rule especially applies to neonates with meconium-stained amniotic fluid (MSAF) and possible depression (i.e., bradycardia, cyanosis, apnea/inadequate breathing).
> **!** Clear the **AIRWAY** rapidly! (see "Suctioning the newborn", p. 66). See Figure 3.5, Table 3.4.

A prospective study, where the indication for cesarean section was frequently made because of postmaturity (prolonged pregnancy) or suspected asphyxia, showed no significant difference between 1-min and 5-min Apgar scores for neonates who were born through either clear or meconium-stained amniotic fluid (MSAF)[69]. Only a few neonates with MSAF seem to develop meconium aspiration syndrome (MAS) under these measures.

Meconium aspiration syndrome (MAS)

Definition

Aspiration of meconium-stained fluid has occured in a then severely depressed, unstable neonate. Laryngoscopy reveals viscous, MSAF/thick mucus behind the vocal cords (i.e., in the trachea).

Epidemiology

Incidence is about 7/1000 (up to 16/1000) live births. Approx. 5% of newborn infants with MSAF develop MAS[70].

Etiology/pathophysiology

The intrauterine passage of meconium rarely occurs before 37 weeks of gestation, but often after the 42nd week of gestation (30%–35%). Meconium passage is often an intrauterine reaction to stress caused by hypoxia (e.g., cord compression in oligohydramnios), acidemia or infection (amniotic infection syndrome, often in premature rupture of the membranes, PROM). Meconium aspiration can happen before or after birth. The worse the 1-min Apgar score, the more likely it is that aspiration has occurred in utero. In preterm infants, MSAF is associated with higher mortality and morbidity and is therefore very concerning[70].

Risk factors for respiratory distress syndrome in neonates with MSAF

- Oligohydramnios
- Pathological cardiotocogram (CTG; fetal heart rate monitoring) indicating fetal hypoxia

---

Neonatal Emergencies: A Practical Guide for Resuscitation, Transport and Critical Care, ed. Georg Hansmann.
Published by Cambridge University Press. © Cambridge University Press 2009.

Management of infants born out of meconium-stained amniotic fluid

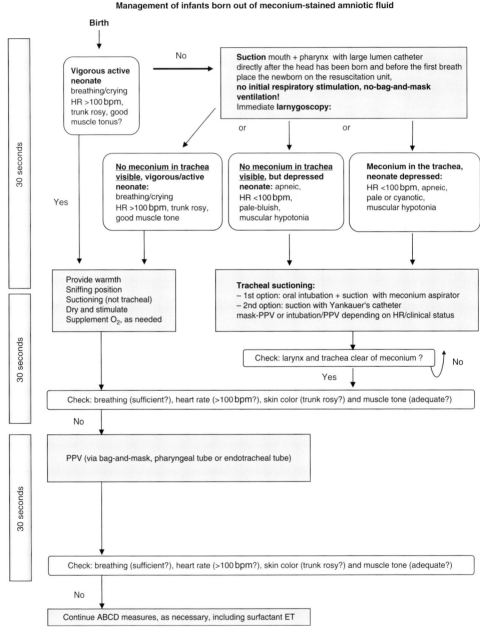

Figure 3.5 Algorithm for the initial management of an infant born out of meconium-stained amniotic fluid (MSAF). Amniotic fluid and/or the newborn's skin are noted to be meconium stained perinatally. Of note, ILCOR (*Resuscitation* 2005; 67:293–303) and the American Academy of Pediatrics (AAP) no longer recommend intrapartal suctioning of newborns with MSAF. This change in the guidelines was based on a single randomized controlled trial primarily conducted in Argentina (with "retrospective consent") that did not show any outcome difference between the "suctioned" and "non-suctioned" group (i.e., MAS rate and neonatal mortality similar; Vain *et al. Lancet* 2004; 364:597–602). However, previous consensus statements requested proven superiority of a new approach in order to change the resuscitation guidelines accordingly (see Resair 2 study and the discussion on room air vs. 100% oxygen). Thus, most of the authors of this handbook and many neonatologists, particularly in Europe but also in Northamerica, still advocate the continuation of (harmless and easy to perform) intrapartal suctioning in cases of MSAF until further evidence becomes available.

Table 3.4 Management of meconium-stained amniotic fluid (CMSAF), meconium aspiration, and meconium aspiration syndrome (MAS)

	Green, slightly viscous amniotic fluid (MSAF), NG vigorous/active	Meconium aspiration (mostly viscous, green amniotic fluid)	Meconium aspiration syndrome (MAS)
Incidence:	• About 13% of all live births • 30%–50% of all postmature newborn infants (>42 weeks of gestation p.m.)	• Likely <5% of all live births • Approx. 25%–30% of all term infants with MSAF	• About 5% of term infants with MSAF • Approx. 7/1000 (~16/1000) of live births in the USA
Definition/ clinical presentation	• Laryngoscopy: no AF/MEC visible in trachea • Newborn vigorous/active, i.e. HR > 100 bpm, RR 40–60 breaths'/min, good muscle tone, and spontaneous movements	• Laryngoscopy: green AF/MEC visible in trachea • Neonate moderately depressed; (still) cardiopulmonary: stable; 1-min Apgar >3 (mostly >6)	• Laryngoscopy: thick, green AF/MEC visible in trachea • Neonate is evidently depressed; cardiopulmonary: unstable; 1-min Apgar ≪7, hypotonic muscle tone, hardly any spontaneous movements.
Procedures in the delivery room	• Before the first breath of the infant, thorough oropharyngeal suctioning! (Suction catheter: Yankauer's or F 18=Ch 18) • Laryngoscopy: no amniotic fluid/MEC visible in trachea • Supplement O_2 • Nasal and gastric suctioning of amniotic fluid! • Continue O_2 supplementation • Stimulation • No intubation • Standard monitoring in the delivery room (pulse oximeter, ABG, blood glucose)	• Before the first breath of the infant, thorough oropharyngeal suctioning (as soon as the head is born)! (Suction catheter: Yankauer's or F 18=Ch 18) • Early cord clamping, place the neonate on the resuscitation table, head facing MD/NP • Supplement O_2 (6–10 l/min) • No initial bag-and-mask ventilation, no inflation, no stimulation • Rapid and brief oro/hypopharyngeal suctioning to improve visualization of vocal cords • Immediate laryngoscopy: "green" AF/MEC visible in trachea • Immediate tracheal suctioning: • Oral intubation and tracheal suctioning with MEC/ET tube adapter ("MEC aspirator") then increase suction (negative pressure) or	• Before the first breath of the infant, thorough oropharyngeal suctioning (as soon as the head is born)! (Suction catheter: Yankauer's or F 18=Ch 18) • Early cord clamping, place the neonate on the resuscitation table • Supplement O_2 (6–10 l/min) • No initial bag-and-mask ventilation, no inflation, no stimulation • Rapid and brief oro/hypopharyngeal suctioning to improve visualization of vocal cords • Immediate laryngoscopy: thick-green AF/MEC visible in trachea or no MEC visible but severely depressed neonate • Immediate tracheal suctioning: • Oral intubation and tracheal suctioning with ET tube adapter ("MEC aspirator," then increase suction or

Table 3.4 (cont.)

Green, slightly viscous amniotic fluid (MSAF), NG vigorous/active

- Tracheal suctioning with Yankauer's catheter (caution: vocal cords!) and often subsequent (nasal or oral) intubation
- In case of intubation and tracheal suctioning: extubation under suctioning (depending on the general condition)
- O_2 supplementation
- Further ABCD measures, as needed
- Nasal and gastric suctioning of amniotic fluid
- O_2 supplementation
- When airways clear—stimulate breathing
- Usually intubation and PPV are not necessary
- Place gastric tube (feeding tube) and leave open to gravity
- Transfer to NICU

Meconium aspiration (mostly viscous, green amniotic fluid)

- Tracheal suctioning with Yankauer's catheter (caution: vocal cords!) and subsequent intubation
- If oral intubation was performed for tracheal suctioning: assess whether neonate is stable enough for extubation under negative pressure/tracheal suctioning or re-intubation (i.e., from oral to nasal, if necessary in the NICU)
- If possible, suctioning ET tube ≠ ventilation tube
- Intubation and PPV are necessary in MAS
- Mechanical ventilation: high F_iO_2 and high rate rather than high PIP
- In term infants, $T_{exp} \gg 0.5$ s
- Further ABCD measures

Meconium aspiration syndrome (MAS)

- Nasal and gastric suctioning of AF
- Place gastric tube and leave it open to gravity! As needed, suction gastric fluid
- Analgesia/sedation and relaxation if ventilator settings high, as indicated
- If general condition remains poor: consider conventional application of surfactant in the delivery room (ET tube position?)

  Caution: pneumothorax
- If in critical condition or before long transport: blood culture and antibiotics IV
- Transfer to NICU

NICU:
- Monitoring
- Closely monitor blood glucose and ABG

Procedures in the neonatal unit

Usual standard monitoring in the nursery (pulse oximeter, capillary or arterial blood gas analysis, blood glucose).

NICU:
- Monitoring

	• Closely monitor blood glucose and blood gas analysis (ABG) • Chest X-ray, laboratory work-up, blood culture intubation and mechanical ventilation, as indicated • Surfactant administration, as needed (then readjustment of F_iO_2, PIP, and PEEP; prepare for chest tube placement) • Antibiotics IV (triple therapy), see pp. 299–301		• Chest X-ray, laboratory work up, BC • Optimize (SIMV or PRVC) ventilation. • Caution: high spontaneous respiratory rate entails short T_E, air trapping and higher risk for pneumothorax! • Analgesia and sedation, as indicated • Muscle relaxant, as indicated (case-by-case basis), more on p. 277
Complications:	• Infection (chorionamnionitis?) • Meconium aspiration, MAS	• Infection (chorionamnionitis?) • Developing MAS, see MAS complications • Higher risk for HIE (cerebral palsy, seizures) and RDS	• Overexpansion of lungs • Pneumothorax (25%) • Pneumomediastinum • Bacterial sepsis (almost always a chemical pneumonitis and secondary bacterial pneumonia) • Secondary surfactant deficiency • PPHN (50%–66% of neonates with PPHN had MSAF)
Outcome:	• 25%–30% of the neonates with MSAF are depressed at birth (meconium aspiration?) and require extended ABCD measures in the delivery room • 5% of those with MSAF develop RDS with or without MAS	• See MSAF • Highest risk for developing MAS for neonates with postnatal depression and for those with very viscous MEC/AF	• Mortality: 3%–12%; in MAS + PPHN up to 80% • High lethality also in preterm infants with MAS (MEC in AF indicates hypoxia!) • MAS is the most common indication for ECMO in respiratory failure

ABG, arterial blood gas; AF, amniotic fluid; BC blood culture; ET, endotracheal; HIE, hypoxic ischemic encephalopathy; HR, heart rate; MA, meconium aspiration; MAS, meconium aspiration syndrome; MEC, Meconium; MSAF, meconium-stained amniotic fluid; NICU, neonatal intensive care unit; PEEP, positive end-expiratory pressure; PIP, peak inspiratory pressure; PPHN, persistent pulmonary hypertension of the newborn; PPV, positive pressure ventilation; PRVC, pressure-regulated volume control; RDS, respiratory distress syndrome; RR, respiratory rate; SIMV, synchronous intermittent mandatory ventilation; T_{exp}, expiration time.

- No intrapartal, oropharyngeal suctioning
- Extremely viscous, MSAF
- Meconium visible behind the vocal cords in laryngoscopy (i.e., Meconium aspiration or MAS)
- 1-min and 5-min Apgar score <7
- Plus several tentative risk factors[70]

Clinical presentation
Usually term or post-term, severely depressed infant, with cardiopulmonary instability/ shock, hypotonic muscle tone and hardly any spontaneous movements. A 1-min Apgar score <7, often <4.

DDx.
The diagnosis of MSAF is often clear if the skin is stained brownish-green; viscous secretion found in the trachea is then almost always meconium. Regardless of the kind of thickened fluid (meconium, other mucous, or blood), the procedure remains the same ($\rightarrow$ tracheal suctioning!).

! If the neonate is depressed and stained with meconium (skin), but no endotracheal meconium is seen by laryngoscopy, then tracheal suctioning should still be performed, because MAS is the most likely diagnosis.

Further differential diagnoses include moderately depressed neonates with MSAF but without aspiration, who suffer from chorioamnionitis (syn. amniotic infection syndrome) and develop pneumonia/sepsis/RDS (see p. 280), or those who are s/p umbilical cord compression (or the like).

Diagnosis in the delivery room
- Pulse oximeters (S_pO_2, HR) – attached both to the right hand/wrist and one leg (monitor for PPHN)
- Arterial blood gas (ABG, pre- and postductal, as indicated)
- Blood glucose (dextrostix, later sodium fluoride/gray top tube)
- Pulse status (all four extremities, start with right arm and right leg)
- Blood pressure (all four extremities, start with right arm and right leg)
- Blood sampling, as necessary (blood cultures, CBC, CRP, IL-6, etc.)

Treatment of a neonate with MAS in the delivery room
- *Prior to the first breath, thorough oropharyngeal intrapartal suctioning at the perineum* (large suction catheter: Yankauer's or 18 F = Ch 18 suction catheter). This is primarily the duty of the obstetrician. Of note, ILCOR and AAP no longer recommend such intrapartal suctioning[71,72]: The ILCOR guidelines 2005 were changed on the basis of a single randomized controlled trial (RCT) primarily conducted in Argentina (with retrospective consent) that did not show any outcome differences between the "suctioned" and "non-suctioned" group (i.e., MAS rate, neonatal mortality)[73]. This change was somewhat surprising because previous consensus statements requested

proven superiority of a new approach in order to change the resuscitation guidelines accordingly (see Resair 2 study[74] and the discussion on room air vs. 100% oxygen). Thus, most of the authors of this handbook, and many neonatologists – particularily in Europe but also in North America – still advocate the continuation of (harmless and easy to perform) intrapartal suctionioning in cases of MSAF until further evidence becomes available

- *Early cord clamping.* The neonate is then placed on the resuscitation table, the head facing the MD/NP in the "sniffing position." Provide O_2 supplementation (6–10 l/min)
- *No initial bag-and-mask ventilation, no inflation, no stimulation of respiration!*
- *Rapid and brief oro-/hypopharyngeal suctioning to improve visualization of vocal cords*
- *Immediate laryngoscopy:* when thick-green amniotic fluid/meconium is visible in the trachea and/or the neonate is depressed: immediate tracheal suctioning – there are two options:
  - Oral intubation and tracheal suctioning (3–5 s while the tube is withdrawn) via an ET tube adapter (then increase the suction; this is the recommended approach), *or*
  - Tracheal suctioning with Yankauer's catheter (caution: vocal cords) and frequently subsequent (oral and nasal) intubation (second choice, if no adapter available)
  - **If no MEC is suctioned from the trachea** → do not carry out further tracheal suctioning, but continue ABCD measures! Consider subsequent (oral and nasal) intubation if breathing is insufficient
  - **If MEC is suctioned from the trachea** → check HR: if HR >80 bpm (>100 bpm) and not dropping, repeat tracheal suctioning via ET tube or Yankauer's catheter
- When the neonate has been orally intubated for tracheal suctioning: assess whether the newborn is stable enough for suctioning and extubation, then repeat intubation/ tracheal suctioning, as indicated. If a nasal ET tube is preferred for mechanical ventilation, evaluate whether the newborn is stable enough for re-intubation (nasal instead of oral, use new tube)
- Significant bradycardia/hypoxemia during or after the first tracheal suctioning: switch to PPV (if necessary, short bag-and-mask ventilation, then rapid intubation). If possible ET tube for suction ≠ ET tube for ventilation (i.e., aim to re-intubate after having suctioned meconium)
- If the general condition has notably improved and the blood gas is acceptable, mechanical ventilation should be avoided by all means. Always chest X-ray in the NICU

! In meconium aspiration syndrome (MAS) intubation is usually required: for mechanical synchronized-assisted ventilation, accept higher F_iO_2 and choose high respiratory rate rather than a high PIP. To prevent air trapping, choose the longest expiration time (T_{exp}) possible, i.e., in term infants $T_{exp} \gg 0.5$ s, and check at the ventilator whether flow comes to baseline at the end of expiration.

- Further ABCD measures, as required
- In arterial hypotension, give 10 (−20) ml/kg volume bolus (NaCl 0.9% or PRBC)
- Nasal and gastric suctioning of amniotic fluid
- Place a gastric tube and leave it open. Gastric suctioning of amniotic fluid, as needed

- An agitated child with an adequate BP should have analgesia/sedation. Muscle relaxation may be indicated for poor lung compliance and very high PIP. These measures are to be taken on a case-by-case basis, since they are not without risk (see Procedure/therapy in the NICU)
- If the general condition remains poor and ventilator settings are high:
  - Consider (repeat) conventional surfactant administration in the delivery room (clarify ET tube position by chest X-ray, be prepared for possible pneumothorax, and adjust PIP)
  - There is currently insufficient evidence to recommend bronchoalveolar lavage with normal saline[70,75] or surfactant[75,76] in the delivery room
- If the general condition is poor or the infant faces a longer transport: administer two antibiotic drugs IV (get blood cultures, then give first dose; see p. X.)
- Foresee complications (e.g., pneumothorax, arterial hypotension, septic shock)

> ❗ Transfer the neonate carefully to the NICU. Administer $D_{10}W$ 3 ml/kg/h IV. Use D_5W during the transport of term/preterm infants with high–normal or elevated blood glucose levels (e.g., after resuscitation/administration of adrenalin).

Monitoring

- *In the delivery room and during transport:*
  - Pre- and postductal S_pO_2 and BP measurement
  - ECG monitoring
- In the NICU:
  - Standard intensive care monitoring
  - Pre- and postductal S_pO_2 and BP measurement
  - $tcPO_2$, $tcPCO_2$ probe
  - Closely monitor ABG, Hct, blood glucose and lactate

> ❗ Measure S_pO_2, ABG (e.g., right arm and UAC) and BP pre- and postductally (right arm/leg) in order to identify significant right-to-left shunt via the ductus arteriosus. If right-to-left shunting is primarily through the patent foramen ovale, then systemic S_aO_2 is low, but there may be no significant difference in S_pO_2 between the right upper and lower extremities. Do not hesitate to perform an echocardiogram.

Diagnosis in the NICU

- Chest X-ray (relatively dense, patchy-nodular, often symmetrical pulmonary consolidations, emphysema with flat diaphragm, or even pneumothorax/pleural effusions)
- Complete microbiological diagnostics:
  - Smears
  - Tracheal secretions
  - Gastric fluid
  - Always obtain blood cultures before administering antibiotics

- ABG, lactate, blood glucose, laboratory work-up including CRP/IL-6, HIV/hepatitis serology, type and screen (cross-matching), electrolytes, creatinine/BUN, coagulation panel
- Ask for maternal HBsAg status and blood type
- Echocardiography when PPHN or poor ventricular function is suspected (see p. 392)
- Head ultrasound

Procedure/therapy in the NICU

- *Supportive therapy:*
  - Minimal handling!
  - Analgesia and sedation for an agitated neonate. Consider muscle relaxation if ventilatory settings are very high. These measures must be taken *on a case-by-case basis*: on the one hand, the respiratory situation may improve (better oxygenation and ventilation → lower PVR and, theoretically, larger ductal left-to-right shunt); on the other hand, particularly in the presence of a borderline BP, systemic vascular resistance (SVR) can drop significantly and may even increase the right-to-left shunt (→ cyanosis, PPHN)
  - Analgesia and sedation: administer morphine 0.1 mg/kg/dose IV q 1–2 h PRN or 0.02–0.05 mg/kg/h. Other non-analgetic option: lorazepam 0.1 mg/kg/dose IV q 6 h PRN; or fentanyl (1–5 µg/kg/min)/midazolam (0.1 mg/kg/h) continuous IV

> **!** Midazolam 0.05–0.2 mg/kg/h IV is often used in NICUs, even though it is not approved for neonatal use. Moreover, a current Cochrane analysis does not recommend midazolam as first-line drug for the sedation of preterm/term infants in the NICU[75].

  - If a muscle relaxant is indicated, use *pancuronium* 0.1 mg/kg/dose IV, then continuously 0.05–0.1 mg/kg/h or 0.1 mg/kg/dose q 1–2 h PRN (adjust the dosage and always watch for adequate analgesia and sedation). Other options: *cis-atracurium* 0.1–0.2 mg/kg/dose IV q 1–2 h PRN (advantages in hepatic/renal insufficiency) or *rocuronium* 0.6–1 mg/kg/dose IV (or 0.6–0.9 mg/kg/h IV)
  - Central venous line/UVC and arterial line (radial artery, UAC)
  - Empiric antibiotic treatment: consider triple combination for severe sepsis (e.g., ampicillin/gentamicin/cefotaxime or meropenem/vancomycin; see pp. 299–301)
  - IV fluids: 80 (–100) ml/kg/day, start with $D_{10}W$
  - Later: chest physiotherapy
- *Respiration/ventilator settings:*
  - Optimize SIMV or PCVR ventilation (see Table 2.10). Caution: high spontaneous respiratory rate means short T_{exp}, air trapping, and increased risk of pneumothorax (if indicated, analgesia and sedation, e.g., morphine IV, see above)
  - In a poor respiratory condition: switch to HFOV (see Table 2.12)
- *Bronchoalveolar lavage/surfactant lavage ("experimental"):* "experimental" surfactant lavage (lucinactant = Surfaxin[®75]):
  - Lavage 1: every side position 20 mg/kg lucinactant (2.5 mg/ml)
  - Lavage 2: every side position 20 mg/kg lucinactant (2.5 mg/ml)
  - Lavage 3: every side position 80 mg/kg lucinactant (higher concentration: 10 mg/ml)

- Safety and efficacy of surfactant lavage in neonates with MAS as mentioned above remain unclear[76], and should be conducted in randomized multicenter trials only
- Lavage with normal saline is no longer recommended, because (1) endogenous surfactant is washed out and (2) the clinical result may be "wet lung"[75]

- *Surfactant replacement therapy*
  - Often required in newborns with MAS[78]
  - Give surfactant 100–200 mg/kg/dose ET (as indicated, fractioned; repeat, if necessary), then adjust F_iO_2, respiratory rate, PIP and PEEP. Be prepared to insert a chest tube in case of pneumothorax
  - Surfactant replacement therapy, if started within 6 h after birth, improves oxygenation and reduces the incidence of air leaks, severity of pulmonary morbidity, and hospitalization time of term infants with MAS[78]
  - In infants with MAS, conventional surfactant administration may reduce the severity of respiratory illness (i.e., RDS) and decrease the number of infants with progressive respiratory failure requiring support with extracorporeal membrane oxygenation. The relative efficacy of surfactant therapy compared to, or in conjunction with, other approaches to treatment, including inhaled nitric oxide, liquid ventilation, surfactant lavage and high-frequency ventilation, remains to be tested (Cochrane meta-analysis, 2007)[79]
- *Pulmonary vasodilatation (see, "Persistent pulmonary hypertension of the newborn (PPHN)", pp. 392–403)*
  - Optimize mechanical ventilation. Correct significant acidosis, if necessary with sodium bicarbonate or THAM. Goals are low–normal P_aCO_2 (35–40 mmHg), high P_aO_2 (>80 mmHg, if possible) and high–normal to mildly alkalotic pH (7.45–7.55) → pulmonary vasodilatation and PVR reduction! Balance the risk and benefits of hypoxia versus lung damage (i.e., is high PIP justified to achieve P_aO_2 goal?)
  - In respiratory failure/PPHN (see p. 392): consider *early NO inhalation* (start with 20 ppm). "It appears reasonable to use inhaled nitric oxide in an initial concentration of 20 ppm for term and near term infants with hypoxic respiratory failure who do not have a diaphragmatic hernia" (Cochrane meta-analysis, 2006)[80]. Whether infants have clear echocardiographic evidence of PPHN or not does not appear to affect outcome[80]
  - Other options for iNO-resistant PPHN (see p. 392): Prostanoids such as treprostinil (Remodulin®) or epoprostenol (Flolan®) IV; phosphodiesterase inhibitors such as sildenafil PO or IV
- *If applicable, extracorporal membrane oxygenation in an experienced center*

Neonatal criteria for extracorporeal membrane oxygenation (ECMO)[81]

General inclusion and exclusion criteria

- Gestational age >34 weeks or birth weight >2000 g (some include those >32 weeks or >1800 g)
- No significant coagulopathy or uncontrolled bleeding
- No major intracranial hemorrhage (>grade II)
- Reversible lung disease with length of mechanical ventilation <10–14 days

- No uncorrectable congenital heart disease (this underlies an ongoing debate; many centers use ECMO s/p non-correcting heart surgery, e.g., single ventricle repair)
- No lethal congenital anomalies (e.g., trisomy 13 or 18)
- No evidence of irreversible brain damage (e.g., severe hypoxic ischemic encephalopathy)

Respiratory entry critera[a]
- Alveolar–arterial oxygen gradient $(AaDO_2)^{b,c}$ >605–620 mmHg for 4–12 h
- Oxygenation index $(OI)^d$ >35–60 for 0.5–6 h
- P_aO_2 <35–60 mmHg for 2–12 h
- Acidosis and shock pH <7.25 for 2 h or with hypotension
- Acute deterioration of P_aO_2 to <30 to <40 mmHg

Neonatal ECMO criteria may slightly differ between large ECMO centers[81,82], and also depend on the underlying cause (e.g., pulmonary vs. cardiac)[83].

Prevention of MAS
Primary prevention is key (also avoiding PPHN; pp. 392–403):
- Detect and prevent prolonged pregnancy (>41 weeks)
- Avoid fetal hypoxia by a quick (then quite often operative) delivery
- Intrapartum suctioning of the oropharynx at the perineum is the primary duty of the obstetrician/midwife (after the head is born)! The neonatal team at the head of the resuscitation unit should organize who will perform laryngoscopy and suctioning of the thick meconium before the first breath. If the earliest timepoint for suctioning is missed, the neonate's risk of morbidity and death will rise significantly
- Of note, based on a single, limited muticenter trial that showed no outcome differences between intranatally and only postnatally suctioned newborns with MSAF (i.e., MAS rate, neonatal mortality[74]), AAP and ILCOR (2005) no longer recommend intrapartum suctioning in babies with MSAF[72,73]. Most of the authors of this handbook, and many neonatologists, particularly in Europe but also in North America still advocate continued effort to perform intrapartum, oropharyngeal suctioning of infants born through MSAF, until further evidence becomes available
- Newborn infants who were born through MSAF but are vigorous (i.e., crying, breathing, moving, HR >100 bpm.) do not require tracheal suctioning. However, meconium-stained newborn infants who are depressed need immediate laryngoscopy and intra-tracheal suctioning without delay (prior to the first breath)

MAS outcome
- See also Table 3.4
- Obvious improvement usually after 24–72 h, clinical recovery often within 7–10 days.
- Antenatal amnioinfusion with normal saline seems to improve neonatal outcome in countries where perinatal monitoring is limited[84]. In clinical settings with standard peripartum surveillance, the current literature does not support the use of amnioinfusion for MSAF[85]

---

[a] 50% of ECMO centers use more than one respiratory entry criterion.
[b] P_{atm} = 760 mmHg at sea level. F_iO_2 is 0.21–1.0 Normal $AaDO_2$ in room air is 5–20 mmHg
[c] $AaDO_2 = [(P_{atm} - 47) \times F_iO_2 - (P_aCO_2 \div 0.8)] - P_aO_2$
[d] $OI = $ (mean airway pressure $\times F_iO_2 \times 100):P_aO_2$

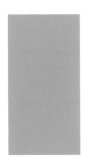

Chorioamnionitis and early-onset sepsis in the newborn infant

Georg Hansmann

Chorioamnionitis

Syndrome
Amniotic infection syndrome

Definition
Chorioamnionitis is defined as an inflammation of the fetal membranes; however, today the term is used to describe an intrauterine, bacterial infection, involving both maternal *and* fetal tissue (choriodecidual compartment, placenta) or exclusively fetal tissue (extra-embryonic membranes, amniotic fluid, umbilical cord).

Epidemiology
Approximately 1%–3% of all live births.

Etiology/pathophysiology
The pathogens identified in chorioamnionitis – at least in premature deliveries – are mostly of low virulence and of maternal (recto-) vaginal origin (*Ureaplasma urealyticum, Myco-plasma hominis, Fusobacterium* spp., *Streptococcus* spp.). Bacterial colonization of the uterus occurs before conception or during the pregnancy (ascending infection). Chorioamnionitis accounts to a great extent for premature births before 30 weeks of gestation, and also contributes to the generally high morbidity and mortality among premature infants: approximately 50% of the neurological long-term morbidity and 70% of the perinatal lethality among newborn infants are found in *preterm* infants[86].

Risk factors for chorioamnionitis
- Interval between rupture of membranes (ROM) and delivery $\geq$18 h (i.e., prolonged ROM)
- Maternal signs of infection before or after delivery:
  - CRP >2 mg/dl
  - WBC >17 000/μl
  - Body temperature $\geq$38.0°C ($\geq$100.4°F)
- Colonization with GBS/other germs in the rectum and urogenital tract
- Reduced function of the maternal or fetal immune system

Neonatal Emergencies: A Practical Guide for Resuscitation, Transport and Critical Care, ed. Georg Hansmann.
Published by Cambridge University Press. © Cambridge University Press 2009.

- Fetal tachycardia: HR >160–180 bpm
- Increased risk for infection in SGA infants (weight <10th percentile) and preterm infants

Maternal symptoms

Maternal symptoms are frequently absent. Relatively unspecific symptoms, such as fever, tachycardia, painful uterus, and foul-smelling amniotic fluid, may occur. WBC/absolute neutrophil count, immature-to-total neutrophil (I:T) ratio and CRP may be elevated.

Prenatal diagnosis

The definitive diagnosis is made by microbiological (positive bacterial culture from amniotic fluid or fetal membranes, umbilical cord or chorionic plate) or is suggested by biochemical (increased IL-6 or IL-8 in the amniotic fluid) tests. For prepartal, genital-rectal smears, see under "early-onset neonatal sepsis." Later on, a positive blood culture obtained from the newborn infant may point to the underlying pathogen.

Prenatal prophylaxis

See later under "Early-onset sepsis in the newborn infant (p. 282)."

Pathophysiology

The result of chorioamnionitis is a *fetal inflammatory response syndrome (FIRS)* which is characterized by bacteria and/or IL-6 in the fetal circulation, and associated with inflammation of the umbilical cord vessels.

Clinical presentation

Clinical sequelae of FIRS are[86]:

In preterm infants:

- Intrauterine growth retardation (IUGR → SGA infant)
- Increased acute neonatal morbidity and mortality (intraventricular hemorrhage (IVH), necrotizing enterocolitis, etc.). The risk for RDS is decreased in FIRS (infection may induce endogenous surfactant production/lung maturity)
- Neurological sequelae (periventricular leukomalacia, IVH, cerebral palsy, polymicrogyria; visual and cognitive sequelae) have not been proven to be associated with FIRS to date
- Chronic lung disease (CLD, bronchopulmonary dysplasia (BPD))
- Early thymic involution
- Development of neonatal sepsis (see p. 282.)

In term infants:

- Low Apgar scores
- Neonatal encephalopathy
- Cerebral palsy (mainly for a combination of chorioamnionitis and asphyxia),
- Neonatal sepsis (see p. 282)

Symptoms and further management

See also under "early-onset sepsis of the newborn infant. p. 282"

> **❗ Characteristics of bacterial infections in the neonatal period**
> - No specific symptoms at the beginning; signs and symptoms resemble systemic inflammatory response (SIRS).
> - There is often no obvious source or entry of the pathogen.
> - Infections often progress quickly to sepsis and septic shock.
> - A prolonged interval without antibiotic therapy increases the risk of shock, meningitis, and poor (neurological) outcome.
>
> **❗** If a baby who required resuscitation in the delivery room continues to be symptomatic (e.g., tachypneic), consider infection as a possible cause and the need for early antibiotic therapy, particularly in infants born preterm[87].

Early-onset sepsis in the newborn infant
Definition
- *Early-onset sepsis in the newborn infant:*
  - Clinical presentation on the 1st to 3rd (up to 7th) day of life
  - Preterm infants are often affected perinatally (the humoral defense system of preterm infants <32 weeks of gestation is remarkably reduced)[88]
  - Case fatality rates for GBS sepsis range from 3% to 5% in term infants but are higher in preterm infants[89]

Other definitions
- *Late-onset sepsis in the newborn infant:*
  - Clinical presentation on the (4th to) 8th to 28th day of life
  - Often occurs in initially healthy, term infants after being discharged from the nursery
  - Seen with Group B streptococci (GBS) and other pathogens. In late-onset and very-late-onset disease, the incubation period from GBS acquisition to disease is unknown. The incidence of GBS declines dramatically after 3 months of age, but up to 10% of pediatric cases occur beyond early infancy, and many but not all of these are infants who were born preterm[89]
- *Nosocomial sepsis in the newborn infant (i.e., acquired in the hospital):*
  - The pathogen derives from the patient's own flora or the germ spectrum of the hospital
  - Presentation between the 4th (−8th) day of life and the day of discharge from the hospital
  - Preterm infants in the NICU with inserted exogenous material (catheters, drains, VP shunts) are particularly affected
  - Often multiresistant pathogens (selection due to use of broad-spectrum antibiotics)
- *SIRS*
  - Systemic inflammatory reaction with cytokine release (especially IL-6, IL-8)
  - Caution: a cytokine burst may also be a stress reaction, e.g., due to prolonged delivery or problems during the initial care/resuscitation
- *Infection:* positive or negative smears/blood culture, elevated biochemical/hematological markers (CRP, IL-6, I:T ratio) and/or clinical signs of infection (so called infectious disease)

- *Bacteremia:* positive or negative smears, and positive blood culture. Positive biochemical/ hematological markers (CRP, IL-6, I:T ratio), and clinical signs of infection may or may not be present
- *Sepsis:* positive or negative smears, positive blood culture plus elevated biochemical/ hematological markers (CRP, IL-6, I:T ratio) plus clinical signs of infection. The term "clinical sepsis" may refer to a condition with significant clinical signs of infection but a lack of biochemical/hematological markers and no positive blood culture

Epidemiology

Incidence of sepsis (early-onset, late-onset, also nosocomial/acquired sepsis) is 1:1500 term infants and 1:250 preterm infants[88]. For details on the pathogens involved, see following text.

Etiology/pathophysiology

Pathogens that cause neonatal infections within the first 3 days of life usually have been acquired from the maternal genital tract or rectum. An infection that begins later is often acquired, either in the nursery from hospital personnel (nosocomial infection, e.g., hand contamination), or in the community from healthy colonized people[89]. In an ill-appearing neonate beyond the third day of life consider late-onset sepsis by GBS and other pathogens as underlying cause.

Clinical presentation

- *Initial symptoms in term/preterm infants often non-specific* (average onset 20 h after birth)
  - Tachypnea, apnea
  - Pale-gray skin color, mottled, cold extremities and prolonged capillary refill >2 s
  - Lethargy/muscular hypotonia/irritability
  - Hyper-/hypothermia
  - Poor feeding/gastric residuals/vomiting, dehydration
  - Distended abdomen/quiet or no bowel sounds
- *Additional clinical signs of infection:*
  - Heart rate >150 bpm
  - Respiratory rate >60 breaths/min
  - Temperature <36.5°C/97.7°F or >37.5°C/99.4°F, body temperature changes (fever not obligatory!)
  - Jaundice

! The clinical evaluation by an experienced NICU nurse should be taken seriously. A statement such as *"The baby does not look well today"* may be a clue to early-onset sepsis. *Do not "wait and watch!"* Neonatal infections, especially in preterm infants, rapidly progress to life-threatening septic shock.

- *Early-onset sepsis often progresses to multi-organ failure*:
  - Pneumonia/respiratory failure, septic shock with arterial hypotension and peripheral vasodilatation (in early stage: warm, well-perfused limbs), disseminated intravascular coagulation (DIC) with petechiae and bleeding, meningitis (in 30%), acute renal tubular necrosis, symmetrical peripheral gangrene[88]

- The course of early-onset GBS sepsis is very variable. In preterm infants RDS and pneumonia predominate, while GBS sepsis in term neonates is often associated with peripheral hypoperfusion and DIC. Septic shock and respiratory failure indicate a poor prognosis. Jaundice, hepatomegaly, petechial purpura and cerebral seizures are late symptoms

Complications

Bacterial meningitis (incidence 0.5/1000 live births and 1.4/1000 preterm infants; mortality approximately 10% in term infants and approximately 30% in preterm infants; mortality up to 50% in meningitis due to coliform bacteria). Meningitis is a common complication if diagnosis and treatment are delayed, and strongly associated with long-term neurological morbidity in survivors. Septic shock with DIC frequently is lethal.

Typical bacterial pathogens in early-onset neonatal sepsis (1st – 3rd – 7th day of life)

- *Group-B-streptococci (GBS, streptococci agalactiae, Gram-positive):*
  - 20%–30% of women of childbearing age are GBS positive (vaginal tract and rectum). This leads to a colonization of the newborn's skin and mucous membranes with GBS in 50% of the infants during birth
  - GBS sepsis (early onset in >90%) is mostly an intrapartum infection. Late-onset GBS sepsis (<10%) usually occurs after birth, may develop beyond the neonatal period, and is often associated with meningitis and neurological sequelae
  - Early GBS disease may present with respiratory distress, apnea, pneumonia, and, less commonly, meningitis. About 1% of the neonates with GBS infection develop fulminant sepsis in the first hours of life[90], frequently leading to neurological sequelae, septic shock, and death
  - Late-onset GBS disease also may present as meningitis, osteomyelitis, septic arthritis, and cellulitis
- *Escherichia coli* (Gram-negative)
- *Listeria monocytogenes* (Gram-positive, listeriosis = transplacental infection; disseminated infection → granulomatosis infantiseptica; not sensitive to cephalosporins)
- *Staphylococcus aureus* (Gram-positive, certain strains may be multiresistant)
- *Enterococcus* (Gram-positive, not sensitive to cephalosporins, frequently multiresistant)
- *Klebsiella* (Gram-negative)
- *Anaerobic bacteria* (mainly *Clostridium*, *Bacteroides*)
- *Other bacteria* may affect neonates with late-onset sepsis, older infants or those with nosocomial infections (e.g., *Staphylococcus epidermidis*, *Pseudomonas* spp.). The local germ spectrum (hospital guidelines) must be taken into consideration!

Pathogens of other sepsis-like infectious diseases (Table 3.5)

- Herpes simplex virus (HSV-2 ≫ HSV-1; intrapartum rather than ascending infections)
- Varicella zoster virus (VZV, caution when mother gets sick 5 days before or within 48 h after delivery)

- Cytomegalovirus (CMV)
- Enterovirus (four groups: coxsackie virus A and B, echovirus, poliovirus): shed from the upper respiratory and GI tract. Infections are typically perinatally acquired from the mother who is ill within a few days of delivery. Peak incidence between July and November. Clinical presentation varies from mild, unspecific febrile illness to life threatening disease (50% mengioencephalitis, 25% myocarditis, 25% sepsis-like syndrome with very high mortality). Note that enterovirus and rotavirus infections (diarrhea) can become epidemic in the NICU
- Other viruses such as RSV, HBV, rubella, etc.
- *Candida* spp. and other fungi
- *Toxoplasma gondii*, etc.

See also Table 3.5, Table 3.6, *Red Book* (American Academy of Pediatrics, 2006)[89], and other standard textbooks[2,91].

Risk factors for neonatal sepsis
- Interval between ROM and delivery $\geq 18\,h$[89]
- ROM before labor has started (=PROM)[92]
- Elevated maternal infection parameters before/during delivery:
  - CRP $>2\,mg/dl$
  - WBC $>17\,000/\mu l$
  - Body temperature $>38.0°C/100.4°F$[89]
- Colonization with GBS/other pathogens in the vaginal or rectal tract
- GBS bacteriuria during the pregnancy[89]
- Previous infant with invasive GBS infection[89]
- SGA infants (weight <10th percentile) and preterm infants (<37 weeks of gestation)[89]
- Reduced function of the maternal or fetal immune system
- Fetal tachycardia: HR $>160–180\,bpm$
- Status post birth asphyxia
- Neonatal co-morbidity (e.g., RDS)
- Steroid treatment of the newborn
- Intravenous lipid infusions

! Meconium-stained amniotic fluid only indicates an increased risk for infection when other risk factors, such as prolonged transition or tachypnea >6 h after birth, are present.

Prenatal diagnostics
Smears and cultures from the genital tract and rectum between the 35th and 37th weeks' gestation to determine GBS status → obstetrician can estimate the likelihood of GBS colonization at the date of delivery.

Table 3.5 Vertical infections of newborn infants (maternal–fetal transmission)

Infection	Symptoms	Measures before and after birth
Rubella (rubella virus)	Cataract, glaucoma, micro-ophthalmos, deafness, mental retardation, heart disease (PDA, PS, myocarditis), interstitial pneumonitis, hepatitis, hepatosplenomegaly, thrombocytopenia, rash (dermal erythropoiesis = "blueberry muffin" lesions)	• Isolation of the newborn, serology, IgM antibodies • No specific therapy available
Cytomegaly (CMV)	Approx. 10% symptomatic at birth: low birth weight, hepatosplenomegaly, thrombocytopenia, jaundice, microcephaly, sensorineural hearing loss, chorioretinitis. Some prenatally infected infants who appear healthy at birth are later found to have hearing loss or learning disability. In preterm infants, postnatal infection (horizontally, via breast milk or transfusions) with sepsis-like clinical presentation may occur	• Diagnostic tests: serology, qPCR (urine), urine culture • Head ultrasound, fundoscopy • Efficacy data on ganciclovir are pending; it may decrease progression of hearing impairment. Consider ganciclovir treatment if newborn has symptoms for more than 2 weeks (not evidence-based) • Although transmission of CMV through human milk has occurred, disease in neonates is uncommon, presumably because of passively transferred maternal anti-CMV IgG. VLBW infants, however, are at greater risk for symptomatic disease. Pasteurization seems to inactivate CMV but reduces the beneficial constituents of human milk; freezing at −20°C only decreases viral titers. If fresh donated milk is needed for infants born to CMV-antibody-negative mothers, providing these infants with milk from CMV-antibody-negative women only may be considered • In preterm infants <1500 g and positive maternal CMV status (IgG), it is controversial whether mother's breast milk should be pasteurized, or whether milk donated by CMV-negative mothers should be pasteurized
Enterovirus–four groups: • Coxsackie virus A • Coxsackie virus B • Echovirus • Poliovirus Coxsackie virus B and echovirus are the most common enteroviruses affecting newborns	Enteroviruses are shed from the upper respiratory and GI tracts. Infections are typically perinatally acquired from the mother, ill within a few days of delivery. Peak incidence between July and November. Clinical presentation varies from mild, unspecific febrile illness to life-threatening disease. Most common are mengioencephalitis (50%), myopericarditis (25%), and sepsis-like syndrome (25%) with very high mortality. Other manifestations include stomatitis, pneumonia, exanthema, paralysis, vomiting/diarrhea, hepatitis, and acute hemorrhagic conjunctivitis. Newborns who acquire infection without	• Diagnosis by PCR (CSF, blood, urine, stool) or culture (nose/throat, blood, urine, stool) • Treatment: if maternal infection is known, delay delivery by 1 week if possible. IgG IV for severe neonatal disease and chronic meningoencephalitis in immunodeficient patients may be used. Initial empiric antibiotic coverage for clinical signs of bacterial sepsis, later neomycin 25 mg/kg/dose q 6 h to suppress the intestinal flora. For experimental-specific therapy, see NIH trial (NCT00031512) on the use of pleconaril in enteroviral neonatal sepsis

maternal antibody are at highest risk for severe disease and death. Incubation period is 3–6 days, except for hemorrhagic conjunctivitis, in which the incubation period is 24–72 h

- Note that enterovirus and rotavirus infections (diarrhea) can become epidemic in the NICU
- Contact precautions (baby) for the duration of illness, and hand hygiene

Herpes simplex (HSV-2 > HSV-1)

Clinical signs occur in first 4 weeks of life. Herpes lesions localized to the eyes, skin, mouth (≈ 1/3). Meningoencephalitis (≈ 1/3). Disseminated disease involving multiple organs (≈ 1/3), with sepsis-like presentation and high mortality. In many neonates with disseminated or CNS disease, skin lesions do not develop or appear late in the course of infection

- Cesarean section with a genital herpes infection. Highest risk with primary infection of the mother (vs. reactivation).
- Isolation of the newborn
- Diagnostic tests: swabs for culture from mouth, nasopharynx, conjunctivae, rectum and specimen from skin vesicles, urine, stool, blood, and CSF (positive culture in first 48 h of life indicates neonatal infection). Direct fluorescent antibody staining of vesicle scrapings, ELISA for HSV antigen. CSF PCR
- Aciclovir 20 mg/kg/dose q 8 h IV × 14 or 21 days (disseminated or CNS disease) for all neonates with HSV infection. Add topical ophthalmic drug (e.g., 1% trifluridine) for (kerato) conjunctivitis
- Maternal HSV: breast feeding is acceptable if no lesions are present on the breasts and if active maternal lesions elsewhere are covered (gown). The mother with stomatitis or herpes labialis should wear a mask until lesions have crusted and dried

Hepatitis B (HBV)

Perinatal transmission rates: in HBs-Ag-positive mothers at least 10%; for acute hepatitis B during the 3rd trimester or positive evidence of HBe-Ag, up to 90%. Rate of premature delivery is increased. Infected newborns are often asymptomatic. In cases of apparent hepatitis → fever, vomiting, elevated LFTs and jaundice ("hepatitis A-like symptoms"). In approx. 1% fulminant hepatitis with high mortality (85%). Coinfection with HDV (caution: fulminant hepatitis), HCV or HIV possible. Incubation period varies (40–180 days). Jaundice appears in 10% of infants at the age of 3–5 months. Approx. 90% of infected neonates develop chronic hepatitis associated with hepatic cirrhosis and hepatocellular carcinoma during childhood

- Serology of all pregnant women: if mother is HBsAg-positive, give hepatitis B immunoglobulin (HBIG) and HBV vaccine to the newborn IM within the first 12 h of life; once vaccinated, breast feeding is possible
- If maternal HBsAg status is unknown → test mother immediately, initiate HBV vaccination of the newborn in the first 12 h of life. Give HBIG within 3 days (BW <2000 g) or 7 days (BW ≥2000 g) of life if (1) HBsAg status is still unknown, or (2) the mother tests positive for HBsAg
- In cases of maternal drug abuse, always initiate HBV vaccination of the newborn within the first 12 h of life and give HBIG, if indicated, in a timely fashion (as above)

Table 3.5 (cont.)

Infection

Hepatitis C (HCV)

Human immunodeficiency virus (HIV)

Symptoms

Vertical transmission rate in HCV-RNA-PCR positive mothers is approx. 5%. Infected newborns usually are asymptomatic. Incubation period varies (40–180 days). An apparent hepatitis may present as fever, vomiting, elevated LFTs and jaundice ("hepatitis A-like symptoms"). Coinfection with HBV or HIV is possible. Progression to chronic hepatitis is probably less common than in adults (<60%–80%), but associated with hepatic cirrhosis and hepatocellular carcinoma during childhood

Mostly asymptomatic after birth. Low birth weight possible. After years: AIDS

Measures before and after birth

- Perinatal medical prophylaxis is not available. Vaginal delivery
- Transient positive HCV-RNA-PCR may occur in non-infected neonates
- It is controversial whether a mother with negative HCV-RNA-PCR may breastfeed. According to current guidelines of the American Public Health Service, maternal HCV infection is not a contraindication to breastfeeding. HCV-positive, HIV-negative mothers should be counseled that HCV transmission by breastfeeding is theoretically possible but has not been documented (controversial topic)
- Treatment of chronic hepatitis C with α-interferon/peginterferon ± ribavirin should be referred to specialists ("experimental")

- Contact pediatric HIV center
- In rich countries, highly active antiretroviral therapy (HAART) has reduced the vertical transmission rates to around 1%–2%. In countries where HAART is not yet routinely available, shorter, less expensive antiretroviral regimens for reducing mother-to-child transmission should be considered, as there is good evidence that the benefits associated with such an intervention outweigh the potential risks. It is not entirely clear which regimen is best but a combination of zidovudine (ZDV=AZT) and lamivudine (3TC) given to mothers in the antenatal, intrapartum, and postpartum periods and to babies for a week after delivery, or a regimen involving a single dose of nevirapine (NVP) given to mothers in labor and babies immediately after birth seems to be effective and feasible. AZT monotherapy is also useful, especially if it includes a long antenatal treatment component
- Where HIV-infected women present late for delivery, post-exposure prophylaxis for the infant with a single dose of NVP immediately after birth plus ZDV for the first 6 weeks of life is beneficial (Cochrane meta-analysis, 2007)[373]

- One successfully prophylactic regimen for non-resistant HIV is as follows: At 32 0/7 weeks' GA, prepartal antiviral therapy for pregnant HIV-positive women. Virus isolation and resistance testing. C-section prior to labor (≈ 35–36 weeks of gestation). Antiviral chemoprophylaxis in the newborn should begin within 6–12 h of birth, e.g., zidovudine (ZDV=AZT) 1.3 mg/kg/dose q 6 h in 60 min IV for 10 days ("reduced Berlin regimen"),[374] or longer ZDV IV prophylaxis (e.g., for infants >35 weeks' GA: ZDV 1.5 mg/kg/dose q 6 h IV for 6 weeks[103]

- Many centers offer outpatient PO chemoprophylaxis for infants of HIV-positive mothers (e.g., for infants ≥35 weeks' GA: ZDV 2 mg/kg/dose q 6 h PO for 6 weeks)[103]

- Many centers now screen all pregnant women with a rapid HIV antibody test (ELISA, "right to refusal"). Routinely, positive results are confirmed by Western immunoblot. If there are concerns about acute infection in an adult (last 1–6 weeks, at most 6 months), send for HIV RNA PCR

- Infants born to HIV-infected women should be tested by HIV DNA PCR during the first 48 h of life (do not use umbilical cord blood for this), and PCR should be repeated at 2 (4–8) weeks and 2–6 months of life. If an infant tests positive, repeat HIV PCR immediately to confirm the results, and start treatment

- An antibody test (ELISA, Western blot) to document seroversion to HIV-antibody-negative status in uninfected infants is recommended at age 12–18 months

- If a high-risk mother with unknown HIV status gives birth, most centers recommend neonatal ZDV prophylaxis (even if maternal HIV antibody test is negative) until HIV PCR in the mother and newborn (first 48 h of life) comes back negative

- HIV-positive mothers must not breastfeed

Table 3.5 (cont.)

Infection	Symptoms	Measures before and after birth

Varicella (VZV)	Fulminant disease possible if the mother has onset of chickenpox 5 days before and up to 48 h after delivery	• qPCR on vesicular fluid or scab, direct fluorescent antibody
		• Post-exposure treatment for:
		  • Newborns whose mother had onset of chickenpox 5 days before and up to 48 h after delivery
		  • Hospitalized preterm infants ≥28 weeks' GA whose mother lacks reliable history of chickenpox or serological protection against chickenpox
		  • Hospitalized preterm infants <28 weeks' GA or ≤1000 g
		• Treatment with:
		  • IV immunoglobulin (VariZIG or IGIV) – not indicated if mother has zoster
		  • Antiviral therapy of the neonate: aciclovir 20 mg/kg/dose q 8 h IV × 8–10 days

Group B streptococci (GBS)	Often asymptomatic. Early stage: pneumonia, sepsis, shock. Late stage: meningitis (see main text)	• Pregnant women: smears at 35–37 weeks' GA, infection parameters and, if indicated, intrapartum antimicrobial prophylaxis (IAP) • Neonate: smears, blood culture, LP optional, CBC, CRP, if possible: IL-6 or IL-8, close monitoring (see algorithm, Figures 3.2 and 3.3). • Early antibiotic treatment of the newborn • See main text
Listeriosis (Listeria monocytogenes)	Early-onset: pneumonia, sepsis, shock. Late-onset: often with meningitis	• Isolation of pathogen/culture (meconium, gastric aspirate, blood, CSF). Gram stain • Treatment with ampicillin plus aminoglycoside IV × 14–21 days or longer. Cephalosporins are ineffective
Syphilis = lues (Treponema pallidum)	Maculopapular skin rash, desquamation, rhinitis, hepatosplenomegaly, periostitis, keratitis	• In the USA, non-treponemal tests (e.g., RPL, VDRL) are used for screening, and treponemal tests (e.g. IgM-FTA-ABS-test) establish the diagnosis. The VDRL test is non-reactive in Lyme disease but positive in syphilis. Some laboratories screen samples using treponemal enzyme immunoassay (EIA) tests • When suspected: IgM-FTA-ABS-test, HIV test, CBC, CRP, ESR, CSF-VDRL/FTA-ABS-test in mother and newborn • When suspected, administer penicillin G IV

Toxoplasmosis (*Toxoplasma gondii*)	Often asymptomatic. Low birth weight, chorioretinitis, intracerebral calcification, hydrocephalus. Generalized form of the disease is possible

- Prenatal: PCR (amniotic fluid, fetal blood), fetal ultrasound (hydrocephalus?). Test maternal serum for IgM: if positive → IgG avidity test. IgM persists for 6–9 (and up to 24) months
- Prepartal therapy of primary infection during pregnancy (controversial): spiramycin (investigational drug); if fetal infection confirmed after 17 weeks' GA or mother acquires infection in 3rd trimester, consider treatment with pyrimethamine/sulfadiazine
- Postnatal: test newborn for serum-specific IgM. WBC, CSF and amniotic fluid to be sent for PCR
- Head ultrasound
- Fundoscopy
- Treat neonate with pyrimethamine/sulfadiazine (often for 1 year)

Tuberculosis (*Mycobacteria*)	Often asymptomatic. Acute stage with pulmonary symptoms, hepatosplenomegaly, etc., but rarely with sepsis-like syndrome

- Placental histology
- Isoniazid (INH) therapy
- No breastfeeding

Table 3.5 compiled/modified from: Pickering LK (ed.) *et al. 2006 Red Book: Report on Infectious Diseases*, 27th edition. Elk Grove Village: American Academy of Pediatrics.
BW, body weight; CBC, complete blood count; CRP, C-reactive protein; CSF, cerebrospinal fluid; ELISA, enzyme-linked immunosorbent assay; ESR, erythrocyte sedimentation rate; GA, gestational age; GI, gastrointestinal; HIV, human immunodeficiency virus; IL, interleukin; LFTs, live function tests; PDA, patent ductus arteriosus; PS, pulmonary valve stenosis; qPCR, quantitative polymerase chain reaction.

Intrapartum antimicrobial prophylaxis (IAP) – indication

As of the time of writing this book, the results of controlled studies on the prophylaxis of neonatal infections do not allow general recommendations. However, for the prevention of neonatal invasive GBS infections, the AAP recommends intrapartum antimicrobial prophylaxis[89] for:

- Positive GBS screening culture from genital tract/rectum of the expectant mother
- Previous infant with invasive GBS disease
- Significant GBS bacteriuria during the current pregnancy
- Unknown GBS status and any of the following:
  - Impending premature delivery (<37 weeks of gestation)[a]
  - Interval between ROM and delivery ≥18 h[a]
  - Maternal fever >38.0°C/100.4 F[a]

> **!** [a]If chorioamnionitis is suspected, broad-spectrum antibiotic therapy that includes an agent known to be active against GBS should replace standard GBS intrapartum antimicrobial prophylaxis.

! Intrapartum antimicrobial prophylaxis (IAP) with any of the following agents[89]:

- Penicillin G, initially 5 million units IV, then 2.5 million units q 4 h IV until delivery, or
- Ampicillin, initially 2 g IV, then 1 g q 4 h IV until delivery
- Cefazoline, initially 2 g IV, then 1 g q 8 h IV, is recommended for women who are allergic to penicillin but at low risk for anaphylaxis, because it has a narrow spectrum of activity and reaches high amniotic fluid concentrations
- GBS resistance to erythromycin (15%–30%) and clindamycin (10%–20%) is common. Women at high risk of anaphylaxis with penicillin whose GBS isolates are clindamycin-susceptible can receive clindamycin 900 mg q 8 h IV until delivery
- Vancomycin 1 g q 12 h IV should be reserved for women at high risk of anaphylaxis for whom GBS isolate susceptibility has not been performed

Epidemiology (early-onset sepsis caused by typical pathogens)

After implementation of guidelines for GBS prevention (screening, IAP), the incidence of early-onset GBS infection dropped by 80% from a rate of 1.7/1000 live births in 1993 to 0.34/1000 live births in 2004. Although the decline was steepest in the mid 1990s, universal screening guidelines in 2002 led to a 33% further decline by 2004[93-94]. However, there are concerns that prepartum administration of ampicillin to pregnant women may lead to selection of drug-resistant gram-negative pathogens, particularly drug-resistant *Escherichia coli* strains[96,97]. *Escherichia coli* sepsis, formerly the second leading cause of early-onset sepsis, is now as common as invasive early-onset GBS disease. *E. coli* sepsis increased from 3.2/1000 (prior to the implementation of guidelines in 1993) to 6.8 cases/1000 live births in 1998–2000 and persisted in 2002–2003; 85% of those *E. coli* infections were ampicillin-resistant (data from the NICHD Neonatal Research Network, reviewed in[98]). Surveillance trends, however, are not sufficient to establish a relationship between GBS prophylaxis and *E. coli* sepsis risk. The NICHD network found that intrapartum antibiotic exposure was not associated with increased odds of non-GBS early-onset sepsis in multi-variable analysis[97].

Recent case series describing invasive early-onset sepsis caused by methicillin-resistant *Staphylococcus aureus* (MRSA) and a growing number of nosocomial MRSA outbreaks among neonates suggest this may be a new pathogen of concern. Other emerging neonatal pathogens include penicillin-resistant *Streptococcus pneumoniae* and coagulase-negative staphylococci[95]. One area requiring close monitoring is the impact of intrapartum vancomycin use because this agent is now recommended in limited circumstances for GBS prevention[95].

DDx.
- RDS of the preterm infant
- Systemic disease involving multiple organs with no response to antibacterial therapy:
  - Infections with virus, fungi, toxoplasmosis, etc.
  - Metabolic disorder
  - Genetic Syndrome
- Ileus of any etiology (p. 437)
- Congenital heart disease with left heart obstruction and duct-dependent systemic perfusion in a state of (pre-) shock (e.g., hypoplastic left heart syndrome, severe aortic valve stenosis, coarctation of the aorta or interrupted aortic arch, see p. 340)
- Tachycardic and bradycardic arrhythmia (e.g., complete heart block, p. 325).

Diagnostic work-up for suspected chorioamnionitis/ early-onset neonatal sepsis in the delivery room
- ABG, lactate, blood glucose, temperature, capillary refill >2 s (?), gray skin color (?)
- Early smears from ears, nose and pharynx are optional (limited). Placental smears (between fetal membranes), smears from umbilical cord vessels (after definitive cord clamping and cord cutting with sterile scissors)
- When risk factors (see p. 285) are present or clinical presentation indicates sepsis: obtain blood culture(s) (aerobic, also anaerobic), from peripheral venous/arterial stick, peripheral venous access (immediately after sterite placement) or UAC/UVC/PICC (when line infection is suspected, obtain two blood cultures from peripheral and central sites, less than 20 min apart, and label tubes accordingly
- Laboratory work-up includes CBC, CRP, IL-6/IL-8, coagulation panel, blood type and screen/cross match
- Request results from maternal, prepartum smears (preferred: cervix)

Procedure/therapy in the delivery room
- ABCD measures (Figure 3.1, p. 222)
- In cases of arterial hypotension and/or poor peripheral perfusion (weak pulse, capillary refill >2 s), administer normal saline 10 ml/kg IV, repeat bolus
- If severe metabolic acidoses persists despite fluid boluses, buffer therapy (guided by ABG and lactate) may be indicated (no colloidal solutions because of possible capillary leak!). Caution: sodium bicarbonate and THAM incompatible with many antibiotics; pp. 58–60)
- If clinical condition poor and strong suspicion of sepsis by perinatal history: after smears and cultures are obtained, slow IV push of two antibiotics (mostly ampicillin plus cefotaxime or ampicillin plus aminoglycoside, pp. 299–301) in the delivery room. Infuse $D_{10}W$ 3 ml/kg/h; use D_5W for infants with high–normal or elevated blood glucose levels

- Figure 3.6, p. 295 shows an algorithm for the management of a neonate s/p maternal intrapartum antibiotic treatment (e.g., penicillin G, ampicillin, cephazolin), to prevent early-onset GBS

Monitoring
S_pO_2 (pulse oximeter), BP, temperature, ET tube position (if intubated) and ECG (optional). If the child is stable → early transfer to the NICU. Check blood gas and glucose prior to departure.

Asymptomatic newborn infants who need close monitoring for ≥48 h, but no routine antibiotic treatment
- Neonates of mothers with unknown GBS status and the following risk factors:
  - Previous infant with invasive GBS infection
  - GBS bacteriuria during this pregnancy
  - Gestational age <37 0/7 weeks
  - Interval between the ROM and delivery ≥18 h
- Well-appearing neonates of GBS-positive mothers who were not treated with intrapartum antibiotics (penicillin, ampicillin, cefazolin) for ≥4 h
- Preterm infants of >32 weeks' gestation also do not need antibiotic treatment if they show no clinical signs of infection

> *!* Close clinical monitoring of newborn infants by RN/NP demands frequent documentation of vital signs (minimum q 4 h). When infection is suspected, a level II or III NICU should be contacted, and diagnostic work-up, antibiotic treatment, and transfer initiated urgently.

Diagnostic work-up in the nursery/NICU
- *Chest X-ray*
- *Complete microbiological diagnostics and diagnostic work-up:*
  - Aerobic (and also anaerobic) blood culture(s) before antibiotic therapy if not yet taken
  - Conjunctival smears when conjunctivitis is apparent
  - If the infant is ventilated: tracheal secretion, ear and nasal smear, gastric fluid, first meconium
  - If the infant is not ventilated: smears of pharynx, nose and ear, gastric fluid, first meconium
  - Urine stix test, urine microscopy, urine culture/cell differentiation (sterile catheterization or suprapubic puncture) when first symptoms occur >48–72 h after birth
  - It is controversial whether a lumbar puncture (LP) should be obtained in an ill-appearing infant who is less than 48 h old and has no neurological symptoms (i.e., no signs for meningitis). If obtained, send CSF for WBC/differential, glucose, protein, Gram stain and culture (consider PCR, e.g., HSV)
  - Further septic work-up includes: CBC with differential and platelets, IL-6 or IL-8, CRP, ABG, lactate, blood glucose, coagulation panel, specific IgM if suspicion

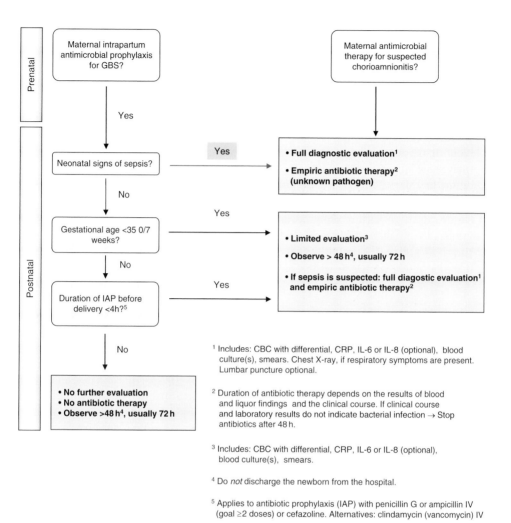

Figure 3.6 Algorithm for the empiric management of a newborn infant following intrapartum antimicrobial prophylaxis to prevent early-onset, invasive B streptococcal (GBS) disease. For intrapartum and postnatal antibiotic therapy see main text. Modified from: American Academy of Pediatrics (2006) Group B streptococcal infections. In: Pickering LK (ed.) *et al.* (2006) *Red Book: Report on Infectious Diseases*, 27th edn., Elk Grove Village: American Academy of Pediatrics.

high, bilirubin total/direct, AST/ALT, albumin, alkaline phosphatase, creatinine, BUN, electrolytes (>6 h after birth), blood type and screen, cross match, if indicated

- CRP increases 4–6 h after onset of inflammation, doubles every 8 h and peaks at about 36–50 h (rapid decline with resolution due to short half-life of 4–7 h). Hence, use serial CRP measurements to rule out infection[98]. For CRP, the false-positive rate is about 8% in healthy neonates. CRP is unreliable in neutropenia

- Combined use of CRP plus IL-6 or IL-8 (both IL with early onset, rapid peak and decline to normal values in approx. 6–8 h) as part of the work-up for bacterial infection reduces unnecessary antibiotic treatment. Current markers are not infallible, however, and do not permit neonatologists to withhold antibiotics in sick infants with suspected infection

- Head ultrasound, eventually head CT
- Ventricular tap for microscopy, Gram stain, and culture is indicated in patients with meningitis not responding to therapy

Pathological laboratory finding of an infant with suspected infection

- Blood: WBC >30 000/µl or <5000/µl, neutrophils <1500/µl, I:T quotient >0.2 (>20% immature granulocytes; gray zone 0.2–0.3), platelets <100 000/µl
- Blood: IL-6 >30 pg/ml (caution: short half-life, peaks at 6 h), IL-8 more than approx. 25 pg/ml (may show longer elevation, i.e., 18–24 h, when measured in lysed RBC), CRP >1 mg/dl on the first day of life, CRP >2 mg/dl plus clinical signs by the second day of life
- ABG with increasing base deficit and PCO_2 (unspecific)
- Serum: drop in serum phosphorus, pathological coagulation, and sudden glucose intolerance are all possible sepsis indicators
- Later: positive smear cultures (after early collection in the delivery room), positive maternal smear culture as well as positive blood cultures of the newborn infant

Lumbar puncture (LP) – indication?

A lumbar puncture is the ultimate diagnostic method for proving bacterial meningitis in the newborn[99]. However, there are no widely accepted recommendations for when LP is to be performed in preterm and term neonates[100], and the need for LP in the first 48 h of life is particularly controversial. In a single retrospective study in neonates and older children (1 day to 16 years), blood cultures were positive in three-quarters of children with meningitis without antibiotic pretreatment, and also positive in two-thirds of meningitis cases with negative CSF culture[101]. CSF cultures became rapidly negative (sterile) in meningococcal (by 0.25–2 h) and pneumococcal meningitis (by 4–10 h) after administration of ≥50 mg/kg of a third-generation cephalosporin, but remained positive in GBS-induced meningitis through the first 8 h after start of parenteral antibiotics[101].

We think the indication for lumbar puncture (LP) in a neonate is given in the following circumstances

- If neurological symptoms (consistent with meningitis) are present – regardless of the infant's age (may consider CNS imaging first if intracranial mass/bleed is likely and risk of herniation with LP would be high)
- If sepsis is suspected after 48 h of life (some centers perform LP regardless of age)
- If CRP is significantly increased (>2.0 mg/dl?) in the first 4 h (?) of life
- If clinical signs (hypotonia, hypotension) or laboratory results (glucose instability, leucopenia) indicate severe sepsis. However, these infants may be too unstable to undergo LP
- When a blood culture of a potential meningitis pathogen is positive (i.e., bacteremia)

! Postpone a lumbar puncture when the preterm/term infant is hemodynamically unstable. If so, antibiotic treatment must begin as soon as possible and prior to any LP. However, keep in mind that for up to 8 h after IV antibiotics are initiated, CSF cultures may still grow GBS, but most likely will be negative in meningitis caused by pneumococci or meningococci[101].

! The Red Book (2006, p. 625)[89] recommends: "if clinical signs in the infant suggest sepsis, full diagnostic evaluation should include LP, if feasible." Blood cultures can be sterile in 15%–38% of newborn infants with meningitis. If an LP has been deferred in a neonate receiving empiric antimicrobial therapy and therapy is continued beyond 48 h because of

---

clinical findings suggesting infection, *The Red Book* (2006)[89] recommends that CSF should be obtained for measurement of WBC/differential, glucose, and protein and for culture.

*For patients outside the neonatal period (29 days to 19 years), a large multicenter study has validated a *Bacterial Meningitis Score Prediction Rule* in the era of conjugate pneumococcal vaccine as an accurate decision support tool. In this study, the risk of bacterial meningitis was very low (0.1%) in patients with none of the criteria described[102].

Pathological CSF findings indicating bacterial meningitis

- Total protein >150 mg/dl (however, up to 170 mg/dl may be normal in preterm infants)
- WBC ≥10/µl (frequently ≫100/µl); usually more cells with Gram negative rods than with GBS. Pleocytosis (neutrophils early) may also be an irritant reaction to CNS hemorrhage
- Evidence of bacterial pathogens by Gram stain (immediate proof!)
- Bacteria are seen in the microscope even without Gram stain (immediate proof!)
- Ratio of CSF glucose/serum glucose often <0.4 in bacterial meningitis
- Rapid antigen tests are available for several pathogens and should be done on CSF
- Positive bacterial CSF culture (unlikely to be due to contamination)

Procedure/therapy in the newborn nursery/NICU

- *Supportive therapy*
  - Monitoring of vital signs, including temperature, $tcPO_2$, $tcPCO_2$
  - Minimal handling
  - Optimize ventilator settings
  - In arterial hypotension → volume expansion: 10–15 ml/kg IV is repeatedly administered (crystalloids and/or packed RBC). Colloidal solutions should not be used, since capillary leak is to be anticipated. When capillary leak is manifest: blood transfusion according to Hct level
  - In persistent arterial hypotension despite sufficient volume expansion: dopamine 2–20 µg/kg/min or norepinephrine 0.1–0.5(–2) µg/kg/min. Do not administer dobutamine alone! Consider a combination of noradrenaline and dopamine
  - Correct anemia, acidosis, and electrolyte and coagulation disorders

! Principles of antibacterial therapy (continued on p. 298)

- Always collect aerobic (and if possible, anaerobic) blood cultures in small, prewarmed bottles *before* the administration of antibiotics! Repeated blood cultures increases the likelihood of bacterial isolation, however neonatal blood volume and antibiotic treatment have to be considered as well
- Obtain blood culture under strictly sterile conditions to prevent iatrogenic contamination
- Indication for lumbar and suprapupic bladder puncture must be considered before initiating antibiotic treatment
- After maternal intrapartum antibiotic prophylaxis (IAP), most cultures of the neonate remain negative, even when the neonate is infected. Request the histology of the placenta, fetal membranes and umbilical cord, as well as the current pathogenic colonization of the mother (GBS smear?)

- IAP may be associated with selection of coagulase-negative *Staphylococci*, *Enterococci*, *Escherichia coli*, *Enterobacter* spp.
- Early antibiotic treatment in an ill-appearing infant with suspected sepsis is key for successful treatment and a beneficial outcome
- The use of appropriate antibiotics for the treatment of specific nosocomial pathogens is important. Remember when initiating antibiotic treatment that cephalosporins are not active against *Listeria* and *Enterococci*, and that Gram-negative pathogens are frequently resistant to ampicillin and its derivatives
- In general, permanent recommendations for certain bacteria and antibiotic combinations do not exist due to the change in colonization and resistance of bacteria. Hence, the choice of antibiotics, dosage, and intervals should be taken from standard textbooks for infectious diseases (e.g., *The Red Book*[89]) but adjusted to the local spectrum of pathogens ("local neonatal drug guidelines")

Initial antibiotic treatment of unknown pathogens during the first week of life (see also pp. 41–62)

Depending on the local spectrum of pathogens, a third-generation cephalosporin (i.e., cefotaxime) should be combined: (1) primarily with ampicillin or piperacillin, (2) together with an aminoglycoside plus ampicillin (ampicillin and piperacillin cover most *Enterococcus* and *Listeria*), or (3) in cases of a new (second) infection, together with piperacillin, instead of the initial combination of ampicillin plus aminoglycoside. Most centers still use the combination of ampicillin plus aminoglycoside (e.g., gentamicin) for the initial treatment of presumed neonatal sepsis in the first week of life. For very preterm infants, severely ill-appearing newborns (±signs of meningitis), and newborns older than 2–7 days, neonatologists may consider drugs with broader coverage and higher CNS penetration (e.g., cefotaxime) for initial treatment. If an infection with *S. epidermidis* or *S. aureus* is likely (e.g., central line, VP shunt, recent MRSA outbreak), vancomycin may be added to the antibiotic regimen. Do not use ceftriaxone in the first 2 months of life!

The updated official recommendations should be taken from most recent drug reference handbooks on pediatric infectious diseases (e.g., Neofax[103]; *Pediatric Dosage Handbook*[104]; *The Red Book*[89]).

Table 3.6 Dosing intervals for commonly used antibiotics (Neofax 2007[103])

Gestational age (weeks p.m.)	Postnatal age (days)	Interval 1	Interval 2	Interval 3	Interval 4	Interval 5
≤29 (or <1200 g)	0–28	q 12 h	q 12 h	q 12 h	q 48 h	q 18 h
	>28	q 8 h	q 8 h	q 8 h	q 24 h	q 12 h
30–36 (≈1200–2700 g)	0–14	q 12 h	q 12 h	q 12 h	q 24 h	q 12 h
	>14	q 8 h	q 8 h	q 8 h	q 12 h	q 8 h
37–44	0–7	q 8 h	q 12 h	q 12 h	q 12 h	q 12 h
	>7	q 6 h	q 8 h	q 8 h	q 8 h	q 8 h
≥45	All	q 6 h	q 6 h	q 8 h	q 8 h	q 8 h

Table 3.7 **Dosing of gentamicin and tobramycin (aminoglycosides)**

Dosing chart A

Birth to 1 month of age

Gestational age (weeks p.m.)	Dose	Interval[a]
<35	3.5 mg/kg/dose	q 24 h
≥35	5 mg/kg/dose	q 24 h

Dosing chart B

>1 month postnatal

Corrected gestational age (weeks p.m.)	Dose	Interval[a]
<35	2.5 mg/kgdose	q 12 h
≥35	2.5 mg/kg/dose	q 12 h

[a]**Special circumstances require modified aminoglycoside dosing:**
1. In infants >1 month of age with renal or cardiac dysfunction (e.g., s/p asphyxia, large patent ductus arteriosus, left ventricular outflow tract obstruction such as hypoplastic left heart syndrome), use 2.5 mg/kg/dose IV q 12 to 24 h.
2. For preterm infants ≤29 weeks postmenstrual age (= corrected gestational age p.m.), some recommend the following dosing regimen[13]: postnatal day 0–7 → 5 mg/kg/dose q 48 h IV, postnatal day 8–28 → 4 mg/kg/dose q 36 h IV, postnatal day ≥29 days → 4 mg/kg/dose q 24 h IV.
3. Avoid aminoglycosides while treating PDA with indomethacin (use ampicillin and cefotaxime).
4. If preterm infants ≤26 weeks GA need to receive aminoglycosides, extend the dosing interval to 36 h to avoid renal failure.

Option 1

Ampicillin:
- Daily dose: 200 mg/kg/day divided in 2–4 single doses slow IV push; see Interval 2
- Initial single dose can be 100 mg/kg/dose IV
- In severe infections (e.g., suspected meningitis), some recommend 100 mg/kg/dose q 6 to 12 h IV, then usually in combination with cefotaxime 150–200 mg/kg/day divided in 3–4 single doses IV (see below) and aminglycoside (e.g., gentamicin, see below)
- Alternatives: piperacillin (150–300 mg/kg/day divided in 2–4 single doses IV) or mezlocillin (150–225 mg/kg/day in 2–3 single doses IV) instead of ampicillin
  plus

Gentamicin (alternatives: tobramycin, netilmicin) – see Tables 3.6 and 3.7, charts A *and* B *for drug dosing*

There are several dosing schemes in the literature (q 12 to 48 h), one of which is given here:
- 3.5–5 mg/kg/dose, q (12 h to) 24 h to 48 h IV infusion over 30 min (depending on gestational age)
- Desired serum trough level: 0.5–1 (–2) µg/ml (mg/l). Samples to be obtained 30 (to 60) min before the third dose. Withhold medication until drug level is known, unless ordered by the doctor. It might be useful to draw trough levels 60 min prior to the next dose in order to get the results back in time
- Desired serum peak level: 5–12 µg/ml (mg/l). Samples should be obtained 30 min after the third dose (infusion) has been completed. In very preterm neonates or in renal insufficiency, determine serum levels both before and after the second dose
- Half-life of gentamicin is 3–7 h. Interval and dosage are individually adjusted to serum levels. Reduce dose and/or prolong interval, if necessary

- Other aminoglycosides: tobramycin or netilmicin (for dosing see gentamicin). Many *Staphylococcus epidermidis* strains are still netilmicin-sensitive. Tobramicin may have the least nephrotoxic, netilmicin the least ototoxic adverse effect
- A common combination is also *piperacillin* (150 mg/kg/day divided into 2–3 single doses IV; when meningitis is suspected, piperacillin up to 300 mg/kg/day divided into 3–4 single doses IV *plus netilmicin* (see dosage of gentamicin)

Option 2

Ampicillin (see above):
- Daily dose 200 mg/kg/day divided into 2–3 single doses slow IV push; (see interval 2 in Table 3.6)
- Initial dose can be 100 mg/kg/dose IV
- High dosage up to 400 mg/kg/day for suspected meningitis (see above)
- Alternative: piperacillin (150 mg/kg/day divided in 2–3 single doses IV) instead of ampicillin plus

Cefotaxime:
- Initial dose: 50 (–75) mg/kg/dose over 5 min slow IV push; (see Table 3.6, interval 2)
- Maintenance dose is 50 mg/kg/dose over 5 min slow IV push
- Total dose: 100–200 mg/kg/day divided in 2–4 single doses IV
- Some use 50 mg/kg/dose q 8 h IV for all newborn infants >2000 g
- Meningitis dose for infants >1 month of age is 50 mg/kg/dose q 6 h slow IV push

! FDA alert (7/2007)

The revisions are based on new information that describes the potential risk associated with concomitant use of **ceftriaxone (Rocephin®)** with calcium or calcium-containing solutions or products. Cases of fatal reactions with calcium–ceftriaxone precipitates in the lungs and kidneys in both term and premature neonates were reported. Hyperbilirubinemic neonates, especially prematures, should not be treated with ceftriaxone (Rocephin®, which displaces bilirubin from albumin-binding sites). The drug must not be mixed or administered simultaneously with calcium-containing solutions or products, even via different infusion lines. Additionally, calcium-containing solutions or products must not be administered within 48 h of the last administration of ceftriaxone.
→ *Do not use ceftriaxone in the first 2 months of life or before the corrected gestational age of 50 weeks p.m.*

If an infection with *S. epidermidis* or *S. aureus* is likely (e.g., central line, VP shunt, recent MRSA outbreak), vancomycin may be added to the antibiotic regimen (occurs in late rather than in early-onset sepsis of the newborn).

Antibiotic treatment of the severely ill term/preterm newborn, or preterm infants <1000 g with a prenatal history indicating bacterial infection (see also pp. 41–62)

Option 1

Combination of: ampicillin + cefotaxime + aminoglycoside IV (dosing see above)

Meropenem:
- 20 mg/kg/dose q 8–12 h IV. For GA ≥36 weeks → q 8 h; for GA <36 weeks → q 12 h. Some use q 12 h-interval dosing on day 0–7 or if <2000 g (regardless of GA)
- Meningitis dose is 30 (−40) mg/kg/dose q 8 h IV. Half-life is 2–3 h, cleared by kidneys

plus

Vancomycin
- 15 mg/kg/dose q 8–12 h IV infusion over 60 min, see interval 5 (Table 3.6)
- Desired serum trough level: 5–10 µg/ml (mg/l); sample must be obtained just before (within 1 h) the third dose. Withhold medication until drug level is known, unless ordered by MD. It might be useful to draw trough levels 60 min prior to next dose in order to get the results back in time
- In preterm neonates or renal insufficiency, determine trough serum level before the second dose; reduce dose and prolong interval, if necessary
- Some experts still recommend obtaining serum peak levels of vancomycin 30 min after the end of the 60-min infusion when treating meningitis (goal: 30–40 µg/ml), but many centers no longer determine peak levels
- Serum half-life is 6–10 h. Interval and dosage are to be adjusted to serum levels
- Vancomycin is active against Gram-positive pathogens, such as coagulase-negative (oxacillin-resistant) *Staphylococci* (*S. epidermidis*), *S. aureus* (including MRSA) and *Enterococci* (*Enterococcus faecalis* > *Enterococcus faecium*). It is also active against a few anaerobic pathogens (clostridia and actinomyces)

Antibiotic regimen in cases of initial treatment failure and unknown pathogen (see also pp. 41–62)

- Request specific information on maternal colonization and peripartum antibiotic prophylaxis if not already done so
- When *infection with anaerobic pathogens* or *necrotizing enterocolitis (NEC)* is suspected: administer antibiotics of the initial treatment + metronidazole 7.5 mg/kg/dose IV infusion over 30 min q 8–48 h (see interval 4, Table 3.6); e.g., ampicillin + gentamicin (or cefotaxime) + metronidazole (some add metronidazole only when bowel is perforated)
- For *likely GBS sepsis/meningitis*: give high-dose ampicillin, (100 mg/kg/dose q 6–12 h; see interval 2, Table 3.6 on p. 298) + aminoglycoside, if this was not implemented in the initial regimen (synergism of aminoglycosides with β-lactam antibiotics). Some centers use Penicillin G alone (150 000 units/kg/dose q 6–8 h IV) for proven GBS sepsis/meningitis if clinical and microbiological response has been documented[89]. For meningitis, some experts believe that a second LP 24–48 h after initiation of antibiotic therapy assists in the management and may be prognostic (if CSF is not sterile, a complicated course can be expected, requiring serial LPs, advanced imaging (e.g., brain MRI) and eventually modification of therapy)[89].

For the treatment of nosocomial infections and infections caused by viruses, fungi or parasites, see additional literature (e.g., *The Red Book*[89]).

1. **Inducible resistance to cephalosporins.** Cephalosporins should not be used as sole treatment for invasive or serious infections by *Enterobacter* spp., *Citrobacter* spp., *Pseudomonas aeruginosa*, *Serratia* spp., or *Providencia* spp., all of which are inducibly resistant to cephalosporins.
2. ***Salmonella* and aminoglycosides.** Despite in vitro susceptibility to aminoglycosides, *Salmonella* spp. are not susceptible in vivo to this class of drugs.
3. ***Pseudomonas* and related species**. *P. aeruginosa* and *Acinetobacter* spp. are usually susceptible to aminoglycosides, but resistant to trimethroprim-sulfamethoxazole (TMP-SMX; Bactrim®/Septra®) despite in vitro susceptibility. *Stenotrophomonas* and *Burkholderia* species on the other hand are resistant to aminoglycosides and often only susceptible to TMP-SMX. Use TMP-SMX very cautiously in infants <2 months of age.
4. **Enterococci and antibiotic resistance.** The following antibiotics are *not* clinically active against enterococci: all cephalosporins, anti-staphylococcal penicillins (e.g., oxacillin), macrolides, clindamycin, and quinolones. Thus, intrinsic resistance to most antibiotic classes necessitates double-agent therapy for synergy and bacterial killing in the treatment of invasive infections. Recommended therapy is ampicillin (vancomycin if ampicillin-resistant) plus gentamicin (or netilmicin) – avoid tobramycin and amikacin. Other antibiotics with activity against enterococcus include piperacillin, penicillin, amoxicillin, and imipenem. Vancomycin-resistant enterococci (VRE) are usually *Entercoccus faecium* and rarely *E. faecalis*. Linezolid is active against most enterococcal isolates, including VRE. Quinupristin/dalfopristin (Synercid®) is active against most *E. faecium*, including VRE, but not against *E. faecalis*. Many of these drugs are not approved for neonatal use (see package inserts).
5. **Listeria.** Listeria are cephalosporin-resistant (as is true for enterococci). Recommended empiric therapy is ampicillin plus aminoglycoside (e.g., gentamicin), consider the addition of rifampicin.
6. **Clindamycin in methicillin-resistant *Staphylococcus aureus* (MRSA) infections:** if MRSA is reported as having susceptibility to clindamycin, a *D-test* (double disc diffusion assay) should be performed to look for inducible macrolide-lincosamide-streptogramin (MLS$_B$) resistance. If the D-test is positive, suspect that MRSA may have inducible clindamycin resistance and consider using vancomycin instead (e.g., long-term treatment for osteomyelitis).

! When the bacterial pathogen is known, adjust the antibiotic treatment to the sensitivities (antibiogram, minimum inhibitory concentration (MIC), minimum bactericidal concentration (MBC)).

Duration of antibiotic treatment

! Do not treat positive smear cultures in the absence of clinical symptoms.

- A maximum of 48 h, when the clinical course and the laboratory findings do not verify the suspected infection
- Usually 3–5 days of treatment for conjunctivitis
- 7 days, when infection is confirmed (evidence of pathogen plus laboratory studies and/or clinical presentation)
- 10 days, when blood culture is positive and/or severe illness

- 14–21 days for meningitis (some suggest treatment for an additional 1 week after the last unremarkable CSF)
- At least 3 weeks IV for osteomyelitis
- Usually 3 weeks IV for fungal infections (for catheter-associated infections, 10 days IV may be sufficient)

Laboratory

Laboratory markers (CBC, CRP, IL-6/IL-8) may be repeated the day after the antibiotic treatment has begun (depending on clinical status/response), or together with a blood draw (e.g., metabolic screening, etc.) on day 3 or 4 of life. The duration of antibiotic therapy is determined by the cause and severity of infection (see above). In severe, invasive infection, some neonatologists prefer to stop antibiotics when a full IV course is completed *and* inflammatory markers (e.g., CRP) have been negative for 1–2 days.

! 12 Steps to prevent antimicrobial resistance

Centers of Disease Control and Prevention's Campaign
1. Vaccinate → Vaccinate at-risk patients
2. Get the catheters out → Remove catheters as soon as possible when not essential
3. Get some culture(s) → Culture before starting empiric therapy
4. Treat to cure → Optimize regimen, dose, route and duration
5. Seek expert input → Consult Infectious Diseases/Infection Control/Pharmacy
6. Know your antibiogram → Use local data to select empiric therapy
7. Know when to say "no" to vanco. . . → Don't treat *Staphylococcus epidermidis* blood culture contaminants
8. Remember that less is often best → Use/switch as soon as possible to an effective narrow-spectrum regimen
9. Don't treat colonization → Treat pneumonia, not the endotracheal tube
10. Quit when you're ahead → Stop antimicrobials when infection is unlikely
11. Isolate the pathogen → Implement and adhere to indicated isolation precautions
12. Break the chain of contagion → Keep your hands clean; stay home when you are sick
    "12 steps" from The Sanford Guide to Antimicrobial Therapy, 2001[106]

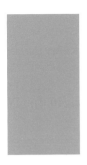

Perinatal hemorrhage

Andrea Zimmermann, Shannon E. G. Hamrick, and Georg Hansmann

Definition

"Asphyxia" (Greek: stopping of the pulse); for details on definition[107] see p. 310.

Etiology/pathophysiology

Common causes are early placental abruption, placenta previa hemorrhage, placental vascular anomalies, trauma (tumor rupture), and hemolytic disease (see chapter on Hydrops fetalis, p. 427). Rapid fetal blood loss dramatically affects fetal perfusion (ischemia) and tissue oxygen supply (hypoxia). Shock symptoms develop when fetal blood loss adds up to approximately 25% of the whole blood volume (total blood volume in the term neonate is approximately 80–85 ml/kg; in the preterm neonate approximately 90–100 ml/kg). Post-asphyxic sequelae such as hypoxic ischemic encephalopathy (HIE), nectrotizing enterocolitis (NEC), hepatic and renal failure are possible (see pp. 310–16).

> *!* If severe (hemorrhagic) anemia is expected, order O Rhesus-negative, <5-days-old packed red blood cells STAT. Cross matching with the maternal serum is useful when time allows, because transfusion of O-Rhesus-negative red blood cells may lead to transfusion reactions due to incompatibility of subgroups. Aim to obtain a neonatal blood sample for blood type and screen/match prior to the first transfusion.

Clinical presentation

- Pale skin color
- Depending on the amount of fetal blood loss and duration of suppressed or interrupted materno-fetal circulation:
  - Initial tachycardia, later bradycardia, finally cardiac arrest
  - Insufficient or absent breathing
  - Arterial hypotension
  - Decreased muscle tone

DDx.

Other causes of asphyxia, hemolytic anemia, feto–fetal transfusion syndrome.

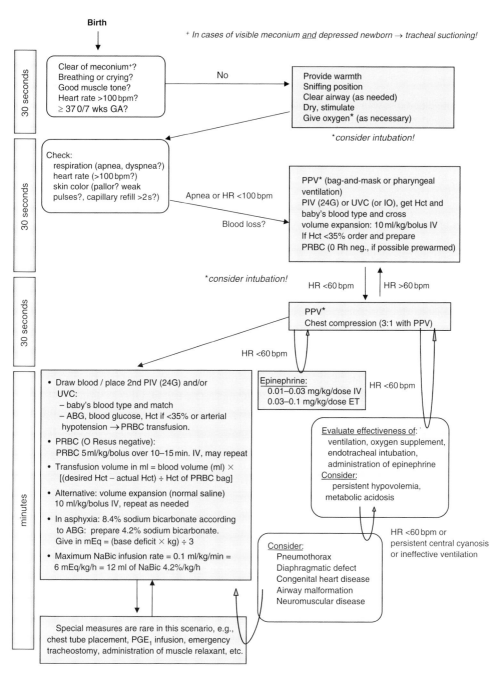

Figure 3.7 Algorithm for the initial management and neonatal resuscitation in early placental abruption/perinatal hemorrhage. If applicable, provide therapeutic hypothermia as soon as possible after the hypoxic-ischemic event (see main text). Hct of PRBC bag is usually 60%–70%. Modified from: American Heart Association (2005) *Guidelines for Cardiopulmonary Resuscitation (CPR) and Emergency Cardiovascular Care (ECC) of Pediatric and Neonatal Patients: Neonatal Resuscitation Guidelines. Pediatrics* **117**(5):e1029–e1038. http://www.pediatrics.org/cgi/content/full/117/5/e1029.

Diagnosis in the delivery room

- ABG (UA, radial artery), blood glucose, spun Hct, CBC and blood type and screen/cross with first blood draw (STAT)

> **!** Acute blood loss with subsequent intravascular hypovolemia can lead to unresponsiveness to expert neonatal resuscitation attempts.
> Remember, acute blood loss does not immediately affect the Hct, therefore a repeat spun Hct is indicated.

Monitoring

S_aO_2, pulse, BP, ECG, temperature, ABG/blood glucose (repeat), eventually CVP via well-placed UVC.

Procedure/therapy in the delivery room (Figure 3.7)

- *ABCD measures/cardiopulmonary resuscitation* when indicated (AHA 2005):
  - Quick action by the team is required, monitor the situation, predict problems
  - Clamp the cord of preterm/term neonates immediately and place them onto the resuscitation unit under thermal radiation
  - Suction pharynx deeply (suction catheter Ch 10) before drying the neonate
  - Immediate bag-and-mask ventilation with F_iO_2 1.0, respiratory rate 60 breaths/min, PIP 20–25 mbar and PEEP 4–5 mbar to obtain chest movements
  - Dry, auscultate, apply standard monitoring (S_aO_2, BP, ECG)
  - Secure airways when breathing is insufficient or absent → endotracheal intubation and intermittent positive pressure ventilation (IPPV)
  - Check position of ET tube (auscultation, watch chest excursions, measure exhaled CO_2) and secure tube
  - Administer chest compressions when HR is <60 bpm
  - Administer epinephrine 1:10 000 0.3–1 ml/kg/dose ET (= 0.03–0.1 mg/kg/dose)
  - Obtain venous access and blood sampling, as required
  - Subsequently 0.1–0.3 ml/kg (= 0.01–0.03 mg/kg/dose) IV, repeat as needed
  - Place gastric tube
- *Volume expansion:* 10 ml/kg/bolus normal saline repeatedly IV until packed red blood cells (PRBC) available
  - Term infants: repeat administration of 10 ml/kg/bolus every (5–)10 min IV until pulse palpable and BP measurable; if BP is low–normal, infuse 10–20 ml/kg/bolus over (30–)60 min IV according to mean arterial pressure (MAP)
  - Preterm neonate with suspected perinatal hemorrhage: repeat administration of 10 ml/kg/bolus every 10–30 min IV until pulse is palpable and BP measurable. If BP is low–normal, infuse 10 ml/kg/bolus over 60–120 min according to MAP
  - If required, give PRBC once available (preferred)
- *Place second peripheral venous line (24G) or UVC or other central venous catheter.* A well-trained team should place *UVC/CVC* early: for infusion and control of volume replacement based on CVP (normal 3–8 mmHg = 2.2–5.9 cmH$_2$O) and BP (MAP ≥ number of weeks' gestation)

- When Hct level is <35% and PRBC are available: *type-O-Rhesus-negative, lysine-free PRBC* (if possible and time allows, PRBC should be cross-matched with maternal serum)
- When Hct ≪30% and shock symptoms are present: transfuse 5 ml/kg O-Rhesus-negative PRBC rapidly over 10–15 min IV, followed by 5–10 ml PRBC/kg/h IV transfusion (when vital signs are acceptable, transfuse 3 ml/kg/h IV)

! 1 ml PRBC/kg body weight elevates the hematocrit by approximately 1 percentage point (assuming Hct of PRBC is approx. 60%– 70%).

- If PRBC are not available: repeat administration of crystalloid volume (e.g., NS) 10 ml/kg/bolus IV (see above)
- *Catecholamine infusions* are rarely indicated after sufficient volume expansion:
  - Insufficient blood pressure with MAP ≪40 mmHg / ≪number of weeks' gestation despite volume expansion: infuse dopamine 5–20 µg/kg/min, epinephrine 0.05–0.1 µg/kg/min or noradrenaline 0.05–1 µg/kg/min via UVC (or other central venous line or intraosseously). In an emergency, infuse dopamine via peripheral venous IV as long as central line (UVC) is not yet established. Dobutamine 5–20 µg/kg/min may be infused via peripheral or central venous access (caution: diastolic BP, tachycardia)
- *Consider buffer therapy with 4.2% sodium bicarbonate (may have to dilute 8.4% sodium bicarbonate 1:1 with sterile water)*
- After 10 min of unsuccessful resuscitation (chest compressions, PPV, epinephrine ET/IV, volume expansion):
  - "Blind" sodium bicarbonate application only in absolute emergency cases, when blood gas analysis not available: give 1–2 mu/kg/dose (= 1–2 mmol/kg/dose), as 4.2% solution over 5–10 min IV
  - In metabolic acidosis with a base deficit greater than –10 mmol/l and PCO_2 <60 mmHg, i.e., adequate ventilation (and perfusion) (see p. 176): the required amount of *8.4% sodium bicarbonate in mEq (= mmol = ml) =* (base deficit × kg body weight) ÷ 3 = ml sodium bicarbonate 8.4% (multiply calculated volume in ml by 2 if using 4.2% solution)
  - Maximum continuous sodium bicarbonate infusion rate: 0.1 mEq/kg/min = 6 mEq/kg/h (= 12 ml of sodium bicarbonate 4.2%/kg/h). Change to THAM infusion if hypernatremia is significant
- $D_{10}W$ 3 ml/kg/h IV (= glucose infusion rate (GIR) of 5 mg/kg/min) according to blood glucose levels; double GIR in presence of hypoglycemia and once a $D_{10}W$ bolus is needed. Use D_5W for transport of term/preterm neonates with elevated blood glucose levels (e.g., after a resuscitation/administration of epinephrine), or reduce $D_{10}W$ infusion rate
- *Transfer the patient quickly.* Inform the admitting NICU about the need for PRBC and the clinical status of the newborn
- Choose a NICU where therapeutic hypothermia is a treatment option

---

! For troubleshooting during neonatal resuscitation, see pp. 88–92, pp. 160–2, Table 2.9.

Monitoring

S_aO_2 (pulse oximeter), BP (desired: MAP $\geq$ number of weeks' gestation), ECG, temperature, and ET tube position. If the child is stable, transfer then early to NICU; blood gas analysis and blood glucose level before departure.

Diagnostic work-up in the NICU

- Chest X-ray:
  - Tube position?
  - Lung inflation?
  - Pneumothorax?
  - Pleural effusion?
  - Pulmonary infiltrate/atelectasis/edema?
  - Heart size?
- Reassessment of hemoglobin and Hct. Signs for hemolytic disease (bilirubin, reticulocyte count)?
- ABG, blood glucose, lactate, chemistry (including ionized calcium, phosphate, magnesium), liver function tests, coagulation panel, blood type and screen/cross. If indicated, advanced metabolic work-up
- Consider early cerebral function monitoring (CFM = aEEG)
- EEG, repeated neurological examinations
- Cranial ultrasonography including color Doppler studies or head CT during the first day of life. Follow-up imaging as necessary for concerns over cerebral edema
- Renal ultrasonography: initial images and progress (Doppler flow, renal vein thrombosis? Parenchymal density?)
- Stool examination for gastrointestinal bleeding
- History? Toxicological screening: urine or meconium
- MRI brain in the first week of life, if indicated

Procedure/therapy in the NICU

- Continue *volume expansion*:
  PRBC transfusion depending on Hct and vital signs

Packed RBC transfusion volume in ml =
[(desired Hct – actual Hct) $\div$ Hct of PRBC bag] $\times$ blood volume (ml)

- Fresh frozen plasma (FFP) if coagulation panel is altered and/or there are signs of bleeding
- Need for platelet transfusion depends on platelet count, gestational age and signs of bleeding
- Avoid persistent pulmonary hypertension of the newborn (PPHN) and maintain adequate perfusion pressure: keep MAP >40 mmHg, aim for adequate oxygenation with P_aO_2 >50 mmHg, pH >7.30
- Normoventilation, no hyperventilation

- Analgesia and sedation, as required
- Buffer therapy with 4.2% sodium bicarbonate, as indicated
- Evaluate fluid status carefully and avoid fluid overload
- Monitor for prerenal failure/renal ischemia
- Check renal function approximately 6–12 h, 24 h, and 48 h after birth. Avoid nephrotic drugs such as aminoglycosides, if possible
- Cerebral function monitoring (CFM = aEEG) within the first few days
- Treatment of post-asphyxial complications (increased risk of cerebral hemorrhage and hypoxic ischemic encephalopathy/periventricular leucomalacia; see 238)
- Consider therapeutic hypothermia.[108–110] See chapter on perinatal hypoxia-ischemia, pp. 314–16
- Catecholamines are rarely indicated when volume expansion is sufficient (see above). If inotropes are needed, myocardial ischemia during a low cardiac output state (and hypoxia) is a likely explanation for mycocardial dysfunction
- Avoid hypo- and hyperglycemia; aim for blood glucose of 60–120 mg/dl, by adjusting GIR
- Check electrolytes including ionized and total calcium, magnesium, phosphorus
- Check liver function (AST, ALT, GGT, albumin) and coagulation panel

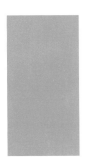

Perinatal hypoxia-ischemia

Shannon E. G. Hamrick, Andrea Zimmermann, and Georg Hansmann

Definition

"Asphyxia" (Greek: stopping of the pulse), i.e., the biochemical and clinical consequences of lack of oxygen and hypercarbia following antepartum or intrapartum interruption of respiration/perfusion. In addition to hypoxia, there is respiratory and metabolic acidosis that can lead to peripheral and pulmonary vasoconstriction and ultimately, if untreated, to myocardial failure, hypotension, and bradycardia.

The term "perinatal asphyxia" should be used with constraint, not only for medical-legal reasons, but also due to the lack of a broadly accepted definition. According to Carter *et al.* (1993)[107], perinatal asphyxia is defined as a combination of:

- Severe umbilical arterial acidosis with a UA pH value <7.00
- Persistently low Apgar score <4 for at least 5 min after birth
- Neurological symptoms, such as seizures, unconsciousness or muscle hypotonia, and
- Cardiac, pulmonary, intestinal or renal dysfunction

The American College of Obstetrics and Gynecology[111] defines an acute intrapartum hypoxic event meeting the following combined criteria as sufficient to cause spastic quadriplegic or dyskinetic cerebral palsy:

- Severe umbilical arterial acidosis with a UA pH value <7.00 and base deficit ≥12 mmol/l
- Early onset of moderate to severe encephalopathy in an infant ≥34 weeks' gestation
- Exclusion of other identifiable etiologies

> **!** It is inappropriate to use the term "birth asphyxia" based on a single low Apgar score[112] or a single low pH value (obtained from the umbilical artery) in the absence of neurological signs or symptoms[113].

Epidemiology

Delayed postnatal adaptation occurs in approx. 5%–10% of all births; thus, in about 2–3/1000 births, birth asphyxia is possible[114].

Etiology/pathophysiology

Impairment of the feto–placental gas exchange:

- *Preplacental*: lack of oxygen supply due to uterine rupture, maternal anemia, shock, embolism, sepsis, respiratory insufficiency, or conditions causing chronic placental insufficiency

Neonatal Emergencies: A Practical Guide for Resuscitation, Transport and Critical Care, ed. Georg Hansmann.
Published by Cambridge University Press. © Cambridge University Press 2009.

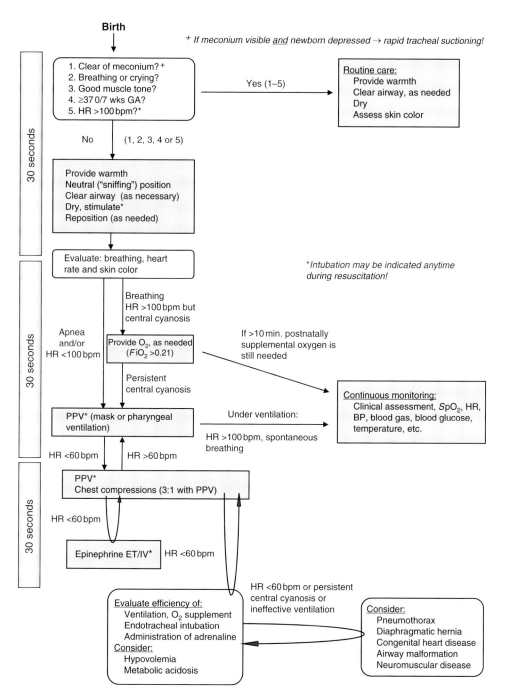

Figure 3.8 Standard algorithm for the initial management and resuscitation of newborn infants, including those s/p perinatal hypoxia-ischemia. If applicable, provide therapeutic hypothermia as soon as possible after the hypoxic event (see main text). Modified from: ILCOR guidelines (2005), *Resuscitation* 2005; 67:293–303 and http://pediatrics.aappublications.org/cgi/content/full/117/5/e978. *Circulation* 2005; 112:IV 188–195 and *Pediatrics* 2006; 117:e1029–1038.

- *Intraplacental*: placental abruption, placenta-previa hemorrhage, severe maternal systemic hypotension
- *Postplacental*: umbilical cord complications, fetal anemia, acute feto–fetal or feto–maternal transfusion, insufficiency of the fetal circulation (i.e., including arrhythmias, hydrops fetalis, multiple births, fetal malformation, sepsis)

> **!** When resuscitating an asphyxiated neonate, the presence of at least three health care providers who are well trained in neonatal resuscitation is necessary: one for airway management, one for chest compressions, drug administration or IV access/umbilical catheter insertion, and one for providing medications and other equipment, monitoring and documentation.

Clinical presentation in the delivery room

Bradycardic, apneic, pale (rather than blue), hypotonic ("floppy") newborn infant. Note that skin pallor or cyanosis may also occur in a neonate who has chronic anemia (blood loss), sepsis or congenital heart disease.

Monitoring

S_pO_2 (pulse oximeter), BP (rough estimate of ideal BP is MAP $\geq$ gestational age in weeks p.m.), temperature, ECG.

Procedure/therapy in the delivery room (Figure 3.8):

- *ABCD measures/cardiopulmonary resuscitation* when indicated[71,115]:
  - Quick action by the team is required, keep track of the situation, predict problems
  - Clamp the cord of preterm/term neonates immediately and place them onto the resuscitation unit, begin to warm and dry the neonate (unless meconium is present in a non-vigorous newborn $\rightarrow$ suction, laryngoscopy)
  - Suction oropharynx including hypopharynx (F 10 = Ch 10)
  - Immediate bag-and-mask ventilation (ventilation has priority over oxygenation). Respiratory rate 60 breaths/min, initial inflation pressure of 20 cmH$_2$O (occasionally as high as 40 cmH$_2$O) (= mbar) to obtain adequate chest expansion. Subsequent pressures should be lower, depending on gestational age. PEEP 3–5 cmH$_2$O. Exception is meconium aspiration that requires rapid intubation (mask PPV is contraindicated)
  - There is currently insufficient evidence to recommend a specific oxygen concentration for neonatal resuscitation[71,116]. Although $F_iO_2 > 0.21$ may be beneficial in cases of pulmonary diffusion impairment and suprasystemic pulmonary vascular resistance (PVR) (e.g., pneumonia/sepsis, meconium aspiration syndrome (MAS), persistent pulmonary hypertension of the newborn (PPHN))[116], there are clinical data from a small randomized controlled trial that room-air resuscitation causes less damage to the heart and kidneys of severely asphyxiated term newborn infants (HR <80 bpm, pale, not responsive, UA $\leq$pH 7.0, 5-min Apgar score 0–5) than 100% oxygen[117]. If S_pO_2

is rapidly improving during initial newborn resuscitation, oxygen supplementation (if provided at all) must be continuously reduced or stopped, since high P_aO_2 levels/oxygen radicals reduce cerebral blood flow[118], induce myocardial and renal tubular damage[117] and promote the development of retinopathy of prematurity (RoP) and bronchopulmonary dysplasia (BPD)/chronic lung disease (CLD) in preterm infants

- Standard monitoring (S_pO_2, BP, ECG, temperature) should be initiated
- When breathing is insufficient or absent, or HR is <100 bpm despite sufficient positive pressure ventilation (PPV) via bag-and-mask or T-piece resuscitator, secure the airway by endotracheal intubation and PPV, check tube position (auscultation, chest excursion, later chest X-ray) and place a gastric tube
- Administer chest compressions when HR <60 bpm (3:1 ratio with PPV)
- Administer epinephrine (1:10 000) 0.01 mg/kg to 0.03 mg/kg/dose IV if HR <60 bpm despite 30 s of efficient chest compressions/PPV, or 0.03–0.1 mg/kg/dose intratracheally via ET tube if no IV access, and repeat administration if needed
- Establish venous access (UVC, PIV, IO) and obtain blood sampling, as needed
- *Volume expansion*: give normal saline (or Ringer's lactate), 10 (–20) ml/kg/bolus IV, generally with the second epinephrine dose, and/or if hypovolemia is suspected. Keep in mind that in perinatal hypoxia, placental vasoconstriction frequently leads to a volume shift towards the placenta. Hence, hypoxic neonates may be intravascularly volume-depleted even if there has been no significant blood loss. If there has been severe blood loss (uterine rupture, early placental disruption, etc., see chapter on perinatal hemorrhage, p. 304 and Figure 3.7), repeated volume bolus and early administration of PRBC (O-Rhesus-negative, if no emergently cross-matched unit against the mother available) are usually needed
- *Place second peripheral venous catheter (24 G) or UVC/central venous line.* A well-trained team should place *UVC* early for IV fluid infusion and CVP monitoring during volume replacement therapy (normal 3–8 mmHg = 2.2–5.9 cmH$_2$O) and BP (MAP ≥ gestational age in weeks p.m.)
- *Place UAC for continuous BP monitoring*
- *Catecholamine infusions* may be rarely indicated: dopamine 5–20 µg/kg/min IV; if ineffective go to epinephrine 0.05–0.1 µg/kg/min IV
- Consider *buffer therapy with 4.2% sodium bicarbonate*:
  - After 10 min of ineffective resuscitation (chest compressions, epinephrine) in spite of adequate ventilation: 2 mEq/kg over 5–10 min IV
  - For documented metabolic acidosis with adequate ventilation (i.e., PCO_2 <60 mmHg) calculated sodium bicarbonate dose in mEq = (base deficit in mEq/l × kg body weight) ÷ 3; re-assess ABG
- *Initial IV fluids*: $D_{10}W$ at 60–80 ml/kg/day (keep blood glucose in goal range 80–120 mg/dl; values up to 150 mg/dl may be acceptable)
- *Initial laboratory studies*: repeat ABG, blood glucose, basic laboratory studies (including ionized calcium, phosphate, magnesium, lactate, electrolytes), blood typing/screening, blood cross-matching, CBC, CRP, blood cultures. Bilirubin, liver function tests, coagulation studies, advanced metabolic screens as indicated

See Table 2.9, "Trouble shooting during neonatal resuscitation," pp. 160–2.

Post-resuscitation intensive care
Diagnosis in the NICU

- Chest X-ray:
  - ET tube position?
  - Lung inflation?
  - Pneumothorax?
  - Pleural effusions?
  - Infiltrates?
  - Pulmonary edema or venous congestion?
  - Cardiac silhouette?
  - Diaphragmatic hernia?
- Early cerebral function monitoring (aEEG = cerebral function monitoring; see chapter on neonatal seizures, p. 317)
- All-lead EEG, repeated neurological examinations
- Neuroimaging: MRI preferred for determining the presence and extent of hypoxic-ischemic injury, ischemic stroke, or congenital brain malformations that could explain an encephalopathy. Also helpful for determining prognosis (see below). If MRI is not available, CT is sensitive enough to determine the presence of hemorrhage or calcifications, and early cerebral edema. Head ultrasound including Doppler flow in the anterior cerebral artery (ACA) helps to determine the degree of cerebral edema initially and in follow-up exams. Head ultrasound may reveal hypodensities indicating hypoxic brain damage (e.g., in the basal ganglia) a few days after birth
- Head ultrasonography may not be sensitive enough to identify parenchymal injury (early). In hypoxic ischemic encephalopathy (HIE), hypodensities may be found in the basal ganglia. Diastolic flow velocity in the ACA is frequently associated with the degree of cerebral edema status post-asphyxia (diastolic velocity may be high in the first few days but then abnormally low later on). Hence, head ultrasonography can be a useful tool in the daily assessment of HIE and cerebral edema
- Follow renal function: urine output, creatinine, blood urea nitrogen (BUN); consider ultrasound to screen for renal-ureteral pathology.
- Toxicological screening (urine or meconium) as indicated

Procedure/therapy in the NICU

- Continue *volume expansion and/or inotropes* depending on BP and clinical scenario

---

! Contraindication for volume expansion: myocardial dysfunction due to arrhythmias or hypoxia ("asphyxial cardiomyopathy").

- Avoid PPHN: aim for adequate oxygenation and perfusion and normal pH, but do not hyperventilate as this can be injurious to brain and lung
- Analgesia and sedation, as needed
- Continue IV fluids in the range of 60–80 ml/kg/day, monitor electrolytes and treat accordingly, especially hypocalcemia or glucose abnormalities. Fluid restriction to

50–60 ml/kg/day may be necessary in syndrome of inappropriate antidiuretic hormone secretion (SIADH) s/p perinatal hypoxia

- Remember the *postasphyxia sequence* can involve the brain, lungs, kidneys, and intestines. Be very cautious when initiating feeds (per nasogastric or orogastric/jejunal tube).
- Control cerebral seizures (see chapter on neonatal seizures, p. 317). If significant seizures occur, load with phenobarbital
- Avoid hyperpyrexia (hyperthermia)

Therapeutic hypothermia in the NICU

- Much attention has been given to therapeutic hypothermia recently, with three randomized controlled trials published in 2005[119–121] and several others to be analyzed/still unpublished (*TOBY, ICE and neo.nEuro.network trials*). Proposed mechanisms of action include decreased metabolism (ATP preservation), inhibition of glutamate release, decreased free radical generation, decreased apoptosis, or reduced inflammatory response[122]. The other important concept is that hypothermia may prolong the therapeutic window, potentially allowing the efficacy of other eventual neuroprotectants.
- Each of the recently published human newborn trials (see below) were multicenter randomized controlled trials. Each initiated cooling within 6 h of life (based on animal data) and continued for 48–72 h, and each had neurodevelopmental follow-up at 12–18 months. None showed significant differences between treatment groups in complications that were clinically relevant (e.g., bleeding, arrhythmias).
- The trial published in *Lancet* by Gluckman *et al.* (the *CoolCap trial*) used selective head cooling (i.e., cool cap), and a strength was the use of aEEG as a stratification criterion. This study showed no difference in the composite outcome of death or severe disability, but a predefined subgroup analysis of the *moderately* affected infants showed a positive effect of hypothermia (OR 0.42 (95% CI 0.22–0.8, $p = 0.009$)[119]. Death or severe disability at 18 months of age was assessed in the CoolCap trial[123]: treatment, lower encephalopathy grade, lower birth weight, greater aEEG amplitude, absence of seizures, and higher Apgar score, but not gender or gestational age, were associated significantly with better outcomes[123].
- The trial conducted by the NICHD (National Institute of Child Health and Human Development) used systemic cooling (i.e., mattress), and described an 18% decrease in the same composite outcome in the hypothermia group (44% vs. 62%, RR 0.72, 95% CI 0.54–0.95, $p = 0.01$) with no significant difference in cerebral palsy in survivors of either group, though more support was withdrawn in the control group[121].
- A smaller trial, designed to test the ability of initiating treatment in the referral hospitals, also used systemic cooling, and also showed a positive effect from hypothermia, with the same composite outcome in 52% of hypothermia-treated newborns and 84% of controls ($p = 0.019$). This study consisted of more severely affected infants, with 77% classified as Sarnat stage 3 (severe), but a high percentage was lost to follow-up[120] (interestingly the target temperature was reached faster in referral patients, though mortality rate was still higher in the outborn population).
- A magnetic resonance neuroimaging study inclusive of 14 infants who received selective head cooling and 20 who received whole-body hypothermia (and 52 controls) determined that both modes of hypothermia reduced basal ganglia/thalamus lesions and this was most significant in patients with moderate injury by aEEG criteria[124].

- The European *neo.nEuro.network study* "Induced hypothermia in asphyxiated new-borns" was terminated early because, "the current evidence of the benefits of therapeutic hypothermia did not justify further randomization" (PI: Georg Simbruner, University of Innsbruck, Austria; personal communication).
- It should be noted that two[120,121] of the three completed RCT[119–121] were published after the ILCOR's guidelines on neonatal resuscitation[71]; the latter made no clear recommendation for or against cooling (by cap or mattress) in birth asphyxia.

> *!* The current clinical data strongly indicate a consistent, robust beneficial effect of therapeutic hypothermia for neonatal post-resuscitation encephalopathy[125,126]. We advocate for therapeutic hypothermia in clinical practice provided the practitioner follows the protocol of one of the published trials[125,126]. Although therapeutic hypothermia appears very promising[122,127,128], residual questions as to the appropriate treatment group, optimal strategy, and long-term effects need to be answered. However, cooling (e.g., whole-body cooling with mattress, 33.5–34.0°C for 72 h) may soon become the standard of care for suspected perinatal asphyxia.

Prognosis

You may anticipate hypoxic ischemic encephalopathy (HIE) when the 5-min Apgar score is <5, endotracheal intubation and/or chest compressions are necessary, and an initial umbilical pH value <7.00 is present[129]. HIE is characterized by neurological symptoms including depressed consciousness, ventilatory disturbances, muscular hypotonia or extreme irritability, and seizures[130]. Note that neonatal encephalopathy is not synonymous with HIE – there are other causes of encephalopathy. The severity and duration of the encephalopathy and the presence of seizures are good clinical markers for estimating prognosis[130,131]. There is currently no perfect *biochemical* predictor of outcome, though magnetic resonance neuroimaging has demonstrated a correlation with outcome[132–134]. Outcome following HIE can include death, cerebral palsy or epilepsy[114,135].

> *!* Both an isolated low 1-min Apgar score and an isolated umbilical arterial acidosis are insufficient to predict neurological outcome.

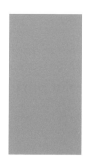

Cerebral seizures

Shannon E. G. Hamrick and Andrea Zimmermann

Definition

Paroxysmal episodes of hypersynchronous neuronal activity[130]. Motor activity, vital signs, and neurobehavior can be affected.

Incidence

Clinically apparent in 1/1000 to 3/1000 term infants, and 1.5/1000 to 5/1000 preterm and term infants[136]. The incidence of electroencephalographic neonatal seizures is unknown.

Pathophysiology

The immature brain is more susceptible to seizures because its γ-aminobutyric acid (GABA) receptors have an excitatory effect, rather than the inhibitory effect seen with maturity[137–139].

Etiology[130,140]

- Hypoxic ischemic encephalopathy:
  - Approx. 50%–60% of cases
  - Within the first 24 h after birth asphyxia, typically before day 3 of life
  - Influencing factors: hypoglycemia, hypocalcemia, intracerebral hemorrhage
- Intracerebral hemorrhage:
  - Approx. 10% of cases
  - Subdural and subarachnoidal hemorrhage, mainly in term neonates,
  - Intraventricular and intraparenchymal hemorrhage, particularly in preterm neonates
  - Arterial cerebral infarction
  - Sinus thrombosis
- CNS infections:
  - Approx. 10% of cases
  - Meningitis, encephalitis, or intrauterine infection
- Congenital brain malformations: approx. 5%–10% of cases
- Metabolic disorders:
  - Hypoglycemia, typically before day 2 of life
  - Hypocalcemia, can be early onset (2–3 days) or late onset (>7 days)
  - Inborn metabolic disorders

Neonatal Emergencies: A Practical Guide for Resuscitation, Transport and Critical Care, ed. Georg Hansmann.
Published by Cambridge University Press. © Cambridge University Press 2009.

- Neurocutaneous disorders (e.g., neurofibromatosis)
- Chromosomal abnormalities
- Neonatal withdrawal syndrome: methadone, morphine, heroin – typically first 3 days
- Vitamin-B_6- (pyridoxine-) dependent seizures
- Benign familiar neonatal seizures

Clinical presentation[130]

There are *four types* of neonatal seizures:

- *Subtle signs of seizures:*
  - Preterm or term
  - Eye deviation or staring, repetitive mouth and tongue movements, rowing/bicycling movements of extremities, apnea
- *Clonic seizures:*
  - Primarily term
  - Rhythmic contractions of an extremity or of the face with or without impaired consciousness
  - Focal or multifocal
- *Tonic seizures:*
  - Primarily preterm
  - Sustained posturing (extension) of an extremity, deviation of the head or eyes, apnea
  - Focal or generalized
- *Myoclonic seizures:*
  - Rare
  - Rapid jerks of extremities
  - Focal, multifocal or generalized
- **Duration of the seizure**: seconds to minutes
- **Concomitant physiological changes**: increase in blood glucose and lactate, decrease in cerebral pH and glucose, increased cerebral blood flow, increased blood pressure

Age at clinical manifestation

- Rarely immediately after birth in the delivery room (occasionally seen with HIE, vitamin-B_6-dependent seizures)
- Predominantly between 12 and 48 h after birth
- Late manifestation >48 h after birth indicates meningitis, benign familiar seizures, or hypocalcemia

DDx.

- Jitteriness = symmetrical tremor of the extremities excluding the facial muscles, cessation on passive flexion, often concomitant in HIE, hypoglycemia, hypocalcemia, drug withdrawal
- Benign neonatal sleep myoclonus – can look like myoclonic seizures
- Apnea of prematurity – apneic seizure is associated with tachycardia

Initial assessment

- Physical examination and history, associated changes in vital signs
- Blood gas, blood glucose, electrolytes, including calcium and magnesium, blood culture

Further studies

- Consider evaluating liver enzymes and renal function, ammonia, lactate, bilirubin, coagulation studies
- Consider lumbar puncture and TORCH (toxoplasmosis, other agents such as varicella zoster virus, rubella, cytomegalovirus, herpes simplex/HIV, syphilis) studies, toxicology screen, serum amino acids and urine organic acids, and chromosomal analysis
- EEG: despite the clinical appearance of a seizure, there may be no ictal activity on EEG especially with subtle and generalized tonic seizures (i.e., electroclinical dissociation[141]). Alternatively, infants can have electroencephalographic seizures without any clinical presentation. However, an EEG is useful for both ictal activity and background activity. Background abnormalities predict risk of seizures and imply a poorer prognosis. An EEG can be particularly helpful in neonates on antiepileptic (especially phenobarbital) and/or muscle relaxing drugs
- aEEG (amplitude-integrated EEG) for CFM (cerebral function monitoring): useful for non-invasive continuous monitoring of electrocortical activity in high-risk neonates, and for potential interventional selection (i.e., induced hypothermia; see chapter on perinatal ischemia-hypoxia, p. 310). A diagnosis of "cerebral seizure" still needs to be made by full-lead EEG (gold standard) because short or focal seizures can be missed[142]. CFM is reliable for detecting the sleep-wake cycle, background patterns (especially at the two ends of the spectrum, i.e., normal and severely abnormal)[143], and generalized ictal activity, all of which might be useful in predicting outcome[144]
- Neuroimaging: essential in determining the etiology of the seizures. Once seizures are controlled, MRI is preferred for determining the presence and extent of hypoxic-ischemic injury, ischemic stroke, or congenital brain malformations. If MRI is not available, CT is sensitive enough to determine the presence of hemorrhage or calcifications. Head ultrasonography may miss subdural or epidural bleeds (always do transtemporal views to evaluate contralateral temporoparietal area), or parenchymal injury

Therapy

! Although a therapeutic intervention may have little or no influence on the extent of the *cause* of brain damage (aside from hypoglycemia) there are emerging data that seizures are associated with worse outcome, even when controlling for the underlying condition[145,146]. On the other hand, animal data have demonstrated that antiepileptic drugs such as phenobarbital, phenytoin, diazepam or clonazepam and valproate, when given in normal clinical doses to neonatal rats, led to apoptotic neuro-degeneration (sole and synergistic toxicity)[147]. Phenobarbital may lead to decreased brain growth and impaired learning[148]. Therefore, the indication for treatment of (often self-limiting) seizures with antiepileptic drugs underlies an ongoing debate. Neurodevelopmental follow-up studies may not only mirror the sequelae of the seizures, but also the side-effects of the medical therapy! The clinical use and benefit of neonatal anticonvulsants is not based on evidence. Randomized controlled trials addressing neurodevelopmental outcome are needed[146,149].

- Maintain adequate ventilation and perfusion. Monitor S_aO_2 (pulse oximetry), BP, ECG, temperature. Consider near-infrared spectroscopy (NIRS) for cerebral oximetry
- Correct metabolic disturbances:
    - Hypoglycemia: $D_{10}W$ 2–4 ml/kg/dose (=0.2–0.4 g/kg/dose) slow IV push over 5–10 min, and follow with continuous $D_{10}W$ infusion at a rate of 5–10 µg/kg/min IV (=3–6 ml $D_{10}W$/kg/min IV)
    - Hypocalcemia: 100 mg/kg calcium gluconate: dilute calcium gluconate 10% 1:1 with D_5W, and give 2 ml/kg/dose slow IV push over 5–10 min under ECG monitoring
    - Hypomagnesemia: 25–250 mg/kg magnesium sulfate IV or IM
    - Hyponatremia: correction determined by underlying etiology of hyponatremia; do not correct hyponatremia rapidly. However, if newborn is actively seizing and severe hyponatremia is the most likely cause, correct more quickly to serum sodium $\geq$125 mmol/l. Aim for sodium correction $\leq$10–15 mmol/l in 24 h
    - Treat underlying conditions (e.g., infection)

Anticonvulsant therapy

Recognizing our treatment is not evidence-based, the standard first-line agent in neonatal seizures is phenobarbital.

Phenobarbital

- Loading dose: 20 mg/kg, slow IV push over 20 min (max 1 mg/kg/min). If necessary, may re-load with an additional 20 mg/kg in 5- to 10-mg/kg aliquots. Monitor blood pressure and breathing
- Maintenance dose: 3–4 (–6) mg/kg/24 h IV or PO, monitor levels[103,150–153]

Unremitting seizures

Lorazepam

- 0.05 mg/kg to 0.1 mg/kg IV in 0.05-mg/kg increments slow IV push over 5–10 min. Monitor breathing; myoclonic jerks may occur with lorazepam treatment in preterm neonates. The half-life in asphyxiated newborns is 40 h; duration of action 3–24 h[103]

Fosphenytoin (expressed in phenytoin equivalents (PE))

- Loading dose 20 mg PE/kg, IM or IV slow push over at least 10 min. For non-emergent loading, use 10–15 mg PE/kg/dose in 30 min IV
- Maintenance dose: 3–5 mg PE/kg q 12 h (or q 24 h) IM or IV slow push (maximum rate 1.5 mg PE/kg/min)
- Flush with saline before and after administration
- Monitor cardiac rhythm and blood pressure, and use with caution in patients with hyperbilirubinemia as fosphenytoin and bilirubin can compete for protein-binding sites, resulting in increased serum phenytoin levels
- Fosphenytoin is preferred over phenytoin because it can be administered more rapidly[103]
- Phenytoin but not fosphenytoin is FDA approved for neonates

- Other agents for consideration (limited clinical data):
  - Midazolam may achieve seizure control in non-responders[154], but paradoxic reactions (agitation, etc.) are common
  - Rectal diazepam 0.5 mg/kg/dose if no IV access (0.2–0.5 mg/kg/dose IV)
  - Clonazepam 0.1 mg/kg/dose IV (not available in the USA)
  - Paraldehyde: consult with pediatric neurology for dosing guidance
  - **Pyridoxine (vitamin B$_6$):** 50–100 mg IV. If pyridoxine deficiency is suspected, one should give treatment under concurrent EEG monitoring[136]
- Other drugs, promising in experimental studies:
  - Bumetanide: loop diuretic that targets chloride transporters, shows potential in animal models, currently under investigation in human newborns[155]
  - Levetiracetam (Keppra®): no neuroapoptosis, available in IV form – NIH trial pending[156]
  - Topiramate (Topamax®): neuroprotective in rat HIE model[157]
- If possible, treat with only one anticonvulsant and lowest possible dose. Randomized controlled trials are underway!
- Consult with pediatric neurology
- If the risk of recurrence is low, and physical examination, neuroimaging and EEG are reassuring, treat for the briefest time possible and do *not* discharge home from NICU on anticonvulsant

Outcome

- Depends primarily on underlying cause
- Long-term treatment with anticonvulsants have been shown to contribute to adverse behavioral and cognitive outcome[140,158]

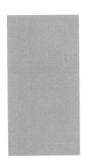

Infants born to mothers on psychoactive substances

Christoph Bührer

Epidemiology

- Abuse of legal psychoactive substances (alcohol, nicotine) during pregnancy is far more common than use of illicit drugs
- Incidence and choice of drugs show strong regional variability. Maternal substance abuse is seen in all socio-economic classes, ages, and races, but there is increased risk in younger women, unmarried women, and women with lower educational achievements
- Many mothers on psychoactive substances use more than one drug. Women on methadone or buprenorphine substitution may still use heroin or other illicits drugs
- Every effort should be made to stop consumption of alcohol, benzodiazepines, phencyclidine, and cocaine during pregnancy and to cut down on smoking cigarettes
- In contrast, avoid withdrawal from opioids (risks of miscarriage in the first trimester, premature labor in the third trimester, fetal distress and fetal intrauterine death close to term)
- Selective serotonin reuptake inhibitors (SSRI) are also commonly prescribed during pregnancy to women with symptoms of depression[159]. Attempts to change an effective medication are contraindicated shortly before and after delivery (mood swings are very common around the time of childbirth, even in women without a history of depression), and women who have been taking a particular SSRI for most of the pregnancy should continue to do so after the baby is born. Women who discontinue antidepressants during pregnancy have about five times the risk for depression relapse than those who continue to take the medications[160]. However, the risk of persistent pulmonary hypertension of the newborn (PPHN) is about sixfold increased in newborns whose mothers used SSRI after 20 weeks of gestation[161], with an overall incidence of approximately 6 to 12 per 1000 exposed women

Perinatal counselling

- Talk openly to the expectant mother about substances she has taken during delivery without blaming her
- Almost all mothers on illicit or prescribed drugs feel guilty about fetal maltreatment
- If a mother has taken opioids explain that evolving withdrawal symptoms may be significant but transient
- A woman on SSRI should be reassured that her psychological well-being as a mother is of paramount importance to the newborn infant. The decision to use or not to use SSRI

Neonatal Emergencies: A Practical Guide for Resuscitation, Transport and Critical Care, ed. Georg Hansmann.
Published by Cambridge University Press. © Cambridge University Press 2009.

is to be made early in pregnancy (or ideally before), and should not be reversed shortly before delivery

Diagnosis and management in the delivery room

- The need for the attendance of a neonatologist during delivery is governed by signs of placental pathology or preterm delivery, not necessarily by drugs or medications taken during pregnancy
- Immediate perinatal problems are not usually caused by substances to which the infant is well adapted, but by placental pathology. Exception: high-dose IV opioids given to a pregnant woman (with or without chronic opioid abuse/substitution) within 4 h of delivery may cause iatrogenic respiratory depression after birth that may require endotracheal intubation and (short-term) mechanical ventilation in the delivery room and the NICU. *Of note, ILCOR (2005) does no longer recommend the use of naloxone in the delivery room* because evidence in the literature on neonatal drug dosing is poor, and health care providers may actually cause *iatrogenic opioid withdrawal syndrome* (seizures!) by administrating naloxone to babies born to women on chronic IV opioids (e.g., heroin) or methadone substitution therapy. Instead, secure the airway, provide adequate ventilation, obtain a full maternal history and monitor these newborns with respiratory depression in the NICU.

> **!** Chronic maternal opioid abuse or methadone substitution during pregnancy does not lead to neonatal respiratory depression, and there is no place for naloxone in these babies (it can precipitate instantaneous and dramatic narcotic withdrawal associated with seizures/status epilepticus). In fact, in 2005, ILCOR abandoned the opioid receptor antagonist naloxone from the delivery room irrespective of chronic opioid abuse/substitution during pregnancy. *"Naloxone is not recommended as part of the initial resuscitation of newborns with respiratory depression in the delivery room. (. . .) There is no evidence to support or refute the current dose of 0.1 mg/kg (IV or IM)."*[71]

- Well babies should stay with the mother after birth but periodically must be assessed for signs of neonatal withdrawal (abstinence) syndrome starting 2–3 h after birth (e.g., Finnegan score, Lipsitz score, or modifications thereof)

> **!** If use of (multiple) illicit drugs is suspected, preserve the infant's meconium for analysis (substances taken during the last months of pregnancy accumulate in meconium). The infant's drug exposure during the previous 2–3 months can also be asssessed from some hair (mother or infant). In contrast, urine screening of the newborn has low sensitivity (high false-negative rate) – only infants with recent exposure will have a positive test.
>
> Any results of neonatal drug screening are to be kept confidential for legal reasons, but may require involvement of social or child protection services later on.

Monitoring

Follow standard protocol for healthy babies. Additional video EEG or SpO_2 monitoring should be reserved for selected cases.

323

Postnatal management in the nursery

- Rooming-in is appropriate unless other medical problems exist
- Start observing infants of opioid-dependent mothers for evidence of neonatal abstinence syndrome between 2–4 h and 7 days of age (heroin withdrawal strikes early; methadone, late)
- Use a standardized score chart (e.g., Finnegan, Lipsitz score, or modifications thereof) to gauge the severity of the neonatal abstinence syndrome. Scores reflect irritability of the central and autonomic nervous systems (restlessness, agitation, tremors, seizures, wakefulness, sweating, vomiting, diarrhea, nasal stuffiness, hyper- or hypothermia, and mottling) and are helpful in guiding therapy[162–164]
- Score jointly with the mother (as it is usually the mother who has been with the baby during the scoring interval). This may increase her acceptance of her baby's condition

Procedure/therapy in the NICU

- Transfer infants with elevated scores (e.g., Finnegan score >8) to the NICU
- Repeat scoring for another 8-h interval (to decide whether medical therapy is indicated). Prophylactic pharmacological treatment is not appropriate
- Infants with opiate withdrawal and elevated scores are given opiates orally (this reduces the time to regain birth weight and reduces the duration of supportive care[165]). The opiate of choice is morphine solution, 0.1 mg/kg every 6 h. Daily adjustments are made according to effect
- For infants with severe symptoms despite treatment with an opiate, add phenobarbital[166]. Phenobarbital loading dose 10 mg/kg, daily maintenance dose 3–5 mg/kg. While opioid withdrawal is best treated with oral morphine solution, withdrawal from benzodiazepines and other $GABA_A$ agonists is best treated by phenobarbital[167]
- Seizures occurring during opioid withdrawal will respond only to morphine, but not to phenobarbital; similarly, seizures occurring during phenobarbital withdrawal will respond only to phenobarbital. Seizure control may need increased dosages
- Symptoms of nicotine and cocaine withdrawal are mild, and no pharmacological treatment is indicated
- Of neonates exposed to SSRI in utero, about 10% show severe, and 20% mild symptoms of a neonatal abstinence syndrome during the first 4 days of life[168] that usually disappear by 2 weeks of age[169]. There is no established treatment of SSRI withdrawal symptoms. Keep in mind that newborns exposed to SSRI have an increased risk of PPHN[161], although the overall risk is quite small
- Emphasis on pharmacological alleviations of symptoms should not detract from establishing effective nursing comfort measures (noise and light control, swaddling, feeding on demand, pacifiers, mittens)
- Start discharge planning early. Mother may need supervision when caring for the baby at home
- Involve social workers and eventually child protection services early (in pregnancy or during the hospital stay)

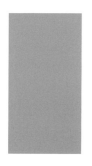

Prenatal and postnatal arrhythmias

Tilman Humpl

Arrhythmias in infants are relatively rare, but they may become evident during pregnancy or early after birth. Transient fetal rhythm disturbances are common and most of these are harmless. However, there are a few arrhythmias that may result in hemodynamic impairment. The diagnostic approach to fetal arrhythmia has changed over time: fetal magnetocardiography has found its role in addition to echocardiography and Doppler imaging.

Fetal arrhythmias[170]

Epidemiology

- Fetal arrhythmias were found in 11% in 433 fetal echocardiographic examinations[171,172]:
  - Approx. 80% supraventricular premature beats
  - 2% atrial fibrillation
  - 15% supraventricular tachycardia (SVT)
  - 4% atrioventricular (AV) blocks
- Malignant fetal arrhythmias 1:5000 (0.2/1000) pregnancies
  - AV nodal re-entry tachycardia
  - Ectopic atrial tachycardia
  - Atrial flutter (AFlu)

Diagnosis

- Intrauterine
  - Echocardiography (M-mode and Doppler)
  - Magnetocardiography (MCG; transabdominal ECG recording has limited value)
- During the second stage of labor (head reaches the small pelvis):
  - Scalp electrodes

Persistent fetal tachycardia

Definition

- HR >180 bpm

Etiology/pathophysiology

- Hypoxia
- Acidosis
- Maternal fever
- Infection/chorioamnionitis

Neonatal Emergencies: A Practical Guide for Resuscitation, Transport and Critical Care, ed. Georg Hansmann.
Published by Cambridge University Press. © Cambridge University Press 2009.

- Myocarditis
- Maternal or fetal anemia
- Maternal medication
- Maternal hormones (e.g., thyroid hormones)
- Transplacental catecholamine transfer between mother and fetus

> **!** Persistent tachycardia may lead to a non-immunological hydrops of the fetus (see chapter on hydrops fetalis, p. 427). However, there is no linear correlation between fetal heart rate and severity of hydrops.

Procedure/therapy

Depends on gestation of fetus, status of the mother, and presence of fetal decompensation. Delivery is the treatment of choice for the baby with fetal tachycardia, but only the fetus with mature lung development should be considered for delivery[170,173].

Re-entry tachycardia

Typical presentation

HR is 240–290 bpm, very abrupt at the beginning and end, relatively regular heart action.

Procedure/therapy

Response to maternal treatment with digoxin.

Atrial flutter

Associated with structural heart disease: hypoplastic left heart syndrome, Ebstein's malformation or cardiomyopathy.

Typical

Regular atrial rate 300–600 bpm with variable AV block (mostly 1:2–1:4), resulting in a ventricular rate less than the atrial rate.

Epidemiology

More common than re-entry tachycardia.

Procedure/therapy

Maternal treatment with digoxin, amiodarone or sotalol.

Fetal bradycardia

Definition

HR <100 bpm.

Etiology/pathophysiology

Perinatal fetal bradycardia is observed by cardiotocography as early decelerations (caused by fetal head compression during uterine contraction, resulting in vagal stimulation and slowing of the heart rate), late decelerations (associated with uteroplacental insufficiency and provoked by uterine contractions), and variable decelerations are most often associated with nuchal cord complications. Some of the common causes are listed below:

- Prolonged cord compression
- Cord prolapse

- Tetanic uterine contractions
- Paracervical block
- Epidural and spinal anesthesia
- Maternal seizures
- Rapid descent
- Vigorous vaginal examination
- Third-degree AV block (= total heart block) in utero. Estimated incidence is 1:15 000–20 000 live births. Approximately 70% of affected fetuses become evident during the last trimester

> *!* Moderate bradycardia of 80–100 bpm is an alarming sign
> Severe prolonged bradycardia of less than 80 bpm that lasts for 3 min or longer should be considered an EMERGENCY indicating severe fetal hypoxia.

Clinical presentation
Persistent bradycardia/third-degree AV block (see below) can lead to a non-immunological fetal hydrops (see p. 427).

Fetus with normal cardiac structure (e.g., exposure to maternal anti-Ro/SSA or anti-La/SSB antibodies). Third-degree AV block may be associated with congenital heart disease (atrial isomerism, L-TGA (transposition of the great arteries), atrioventricular septal defect).

Procedure/therapy
Optimal management of immune-mediated congenital heart block remains highly controversial[174]. Treatment options include dexamethasone, terbutaline, intravenous immunoglobulin (IVIG).

Postnatal arrhythmias

> *!* In the first week of life up to 5% of all neonates exhibit some disturbance in heart rate or rhythm.

Postnatal arrhythmias in term and near-term newborn infants
Etiology
- Premature atrial contractions (10%–35%)
- Sinus pauses (72%)
- Absent sinus rhythm: in 35% of newborns (25% junctional rhythm, 4% supraventricular tachycardia)[175]

Diagnosis
- Palpation of peripheral pulse and cardiac auscultation
- Standard 12-lead ECG
- 24-h ECG
- Echocardiography (rule out congenital heart disease)
- Blood glucose
- Serum electrolytes (including ionized calcium, magnesium, phosphorus)

Postnatal arrhythmias in preterm and growth-restricted newborn infants

Etiology

- Frequently premature atrial contractions (2%–33%)
- Junctional rhythm (18%–70% of preterm neonates)
- Sinus arrhythmia in almost all preterm neonates[175]

Diagnosis

As for postnatal arrhythmias in term and near-term newborn infants.

❗ Normal sinus rhythm:

- HR stable (variation associated with breathing is physiological)
- HR appropriate for age (term newborn infants 100–160 bpm, preterm newborn infants 100–180 bpm)
- P waves precede each QRS complex with regular PR interval (may be prolonged in first-degree AV block)
- P axis between 0 and +90 degrees (i.e., P waves upright in lead II and inverted in aVR)

Premature atrial contractions

Definition

Premature P-waves with a different morphology. QRS is narrow, T waves are often discordant.

Procedure/therapy

Observe and refer to pediatric cardiologist. Usually benign.

Premature ventricular contractions

Definition

Wide and unusual QRS complex occurring before the next expected QRS complex in a regular rhythm (no premature P wave preceding the premature QRS complex).

Procedure/therapy

Commonly seen in up to 20% of healthy neonates. Rule out asymptomatic VT, structural or functional cardiac disease (echocardiography), or prolonged QT interval.

Tachycardic arrhythmias (Figure 3.9; see also Figure 3.10)

Definition

The most common types of postnatal tachycardiac arrhythmias are:

- Sinus tachycardia: regular HR >160 bpm
- *Transient* neonatal sinus tachycardia: HR 180–190 bpm, frequently seen in healthy term newborns (HR hardly ever >220–240 bpm)
- *Persistent* tachycardia (identification of P waves may be difficult)

Etiology

- Hypovolemia
- Elevated core temperature (check incubator temperature!)
- Hyperthyroidism

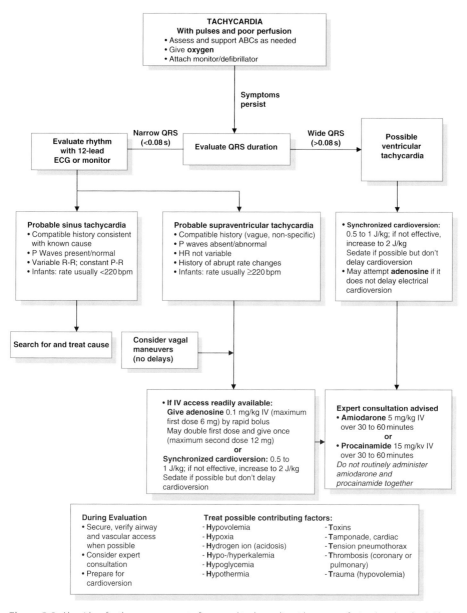

TACHYCARDIA
With pulses and poor perfusion
- Assess and support ABCs as needed
- Give **oxygen**
- Attach monitor/defibrillator

Symptoms
persist

Narrow QRS
(<0.08 s)

Evaluate rhythm
with 12-lead
ECG or monitor

Evaluate QRS duration

Wide QRS
(>0.08 s)

Possible
ventricular
tachycardia

Probable sinus tachycardia
- Compatible history consistent
  with known cause
- P Waves present/normal
- Variable R-R; constant P-R
- Infants: rate usually <220 bpm

Probable supraventricular tachycardia
- Compatible history (vague, non-specific)
- P waves absent/abnormal
- HR not variable
- History of abrupt rate changes
- Infants: rate usually ≥220 bpm

- **Synchronized cardioversion:**
  0.5 to 1 J/kg; if not effective,
  increase to 2 J/kg
  Sedate if possible but don't
  delay cardioversion
- May attempt **adenosine** if it
  does not delay electrical
  cardioversion

Search for and treat cause

Consider vagal
maneuvers
(no delays)

- **If IV access readily available:**
  Give **adenosine** 0.1 mg/kg IV (maximum
  first dose 6 mg) by rapid bolus
  May double first dose and give once
  (maximum second dose 12 mg)
  or
  Synchronized cardioversion: 0.5 to
  1 J/kg; if not effective, increase to 2 J/kg
  Sedate if possible but don't delay
  cardioversion

Expert consultation advised
- **Amiodarone** 5 mg/kg IV
  over 30 to 60 minutes
  or
- **Procainamide** 15 mg/kv IV
  over 30 to 60 minutes
  Do not routinely administer
  amiodarone and
  procainamide together

During Evaluation
- Secure, verify airway
  and vascular access
  when possible
- Consider expert
  consultation
- Prepare for
  cardioversion

Treat possible contributing factors:
- **H**ypovolemia
- **H**ypoxia
- **H**ydrogen ion (acidosis)
- **H**ypo-/hyperkalemia
- **H**ypoglycemia
- **H**ypothermia

- **T**oxins
- **T**amponade, cardiac
- **T**ension pneumothorax
- **T**hrombosis (coronary or
  pulmonary)
- **T**rauma (hypovolemia)

Figure 3.9 Algorithm for the management of neonatal tachycardia with poor perfusion (weak pulses). Please note: Neonates with ventricular tachycardia may have a narrow QRS complex. Modified from: Ralston M *et al. PALS Provider Manual.* Dallas, TX: American Heart Association, 2006.

- Hypoxia
- Pain
- Anemia
- Medications
  - Atropine
  - Pancuronium

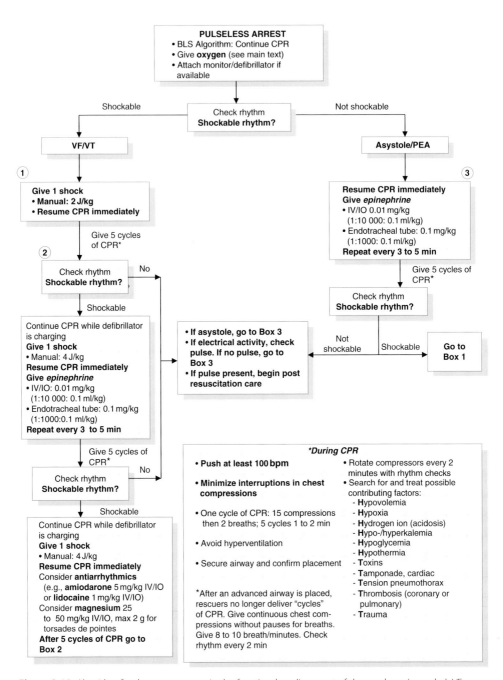

Figure 3.10 Algorithm for the management in the functional cardiac arrest of the newborn (no pulse). VF = ventricular fibrillation, VT = Ventricular tachycardia, PEA = pulseless electrical activity. Of note, PALS recommends the use of epinephrine in 1:1000 dilution for ET drug administration whereas NRP recommends 1:10 000 dilution. PALS and NRP (Fig. 3.8) algorithms differ (e.g. compression/PPV ratio). Please note: neonates with ventricular tachycardia may have a narrow QRS complex. Modified from: Ralston M *et al. PALS Provider Manual.* Dallas, TX: American Heart Association, 2006.

- Catecholamines
- Methylxanthine (theophylline, caffeine), and other medications with chronotropic or dromotropic effects

Supraventricular tachycardia (SVT)

Epidemiology Most common arrhythmia in infants. Incidence is 1:250 to 1:1000 infants.

Etiology
- Ectopic focus
- Re-entry tachycardia
- Accessory bundle (>75% of infants), e.g., Wolff–Parkinson–White syndrome

Pathophysiology Usually tolerated by the newborn, however after 24–72 h, sometimes signs of myocardial failure (decrease of cardiac output by shortened diastole, leading to impairment of coronary blood flow and myocardial perfusion), and rarely cardiogenic shock.

Clinical presentation Paroxysmal (sporadic) occurrence is possible. Pallor, cyanosis, agitation, poor feeding, vomiting, tachypnea, and persistent crying. Structural heart disease in 8%–25% (most common: Ebstein's anomaly, congenitally corrected transposition of the great arteries, tricuspid atresia, cardiac rhabdomyoma). There is a 20% risk of recurrence, which drops significantly after 1 year of age.

Diagnosis
- Sudden onset
- HR usually >240–300 bpm
- Fixed R-R interval
- Constant and narrow QRS complexes, P waves often indistinguishable
- P waves can be negative
- No change in HR with activity or crying

DDx Sinus tachycardia with a HR <240 bpm, variability of the HR, etc.

Diagnostic work-up
- Electrolytes (including ionized calcium, magnesium, phosphorus), ABG, blood glucose
- 12-lead ECG including right precordial leads
- Eventually echocardiogram when stable

Procedure/therapy Aim: decelerate AV conduction to decrease ventricular rate. Refer to pediatric cardiology:
- *Acute therapy:*
  - Short (4–6 s) application of ice pack or ice water to the forehead, i.e., "diving reflex" (more successful than other vagal maneuvers, e.g., carotic sinus massage; massage of eye ball is obsolete)
  - Avoid: apnea, aspiration and longer ice pack application (possible fat tissue necrosis)
  - Adenosine IV with ECG recording (→ transient AV block and sinus bradycardia by changing the conduction in potassium and calcium channels; see Figure 3.11) and defibrillator/cardioverter standby (see below)
  - Establish venous access. Use central line if present, otherwise give drug through peripheral venous access (preferably on the right arm)
  - *Adenosine (stock solution 3 mg/ml):*
    - PIV (right arm) / central IV line/IO

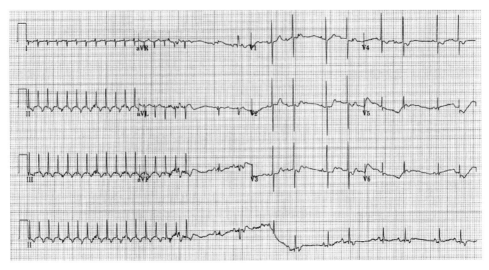

Figure 3.11 Supraventricular tachycardia and its pharmacological conversion to normal sinus rhythm by adenosine IV administration. Adenosine-induced transient AV block and sinus bradycardia, followed by normal sinus rhythm, is best seen in lead II (last row).

- First dose 0.1 mg/kg/dose rapid IV push (use 1/2 dose e.g. in patients status post heart transplantation)
- Second dose 0.2 mg/kg/dose rapid IV push (PALS 2006)[176]
- Adenosine should always be followed by rapid flush with 5–10 ml normal saline. Half-life of adenosine is very short (1–5 s). Use central IV line if available

Adenosine (stock 3 mg/ml, diluted 1:5) – emergency dosing chart

Body weight	First dose	Second dose	Third dose
1.5–2.5 kg	0.2 mg ≅ 0.3 ml *(1:5 dilution)*	0.3 mg ≅ 0.5 ml *(1:5 dilution)*	0.45 mg ≅ 0.75 ml *(1:5 dilution)*
2.5–3.5 kg	0.3 mg ≅ 0.5 ml *(1:5 dilution)*	0.45 mg ≅ 0.75 ml *(1:5 dilution)*	0.6 mg ≅ 1 ml *(1:5 dilution)*

Legend: Doses (in ml) for adenosine (stock = 3 mg/ml), diluted 1:5 (then 0.1 ml = 60 µg)

- If first adenosine dose unsuccessful or only has transient effect in a stable patient, repeat single dose after 2 min and increase dose by 0.05–0.1 mg/kg/dose (see Table above). Usual maximum single dose is 0.25 mg/kg
- *Rules of thumb for the use of adenosine:*
  - Perform synchronized cardioversion if patient unstable or three doses of adenosine IV if unsuccessful
  - Use central IV line if available
  - PIV should be as close as possible to the heart (right arm preferred)
  - ECG monitoring + documentation
  - Have defibrillator/cardioverter at the bedside when giving adenosine IV

- *What to do after the first dose of adenosine IV:*
  - SVT converts usually 15–25 s after adenosine injection. If not and patient is hemodynamically stable, consider second and third dose of adenosine (see above)
  - If atrial flutter is the cause, P waves become apparent after administration of adenosine. Caution – adverse effects of adenosine: rarely arrhythmia (atrial fibrillation/flutter, ventricular fibrillation; caution: do not use in known Wolf–Parkinson–White syndrome), bronchospasm, arterial hypotension, flush. Be prepared for resuscitation and cardioversion
  - Cardioversion 0.5 J/kg
  - Transesophageal pacing (controversial): special equipment and experience are necessary
  - Analgesia and sedation as indicated
  - Transfer to NICU after acute treatment (if not yet done)

> *!* Digoxin is not effective in the acute situation of SVT.

- *Long-term treatment:*
  - Refer to pediatric cardiology
  - For recurring SVT, may consider digoxin (caution: possible overdose), β-blocker (propanolol, atenolol, sotalol), propafenone, or amiodarone

Ventricular tachycardia (VT, VTach)

Epidemiology Relatively uncommon in neonates.

Definition
- Non-sustained VT: up to a duration of 30 s
- Sustained VT: duration longer than 30 s

In typical VT HR is mostly 120–200 bpm, P waves are absent or dissociated (in rare cares 1:1 retrograde VA conduction), broad QRS complexes with different morphology from sinus QRS (caution: in the newborn QRS may not be very broad, however in most cases >0.08 s), altered QRS morphology (monomorphic or polymorphic), T waves are discordant with QRS (Figure 3.12).

Etiology/pathophysiology
- Cardiomyopathies
- Myocarditis
- Potassium imbalance (particularly hypokalemia)
- Maternal cocaine or heroin abuse
- Congenital heart disease (e.g., severe aortic stenosis, coronary anomalies, e.g., anomalous origin of the left coronary artery from the pulmonary artery or ALCAPA)
- Cardiac tumors
- Coronary embolism/ischemia
- Air embolism (central catheter!)

Diagnosis/work-up 12-lead ECG (eventually 24-h ECG). Electrolytes (including ionized calcium, magnesium, phosphorus), ABG, blood glucose

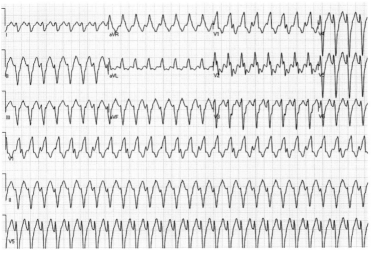

Figure 3.12
Ventricular tachycardia. Key features: HR <200 bpm, absent or dissociated P waves (in rare cares 1:1 retrograde VA conduction), broad QRS complexes (caution: in the newborn QRS may not be very broad, however in most cases >0.08 s), altered QRS morphology (monomorphic or polymorphic), T waves are discordant with QRS.

DDx. SVT, junctional tachycardia, atrial flutter with aberrant conduction, sinus tachycardia with aberrant conduction.

Clinical presentation Minimal symptoms despite tachycardia – most children will be symptomatic (lethargy, tachypnea, pale, mottling or cyanosis)
Hemodynamic effects:

- Impaired diastolic filling of the ventricle and diminished coronary artery flow →
  decrease in cardiac output and myocardial ischemia

> *!* *Persistent* ventricular tachycardia is an EMERGENCY.

Procedure/therapy Immediate referral to pediatric cardiology! In arterial hypotension/
unconsciousness/apathy: synchronized cardioversion with 1–2 J/kg.

Rare types of tachycardia
Junctional ectopic tachycardia (JET)
- Automatic rhythm arising from AV node or bundle of His
- Narrow QRS
- Ventricular rate higher than atrial rate
- AV dissociation
- Congenital/familial or postoperative (cardiac)
- Difficult to treat. Cool core temperature to 34°C (intubate and provide fedation/analgesia)

Accelerated baseline idioventricular rhythm = ectopic focal tachycardia:
- Slower heart rate (mostly only 10% above normal sinus rhythm)
- Change of sinus rhythm and ventricular rhythm
- AV dissociation
- Usually no hemodynamic effect
- Neonates are asymptomatic, specific treatment is not necessary

Bradycardic arrhythmias (Figure 3.13; see also Figure 3.10)

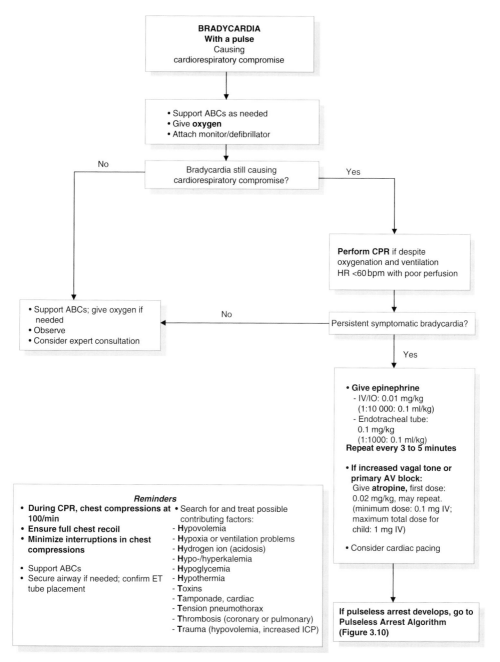

Figure 3.13 Algorithm for the management of neonatal bradycardia. Of note, PALS recommends to use epinephrine 1:1000 dilution for ET drug administration (NRP recommends 1:10 000). PALS and NRP (Figure 3.8) algorithms differ (e.g., compression/PPV ratio). Modified from: Ralston M *et al. PALS Provider Manual.* Dallas, TX: American Heart Association, 2006.

Sinus bradycardia

Definition Regular HR <100 bpm (while awake) / <80 bpm (resting or sleeping). Transient versus persistent bradycardia may be differentiated.

Etiology
- Increased intracranial pressure, increased vagal tone:
  - Pharyngeal stimulation (tube feeding, suctioning)
  - Gastric distension
  - Obstruction of the upper airways
  - Valsalva maneuver, e.g., while crying and straining (e.g., defecation)
  - Drugs (via placenta or breast milk)
- Hypothermia
- Hypothyroidism
- Hydrocephalus

Procedure/therapy Most bradycardias in the newborn are transient and benign with apnea/ cyanosis → bag-and-mask ventilation. When persistent, atropine: 0.1 mg IV. Intermittent bradycardia with apnea is common in a premature baby.

Long QT syndrome (LQTS)

Typical QTc >0.45 s, positive family history (sudden cardiac death, syncope)

Clinical presentation Syncopy, seizures, hemodynamic failure, pathological audiometry (otoacoustic emissions and auditory evoked potentials), implicated in the pathogenesis of sudden infant death syndrome in approximately 10% (?). Potentially triggered by drugs (e.g., doxapram). Estimated incidence is 1:5000–10 000.

> **!** Longer bradycardic episodes may be caused by (recurrent) apnea.

Diagnosis Electrolytes (including ionized calcium, magnesium, phosphorus), 12-lead ECG, 24-h ECG. Clinical diagnosis: genetic testing for known mutations. Clinical association: congenital heart block 5%, congenital deafness 5%, congenital heart disease 12%. Jervell and Lange–Nielsen syndrome: autosomal-recessive form of LQTS (congenital deafness). Romano–Ward syndrome: autosomal-dominant form of LQTS.

Procedure/therapy Transfer to NICU, immediate referral to pediatric cardiology.

Atrioventricular block (AVB)

First-degree AV block (delayed AV conduction) **Definition:** Prolonged PR interval (for age and HR). Upper limit for the newborn on the first day of life: PR interval 160 ms, 140 ms thereafter.
Incidence: 6% of all healthy newborns.
Cause: congenital heart diseases (e.g., AVSD, ASD, Ebstein's anomaly), drugs (e.g., digoxin), trauma/ischemia after heart surgery.

Second-degree AV block (intermittent loss of AV conduction)
- Mobitz type I (Wenckebach phenomenon)
  - **Definition**: Gradual lengthening of PR interval followed by a P wave without a subsequent QRS complex ("dropped beat"). PR interval increases with successive beats, until the conduction fails, i.e., P wave lacks a subsequent QRS complex ("dropped beat"). The pause resulting in the rhythm is shorter than a doubled P-P interval

- **Etiology** Occurs typically in patients with an increased vagal tone or during sleep
- **Therapy** not necessary
- **Mobitz type II**
  - **Definition:** Intermittent failure of AV conduction ("all or none"), no prolongation of the PR interval. 2:1, 3:1 or 4:1 AV block (P/QRS ratio)
  - **Etiology:** Heart disease (e.g., myocarditis, cardiomyopathy, congenital heart disease)
  - **Clinical presentation:** Caution: possible transition to third-degree AV block
  - **Procedure/therapy:** Transfer to NICU, observe (cardiac monitor). Refer to pediatric cardiology. Permanent pacemaker implantation may be necessary (rarely required)

Third-degree AV block (syn. complete heart block, CHB)

- **Definition:** Complete failure of AV conduction, P-waves have no relation to QRS complexes (Figure 3.14)
- **Etiology:** Frequently seen in association with maternal systemic lupus erythematosus (SLE), Sjögren's syndrome or other collagenoses. Maternal anti-Ro/SSA and anti-La/SSB antibodies are able to cross the placenta and damage the cardiac conduction system of the fetus. Other distinctive features in these affected neonates are: skin changes, liver dysfunction, leucopenia, thrombocytopenia, hemolytic anemia. Of the neonates born to mother with SLE 6%–20% have congenital heart disease
  - Risk of third-degree AV block when maternal anti-Ro/SSA and anti La/SSB antibodies are present: 1%–2%[173]. Third-degree AV block occurs in up to 20% of siblings subsequently born to infants with congenital third-degree AV block[177]
  - Maternal SLE and neonatal third-degree AV block: requires permanent pacemaker implantation in 50% of cases. Mortality in the neonatal period is over 15%[178,179], recurrence rate for third-degree AV block in subsequent pregnancies is 10%–15%
  - Associated with congenital heart disease, e.g., heterotaxy syndrome, l-TGA
- **Epidemiology**
  Estimated incidence of isolated third-degree AV block: 1:15 000 to 1:20 000 (0.05–0.07/1000) pregnancies[180]

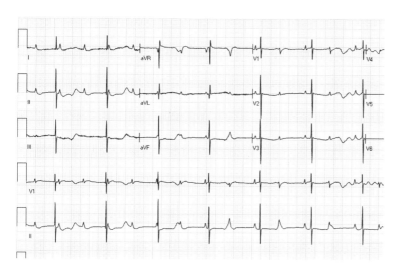

Figure 3.14
Complete heart block (third-degree AV block). Key features: complete failure of AV conduction, P-waves have no relation to QRS complexes (see lead II, last row).

- **Prenatal diagnosis**

  Detection in the fetus by echocardiography between 18 and 24 weeks of gestation[181]: evaluation of cardiac rhythm and function, hydrops? Non-immunological hydrops (p. 427) is associated with structural heart disease or arrhythmia (20%–50%).

- **Prenatal therapy**[182]

  - Dexamethasone
  - IVIG
  - Plasmapheresis
  - Beta$_2$ sympathomimetics (e.g., terbutaline) during pregnancy (may increase fetal heart rate and eventually delay the development of fetal hydrops)
  - Frequently cesarean section (before the expected date) may be necessary, since fetal heart rate monitoring during the vaginal delivery is difficult

- **Clinical presentation**

  HR may rise for a short time immediately after birth – possibly due to the increased release of endogenous catecholamines – but may return to bradycardic baseline after a few hours.

- **Diagnosis/monitoring**

  S_aO_2, ECG, BP, blood gas analysis, blood glucose, electrolytes

- **Procedure/therapy in the delivery room/NICU**

  - Isoprenaline 0.2–0.6 µg/kg/min IV[178]
  - Emergency pacemaker treatment in the delivery room is rarely necessary (→ pediatric cardiologist). If indicated, temporary placement of transesophageal or transcutaneous pacemaker
  - Early arrangements with a pediatric heart center
  - Indication for permanent pacemaker implantation because of underlying cardiac disease as follows:
    - Persistent heart rate <55 bpm
    - Cardiac failure or structural heart diseases (e.g., in congenitally corrected transposition of the great arteries, heterotaxy syndrome)
    - Cardiomegaly with impaired ventricular function
    - Broad QRS complexes
    - Prolonged QTc interval
  - Rule out congenital heart disease (→ echocardiography)

- **Prognosis**

  About 50% of these infants require a permanent pacemaker, mostly within the first month of life. Mortality is relatively high, about 20%[177]. The prognosis of third-degree AV block (= total heart block) + fetal hydrops is very poor

Secondary ECG changes/arrhythmias
Hyperkalemia

- Peaked, tent-like T waves
- Disappearance of P waves
- Prolonged PR interval
- Prolonged QRS complexes

- Ventricular fibrillation
- Cardiac arrest

Hypokalemia
- Prominent U wave
- Flattened or biphasic T waves
- ST-segment depression

Hypocalcemia
- Prolonged QT interval

Hypercalcemia
- Shortened ST segment without affecting the duration of the T wave

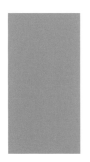

Critical congenital cardiovascular defects

Georg Hansmann and Tilman Humpl

Basic approach to cardiovascular defects in neonates and young infants

Acyanotic and cyanotic cardiovascular defects

Acyanotic cardiovascular defects (approx. 80%)

- *With left-to-right shunt*[175]:
  - Atrial septal defect (ASD I; ASD II, as isolated lesion: approx. 5%–10% of all congenital heart defects), sinus venosus defect
  - Ventricular septal defect (VSD, as isolated lesion: approx. 15%–20% of all congenital heart defects)
  - Atrioventricular septal defect (AVSD, syn.: AV canal; accounts for about 2% of all congenital heart defects)
  - Patent ductus arteriosus (PDA; in 5%–10% of all term newborns with congenital heart defects)
- *With valvular, sub- or supravalvular obstruction*[175]:
  - Aortic stenosis (AS, approx. 3%–6% of all congenital heart defects: valvular, sub- or supravalvular)
  - Pulmonary stenosis (PS, approx. 8%–12% of all congenital heart defects: valvular, sub- or supravalvular)
  - Coarctation of the aorta (CoA, approx. 8%–10% of all congenital heart defects; 30% of girls with Turner's syndrome have CoA)
  - Interrupted aortic arch (IAA, Types A–C, approx. 1% of all symptomatic infants with congenital heart defects; 22q11 microdeletion syndrome in more than 15% of patients with IAA)
  - Mitral stenosis
  - Tricuspid stenosis
- *With valvular regurgitation*[175]:
  - Aortic valve regurgitation (syn. insufficiency; abbrev.: AR, AI)
  - Pulmonary valve regurgitation (abbrev. PR, PI)
  - Mitral valve regurgitation (abbrev. MR)
  - Tricuspid valve regurgitation (abbrev. TR, TI)

Neonatal Emergencies: A Practical Guide for Resuscitation, Transport and Critical Care, ed. Georg Hansmann.
Published by Cambridge University Press. © Cambridge University Press 2009.

Cyanotic cardiovascular defects (approx. 20%)

- *With increased pulmonary blood flow*[175,183]:
  - Single ventricle (double-inlet ventricle: in 80% double-inlet *left* ventricle)
  - Hypoplastic left heart (HLH)
  - TGA + VSD without pulmonary stenosis (PS)
  - TGA without VSD/pulmonary stenosis (severe cyanosis)
  - Double-outlet right ventricle (DORV) + subpulmonary VSD without PS (often associated with sub AS, CoA, IAA) = Taussig–Bing malformation (hemodynamically similar to d-TGA + VSD → results in cyanosis)
  - Tricuspid atresia (TA) + VSD + TGA without PS (type IIc or III)
  - Total anomalous pulmonary venous return (TAPVR, mild-moderate cyanosis)
  - Truncus arteriosus
- *With decreased pulmonary blood flow*[175,184]:
  - TGA + pulmonary stenosis (LVOTO)
  - Single ventricle (double-inlet ventricle) with pulmonary stenosis
  - Tricuspid atresia (TA, exemptions see above)
  - Pulmonary atresia with intact ventricular septum (PA/iVS) and hypoplastic right ventricle
  - Tetralogy of Fallot (ToF), PA/VSD
  - DORV + subaortic VSD + pulmonary stenosis = Fallot's type DORV
  - Truncus arteriosus (TAC) with hypoplastic pulmonary artery
  - Severe Ebstein's anomaly

Duct-dependent and duct-independent cardiovascular defects

Duct-dependent cardiovascular defects can be divided into three groups

Reported percentages are related to all critical (symptomatic) cardiac defects during the first month of life:

- *Duct-dependent cardiovascular disease with critical left heart obstruction (≈35%–45%):*
  - Critical aortic stenosis of the newborn (AoVS)
  - Aortic atresia (HLH)
  - Coarctation of the aorta (CoA)
  - Interrupted aortic arch (IAA)
  - Shone's complex
- *Duct-dependent cardiovascular disease with critical right heart obstruction (≈20%):*
  - Critical pulmonary stenosis of the newborn (PaVS)
  - Pulmonary atresia (PaVA) with or without VSD
  - Extreme types of tetralogy of Fallot (ToF)
  - Tricuspid atresia (TA)
  - Ebstein's anomaly (some cases)
- *D-Transposition of the great arteries (≈25%–30%):*
  - d-TGA without VSD with a restrictive (too small) PFO/ASD
  - d-TGA without VSD, but a large PFO/ASD
  - d-TGA with VSD

- d-TGA with (or without) VSD and pulmonary stenosis (LVOTO)
- d-TGA with (or without) VSD and (sub-) aortic stenosis (RVOTO)

Duct-independent cardiovascular defects
- Most congenital cardiovascular defects not listed in the classification above
- See further literature[175,185]
- See pp. 348–50

Special subgroup: total anomalous pulmonary venous return (TAPVR, duct-independent)

> **!** None of these cardiovascular defects can be diagnosed accurately in the delivery room without echocardiography – perhaps with the exception of a preductal coarctation of the aorta with a high BP gradient. Establishing the final diagnosis is not expected from the neonatal/transport team. However, it is important to classify cardiac emergencies, i.e., when they occur and to discuss the underlying pathophysiology.

The specific management of PDA of the preterm newborn infant, and congenital cardiovascular diseases of the neonatal period and early infancy (critical AoVS, HLH, CoA, IAA, critical PaVS, PaVA/IVS, ToF, TA, d-TGA, and sometimes AVSD, TAPVR) will be discussed separately (for cardiac arrhythmias, see p. 325; for PDA, see p. 380; for PPHN, see p. 392). For standard echocardiographic transducer positions, see Figure 3.15)

Management of cardiovascular emergencies in neonates and young infants
Pre- and postnatal cardiac arrhythmias
See, pp. 325–39

Sudden closure of the ductus arteriosus (see, Algorithm, Figure 3.16)
Cardiovascular defects with duct-dependent systemic blood flow
Etiology
- AoVS, HLH, IAA, preductal CoA

Clinical presentation
- *Shock during the first (or second) week of life as a primary symptom:*
  - Pale-grayish skin color
  - Cool extremities, capillary refill >2 s, weak or absent pulses (especially in lower extremities)
  - Pulmonary edema may be present
  - Hepatomegaly may be present
  - CoA may become symptomatic as late as at 4 weeks of life
- With significant left heart obstruction (CoA, IAA, AoVS): "differential cyanosis" as a sign of a ductal right-to-left shunting may occur
- Acidosis

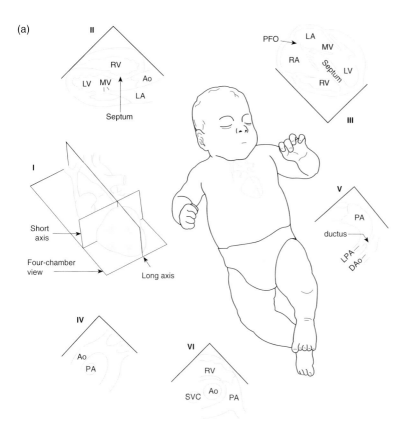

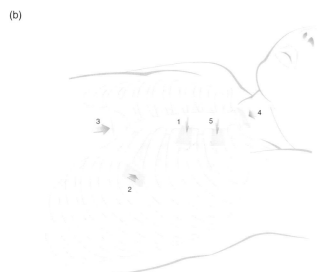

Figure 3.15 Routine position of ultrasound probes, standard echocardiographic views (a), and an illustration of ultrasound probe-positions (b).
1 = 2nd to 4th intercostal space; left parasternal long axis view = II, short axis view = VI.
2 = 5th intercostal space in midclavicular line, apical four-chamber view = III.
3 = subxiphoid and subcostal four-chamber view = III.
4 = jugular = IV.
5 = 2nd intercostal space, high left parasternal short axis view = V ("ductal view").
RA, right atrium; RV, right ventricle; LA, left atrium; LV, left ventricle; MV, mitral valve; PFO, patent foramen ovale; Ao, aorta; DAo, descending aorta; PA, pulmonary artery; LPA, left pulmonary artery; SVC, superior vena cava.

Postnatal management of critical, duct-dependent cardiovascular defects

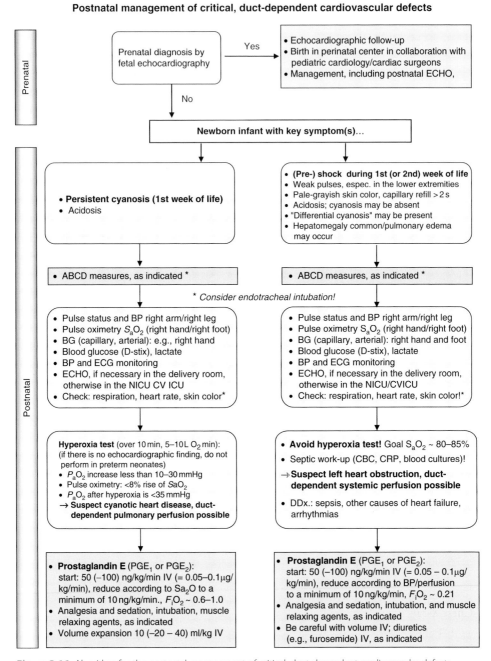

Figure 3.16 Algorithm for the postnatal management of critical, duct-dependent cardiovascular defects.

DDx. Sepsis (especially for HLH), arrhythmias (p. 325), heart failure)

Diagnosis in the delivery room/nursery

- Pulse oximeter (HR, S_pO_2)
- BP (right arm/left arm/one leg or all four extremities)

- Pulse status (all four limbs)
- Preductal blood gas analysis (arterial, if possible), blood glucose, lactate
- Body temperature
- Avoid hyperoxia test, use room air when S_pO_2 >85%, even lower S_pO_2 goal when (prenatal) diagnosis of left heart obstruction is confirmed by echocardiography ($\approx$75%–80%)
- Blood tests including: CBC, CRP, coagulation profile, blood culture, type and screen/cross
- Echocardiography (rarely in delivery room, more commonly in ICU/nursery)

Therapy in the delivery room/nursery
- *Use oxygen with caution:* oxygen increases pulmonary blood flow and hence lowers systemic perfusion (systemic blood flow)! After initial care/resuscitation, aim for a F_iO_2 of 0.21 (even after intubation). In neonates with HLH: aim for P_aO_2 of 40 mmHg and S_aO_2 75% (when peripheral perfusion is poor, only a preductal arterial blood gas is reliable). HLH is frequently diagnosed prenatally
- *Prostaglandin E_1 (PGE$_1$):* start with 50 ng/kg/min (= 0.05 µg/kg/min) continuous IV; maximum dosage is 100 ng/kg/min (=0.1 µg/kg/min), however some set the PGE$_1$ maximum as high as 400 ng/kg/min[175]). When peripheral (systemic) perfusion has improved with PGE$_1$, attempt to reduce infusion step-by-step to the minimum required to keep the ductus open (in general, do not go lower than 10 ng/kg/min = 0.01 µg/kg/min). Caution: apnea, hypotension, fever, bradycardia are side-effects of PGE$_1$
- *Intubation, as indicated:* provide analgesia and sedation; administer muscle relaxing agent, as needed. If anticipated transport time is longer than 30 min and continuous infusion of PGE$_1$ is required, consider intubation; otherwise, be prepared for intubation during transport
- *Use volume – if at all – with caution* until the cardiac function is evaluated by echocardiography (e.g., normal saline 5–10 ml/kg/bolus).
- *Administer diuretics to decrease preload* (e.g., furosemide 0.5–1 mg/kg/dose; rarely indicated in the delivery room)

Monitoring Pre- and postductal S_aO_2 (pulse oximeter), blood pressure, ECG; check ET tube position, as indicated. Determine ABG/CBG and blood glucose prior to departure.

Diagnosis in the NICU/PICU/cardiac ICU
- ABG, lactate, blood glucose, blood chemistry (including: CRP (IL-6), creatinine, urea, liver enzymes, coagulation panel, CK, troponin), HIV/hepatitis serology, type and screen/cross. If sepsis is considered as a differential diagnosis, extended septic work-up (additional blood culture(s), LP, bladder puncture)
- Chest X-ray
- Transthoracic echocardiography
- ECG
- Request maternal HBs Ag status and blood group
- Newborn metabolic screening test (>48 h post partum), and chromosomal analysis, as indicated

Procedure/therapy in the NICU/PICU/cardiac ICU
- Adjust PGE$_1$ depending on clinical status, systemic perfusion, P_aO_2, S_pO_2 and echocardiography (ductus patent? shunt volume?)

- (Usually) central venous access (UVC, internal jugular vein, subclavian vein, femoral vein), consider arterial line (UAC, radial artery, femoral artery)
- Inotropes/vasopressors (e.g., dopamine, milrinone, epinephrine) may be required, depending on BP and cardiac function. Avoid inotropes/vasopressors in significant LV obstruction (AoVS, hypertrophied obstructive cardiomyopathy)
- Cardiac catheterization ± intervention may be indicated:
  - In severe AoVS → balloon valvuloplasty
  - In HLH with restrictive PFO/ASD → enlargement of PFO/ASD
- Furosemide (0.5–1 mg/kg/dose IV) to decrease preload
- Broad-spectrum antibiotics IV, as indicated
- For specific treatment of most common critical cardiac defects in the newborn period, see p. 350–79.

In duct-/shunt-dependent critical heart disease, think of a **fluid-filled U-shaped tube**:

*When PVR ↓ then pulmonary blood flow ↑ and systemic blood flow ↓ (to be avoided in left-sided obstructions such as hypoplastic left heart syndrome).

*When PVR ↑ then pulmonary blood flow ↓ and systemic blood flow ↑. In HLH/single ventricle with generally high pulmonary and low systemic blood flow, the goal of balanced Qp/Qs (1:1) may be achieved by optimizing ventilation (pH 7.35, $PaCO_2$ 45–50) or by reducing F_iO_2 <0.21 (0.18–0.20) through the addition of nitrogen or carbon dioxide to the inspiratory gas mix.

Cardiovascular defects with duct-dependent pulmonary blood flow

Etiology Pulmonary atresia (PaVA), critical pulmonary valve stenosis (PaVS), extreme types of ToF (ToF with very severe PS = functionally pulmonary atresia), hypoplastic right heart/tricuspid atresia (TA). Significant cyanosis also in d-TGA with restrictive (very small) PFO/ASD and intact ventricular septum (so-called "simple TGA").

Clinical presentation
- *Central cyanosis during the first week of life is a key symptom*
- Acidosis
- Signs of right-sided congestion/RV failure (e.g., hepatomegaly, peripheral edema) may be present. Congestive heart failure (e.g., tachypnea/dyspnea, pulmonary edema, hepatomegaly) can develop in d-TGA with an intact ventricular septum ("simple TGA") and (earlier) in the less cyanotic d-TGA with VSD/large PDA

! Differential diagnosis of central cyanosis

- Cardiovascular: d-TGA, HLH, critical PaVS/PaVA, ToF, TA, PDA + PS, Ebstein's anomaly, and others
- Pulmonary: pneumothorax, RDS/atelectasis, pleural effusion, congenital diaphragmatic hernia, PPHN
- CNS: perinatal asphyxia, withdrawal reactions to analgesia and sedation, intrauterine fetal stress
- Hematologic and metabolic disorders: polycythemia, methemoglobinemia (i.e., normal P_aO_2, increased methemoglobin)
- Peripheral cyanosis, e.g., in septic shock and hypothermia

Diagnosis in the delivery room/nursery
- Pulse oximeter (HR, S_aO_2)
- BP (right arm/leg)
- Pulse status
- Preductal BG (arterial, if possible), BS, lactate
- Body temperature
- Hyperoxia test
- Blood work, including coagulation, type and screen/cross, blood cultures, as indicated
- Echocardiography, if possible

! The very young newborn who exhibits severe cyanosis (in the first hours of life) is likely to
have one of the following: transposition of the great arteries, pulmonary atresia, or Ebstein's
malformation[186]. However, other defects are in the DDx (p. 341).

Therapy in the delivery room/nursery
- *Prostaglandin E_1 (PGE$_1$):* start with 50 ng/kg/min (=0.05 µg/kg/min) IV (maximum dosage 100 ng/kg/min = 0.1 µg/kg/min); when peripheral perfusion has improved with PGE$_1$, attempt to reduce step-by-step to a minimum required dose to keep ductus sufficiently open, but generally not lower than 10 ng/kg/min (=0.01 µg/kg/min) IV. Caution: apnea, hypotension, bradycardia are side-effects of PGE$_1$!
- *Oxygen supplemention* depends on the S_aO_2 (caution: iatrogenic closure of the patent ductus with high F_iO_2 is theoretically possible). If intubation is indicated, provide analgesia and sedatives, and possibly muscle relaxants. For an anticipated transport time of longer than 30 min and continuous infusion of PGE consider intubation; otherwise, consider and be prepared for intubation during the transport
- *Volume IV:* Start with normal saline 10 ml/kg/bolus IV. Bolus increases the cardiac stroke volume to a certain extent, and thus the flow through the ductus arteriosus (right-to-left shunt). Be careful with volume in (de-) compensated heart failure! However, in an emergency such as d-TGA without VSD and restrictive PFO (before BAS = balloon atrial septostomy), the amount of volume needed in order to achieve some shunt volume (PFO/ASD and ductus) may be quite high (total ≈ 25–50 ml/kg IV)
- *4.2% sodium bicarbonate* (0.5 mEq/ml = 0.5 mmol/ml), need in mmol = (negative BE × kg) ÷ 3. If 8.4% stock solution is used, always dilute 1:1 with sterile water to final concentration of 0.5 mEq/ml

---

! Patients with d-TGA, intact ventricular septum and very small (restrictive) atrial communication or those with ToF/PA may not improve their S_aO_2 after intubation and PPV with F_iO_2
1.0, because the major problems are insufficient blood mixing in d-TGA (depending on
atrial defect, ductus?) or insufficient lung perfusion in ToF/PA.

! PPV and PEEP increase intrathoracic pressure (may improve systemic BP generation) but
decrease cardiac venous return and pulmonary blood flow.

Monitoring Pulse oximeter, blood pressure, ECG. Determine the actual BG and BS before departure. Check ET tube position, as indicated.

347

Diagnosis in the NICU/PICU/cardiovascular ICU
- ABG, lactate, blood glucose, blood chemistry (including: CRP (IL-6), creatinine, urea, liver enzymes, coagulation panel, CK, troponin), HIV/hepatitis serology, type and screen/cross. If sepsis is considered as a differential diagnosis, extended septic work-up (additional blood culture(s), LP, suprapubic bladder puncture)
- Chest X-ray (in d-TGA: cardiomegaly may be present, "egg-shaped heart," increased lung vascular markings)
- Transthoracic echocardiography
- ECG
- Request maternal HBs-Ag status and blood group
- Newborn metabolic screening test ($>48\,h$ post partum), chromosomal analysis, as indicated

Procedure/therapy in the NICU/PICU/cardiovascular ICU
- Adjust PGE_1 dose to clinical presentation, systemic perfusion, S_aO_2 and echocardiography
- Usually obtain central venous access (UVC, internal jugular vein, subclavian vein, femoral vein) and consider arterial line (UAC, radial artery, femoral artery)
- If indicated, initiate/continue buffer therapy (sodium bicarbonate)
- Cardiac catheterization $\pm$ intervention, may be indicated:
  - Balloon valvuloplasty for significant PS
  - Balloon atrial septostomy (Rashkind procedure) in TGA and restrictive PFO/ASD
  - (See Figure 2.41)
- Vasopressors/inotropes (norepinephrine (noradrenaline), dopamine) may be required to increase systemic vascular resistance (SVR) and thus pulmonary blood flow
- Broad-spectrum antibiotic coverage (after cultures), as indicated
- For specific therapy of most common critical cardiac defects in the newborn period, see p. 344

> **!** Avoid vasopressors/inotropes (catecholamines) in outflow tract obstructions (e.g., Tetralogy of Fallot) and lesions that depend on a balanced Q_p:Q_s ratio (e.g., HLH).
> **!** Avoid (further) increase of pulmonary blood flow in left-sided obstructions (HLH, CoA, IAA, AoVS) and d-TGA with restrictive atrial defect.

Congestive heart failure with falling pulmonary vascular resistance (PVR) and subsequently increased left-to-right shunt (4th to 6th week of life)

Etiology
Large VSD, AVSD, large PDA (mostly in preterm infants – congestive heart failure often occurs after improvement of RDS or BPD/CLD), TAC, complex cardiovascular diseases without obstruction between ventricle and PA (e.g., DORV + subaortic VSD without PS).

Pathophysiology
Large left-to-right shunt without pulmonary stenosis $\rightarrow$ cardiac failure.

Clinical presentation
- *Signs of heart failure with (pre-)shock is a key symptom between the 4th and 6th week of life:*
  - Pale-grayish skin color
  - Cool extremities, capillary refill >2 s, weak pulses
  - Tachypnea
  - Increased work of breathing
  - Poor feeding
  - Diaphoresis with feeds
  - Failure to thrive
  - Pulmonary edema may be present
  - Hepatomegaly may be present
- Acidosis (mixed or primarily respiratory)

! Differential diagnosis of heart failure in neonates and young infants:

- Arrhythmias (pp. 325–39: SVT, atrial fibrillation/flutter)
- Structural heart disease (see above); DDx depends on the time of manifestation:
  1. Ventricular failure (often) as early as on the 1st day of life: HLH, severe TI, transient myocardial ischemia, large AV fistula
  2. Ventricular failure in the first week of life: TGA, preterm infants with large PDA and relatively low PVR, TAPVC
  3. Ventricular failure during the 1st to 4th week: severe AoVS or PaVS, IAA, CoA
- Transient myocardial ischemia after perinatal hypoxia-ischemia ("birth asphyxia")
- Cardiomyopathy (e.g., diabetic fetopathy)
- Myocarditis (rare)
- Volume overload (e.g., very late cord clamping, PRBC transfusion, IV fluids, TTTS)
- Severe anemia (e.g., hydrops fetalis, TTTS, perinatal hemorrhage)
- Metabolic causes (e.g., hypoglycemia, hypocalcemia)
- Sepsis (increased cardiac output, warm extremities)

Diagnosis in the emergency room (ER)/NETS/clinical practice/nursery
- Pulse oximeter (HR, S_pO_2)
- BP (right arm, left arm, one leg)
- Pulse status (all four extremities)
- Preductal blood gas analysis (arterial, if possible), blood glucose, lactate
- Body temperature
- Avoid hyperoxia test (!)
- Blood work, including coagulation, blood culture, type and screen/cross
- Echocardiography, as indicated

Therapy in the ER/NETS/clinical practice/nursery:
- *Use oxygen with caution:* oxygen may cause increase of pulmonary blood flow, and at the same time decreases systemic blood flow!
- *No prostaglandin E_1*

- *Endotracheal intubation* may be indicated in an unstable neonate/infant. Should the transport time take longer than 30 min and cardiopulmonary status is borderline, consider intubation as well
- *Restrict volume/fluids IV*
- *Administer diuretics to decrease preload* (e.g., furosemide 0.5–1 mg/kg/dose IV)

Monitoring
Check ET tube position, if needed. Pulse oximeter, blood pressure and ECG. Determine the actual BG and BS before initiation of transport.

Diagnosis in the NICU/PICU/cardiovascular ICU
- ABG, lactate, blood glucose, blood chemistry (including: CRP (IL-6), creatinine, urea, liver enzymes, coagulation panel, CK, troponin), HIV/hepatitis serology, type and screen/cross. If sepsis is considered as a differential diagnosis, extended septic work-up (additional blood culture(s), LP, suprapubic bladder puncture)
- Chest X-ray
- Transthoracic echocardiography to establish diagnosis (Figure 3.14a,b),
- ECG
- Request maternal HBS-Ag status and blood type
- Newborn metabolic screening test (>48 h post partum; might have to repeat later on when enteral intake is adequate); chromosomal analysis, as indicated

Procedure/therapy in the NICU/PICU/cardiovascular ICU
- If indicated: central venous access (UVC, internal jugular vein, subclavian vein, femoral vein) and consider arterial line (UAC, radial artery, femoral artery)
- If indicated: cardiac catheterization (rarely)
- Administer furosemide to decrease the preload (0.5–1 mg/kg/dose IV every 6–12 h)
- Consider milrinone, ACE inhibitor
- Cardiology consult
- If indicated: broad-spectrum antibiotic coverage
- For specific treatment of the frequent critical cardiac diseases in the newborn, see below

Specific approach to critical cardiovascular defects in neonates

Within this chapter, the most common congenital cardiovascular defects will be briefly discussed. With the advances in prenatal ultrasound, cardiac defects are being diagnosed earlier and more accurately[187]. The diagnosis of complex defects may lead to a termination of pregnancy or to a planned delivery in a center with expert experience in neonatology, pediatric cardiology, and pediatric cardiac surgery. Low-birth-weight or preterm infants with congenital heart disease require a meticulous management approach[188].

Due to the complexity of congenital cardiac defects, it is beyond the scope of this book to give a broad and detailed description of anatomy, hemodynamics, treatment, and outcome. Detailed information can be obtained from the standard textbooks on pediatric cardiology and pediatric cardiac critical care[175,185,189]. If a cardiovascular defect is suspected, a pediatric cardiologist must be consulted as soon as possible.

Critical aortic valve stenosis (AoVS)

Definition
Obstruction of the LVOT at the level of the aortic valve. Group: ductal-dependent cardiac defect with critical left-sided obstruction. Classification of aortic stenosis (AS):

- *Valvular:* approx. 70% of aortic stenosis
- *Subvalvular:* approx. 25% of aortic stenosis
- *Supravalvular:* approx. 5% of aortic stenosis (associated with William–Beuren syndrome).

Epidemiology
- Rare

Etiology/pathophysiology
- *Valvular:* stenotic valve, often a bicuspid with thickened cusps and fused commissures. Hypoplasia of the LV and endocardial fibroelastosis are possible. The arterial duct shunts primarily right-to-left. Increasing LV afterload (valvular stenosis, postnatal rise in SVR) leads to decompensation of the LV and fall of cardiac output with possible further decrease of critical coronary perfusion. The closure of the arterial duct may decrease systemic perfusion and symptoms of (pre-) shock arise (see below)
- *Subvalvular:* Obstruction is often absent in early life and becomes evident in childhood
- *Supravalvular:* Localized or diffuse narrowing of the aortic lumen directly above the aortic valve. Symptoms rarely develop in infants but appear frequently in childhood

Clinical presentation
Neonates with critical valvular AS usually present during the first days to weeks of life:

- Shock
- Pallor
- Cardiac failure
- Weak peripheral pulses, capillary refill >2 s
- Tachypnea and dyspnea (at first when stressed, then while at rest)
- (Mostly) no or only mild cyanosis
- Absent (or very faint) heart murmur (systolic murmur may be louder with the improvement in LV function; ejection click may be heard)

DDx.
Sepsis, other cardiac defects with critical left-sided obstruction (HLH, CoA, IAA).

Diagnosis in the delivery room/nursery
Typically symptoms become evident or progress in the nursery or at home:

- Clinical examination, especially auscultation and checking the pulse status
- BP, ECG, S_aO_2
- Signs of sepsis (?), capillary refill (>2 s?)
- Body temperature
- Blood gas, lactate, blood glucose, CBC, chemistry, blood cultures, as indicated
- Echocardiography, as indicated

Therapy in the delivery room/nursery
- PGE continuous IV infusion: start with 50–100 ng/kg/min ($=0.05(-0.1)$ µg/kg/min)
- Avoid catecholamines (increase of myocardial O_2 consumption); if necessary, use epinephrine or dopamine
- Diuretics
- Sedation and intubation, as indicated; (mild) ventilation (no hyperventilation, because pulmonary blood flow will increase and systemic perfusion will decrease)

Monitoring
Pulse oximetry, ECG, blood pressure. Determine actual BG and BS before transport. Check ET tube position, as indicated.

Diagnosis in the NICU/PICU/cardiac ICU
- Chest X-ray (may show pulmonary edema and enlarged heart)
- ABG, lactate, blood glucose, CBC, chemistry, coagulation panel, urine diagnostics (stix, microscopy), blood culture, HIV/hepatitis serology, type and screen/cross match, as indicated
- Echocardiography
- ECG: LVH; repolarization disorder and arrhythmias may be present
- Complete microbiological work-up, if necessary: smears, tracheal secretion, gastric juice, blood culture(s)
- Cardiac catheterization, as indicated

Procedure/therapy in the NICU/PICU/cardiac ICU
- Continue PGE infusion, adjust dose according to clinical presentation and findings of echocardiogram
- Catheter-based interventional balloon valvuloplasty – if feasible according to anatomical features (subsequent aortic insufficiency is frequent with improvement of LV function)[190]. Patients may need PGE IV for several days after balloon dilation.
- Surgical valvulotomy
- Or: Norwood procedure (palliative approach)

Hypoplastic left heart (HLH)
Definition
- Heterogeneous group of cardiac malformations characterized by complex spectrum of anatomic defects:
  - Aortic valve stenosis or atresia
  - Hypoplasia of the ascending aorta/aortic arch
  - Mitral valve stenosis or atresia
  - Hypoplasia of the LV
- Group: ductal-dependent defects with critical left-sided obstruction (Figure 3.17)

Epidemiology
0.164/1000 live births[191]; approx. 1% of all cases of congenital cardiac defects; includes approx. 9% of all cases of congenital cardiac defects that become apparent in the neonatal period; the most frequent cause of cardiac death in the first month of life.

Etiology/pathophysiology

Small LA, reasonable size to minuscule LV, PFO/ASD with left-to-right shunt. During intrauterine life the blood flows reversely through the ascending aorta, coronary arteries, and CNS. The dominant RV pumps blood to both the lungs (via the pulmonary artery) and to the systemic circulation through the descending aorta (via arterial duct). After birth, there is little change, as long as the arterial duct remains open.

Associated cardiac anomalies are uncommon but include: intact atrial septum (emergency: → perform BAS), TAPVR, levo-atrial cardinal vein, complete AVSD, TGA, IAA.

Problems

First, closure of the arterial duct; Second, after birth SVR > PVR, leading to shock and metabolic acidosis.

Clinical presentation in the first hours to days of life:

- Mild cyanosis
- Tachycardia
- Respiratory distress (moist rales may be heard over the lungs)
- Advanced heart failure with severe myocardial dysfunction (ischemia)
- Hypoxia and *shock,* namely:
  - Poor to absent peripheral pulse
  - Tachycardia
  - Cold sweat
  - Capillary refill >2 s
  - Tachydyspnea
  - Cyanosis
  - Usually no (or very faint) heart murmur, sometimes gallop rhythm
  - Hepatomegaly
- Rapidly evolving *pulmonary edema* (S_aO_2 ≪80%) is possible, especially when LA "decompression" through PFO/ASD is not preserved (intact atrial septum)

DDx.

Sepsis, other cyanotic cardiac defects, PPHN, pulmonary diseases. The diagnosis HLH is often already known before birth (prenatal echocardiography).

Prenatal diagnosis

Fetal echocardiography is quite sensitive for prenatal diagnosis of HLH (and other LVOTO).

Diagnosis in the delivery room/nursery

Typically, symptoms begin or become aggravated when the arterial duct closes (or narrows):
- Auscultation, pulse status
- BP, S_aO_2, ECG
- Capillary refill
- Blood gas, lactate, blood glucose, CBC, chemistry, blood cultures, as indicated
- Body temperature
- Echocardiography, as indicated

Therapy in the delivery room/nursery
- *PGE_1 continuous IV infusion:* start with 50 (–100) ng/kg/min = 0.05 (–0.1) µg/kg/min *(goal: to secure systemic circulation by keeping the ductus open)*
- *Increase pulmonary vascular resistance (goal: to improve systemic perfusion)*

> **!** After stabilizing the neonate, avoid oxygen supplement (i.e., after the initial care, aim for a F_iO_2 of 0.21 – even after intubation).

- Desired parameters:
  - P_aO_2 40 mmHg
  - P_aCO_2 40 mmHg
  - S_aO_2 70%–75% (transcutaneous measurements are not always reliable, especially with cold extremities)
- With increased pulmonary blood flow ($S_aO_2 \gg 75\%$):
  - Reduce ventilation, allow P_aCO_2 to increase up to 50 mmHg/pH 7.25–7.3
  - Consider CO_2 supplementation via the inspiratory gas
- No buffer therapy for BE of –2 to –5 mmol/l (i.e., only in severe metabolic acidosis)

Monitoring
Pulse oximetry, ECG, blood pressure. Determine actual BG, lactate and BS before departure. Check ET tube position, as indicated.

Diagnosis in the NICU/PICU/cardiovascular ICU
- Chest X-ray (may show pulmonary edema and moderate cardiomegaly)
- ABG, lactate, blood glucose, CBC, chemistry, coagulation panel, urine diagnostics (stix, microscopy), blood culture, HIV/hepatitis serology, type and screen/cross match, as indicated
- After stabilization of the newborn: echocardiography to establish the diagnosis (Figure 3.17), rule out or diagnose other malformations (i.e., complete echocardiography, abdominal and cerebral ultrasound)
- ECG: right axis deviation, right ventricular hypertrophy (RVH), no LV forces
- Complete microbiological diagnosis, if necessary: smears (limited significance), tracheal secretion, gastric aspirate, blood culture(s)

Procedure/therapy in the NICU/PICU/cardiovascular ICU
- Continue PGE_1 infusion, adjust dose according to clinical presentation and findings of the echocardiogram
- Optimize ventilation:
  - If high saturations and/or increasing lactate (frequent checks): intubate and ventilate on a lower rate with mildly elevated CO_2 and mildly acidotic pH (resulting in a decrease of pulmonary blood flow and an increase in systemic blood flow). Desired parameters: pH 7.25–7.35, P_aO_2 40 mmHg, P_aCO_2 45–50 mmHg, S_pO_2 70%–75% (caution: transcutaneous measurement is not always reliable, especially with cold extremities). If the pulmonary blood flow is too high

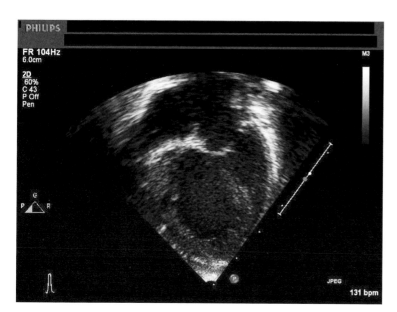

Figure 3.17
Hypoplastic left heart. Echocardiography, four-chamber view. Hypoplastic mitral valve, small left ventricle, patent foramen ovale/atrial septal defect with left-to-right shunt (not shown). The dominant right ventricle pumps blood to both the lungs (via pulmonary artery) and the systemic circulation (i.e., descending aorta via patent ductus arteriosus).

(saturation >85%–90% = "overcirculation"), consider CO_2 supplementation via inspiratory gas or afterload reduction with milrinone (0.33–0.99 µg/kg/min)

- Reduction of systemic vascular resistance with continuous nitroglycerine or milrinone infusion may be necessary (rarely required in the delivery room)
- After stabilization of the newborn: discuss possible treatment options with parents

Surgery

- Staged palliation[192,193]
  - Standard *Norwood operation* (within the first week of life) that includes creation of a neo-aorta and a aortopulmonary shunt or modified Blalock–Taussig shunt as a source of pulmonary blood flow. *Bidirectional cavopulmonary connection* (approx. 3–6 months of age). *Fontan* (approx. 1 year of age). Survival rate: approx. 60%–85% after surgical correction in three stages; unknown morbidity; longer/frequent hospitalization), *or*
  - *Sano modification* (within the first week of life) using a RV-PA conduit as a source of pulmonary blood flow. *Bidirectional cavopulmonary connection* at approx. 3–6 months of age. *Fontan* (approx. 1 year of age). Survival rate: approx. 60%–85% after surgical correction in three stages; unknown morbidity; longer/frequent hospitalization), *or*
  - *"Hybrid procedure"* (within the first week of life): stenting of the arterial duct and bilateral pulmonary artery banding. Advantage: no cardiopulmonary bypass during the newborn period. More complex surgery at second stage (*bidirectional cavopulmonary connection* that includes creation of a neo-aorta and aortic arch augmentation at approx. 3–6 months of age). *Fontan* (approx. 1 year of age)
- *Orthotopic heart transplantation* (transfer to a transplant center: risk of decompensation leading to death while on the waiting list; risk of graft rejection). Survival approx. 80%
- *Alternative option: no therapy* (especially valid in neonates with severe associated malformations or chromosomal abnormalities)

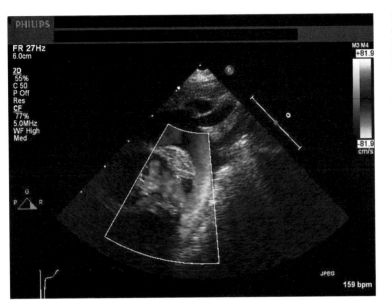

Figure 3.18 Patent ductus arteriosus (PDA) with right-to-left shunting (pulmonary artery → ductus → aorta) in a patient with coarctation of the aorta (CoA). See color plate section for full color version.

Fetal advanced therapy

- Very few centers worldwide have significant experience with prenatal interventions in left heart obstruction such as HLH and severe aortic valve stenosis (→ balloon dilatation).

Coarctation of the aorta (CoA)

Definition

Localized lesion with a shelf of infolding of the aorta into the lumen, typically opposite the arterial duct, leading to a significant narrowing of the aortic lumen; belongs to the group of cardiac defects with left-sided obstruction. The severely symptomatic CoA is a duct-dependent defect, with the ductus shunting primarily right-to-left (PA → ductus → aorta; see Figure 3.18).

Epidemiology

- 0.239/1000 live births[194], approx. 7%–10% of all congenital defects; boys:girls = 2:1.
- Approx. 30% of female patients with Turner's syndrome present with CoA

Pathophysiology

Obliteration of the arterial duct decreases right-to-left shunting to the systemic circulation, leading to (1) severe obstruction of the aorta with a restriction of the antegrade flow and (2) shock/acidemia, pre-renal failure.

Concomitant defects/associated malformations: bicuspid aortic valve (up to 85%), aortic hypoplasia, mitral valve anomaly, VSD, PDA, TGA, DORV, and HLH.

Clinical presentation

Symptoms develop mostly during the first 3–6 weeks of life:

- Heart failure
- Tachydyspnea
- Sweating

- Increased efforts while feeding
- Failure to thrive
- Cold lower extremities with poor peripheral perfusion
- Poor femoral pulse (compared with brachial pulses)
- Decreased urine output or anuria
- Acidosis, shock
- Gallop rhythm
- No generalized cyanosis; S_aO_2 difference between right arm/leg may be present
- No heart murmur in approx. 50% of patients, otherwise non-specific systolic ejection murmur
- Systolic blood pressure gradient between the right arm and leg >10–$15\,mmHg$ (provided the cardiac function is still preserved)

DDx.
IAA and other cardiac defects with left-sided obstruction; sepsis, renal insufficiency of other origin (e.g., renal/bladder outflow obstruction).

Diagnosis in the delivery room/nursery
Usually with (the beginning of) the closure of the arterial duct. Symptoms usually become evident when the newborn is in the nursery room or (more frequently) already at home:
- Pulse status
- BP on the right arm/leg
- "Differential cyanosis" may be present (p. 125)
- Decreased urine output, anuria
- Capillary refill
- Body temperature
- Blood gas, lactate, blood glucose, CBC, chemistry, blood cultures, as indicated
- Echocardiography, as indicated

Therapy in the delivery room/nursery
- Try continuous IV infusion of PGE_1 to reopen the ductus arteriosus: start with 50 (–100) ng/kg/min = 0.05 (–0.1) µg/kg/min
- Correct acidosis according to BG
- Consider oxygen supplementation, intubation and ventilation but keep F_iO_2 low (to prevent lowering of pulmonary vascular resistance)
- Diuretics
- Consider catecholamines for reduced cardiac function (e.g., dopamine)
- Contact a pediatric cardiology center

Monitoring
Pulse oximetry (right arm), ECG, blood pressure (right arm). Check BG and BS before departure. Check ET tube position, if indicated.

Diagnosis in the NICU/PICU/cardiac ICU
- Monitoring of blood pressure gradient (right arm/leg)
- Measure S_aO_2 by pulse oximetry on right arm/leg

- Fluid balance
- Echocardiography
- Chest X-ray: cardiomegaly, increased pulmonary vascular markings, pulmonary edema
- ECG: RVH, but LVH is rare
- ABG, lactate, blood glucose, CBC, chemistry, coagulation panel, urine diagnostics (stix, microscopy), blood culture, HIV/hepatitis serology, type and screen/cross match, as indicated
- Complete microbiological work-up, as indicated: smears (limited significance), tracheal secretion, gastric aspirate and blood culture(s), as indicated
- Cardiac catheterization, as indicated

Procedure/therapy in the NICU/PICU/cardiovascular ICU
- Continue PGE_1 infusion, adjust dose according to clinical presentation and the echocardiography findings
- Ventilation with lowest F_iO_2 possible, as indicated; diuretics and catecholamine, as required
- When in shock: decision for urgent surgery[195,196] versus stabilization (ventricular function?) must be made (e.g., resection of the stenotic area, subclavian flap, end-to-end anastomosis)

Interrupted aortic arch (IAA)
Definition
Complete interruption of the aortic lumen and anatomic discontinuation between two segments of the aortic arch; belongs to the group of ductal-dependent cardiac defects with critical left-sided obstruction.

Classification (according to site of interruption; see Figure 3.19):
- *Type A*: interruption just distal to the left subclavian artery near the isthmus (20%–35%)
- *Type B*: interruption between left subclavian artery and left common carotid artery (60%–80%). Aberrant right subclavian artery (arteria lusoria) is common in Type B
- *Type C*: interruption between the left common carotid artery and innominate artery (<5%)

Epidemiology
Very rare. 0.003/1000 of live births[191]; comprises approx. 1% of all critically ill infants with congenital cardiac defects.

Etiology/pathophysiology
Discontinuity between the ascending and descending aorta → closure of the arterial duct leading to shock/hypoxia, pre-renal failure
Concomitant defects/associated malformations:
- 95% of the patients have other cardiac deformities: large VSD (90%), TAC (10%), bicuspid aortic valve (60%)
- Microdeletion 22q11 (DiGeorge syndrome) is present in 16%–63% of patients with IAA, in 50–90% of patients with Type B IAA, but rarely seen in Type A and Type C IAA.

Clinical presentation
- Heart failure
- Respiratory distress

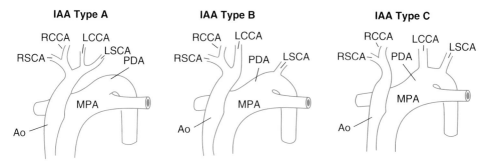

Figure 3.19 Interrupted aortic arch (IAA). Type A: interruption just distal to the left subclavian artery near the isthmus (20%–35%). Type B: interruption between left subclavian artery and left common carotid artery (60%–80%). Aberrant right subclavian artery (lusoric artery) is common in Type B (in this case preductal S_pO_2 to be measured at the right ear lobe). Type C: interruption between the left common carotid artery and innominate artery (5%). Ao, aorta; LCCA, left common carotid artery; LSCA, left subclavian artery; MPA, main pulmonary artery; PDA, patent ductus arteriosus; RCCA, right common carotid artery; RSCA, right subclavian artery.

- Metablic acidosis
- Cyanosis
- "Differential cyanosis" (S_aO_2 difference between the right arm/leg) may be present
- Poor peripheral pulse, capillary refill >2 s
- Blood pressure gradient between the right arm and leg may be present
- Shock symptoms may be present

DDx.
- Coarctation of the aorta (CoA)

Diagnosis in the delivery room/nursery
- Clinical examination
- Non-specific murmur
- Diminished femoral pulses
- BP of the right arm/leg
- "Differential cyanosis" may be present
- Anuria (?), capillary refill
- Body temperature
- BG, BS, lactate and blood work and blood cultures, as indicated
- Echocardiography, as indicated

Therapy in the delivery room/nursery
- PGE$_1$ continuous IV infusion: start with 50 (–100) ng/kg/min ($=0.05$ (–0.1) µg/kg/min)
- Correct acidosis according to ABG ("do not overtreat in mild acidosis," consider buffer therapy for base deficit >-5 mmol/l)
- Consider intubation and ventilation. In pulmonary edema: ventilation with elevated PEEP, maintain low F_iO_2 in order not to reduce the pulmonary resistance. Avoid hyperventilation (otherwise PVR will drop and ionized calcium will decrease further; caution: tetany/seizures in DiGeorge syndrome!)
- Consider the use of catecholamines (e.g., dopamine)
- Contact pediatric cardiology center

Monitoring

Pulse oximetry, ECG, blood pressure. Determine actual BG and BS before the departure. Check ET tube position, as indicated.

Diagnosis in the NICU/PICU/cardiovascular ICU

- Chest X-ray:
  - Cardiomegaly
  - Increased pulmonary vascular markings
  - Pulmonary edema
  - In thymus aplasia: narrowed upper mediastinal space
- Echocardiography
- Complete microbiological diagnostic/septic work-up, as indicated
- ABG, lactate, blood glucose, CBC, chemistry, coagulation panel, urine diagnostics (stix, microscopy), blood culture, HIV/hepatitis serology, type and screen/cross match, as indicated
- Close monitoring of calcium until microdeletion 22q11 is ruled out
- When transfusing: have blood components irradiated (if not routine at your institution); in patients with DiGeorge syndrome do not transfuse citrate red blood cells (this may worsen hypocalcemia by chelate formation)
- Consider cardiac catheterization: to establish the diagnosis and to determine further cardiac malformations
- Chromosomal analysis, fluorescence in situ hybridization (FISH) to diagnose microdeletion 22q11

Procedure/therapy in the NICU/PICU/cardiovascular ICU

- Continue PGE_1 infusion, adjust dose according to clinical and echocardiography
- Ventilation, as indicated, with the lowest F_iO_2, diuretics; catecholamines, as indicated (see above)
- Depending on the anatomy: primary corrective surgery[197]

Critical pulmonary stenosis (PS)

Definition

Obstruction of RVOT at the level of the valve; belongs to the group of duct-dependent cardiac defects with critical right-sided obstruction. Variants of PS include valvular, infundibular (subvalvular) and supravalvular stenosis, and a combination thereof (see Figure 3.20).

Epidemiology

- Isolated form is rare

Etiology/pathophysiology

In *critical valvular* PS, fused leaflets with a central opening of varying diameter. RV size is small (hypoplastic) to normal. Coexisting cardiac conditions are possible but not common.

Clinical presentation

Presentation of neonate with *critical PS*:

- Critically ill
- Hypoxemia

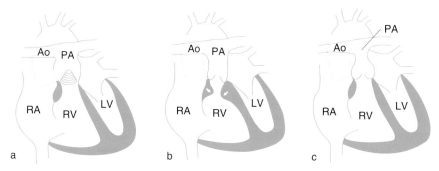

Figure 3.20 a–c Variants of pulmonary stenosis (PS). (a) Valvular stenosis. (b) Infundibular (subvalvular) stenosis. (c) Supravalvular stenosis. RA, right atrium; RV, right ventricle; Ao, aorta; PA, pulmonary artery; LV, left ventricle.

- Tachycardia
- Cyanosis (absent if atrial septum is intact)
- Tachydyspnea
- Hepatomegaly
- Feeding problems
- 2/6–5/6 systolic murmur on the left side of the sternum (may be heard also partly at the back; the louder and longer the heart murmur, the greater the degree of the stenosis)

DDx.
- Sepsis, other cyanotic cardiac defects (HLH), PPHN, lung diseases

Diagnosis in the delivery room/nursery
Rare, because clinical presentation and findings of auscultation are only apparent when the arterial duct closes:
- Clinical examination, especially auscultation and pulse status
- S_aO_2 and BP of the right arm/leg
- Capillary refill
- BG, lactate, BS, blood work-up
- Echocardiography, as indicated

Therapy in the delivery room/nursery
- Continuous PGE_1 infusion: start with 50 ng/kg/min (= 0.05 µg/kg/min)
- Correct acidosis according to BG
- Consider intubation and ventilation
- Are catecholamines necessary? If yes, then choose dopamine, epinephrine or norepinephrine
- Contact a pediatric cardiology center and transfer the newborn

Monitoring
Pulse oximetry, ECG, blood pressure. Determine actual BG and BS. Check ET tube position, as indicated.

Diagnosis in the NICU/PICU/cardiovascular ICU

- Echocardiography: estimation of the gradient across the stenosis by Doppler:
  - A gradient up to 40 mmHg: mild stenosis
  - A gradient of 40–70 mmHg: moderate stenosis
  - A gradient >70 mmHg: severe stenosis
- Chest X-ray: prominent PA branch (post stenotic dilatation), in a severe PaVS, pulmonary vascular markings are diminished; cardiomegaly may be present
- ECG: right atrial enlargement, RVH
- ABG, lactate, blood glucose, CBC, chemistry, coagulation panel, urine diagnostics (stix, microscopy), blood culture, HIV/hepatitis serology, type and screen/cross match, as indicated

Procedure/therapy in the NICU/PICU/cardiovascular ICU

- Continue PGE_1 infusion, adjust dose according to clinical presentation and echocardiographic finding
- Ventilation with an appropriate F_iO_2, as indicated (see above)
- Transcatheter therapy: balloon dilatation if the gradient is >40–50 mmHg. Follow-up! Pulmonary insufficiency is a possible outcome
- Re-intervention or surgical procedure may be required[198]

Pulmonary atresia with intact ventricular septum (PA/IVS)

Definition

Membranous or muscular obstruction of the RVOT. Belongs to the group of duct-dependent cardiac defects with critical right-sided obstruction (Figure 3.21).

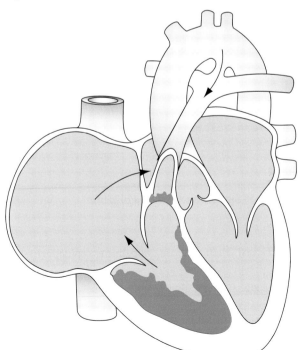

Figure 3.21 Pulmonary atresia with intact ventricular septum (PA/IVS). Anatomy and shunts. PA/IVS, atrial septal defect/patent foramen ovale (ASD/PFO) with right-to-left-shunt, patent ductus arteriosus (PDA) with left-to-right shunt, RV hypertrophy (RVH) and small right ventricular (RV) chamber (high RV pressure), (possible) tricuspid regurgitation (TR) and right atrial enlargement. Cross-sections of the right and left ventricular outflow tracts are angled to the cross-sections of the ventricles in order to visualize the subvalvar, valvar, and supravalvar regions (aortic and pulmonary valve).

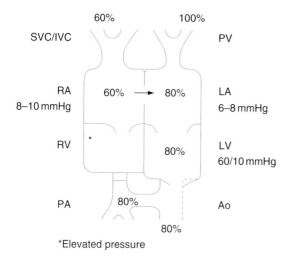

Figure 3.22 Pulmonary atresia with intact ventricular septum (PA/IVS). Hemodynamics and blood oxygen saturations. Obligatory shunt through the atrial septal defect (ASD) (right-to-left). SO_2 in percent, pressure in mmHg. Oxygen saturations (SO_2) in the pulmonary artery (PA) and aorta (Ao) are equal. SVC/IVC, superior/inferior vena cava; RA, right atrium; RV, right ventricle; PV, pulmonary veins.

Epidemiology
- 0.083/1000 of live births[194]; approx. 1% of all the congenital cardiac defects
- Is present in approx. 3% of critically ill neonates with congenital cardiac defects

Etiology/pathophysiology
The arterial duct is the main source of pulmonary blood flow. The systemic venous return passes from the RA through an obligatory interatrial connection (PFO/ASD) to the LA (right-to-left shunt). Therefore, blood mixing with various oxygen saturations may be found (Figure 3.22). The right-to-left shunt results in LV volume overload and central cyanosis. The anatomical spectrum ranges from a well-developed RV (feasible for anatomical biventricular repair) to a severely hypoplastic RV with suprasystemic pressure; coronary anomalies (sinusoidal vessel, stenosis) may be present ($\rightarrow$ RV-dependent coronary circulation). The reduction of RV systolic pressure (RVSP) may lead to myocardial ischemia/infarction and sudden cardiac death.

Clinical presentation
The clinical condition of the newborn is severely compromised:
- Severe cyanosis
- Acidosis
- Tachydyspnea
- Hepatomegaly
- Auscultation: PDA murmur, and a holosystolic thrill may be present
- 90% of neonates with PA/IVS present within the first 3 days of life

DDx.
- Sepsis, other cyanotic cardiac defects, PPHN, lung diseases

Diagnosis in the delivery room/nursery
- Clinical examination, especially auscultation, pulse status
- S_aO_2 and BP right arm/leg
- Capillary refill
- ABG, lactate, BS
- Echocardiography, as indicated; otherwise hypoxia test

Therapy in the delivery room/nursery
- PGE_1 continuous IV infusion: start with 50 (–100) ng/kg/min = 0.05(–0.1) µg/kg/min
- Correct acidosis according to BG
- Consider intubation and ventilation. An increase of systemic vascular resistance (SVR) and pulmonary blood flow may be achieved by increasing F_iO_2. Moderate hyperventilation is an option
- Contact a pediatric cardiology center and transfer the newborn

Monitoring
Pulse oximetry, ECG, blood pressure. Determine actual BG and blood glucose before departure. Check ET tube position, as indicated.

Diagnosis in the NICU/PICU/cardiovascular ICU
- Echocardiography
- Chest X-ray: diminished pulmonary vascular markings ("black lung"), PA branch is concave, cardiomegaly may be present due to enlargement of RA
- ECG: RAH, absent right forces
- ABG, lactate, blood glucose, CBC, chemistry, coagulation panel, urine diagnostics (stix, microscopy), blood culture, HIV/hepatitis serology, type and screen/cross match, as indicated
- Cardiac catheterization: to determine or to rule out coronary anomalies
- Chromosomal analysis, FISH to diagnose a microdeletion 22q11

DDx.
Severe cyanosis in the first few hours to days of life is common in d-TGA/IVS, tricuspid atresia, Ebstein's anomaly, and PA/IVS. Pulmonary atresia with VSD (PA/VSD; see Figure 3.23) usually presents with less severe central cyanosis.

Procedure/therapy in the NICU/PICU/cardiovascular ICU
- Continue PGE_1 infusion, adjust dose according to the clinical presentation and echocardiographic finding
- Ventilation with a high F_iO_2 may be required (see above)
- Catheter-based interventional opening of the pulmonary valve is possible frequently[199]
- In some cases a systemic-to-pulmonary shunt (modified Blalock–Taussig shunt) is indicated in severe RV hypoplasia and major coronary abnormalities

Tetralogy of Fallot (ToF)
Definition
A combination of:
- RVOT (infundibular 45%, PaVS 10%, infundibular + valvular 30%, PaVA 15%)
- Large perimembranous VSD, which usually equalizes the pressure in the ventricles
- Aorta overrides the VSD (variable)
- Right ventricular hypertrophy (RVH) as a result of RVOTO (Figures 3.23, 3.24, 3.25)

ToF belongs to the group of cardiac defects with critical right-sided obstruction; pulmonary blood flow is supplied by the aterial duct and/or the central pulmonary artery. In patients with atretic pulmonary arteries, the pulmonary blood flow is supplied by major aorto-pulmonary collateral arteries (MAPCAs) (Figure 3.26).

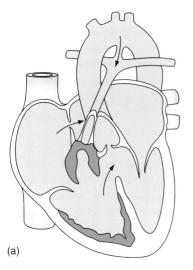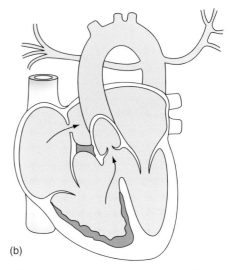

Figure 3.23 Pulmonary atresia with ventricular septal defect (PA/VSD). Anatomy and shunts. **(a)** Pulmonary atresia, ASD/PFO with right-to-left-shunt, PDA, VSD with predominant right-to-left shunt. **(b)** Pulmonary atresia with absent central pulmonary arteries and major aorto-pulmonary collaterals (MAPCAs) from the descending aorta, VSD, ASD/PFO. Cross sections of the right and left ventricular outflow tracts are angled to the cross sections of the ventricles in order to visualize the subvalvar, valvar and supravalvar regions (aortic and pulmonary valve).

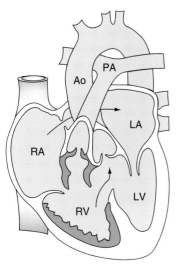

Figure 3.24 Tetralogy of Fallot (ToF). Anatomy and shunts. ToF is characterized by the combination of (1) perimembranous ventral septal defect (VSD; here shown with predominant right-to-left shunt → cyanosis), (2) the aorta widely overriding the VSD (aorta normally overrides the septum to some extent), (3) valvular and subvalvular (infundibular) pulmonary stenosis (PS), (4) right ventricular hypertrophy (RVH). Also shown: atrial septal defect/patent foramen ovale (ASD/PFO) (here mainly with right-to-left shunt); the main pulmonary artery (PA) is present. Cross sections of the right and left ventricular outflow tracts are angled to the cross sections of the ventricles in order to visualize the subvalvar, valvar and supravalvar regions (aortic and pulmonary valve).

Epidemiology
- 0.21/1000[191] to 0.26/1000 of live births[194]; includes approx. 10% of all congenital cardiac defects
- Most frequent cardiac defect detected beyond the neonatal period

Etiology/pathophysiology
Depending on the degree of RVOTO, there are two types:
- Acyanotic ToF ("pink Fallot")
- Cyanotic ToF ("blue Fallot")

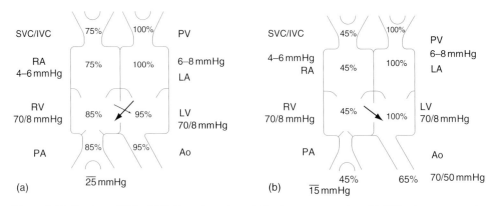

Figure 3.25 Tetralogy of Fallot (ToF). Hemodynamics and blood oxygen saturations. **(a)** Mild pulmonary stenosis, bidirectional shunt through ventricular septal defect (VSD), predominant left-to-right shunting leads to higher left ventricular (LV) and higher right ventricular (RV) saturations (acyanotic ToF, "pink Fallot"). **(b)** Significant pulmonary stenosis, leading to right-to-left shunting (RV → LV) with systemic arterial desaturation and further decrease of mixed venous saturation (cyanotic ToF, "blue Fallot"). SO_2 in percent and pressure in mmHg. Note that systolic pressures are equal in RV, LV and aorta (a and b).

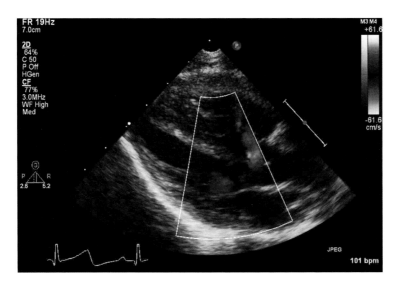

Figure 3.26 Tetralogy of Fallot (ToF). Echocardiography, long axis view. Key features of ToF include: (1) perimembranous ventricular septal defect (VSD), (2) the aorta overriding the VSD (aorta normally overrides the intact septum to some extent), (3) valvular and subvalvular (infundibular) pulmonary stenosis (PS; not shown in this view), (4) significant right ventricular hypertrophy (RVH). See color plate section for full color version.

A hypoxic spell is most likely caused by a muscular spasm of the infundibulum (subvalvular); it leads to an aggravation of the RVOTO (Q_p) and also to a right-to-left shunt through the VSD. Neonates can be asymptomatic and then may develop gradually increasing cyanosis or cyanotic spells.

Clinical presentation

- *Extreme types of ToF* (= ToF with pulmonary atresia; PaVA is present in approx. 15% of all types of ToF): Symptoms may already be present during the neonatal period or on the first day of life, with tachypnea, cyanosis, and hypoxic spells. In the newborn with ToF and PaVA, the pulmonary blood flow is duct-dependent

- *Typical hypoxic spell:*
  - Hyperventilation (fast and deep)
  - Irritability
  - Prolonged crying
  - Increasing cyanosis, somnolence
  - Systolic ejection murmur (RVOTO) becomes fainter and shorter

> **!** Hypoxic spells in children with ToF usually occur during the 3rd to 6th month of life. However, neonates with severe RVOTO/pulmonary atresia may become symptomatic as early as during the first few days of life. Spells frequently occur in the morning, while waking up, after feeding, while crying/screaming or during defecation.
>
> **!** Cyanosis may be absent in anemic neonates and infants with ToF (e.g., at age 2–4 months).

- *Heart murmurs and cyanosis*
  - Cyanotic ToF: holosystolic VSD murmur and a rough ejection murmur (RVOTO) along the left sternal border of the 2nd to 4th intercostal space: the more narrow the RVOT, the more faint, short, and soft the systolic murmur. In cyanotic neonates with PaVA, a systolic ejection murmur can be heard instead of a ductal murmur
  - Acyanotic ToF: a long systolic murmur along the left sternal border may be heard; signs of cardiac failure may be present; there is no cyanosis as a newborn, but an increasing cyanosis during the first year of life

Complications
Seizures, cerebrovascular insult, lethal hypoxic spell (rare!); further complications of cyanotic cardiac defects, such as endocarditis, brain abscess, coagulopathy, growth retardation.

DDx.
Cerebral seizures (caution: a seizure can be triggered by hypoxemia), aspiration, acute closure of the shunt in children after cardiac surgery.

Diagnosis in the delivery room/nursery
- Clinical examination, especially auscultation, pulse status
- S_aO_2 and BP on the right arm/leg
- Capillary refill
- Blood gas, lactate, glucose
- Echocardiography, as indicated

Therapy in the delivery room/nursery
Acyanotic ToF
No treatment necessary, confirm diagnosis by echocardiography (if result of prenatal echocardiogram is available). Elective repair at 6 months of age (refer to pediatric cardiology).

Cyanotic ToF with hypoxic spells
- Administer oxygen
- PGE_1 continuous IV infusion: start with 50 (–100) ng/kg/min = 0.05 (–0.1) µg/kg/min
- Bring the infant's knees up to their chest (to increase the venous return to the RV, and promote blood flow to the lungs); prevent aspiration; minimal handling
- Correct acidosis according to the ABG

> **!** Avoid catecholamines in tetralogy of Fallot – they may worsen the RVOT obstruction.

- Avoid intubation and ventilation, if possible. Increase peripheral resistance. Oxygen supplementation; hyperventilation may be advantageous
- Contact the pediatric cardiology center and transfer the newborn

Monitoring
Pulse oximetry, ECG, blood pressure. Determine current blood gas analysis and blood glucose concentration before departure. Check ET tube position, as indicated.

Diagnostics in the NICU/PICU/cardiovascular ICU
- Determine BG before and during correction of acidosis
- ABG, lactate, blood glucose, CBC, chemistry, coagulation panel, urine diagnostics (stix, microscopy), blood culture, HIV/hepatitis serology, type and screen/cross match, as indicated
- Chest X-ray. Cyanotic ToF: no cardiomegaly, decreased pulmonary vascular markings, "black lung" in PaVA, "boot-shaped heart" by hypoplastic PA, concave PA and elevated apex
- Echocardiography for exact diagnosis (see Figure 3.25). Caution: coronary anomalies; right aortic arch is present in 25% cases of ToF
- ECG: QRS axis $+120°$ to $150°$, (right axis deviation), RVH, biventricular hypertrophy may be present in acyanotic ToF
- Chromosomal analysis, FISH to diagnose microdeletion 22q11

Procedure/therapy in the NICU/PICU/cardiovascular ICU
- Continue with PGE_1 infusion (in symptomatic neonates), adjust dose depending on clinical presentation and echocardiography
- In cases of a hypoxic spell, bring the knees to the chest; minimal handling
- Administer oxygen; limit intubation attempts
- Analgesia and sedation: if there is no venous access $\rightarrow$ chloral hydrate 40–60 mg/kg PR or morphine 0.1–0.2 mg/kg SC/IM or 0.05 mg/kg IV
- Careful volume expansion: 5 ml/kg IV, repeat as indicated
- Is further treatment necessary?
- Correct metabolic acidosis
- In an emergency case, some authors recommend beta adrenergic antagonists to decrease the spasm of the infundibulum:
  - Esmolol (short half-life) 0.5 mg/kg slow IV push, then a continuous IV infusion 50–75–100 µg/kg/min (watch BP and blood glucose)
  - Propanolol (0.01–) 0.05 (–0.25) mg/kg slow IV push
- Transfer infant with symptomatic ToF immediately to the cardiac ICU. Emergency surgery may be indicated: systemic-to-pulmonary artery shunt (modified Blalock – Taussig shunt) versus (primary) correction[200]
- Propanolol (0.5–1.5 mg/kg every 6 h PO) as a medical management to decrease spells until surgery is performed

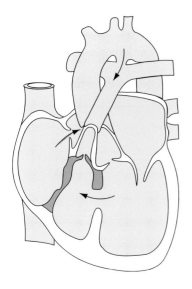

Figure 3.27 Tricuspid atresia (TA). Anatomy and shunts. A combination of TA, VSD, pulmonary stenosis, small RV, PDA, ASD/PFO (= TA type Ib or Ic) is shown here. Because of the complete mixture of blood in the LV and due to the perfusion from the LV (RV is hypoplastic) into both systemic and pulmonary circulations, the SO_2 values in the aorta and pulmonary artery are identical. The pulmonary arteries may be hypoplastic, depending on the extent of the pulmonary valve stenosis. Cross-sections of the right and left ventricular outflow tracts are angled to the cross sections of the ventricles in order to visualize the subvalvar, valvar and supravalvar regions (aortic and pulmonary valve).

Tricuspid atresia (TA)

Definition
Absence of a connection between the RA and RV; usually hypoplastic RV; belongs to the group of cardiac defects with a critical right-sided obstruction; mostly ductal dependent (exemptions are Type IIc and Type III: with transposition of the great arteries, a large VSD and absent PS → pulmonary blood flow is usually increased, therefore there is no dependence on the arterial duct) (Figure 3.27).

Epidemiology
- Rare. 0.039/1000[194] to 0.057/1000[191] live births; comprises approx. 1.2% of all congenital cardiac defects

Etiology/pathophysiology
Classification, modified after Edwards and Burchell:
- *Type I:* normal position of the great arteries (approx. 70%):
  - A: intact ventricular septum and pulmonary atresia
  - B: small VSD and pulmonary valve stenosis (approx. 50%)
  - C: large VSD and pulmonary valve stenosis
- *Type II:* d-transposition of the great arteries (approx. 30%):
  - A: intact ventricular septum and pulmonary atresia
  - B: VSD and pulmonary valve stenosis
  - C: VSD without pulmonary valve stenosis (approx. 20%)
- *Type III:* l-transposition of the great arteries (approx. 3%):
  - Frequently large VSD
  - Subvalvular pulmonary or aortic stenosis may be present

Systemic venous blood flow through the atrial defect from RA to LA (right-to-left-shunt) leads to volume overload and dilatation of LA and LV (Figure 3.27). Because of the complete mixture of blood in the LV and due to the perfusion from the LV (RV is hypoplastic) into both systemic and pulmonary circulations, the SO_2 values in the aorta and pulmonary artery are identical. The pulmonary arteries may be hypoplastic, depending on the extent of the pulmonic valve stenosis.

Concomitant defects: PFO/ASD (>80%), VSD, PDA, CoA (especially when transposition is present), persistent left superior vena cava (LSVC).

Clinical presentation
- Significant cyanosis immediately after birth
- Tachydyspnea
- Hepatomegaly
- Signs of heart failure
- 2/6–3/6 left parasternal systolic murmur (VSD)

DDx.
Other cyanotic cardiac defects (HLH), sepsis, PPHN, lung diseases.

Diagnosis in the delivery room/nursery
- Blood gas, lactate, glucose, blood culture, etc., as indicated
- Echocardiography, as indicated, otherwise: hyperoxia test

Therapy in the delivery room/nursery
- Administer oxygen
- PGE_1 continuous IV infusion: start with 50 (–100) ng/kg/min = 0.05 (–0.1) µg/kg/min
- Intubation and ventilation, as indicated
- Correct acidosis according to BG
- Contact pediatric cardiology and transfer the newborn

Monitoring
Pulse oximetry, ECG, blood pressure. Check ET tube position. Determine actual BG, lactate and BS before departure.

Diagnosis in the NICU/PICU/cardiovascular ICU
- Chest X-ray: RA and LV are enlarged, "boot-shaped heart" due to concave PA. Elevated apex may be present, mostly with diminished pulmonary vascular markings (exemptions: transposition of the great arteries, large VSD)
- Echocardiography: RV hypoplasia, TA, LV enlargement, VSD, atrium septum protrudes to the left (PFO/ASD size? PS? TGA? Subaortic valve stenosis? Has the aortic arch been visualized?)
- ABG, lactate, blood glucose, CBC, chemistry, coagulation panel, urine diagnostics (stix, microscopy), blood culture, HIV/hepatitis serology, type and screen/cross match, as indicated
- ECG: LVH, RAH, QRS axis: left axis deviation

Procedure/therapy in the NICU/PICU/cardiovascular ICU
- Continue/start PGE_1 infusion, adjust dose to clinical presentation and echocardiographic finding
- Correct acidosis according to BG

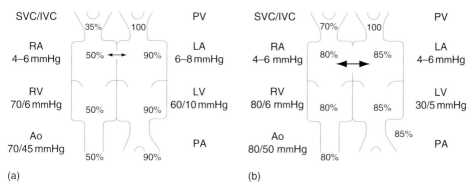

Figure 3.28 d-Transposition of the great arteries (d-TGA) without VSD. Hemodynamics and blood oxygen saturations. (a) d-TGA with poor mixing. (b) d-TGA with good mixing at the atrial level. SO_2 in percent (within the diagram), pressure in mmHg (outside the diagram). PA, pulmonary artery; Ao, aorta; SVC/IVC, superior/inferior vena cava; RA, right atrium; RV, right ventricle; LA, left atrium; LV, left ventricle; PV, pulmonary veins.

- Balloon atrioseptostomy (Rashkind maneuver), if atrial communication is not large enough
- Check for heart failure
- Surgery is performed in multiple steps: systemic-to-pulmonary shunt (modified Blalock–Taussig shunt), bidirectional Glenn surgery (bidirectional cavo-pulmonary connection (BCPC)), modified Fontan surgery (total cavo-pulmonary connection (TCPC))[201]

d-Transposition of the great arteries (d-TGA)
Definition
Complete transposition of the great arteries is defined as a concordant connection at the atrioventricular level and a discordant connection at the ventriculoarterial level, with the pulmonary artery arising posteriorly from the morphological left ventricle and the aorta anterior to the morphological right ventricle.

Epidemiology
- 0.215/1000 live births[191]; includes approx. 5% of all congenital cardiac defects[175]; 2/3 of the patients are males

Etiology/pathophysiology
Systemic venous, deoxygenated blood flows through the RA → RV into the aorta; well oxygenated blood flows from the lungs through the LA → LV into the pulmonary artery; thus, the systemic and pulmonary circulations are arranged in parallel rather than in series (Figure 3.28).

> **!** A communication between the two circulations (at the atrial and/or ventricular level and/or through the arterial duct) is essential for survival.

Concomitant defects
VSD (up to 50%; ranging from very small, thus hemodynamically/clinically irrelevant, to very large and mostly hemodynamically/clinically relevant), ASD II, underdevelopment of

the right ventricle with a small tricuspid valve (this constellation often involves CoA), LVOTO, coronary anomalies.

Clinical presentation
- Generalized cyanosis with flow restriction of the PFO and/or the PDA
- In spite of O_2 supplementation P_aO_2 remains <30 mmHg
- Symptoms of shock with metabolic acidosis

Diagnosis in the delivery room/nursery
Diagnosis in the delivery room is rare; symptoms with closure of the PDA (6–48 h post partum):
- Blood gas analysis, lactate, blood glucose, and lactate, as indicated
- Echocardiography, as indicated; hyperoxia test only if echocardiography (Figure 3.29) not available (caution: iatrogenic induction of PDA closure is possible)

Therapy in the delivery room/nursery room
- PGE_1 continuous IV infusion: start with 50 (–100) ng/kg/min = 0.05 (–0.1) µg/kg/min
- Fractioned volume expansion (5–10–15 ml/kg/bolus IV), repeat, as indicated
- Correct acidosis according to BG
- Be cautious with oxygen (iatrogenic PDA closure). Exemptions: severe cyanosis of the neonate whose arterial duct has already closed, or a cyanotic neonate with a very large open patent duct (but a restrictive PFO/ASD) before or after an effective balloon atrial septostomy
- Consider intubation and ventilation, as indicated
- Are catecholamines (e.g., dopamine) indicated?
- Contact a pediatric cardiology department that provides catheter interventions. Transfer the newborn as soon as possible!
- Physician trained in BAS (Rashkind procedure) may come to the newborn if transport is the limiting factor

> **!** Patients with d-TGA without VSD and a very small (flow restrictive) atrial septal communication (see Figure 3.29a) will not necessarily improve their arterial S_aO_2 after intubation and F_iO_2 of 1.0 because of the insufficient blood mixing/shunt (atrial septal defect, patent arterial duct?).
>
> **!** The amount of IV volume administration in d-TGA patients can be significant (up to 20–50 ml/kg IV, fractioned). Typical situation: severe cyanotic neonate without prenatal diagnosis.

Monitoring
Pulse oximetry, ECG, blood pressure. Determine actual BG, lactate and BS before departure. Check ET tube position, if necessary.

Diagnosis in the NICU/PCU/cardiovascular ICU
- Chest X-ray: "egg-shaped heart" with a narrow upper mediastinum, cardiomegaly may be present with increased pulmonary vascular markings
- Echocardiography (see Figure 3.29):

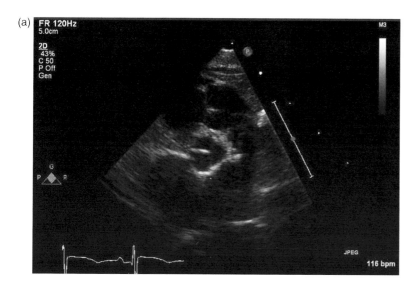

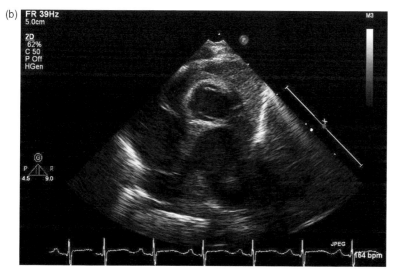

Figure 3.29 d-Transposition of the great arteries (d-TGA) without VSD. Echocardiography, atrial communication, subcostal view. Left atrium (LA), shunt through atrial septum, right atrium (RA, closest to the transducer) and inferior vena cava (IVC) are shown. **(a)** *Normal anatomy, short axis view*: central aorta with pulmonary artery (PA) crossing anteriorly, so-called circle (aorta) and sausage (PA). **(b)** *d-TGA, short axis view*: transversal views of both aorta and PA, with aorta right and anterior of the PA, so-called double circle image typical for d-TGA. **(c)** *Small, restrictive ASD/PFO, little left-to-right atrial shunting, systemic arterial desaturation* (severe cyanosis; SO_2 in the aorta approx. 30%–50%.). (See plate section for full color version). **(d)** *Unrestrictive ASD after balloon atrioseptostomy* (BAS = Rashkind procedure), SO_2 in the aorta ≈80%. See color plate section for full color version.

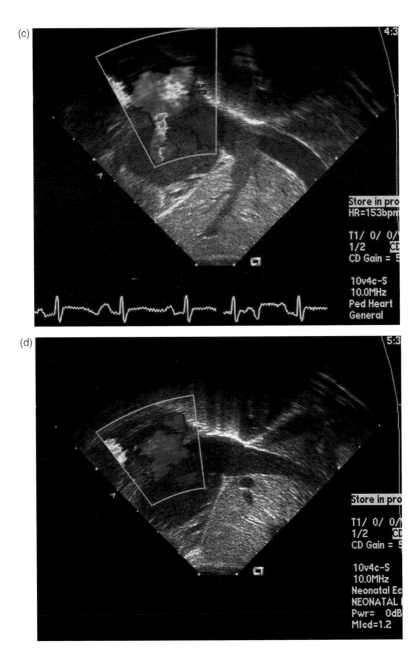

(c)

(d)

Figure 3.29 (cont.).

- Parasternal long axis view: the great arteries lie parallel to each other with the pulmonary artery posterior (PA); the PA branches posteriorly towards the lungs
- Parasternal short axis view: a "double circle" is seen instead of the normal constellation "circle (aorta) and sausage (PA)"
- Subcostal view: evaluate for restriction of ASD/PFO and left-to-right atrial shunting (pressure gradient?)

- Complete microbiological work-up: smears, tracheal secretions, gastric fluid aspirate and blood cultures, if indicated
- ABG, lactate, blood glucose, CBC, chemistry, coagulation panel, urine diagnostics (stix, microscopy), blood culture, HIV/hepatitis serology, type and screen/cross match, as indicated

DDx.
Lung disease, PPHN, other cyanotic cardiac defects, e.g., double-outlet right ventricle (DORV) with a subpulmonary VSD (= Taussig – Bing malformation). If cardiac failure is predominant (TGA with VSD or a large PDA), consider the following differential diagnoses: cardiac arrhythmias, pericardial effusion, other cardiac defects, metabolic disorder, and others.

Procedure/therapy in the NICU/PICU/cardiovascular ICU
- Start/continue PGE$_1$ IV infusion: start with 50 (–100) ng/kg/min = 0.05 (–0.1) µg/kg/min, and adjust dosage according to clinical status and echocardiography
- A neonate with "simple TGA" (d-TGA without VSD) may be hypoxemic and seriously ill. These infants benefit from a balloon atrioseptostomy (Rashkind procedure) if the atrial communication is not large enough (see Figure 3.29c). After balloon atrioseptostomy (see Figure 3.29d) S$_a$O$_2$ usually improves significantly with a minimal or absent pressure gradient between LA and RA. Adjust ventilation parameters according to ABG
- Surgery: arterial switch operation (anatomical correction according to Jatenne – usually performed on days 5–10 of life)[202]; d-TGA with VSD and severe PS: Rastelli procedure (intracardiac tunnel, LV through the VSD to the aorta and a connection from RV to PA)
- Neonates with d-TGA and a (larger) VSD (Figure 3.30) are less cyanotic, but may develop cardiac failure and pulmonary vascular disease (3rd to 4th month of life), if diagnosis was not established during the neonatal period

Atrioventricular septal defect (AVSD)
Syndrome
- Endocardial cushion defect, AV canal

Definition
- Incomplete development of the endocardial cushion and the atrioventricular septum

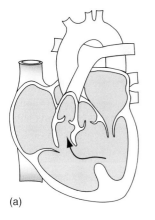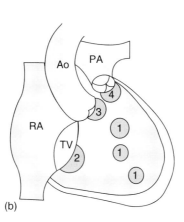

Figure 3.30 Classification of ventricular septal defects (VSDs). **(a)** VSD with left-to-right shunt. **(b)** View on the interventricular septum from the right ventricle. 1 = Muscular VSDs; 2 = inlet VSD (perimembranous VSD); 3 = subaortic VSD (perimembranous VSD); 4 = subpulmonary VSD (perimembranous VSD). RA, right atrium; Ao, aorta; TV, tricuspid valve; PA, pulmonary artery.

(a)   (b)

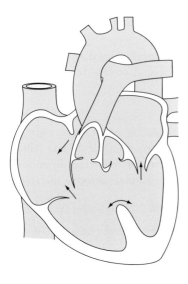

Figure 3.31 Atrioventricular septal defect (AVSD, syn. AV canal, endocardial cushion defect). Anatomy and shunts. Ostium primum ASD (ASD I), VSD in the inlet part of the ventricular septum, common (undivided) AV valve annulus; or separate valves: left AV valve with a cleft in the anterior leaflet. Defect leads to intracardiac shunts and AV valve regurgitation. Cross-sections of the right and left ventricular outflow tracts are angled to the cross sections of the ventricles in order to visualize the subvalvar, valvar and supravalvar regions (aortic and pulmonary valve).

Epidemiology
- 0.12/1000[191] to 0.36/1000 live births[194]; represents 2% of all congenital cardiac defects
- AVSD is present in approx. 40% of all children with Down syndrome and approx. 30%–40% of all patients with AVSD are children with Down syndrome

Etiology/pathophysiology
- Differentiation: partial or complete AVSD with ventricular balance or imbalance
- Forms and categories (Figure 3.31):
  - Ostium primum ASD (ASD I)
  - VSD in the inlet part of the ventricular septum (Figure 3.30)
  - Common (undivided) AV valve annulus; or separate valves: left AV valve with a cleft in the anterior leaflet
  - Results in intracardiac shunts, AV valve regurgitation

Clinical presentation
- Signs of heart failure with tachydyspnea, tachycardia, hepatomegaly; recurrent lung infections (upper lung), failure to thrive

DDX.
- VSD

Diagnosis in the delivery room/nursery room
- Medical history
- Blood gas, glucose, lactate, basic labs (including: thyroid hormone status in infants with Down syndrome)

! There is a high prevalence of AVSD (= AV canal) in infants with Down syndrome. Echocardiography should be considered early in life.

Monitoring
- Pulse oximetry, ECG, blood pressure. Determine actual BG, lactate and BS before departure

Procedure/therapy in the delivery room/nursery
- Do not administer PGE_1!
- Contact a pediatric cardiology department for evaluation and treatment

Diagnosis in the NICU/PICU/cardiovascular ICU
- Chest X-ray: cardiomegaly, increased pulmonary vascular markings, possibly prominent PA
- Echocardiography: see finding above
- ECG: Superior QRS axis in CAVSD = CAVC (DDx: e.g., tricuspid atresia)
- ABG, lactate, blood glucose, CBC, chemistry, coagulation panel, urine diagnostics (stix, microscopy), blood culture, free tri-iodothyronine (T_3), free thyroxine (T_4), thyroid stimulating hormone (TSH), HIV/hepatitis serology, type and screen/cross match, as indicated
- Complete microbiological work-up; septic work up, as indicated

Procedure/therapy in the NICU/PICU
- Medical therapy of heart failure: diuretics, angiotensin converting enzyme (ACE) inhibitors
- Surgical correction most commonly between the age of 4 and 8 months (or earlier, if conservative therapy fails)[203]

Total anomalous pulmonary venous return (TAPVR)
Definition
- All pulmonary veins connect to the systemic venous system (and not to the left atrium)

Epidemiology
- 0.083/1000 live births[194]; as an isolated malformation: 0.058/1000 live births[191]

Etiology/pathophysiology
Failure of the development of the common pulmonary vein. Classic form: the pulmonary veins of both lungs drain behind the left atrium into a confluence, which connects either into a systemic vein or into the right atrium, or both.

Concomitant defects: obligatory PFO/ASD II. Associated with complex congenital cardiac defects (e.g., heterotaxy syndromes).

Different TAPVR types
- *Supracardiac (50%)* connection to:
  - Brachiocephalic vein
  - (Right) superior vena cava
  - (Right) azygos vein
  - (Left) hemiazygos vein
  - Left persistent superior vena cava
- *Cardiac (20%)* connection to:
  - Coronary sinus
  - Right atrium

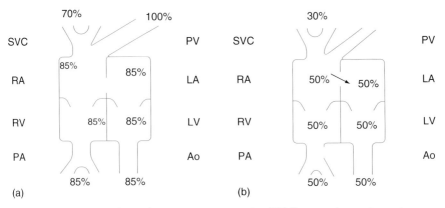

Figure 3.32 Total anomalous pulmonary venous connection (TAPVC; syn. total anomalous pulmonary venous return, TAPVR). Hemodynamics and blood oxygen saturations. (**a**) Supracardiac – without obstruction. Similar to large ASD, increased blood flow through RA/RV with some shunting to LA/LV causing mild desaturation. (**b**) Supracardiac – with obstruction, causing pulmonary edema/congestion, leading to desaturation of pulmonary venous return. Mixing in RA with systemic return (SVC/IVC) → further desaturation of systemic blood.

- *Infracardiac (20%)* connection to:
  - (Supradiaphragmal): inferior vena cava
  - (Infradiaphragmal): inferior vena cava, portal vein, left gastric vein,
- *Mixed (10%)*

Hemodynamics of TAPVR without obstruction are similar to those of a large VSD: the blood flow is determined by both the size of the atrial defect and the compliance of the RV. A small PFO/ASD and gradual decrease in pulmonary vascular resistance after birth may result in volume overload of RA, RV, and the pulmonary artery (Figure 3.32a).

Hemodynamics of TAPVR with obstruction are similar to those of mitral stenosis: both pulmonary venous and pulmonary arterial pressure are raised, leading to reduced pulmonary blood flow and a severe right-to-left shunt at the atrial and ductal level (cyanosis). The obstruction of the venous lung drainage results in an increase in pulmonary venous pressure, pulmonary edema, and (tachy-)dyspnea (Figure 3.32b).

> **!** An interatrial communication via PFO/ASD is essential for the survival of an infant with TAPVR.

Clinical presentation
Infants with TAPVC are usually clinically stable; they may develop mild to severe cyanosis (usually while feeding), (tachy-) dyspnea and failure to thrive; also hepatomegaly and rales over the lungs. Usually there is no heart murmur. Clinical signs depend on the severity of obstruction: most of these newborns develop symptoms within the first 7 days of life.

DDx.
Sepsis, other cyanotic cardiac defects (HLH), pulmonary diseases, PPHN.

Diagnosis in the delivery room/nursery room
Symptoms may begin in the nursery room:
- Auscultation (moist rales?)
- ABG, lactate, blood glucose, blood culture, basic lab work, as indicated

- Pulse oximetry (S_aO_2)
- Pulse status
- Blood pressure

Therapy in the delivery room
- Supplementary oxygen
- Do not administer PGE_1!
- Start diuretics (when diagnosis is known), correct acidosis according to blood gas

> **!** Catecholamines can aggravate pulmonary edema in patients with obstructive TAPVR.

- Intubation and ventilation with a low rate and high PEEP (>4 mmHg, especially in pulmonary edema)
- Contact pediatric cardiology/pediatric cardiac surgery: TAPVC with obstruction is an EMERGENCY!

Monitoring
Pulse oximetry (S_aO_2, HR), ECG, blood pressure; ABG, lactate and blood glucose; check ET tube position, if necessary.

Diagnosis in the NICU/PICU/cardiovascular ICU
- Chest X-ray: hazy ground-glass appearance, normal heart size; classic "snowman appearance" in supracardiac drainage (due to the partly dilated right superior vena cava, vena verticalis and left innominate vein) is rare during the first 4 weeks of life
- ECG: RA enlargement, RV hypertrophy, right axis deviation
- Echocardiography: large RV with a "relatively underfilled LV," large RA/small LA, leftward deviation of the interatrial septum. Concomitant defects? Heterotaxy syndrome?
- ABG, lactate, blood glucose, CBC, chemistry, coagulation panel, urine diagnostics (stix, microscopy), blood culture, HIV/hepatitis serology, type and screen/cross match, as indicated
- Complete microbiological work-up; septic work-up, as indicated
- Possibly: cardiac catheterization

Procedure/therapy in the NICU/PICU/cardiovascular ICU
- Supplementary oxygen, administer diuretics, correct acidosis according to BG
- Low-frequency ventilation and increased PEEP (>4 mmHg, especially if pulmonary edema is present). With increased pulmonary vascular resistance: hyperventilation and increased F_iO_2, inhaled nitric oxide (iNO) may not be helpful. PGE improves systemic output at the expense of pulmonary blood flow and oxygenation
- Consider extracorporeal membrane oxygenation (ECMO) for presurgical stabilization
- Rule out cardiac (and other somatic) malformations
- Surgical correction by connecting the pulmonary veins to LA[204]

> **!** Obstructive TAPVR is a surgical EMERGENCY and requires immediate correction.

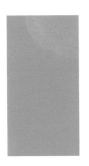

Patent ductus arteriosus of the preterm infant

Georg Hansmann

Definition

A patent ductus arteriosus (PDA) in the first 3 days of life is a physiological shunt connection (PA – aorta) in healthy term and preterm newborn infants[205]. In contrast, a persistently patent ductus arteriosus in preterm infants can become a clinical problem, e.g., during the recovery period from respiratory distress syndrome (RDS). With the improvement of ventilation and oxygenation, pulmonary vascular resistance (PVR) decreases early and rapidly (starting within the first hours of life), especially in preterm infants <1000 g (ELBW)[205]. Subsequently, the left-to-right shunt through the ductus arteriosus (aorta → DA → PA) and optionally the patent foramen orale (PFO) (RA → LA) increases, as does the pulmonary blood flow, leading to (interstitial) pulmonary edema and overall worsening of respiratory status. PDA of the preterm infant is frequently not symptomatic before day 4 of life.

Epidemiology

- 31% of preterm infants with a birth weight (BW) of 501–1500 g have a PDA
- A significant PDA associated with heart failure is found in 15% of preterm infants weighing less than 1750 g[175]
- A significant PDA that may require treatment during the neonatal period occurs in approximately 60% of preterm infants weighing less than 1000 g

Etiology/pathophysiology

In term neonates, a postnatal increase in P_aO_2 and a decrease in prostaglandin E (PGE), nitric oxide (NO), and other vasodilator substances induces constriction of ductal vascular smooth muscle cells and consequently functional closure of the ductus. This results locally in a "hypoxic zone" and triggers neointimal proliferation ("vascular remodeling") and thus anatomical DA closure. However, in preterm infants, the sensitivity for oxygen is reduced, while that for PGE and NO is increased[206]. This is why the physiological DA closure (day 1–3) often does not occur promptly in preterm infants <1500 g (VLBW). In addition to NO and PGE, oxygen-sensitive Kv channels[207] and Rho/Rho-kinase pathways[208] may also be involved in regulating DA closure.

A so-called winking ductus, which closes and opens periodically, is actually not very common in preterm infants – with the exception of very preterm infants <1000 g after pharmacological DA closure[205].

Due to the immaturity of vascular musculature, the pulmonary vascular resistance (PVR) decreases earlier and faster in preterm infants (particularly those <1000 g) than in term infants. With the improvement of RDS, pH and P_aO_2 rise, leading to a rapid fall in

Neonatal Emergencies: A Practical Guide for Resuscitation, Transport and Critical Care, ed. Georg Hansmann.
Published by Cambridge University Press. © Cambridge University Press 2009.

PVR and pulmonary artery pressure (PAP). Depending on the severity of lung disease and the associated PVR elevation, a significant drop in PVR may be observed either in the first week of life (e.g., improvement of RDS) or after several weeks under mechanical ventilation (bronchopulmonary dysplasia/chronic lung disease (BPD/CLD)). When pulmonary blood flow is unrestricted (i.e., no right ventricular outflow tract obstruction (RVOTO)), the ductal left-to-right shunt (aorta → DA → PA→ LA→ LV) increases, which can lead to *volume overload and LV dysfunction.*

The increased pulmonary blood flow can result in pulmonary hypertension (shear stress → endothelial dysfunction), interstitial/alveolar pulmonary edema, and decreased lung compliance; this in turn will lead to higher ventilator settings (PIP and F_iO_2), and ultimately to BPD/CLD. In ELBW and VLBW infants, the latter is often combined with myocardial dysfunction that – together with a ductal steal phenomenon (aorta → PA ≈ functional aortic insufficiency) – will worsen systemic perfusion. Therefore, these preterm infants <1500 g are very susceptible to hypoperfusion of vital organs, which is frequently associated with one (or a combination of) the following *co-morbidities:*

- Cerebral ischemia/ICH/PVL,
- Necrotizing enterocolitis
- (Pre-) renal failure
- Myocardial ischemia/infarction

Clinical presentation

- Respiratory deterioration: (1) Re-intubation/second course of PPV; (2) increase in ventilator settings; or (3) first intubation/mechanical ventilation on days 2–5 of life or later (rare)
- Heart murmur (in 75%, mid-systolic; only in 25% with an additional diastolic component = so-called machinery murmur) *plus* a precordial thrill (acceptable specificity, weak sensitivity). If present, it appears 3–7 days later than the positive echocardiographic finding of a large left-to-right shunt
- All clinical signs such as tachycardia, wide pulse pressure with a low diastolic BP, apical mesodiastolic murmur (functional mitral valve stenosis as a sign of an excessive hemodynamic load of the LA), gallop rhythm (sign of cardiac failure), and hepatomegaly are neither specific nor reliable – especially in (ventilated) preterm infants with VLBW (<1500 g)[205]

! In preterm infants <32 weeks' gestation, the presence of a significant/symptomatic PDA should always be kept in mind.
   A hemodynamically significant PDA is not a single entity: it often brings respiratory, cerebral, gastrointestinal, and renal problems and may occur in the context of congenital heart disease (see DDx below).

DDx.

- Congenital heart disease with duct-dependent pulmonary perfusion, e.g., pulmonary valve atresia or severe pulmonary valve stenosis (caution: cyanosis can be absent if the ductus arteriosus is large); cardiovascular disease with increased pulmonary blood flow and predominant heart failure (truncus arteriosus, total anomalous pulmonary venous return, TGA + VSD, DORV + VSD and no PS, tricuspid atresia + VSD + TGA without pulmonary stenosis); acyanotic cardiovascular disease with LV dysfunction (e.g., aortic valve stenosis, coarctation of the aorta, interrupted aortic arch)

- Other causes of respiratory distress syndrome (primary RDS; secondary surfactant deficiency due to perinatal hypoxia/asphyxia, pneumonia/sepsis or aspiration syndrome), BPD/CLD, wet lung/transient tachypnea of the newborn, malformations (especially those of the upper and lower respiratory tract), pneumothorax, pleural effusion/chylothorax

Prior to transfer (NETS)

ABCD measures, as indicated. Depending on the gestational age, birth weight and RDS symptoms, arrange rapid transfer to a NICU (and adjacent cardiac surgery). In general, avoid interhospital transport of VLBW infants! Intubate before transfer, as indicated.

Monitoring

S_pO_2, BP, ECG. ET tube position, if intubated. Determine current blood glucose, lactate, and ABG prior to departure.

Diagnosis in the NICU

Echocardiography: Gold standard to rule out duct-dependent cardiovascular disease. For standard echocardiographic transducer positions see Figure 3.15.

- Partial or total ductal left-to-right shunt is detectable within and often beyond 24 h of age. Large left atrium (LA), large pulmonary veins. Many centers perform echocardiography at $\approx$24 h of age in preterm infants $\leq$30 weeks' gestation, or in preterm infants with clinical signs for symptomatic PDA (Figure 3.33). Scheduling of follow-up echocardiograms is based on symptoms, hemodynamic relevance in the initial echocardiographic study, and planned/performed treatment interventions
- Ultrasonography (U/S), particularly head U/S, including cerebral and mesenterial Doppler measurement of maximum systolic velocity (V_{max}) and end-diastolic velocity (V_{ed}) as well as resistance index. With a large PDA, there is frequently absent or minimum diastolic flow, or even reverse flow in the aorta and cerebral arteries (e.g., anterior cerebral artery, ACA). The ACA resistance index alone is not sufficient to evaluate PDA – it can be falsely normal!
- Chest X-ray: non-specific, often cardiomegaly, pulmonary edema may be present
- ECG: non-specific, abnormal repolarization may be present
- ABG, blood glucose and lactate, laboratory work-up including coagulation panel, prior to surgery HIV/hepatitis serology, blood type and screen/cross, if indicated septic work-up
- Request for maternal HBs-Ag status and blood type, Coombs test
- Newborn screening for metabolic disorders (>48 h after birth)

Differential diagnosis and pitfalls in evaluating and treating preterm infants with PDA

- When the systolic murmur becomes faint or disappears, it does not mean that the ductus arteriosus is in the process of obliteration (closure). Instead, LV function may

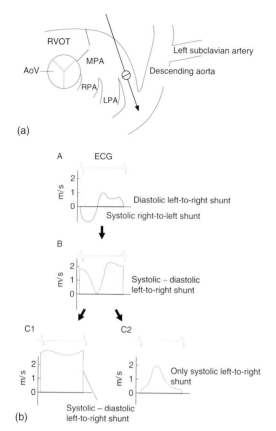

Figure 3.33 Hemodynamics in patent ductus arteriosus (PDA) of the preterm infant (echocardiography). The positioning of the Doppler probe in the high left parasternal axis view ("ductal view") (a) to demonstrate the changes in ductal flow, (b) in the first days of life of a healthy term infant (C1), and in a term/preterm infant with PDA and respiratory distress (C2) by using a PW Doppler. In color Doppler, a ductal left-to-right shunt (LRS) appears as a "red flag" (flow towards the probe) at the left side of the pulmonary artery (LPA). bA Bidirectional ductal flow immediately after birth: systolic right-to-left shunt, diastolic left-to-right shunt. bB Decreased pulmonary arterial pressure (PAP) in relation to the aortic pressure a few hours after birth. bC1 In a healthy neonate, PAP drops with closure of the ductus arteriosus. The flow velocity is high (constriction of the duct) in a systolic–diastolic left-to-right shunt (aorta → PA). bC2 In a sick term/preterm neonate with a patent ductus arteriosus (PDA), a systolic left-to-right shunt with great volume shift towards the lungs develops (aorta → PDA → PA → LA dilatation). In diastole, PAP is close to the aortic pressure. This explains why a diastolic murmur cannot be heard over a great ductal left-to-right shunt (i.e., no diastolic pressure gradient). RVOT, right ventricular outflow tract; AoV, aortic valve (horizontal); MPA, main pulmonary artery; RPA, right pulmonary artery; LPA, left pulmonary artery. Modified from Skinner J. Diagnosis of patent ductus arteriosus. *Semin Neonatol* 2001; 6:49–61.

have worsened and PAP may have reached ≈ near systemic pressure, that there is no longer an audible pressure gradient across the PDA. If in doubt, perform an echocardiogram.

- The intensity of a systolic murmur can be caused by increased ductal flow after a volume bolus IV, anemia or an early, rapid fall of pulmonary vascular resistance (especially in preterm infants <1000 g). The latter refers to a *remaining patent ductus* and conveys a greater shunt volume into the lungs → interstitial pulmonary edema/impairment of pulmonary compliance. After extubation, decompensation in the absence of CPAP/PEEP is possible, even without previous clinical signs of a significant ductal left-to-right shunt (the so-called *silent dangerous ductus*)

- A so-called *winking ductus*, which closes and opens periodically, is rare, but frequently observed in ELBW preterm infants after medically induced closure of the duct[205]

- If the left ventricle had been hyperdynamic initially (common in PDA) and now has "normal" (or slightly decreased) LV function, it should be taken as a warning sign of imminent heart failure, especially when all other echocardiography parameters indicate a large ductal left-to-right shunt (i.e., LV volume overload)

- When the resistance index (RI = $(V_{max} - V_{ed}) \div V\,max$) in the cerebral (ACA) or abdominal (coeliac trunk) U/S Doppler becomes normal, this does not necessarily mean that the ductal steal, i.e., ductal left-to-right shunt (aorta $\rightarrow$ DA $\rightarrow$ PA), is diminished. Instead, a decreased maximal systolic velocity (V_{max}) and impaired LV function may be present. Always document absolute flow velocities (not only indices) and interpret them in the right context (i.e., the patient's clinical status)

- When a large PDA is diagnosed by echocardiography, the following diagnoses are easily overlooked:
  - CoA (lower limb pulses present and strong? Could you see the complete aortic arch? Is there an exclusive left-to-right shunt across the duct, or is the shunt bidirectional or predominantly right-to-left (PA $\rightarrow$ DA $\rightarrow$ aorta)?
  - Pulmonary atresia or stenosis (PaVA/PaVS: 100% S_aO_2 possible, PV opening normal?)
- Further pitfalls when doing an echocardiogram for presumed PDA:
  - The "PDA" actually is a diastolic turbulence caused by (1) aortopulmonary collaterals in chronic lung disease or congenital heart disease, (2) an aortopulmonary window or (3) an abnormal coronary artery
  - The LV is hyperdynamic in the presence of a large ductal left-to-right shunt. If not, then aortic stenosis, CoA or arterial hypertension (high after load) certainly must be ruled out

---

! When is a PDA hemodynamically significant and when does it require closure?

There are no stringent criteria for the need for PDA closure to date. If the size of the PDA is bigger than or just as big as the pulmonary artery on the second day of life, then early pharmacological or surgical treatment should certainly be initiated. A ratio of the diameter of the LA to that of the aorta >1.3 (1.1) in the parasternal long-axis view, or a resistance index (RI) >0.9 on cerebral Doppler (ACA) is often considered as a sign of a significant shunt. Pharmacological or surgical intervention for a significant PDA should be pursued *before* symptoms of cardiac or respiratory failure become apparent.

Procedure/therapy in the NICU

- *Supportive treatment:*
  - Monitor vital signs including temperature (36.6–37.2°C/ 97.8–98.9°F), tcPO_2, tcPCO_2
  - Minimal handling
  - Optimize ventilator/respiratory status, especially oxygenation (caution: hypoxia increases PGE synthesis); administer analgesia and sedation, when indicated
  - Treat anemia (aim for Hct >45%) and correct electrolyte disorders
  - Give vitamin K IV (if not yet administered)
  - Fluid restriction over 24 h when the renal function is normal (up to a maximum of 48 h): depending on body weight/gestational age, creatinine and urine output. Give 70–100 ml/kg/day on the second day of life, then increase to a maximum of 130 ml/kg/day, which may be reached by day 7 of life. Caution: NEC + renal failure!
  - Diuretics (controversial)

> ! Fluid restriction before but not during pharmacological treatment of PDA (i.e., indomethacin or ibuprofen): among other sequelae, renal failure/oliguria is common.
>
> ! Avoid the use of furosemide (Lasix®) in preterm infants with PDA as it may increase prostaglandin synthesis.

Closure of the ductus arteriosus

Most of the RCTs from the 1980s evaluated **three specific treatment approaches** for closure of the ductus arteriosus (most commonly: pharmacological treatment with indomethacin)[209].

- Prophylactic treatment, to be started in the first 24 h of life (e.g., indomethacin IV)
- "Pre-symptomatic" treatment, when PDA has been found to be large by echocardiography or when the first clinical signs occur (usually day 2–3, sometimes later)
- Specific treatment when PDA and its shunt volume have been found to be hemodynamically relevant by echocardiography (mostly a so-called symptomatic PDA)

> ! Until now, none of these pharmacological approaches has been shown to improve long-term *pulmonary* outcome[209].

Pharmacological ductus closure with cyclooxygenase (COX) inhibitors

Current evidence and areas of uncertainty

Neurological outcome

- Although indomethacin is known to cause profound reduction in cerebral perfusion, an RCT using neuroimaging showed that low-dose indomethacin reduces the incidence of intracranial hemorrhage (ICH)[210].
- Later, the *Trial of Indomethacin Prophylaxis in Preterms (TIPP)*[211], a larger RCT with neurological function as a primary endpoint, confirmed the neuroimaging result but failed to find a benefit in its primary outcome (improved survival/neurodevelopmental outcome).
- A *Cochrane meta-analysis (Fowlie and Davis, 2003)*[30] concluded that "there is no evidence to suggest either benefit or harm in longer term outcomes including neurodevelopment," and did not recommend prophylactic use of indomethacin.
- However, others criticized that the primary outcome's anticipated effect size ($\geq 20\%$) in the TIPP trial was too large; a smaller effect size ($<3\%$) would have been more appropriate based on the incidence of ICH in that particular population and its association with neurodevelopmental outcome[212].
- A group from Yale (Ment *et al.*, 2004)[213] re-evaluated their original trial from 1994 and found that indomethacin-treated boys had significantly less intracranial hemorrhage and higher scores in one neurocognitive test than girls, suggesting that the effect of indomethacin was gender specific. A review of the TIPP data set suggested a weak differential treatment effect of indomethacin by sex[31]. However, the nature of the interaction was qualitatively different than that observed by Ment *et al.* (2004)[213]: In the TIPP study, a negative effect of indomethacin in females was a more prominent observation than a positive effect in males[31].

385

Pulmonary outcome

- It should be noted that there is an ongoing controversy about whether ibuprofen treatment[214] or indomethacin prophylaxis (see TIPP trial[215]) increases the incidence of BPD/CLD in ELBW infants without PDA. *So far, treatments that successfully close a PDA have not resulted in a reduction of BPD*[216,217]. The uncertainty about the benefits and risks of the use of COX inhibitors can only be resolved by performing randomized, controlled trials, and these trials should include a placebo group in which treatment of a PDA is offered to infants in very limited circumstances only[216].

- *Cochrane meta-analysis (Ohlsson* et al., *2005)*[214] *entitled "Ibuprofen for the treatment of patent ductus arteriosus in preterm and/or low birth weight infants,"* states that there is "… no statistically significant difference in the effectiveness of ibuprofen compared to indomethacin in closing the PDA. Ibuprofen reduces the risk of oliguria. However, ibuprofen may increase the risk for CLD, and pulmonary hypertension has been observed in three infants after prophylactic use of ibuprofen."

- *Cochrane meta-analysis (Shah and Ohlsson, 2006)*[218] *entitled "Ibuprofen for the prevention of patent ductus arteriosus in preterm and/or low birth weight infants,"* states "Prophylactic use of ibuprofen reduces the incidence of PDA, the need for rescue treatment with cyclo-oxygenase inhibitors and surgical closure. However, in the control group, the PDA had closed spontaneously by day three in 60% of the neonates. Prophylactic treatment therefore exposes a large proportion of infants unnecessarily to a drug that has important side effects (mainly involving the kidneys) without conferring any important short term benefits. Prophylactic treatment with ibuprofen is not recommended. Until long-term follow-up results are published from the trials included in this review, no further trials of prophylactic ibuprofen are recommended."

- *Cochrane meta-analysis (Herrera* et al., *2007)*[219], *entitled, "Prolonged versus short course of indomethacin for the treatment of patent ductus arteriosus in preterm infants,"* states, "Implications for practice: prolonged indomethacin course does not appear to have a significant effect on improving important outcomes, such as PDA treatment failure, CLD, IVH, or mortality. The reduction of transient renal impairment does not outweigh the increased risk of NEC associated with the prolonged course. Based on these results, a prolonged course of indomethacin cannot be recommended for the routine treatment of PDA in preterm infants. Implications for research: there is a paucity of data on optimal dosing and duration of indomethacin therapy for the treatment of PDA, in particular for extremely low birth weight (ELBW) premature infants. It is likely that a single standard indomethacin regimen is not the ideal for every premature infant. Therefore, individual patient response should be considered and evaluated, in particular in ELBW infants."

Risks and benefits with the use of COX inhibitors in VLBW infants

! Indomethacin decreases the rate of intracranial hemorrhage (e.g., intraventricular hemorrhage) in VLBW infants, however, the clinical relevance of this finding is unclear.

! On the basis of the current data, *there is no role for ibuprofen prophylaxis in VLBW infants at risk for PDA*[214,218].

! Given the *high spontaneous PDA closure rate in very preterm infants* (≈60%–70% by day 3), prophylaxis with either indomethacin or ibuprofen exposes a large proportion of infants unnecessarily to a drug class that has important side-effects (mainly involving the kidneys) without conferring any important short term benefits[218].

! If one finds the reduction in serious ICH a sufficient justification for prophylactic use (even without certainty about long-term benefits; see TIPP Trial), then selective use in populations in which the rate of ICH is high (i.e., ELBW) may be reasonable[216]. Hence, *many centers reserve indomethacin prophylaxis for selected patients at very high risk for ICH, although the exact criteria are subject of an ongoing debate* (Boys <28 0/7 weeks' gestation p.m.? Girls at all? Or girls only when <26 0/7 weeks' gestation?)

! There is still no consensus as to whether (and when) indomethacin or ibuprofen should be used for the early treatment of PDA ($\geq$24–72 h of life) in very preterm infants[214,220], in terms of acute side-effects, intact survival and long-term morbidity. There are no current data on whether this decision should depend on the renal function of the preterm infant, e.g., the urine output or serum creatinine on the second/third day of life[220].

! Conservative treatment of PDA (fluid restriction, ventilator adjustment; see below) may be an alternative for a subgroup of VLBW infants with PDA[221].

How do COX-2 inhibitors prevent intracranial hemorrhage (ICH)?
This question has remained unanswered for decades. Recently, Ballabh *et al.* (2007) demonstrated that prenatal COX-2 inhibition decreases angiopoietin-2 and vascular endothelial growth factor levels as well as germinal matrix endothelial proliferation, and lowers the incidence of germinal matrix hemorrhage (GMH = IVH grade I) in premature rabbit pups[25]. The authors speculate that by suppressing germinal matrix angiogenesis, prenatal COX-2 inhibitors (celecoxib) or VEGF receptor 2 blockers (ZD6474) may be able to reduce both the incidence and the severity of GMH in susceptible premature infants[25]. However, there are currently no human data to support this hypothesis.

Indications for pharmacological closure of PDA with COX inhibitors

- There is a clear indication for rapid therapeutic closure of the arterial duct in preterm neonates with ELBW, large left-to-right shunt, and poor pulmonary function

- The indication for ductal closure is not certain if the shunt is small or when only slight respiratory problems are present

- In many hospitals, only a symptomatic PDA is treated (pulmonary deterioration/ stagnation, heart failure, decrease in the cerebral or mesenterial diastolic blood flow)

- Prophylactic indomethacin (e.g., 0.1 mg/kg IV during the first 24 h after birth, continued every 24 hours up to the fifth day) does not improve respiratory status. However, it reduces the incidence of intracranial hemorrhage (e.g., IVH)[209,211], and might improve long-term neurological outcome in boys (600–1250 g)[213]

! Based on the current clinical data, there are no benefits and possibly harm with both early use of ibuprofen (prophylaxis, treatment) in the first 24 h of life (e.g., pulmonary hypertension)[218], and prolonged courses of indomethacin for PDA treatment (e.g., NEC)[219].

Prerequisites and exclusion criteria for ibuprofen or indomethacin treatment

- Establish the diagnosis of PDA and rule out duct-dependent congenital heart disease by echocardiography (or MRI)
- Rule out abnormal coagulation
- Confirm adequate renal function (urine output, creatinine, urea): COX inhibitors are contraindicated when serum creatinine >2.0 mg/dl or urine output <0.8 ml/kg/h in the previous 8 h (not evidenced-based)
- CBC, CRP: rule out thrombocytopenia (<60 000/μl) and infection (controversial contraindication)
- Transcranial ultrasonography (including U/S Doppler with cerebral and mesenterial V_{max}/V_{ed} and RI)
- Progressing and/or severe intracranial hemorrhage (controversial contraindication)
- Severe hyperbilirubinemia close to exchange transfusion threshold ($\rightarrow$ release of bilirubin)
- Do not administer dexamethasone when giving COX inhibitors (be careful with steroids in general; if necessary, hydrocortisone preferred vs dexamethasone in newborn infants)
- Assess occult bleeding: screen with urine stix (U/A dip/microanalysis) and hemoccult testing, as long as pharmacological treatment is ongoing (NEC?)

Ibuprofen IV treatment for PDA closure

- First dose: 10 mg/kg/dose IV infused over 30 min on the first day of treatment $\rightarrow$ 24-h intervals
- Second dose: 5 mg/kg/dose IV infused over 30 min on the second day of treatment $\rightarrow$ 24-h intervals
- Third dose: 5 mg/kg/dose IV infused over 30 min on the third day of treatment $\rightarrow$ 24-h intervals

Ibuprofen failure: repeat either ibuprofen dosage scheme (see above) or switch to indomethacin treatment (see below).

Indomethacin IV treatment for PDA closure (indomethacin prophylaxis is performed in some centers for infants <26–28 weeks GA p.m. at 12–15 h of life; some centers give prophylactic indomethacin only to boys)

- Three initial doses: first = 0.2 mg/kg/dose IV, second = 0.1 mg/kg/dose IV (24 h after the first dose), third = 0.1 mg/kg/dose IV (24 h after the second dose)
- Serum creatinine and platelet count should be checked before second and third doses
- Just prior to the third indomethacin dose, obtain an echocardiogram
- If there is echocardiographic evidence of patency of the ductus (even if there are no clinical signs), some neonatologists give fourth, fifth, and sixth doses of indomethacin (0.1 mg/kg/dose IV at 24-h intervals). Repeat echo cardiogram after the sixth dose.

It is debatable whether prolonged low-dose indomethacin (6×0.1 mg/kg IV every 12 h) is associated with fewer cases of creatinine retention and a higher rate of PDA closure at the same time[222]. However, a recent Cochrane meta-analysis concluded that the reduction of transient renal impairment does not outweigh the increased risk of necrotizing enterocolitis

(NEC) associated with the prolonged course[219], and discourage the prolonged use of indomethacin for the treatment of PDA.

> ! Always draw up the exact amount of indomethacin or ibuprofen, and make sure that the patient receives the full drug dose (e.g., flush with a continuous infusion of D_5W, as drug may remain in the infusion tubing).

Adverse effects of COX inhibitors
- Renal insufficiency/oliguria: with indomethacin in $\approx 19\%$ (has a stronger effect on COX-1), with ibuprofen in $\approx 7\%$[220]
- Adverse and independent effects of indomethacin prophylaxis on the need for supplemental oxygen and on weight loss by the end of the first week of life may increase the risk of BPD/CLD in ELBW infants without PDA[215]
- Probably higher incidence of BPD/CLD in VLBW infants with PDA s/p ibuprofen treatment
- Probably higher incidence of pulmonary hypertension in VLBW infants s/p ibuprofen prophylaxis
- Feeding intolerance
- Occult blood in the stool
- NEC risk is increased: especially, when oliguria occurs. NEC twice as often with indomethacin when compared to ibuprofen (trend)[220]
- Occasionally hematuria
- "Asymptomatic" perforation of the intestines
- Thrombocytopenia (4%)

Ibuprofen versus indomethacin
- The rate of the primary ductal closure is similar for both drugs: 66%–80%. Successful secondary closure after a second course of indomethacin was found in 1/4 to 1/3 of the patients with primary treatment failure
- Advantages of ibuprofen when compared to indomethacin: ibuprofen does not reduce either gastrointestinal or cerebral perfusion, and has fewer negative effects on renal perfusion (oliguria 7% vs. 19%). There is probably no significant difference in the rate of BPD/CLD; however, in the largest prospective study at present, NEC was diagnosed twice as often with indomethacin treatment (trend)[220]
- When indomethacin is infused slowly, i.e., over 6 h IV, it may have fewer renal side-effects (caution: this observation has not been studied systematically in a randomized controlled trial)
- Prophylactic indomethacin decreases the rate of intracranial hemorrhage (ICH) in preterm infants (males only?)
- At present, ibuprofen is as affordable as indomethacin. Costs for indomethacin are many times higher in the USA when compared to Canada, Europe, and Australia[223]

Pharmacological treatment failure (indomethacin, ibuprofen)
In one of the largest prospective studies performed to date, high-frequency oscillatory ventilation (HFOV) was associated with lower rates of PDA closure. Severe immaturity

(<27 weeks' gestation) and high pulmonary arterial pressure were associated with failure of pharmacological treatment with indomethacin or ibuprofen[220].

Surgical ligation of the ductus arteriosus

- Preoperative procedures:
  - Secure peripheral venous access; central venous line, when indicated
  - Type and screen/cross, order PRBC; coagulation panel
  - Additional radiant warmer: monitor body temperature closely
  - Before/during surgery: mechanical ventilation (IPPV/IMV), administer analgesia and sedation
- Postoperative procedures: chest X-ray, blood glucose, ABG, hematocrit, echocardiography

> *!* During and after surgery, acute hemodynamic changes may occur. When the PDA is closed, SVR increases rapidly and may lead to a LV dysfunction due to increased afterload; consider echocardiogram and dopamine IV (as indicated).

Surgical versus pharmacological PDA closure

- Operation can be done in the NICU when treatment with cox inhibitors is contraindicated or fails
- Beyond the fourth week of life, the success rate of pharmacological treatment falls rapidly. Therefore, surgical closure of a (symptomatic) PDA is usually done 3–4 weeks after birth
- Advantage: secure and definitive closure of the ductus arteriosus
- Low morbidity and mortality in experienced centers
- Common adverse events s/p PDA ligation are recurrent laryngeal nerve damage, chylothorax (thoracic duct injury), pneumothorax, and a period of LV dysfunction immediately following ligation. Infants whose ductus arteriosus is ligated may be at greater risk for poor developmental outcome compared with infants treated medically. Unfortunately, there have been no recent controlled trials comparing outcomes following ligation with outcomes following either placebo or medical treatment. Therefore, the risks and benefits of surgical PDA ligation are unknown[217]

Conservative treatment of PDA (no drugs, no surgery)

Recently, Vanhaesebrouck *et al.* (2007)[221] prospectively studied a total of 30 neonates ≤ 30 weeks' gestations; (46% boys, 54% girls; mean gestational age 26.6 weeks with range 25–30 weeks; mean birth weight 994 g (600–1484 g)). All infants with PDA were treated following a standard protocol as soon as the diagnosis of a hemodynamically important PDA had been made (echocardiography 48–72 h after birth: ductus arteriosus diameter >1.4 mm, assessed with color Doppler). First, conservative treatment consisting of fluid restriction (maximum 130 ml/kg/day beyond day 3) and adjustment of ventilation by lowering inspiratory time to as low as 0.35 s, and giving higher PEEP (as high as 4.5 mbar ($=$cmH$_2$O); usual practice included inspiratory time 0.4–0.45 s and PEEP 3.5–4.0 mbar). Second, infants with a PDA that did not show clinical improvement and/or deterioration, and who had continuing need for ventilatory support, would undergo ductal ligation.

The investigators did not use any medication for prophylactic or therapeutic treatment of PDA. Ten neonates (33%) developed a clinical important PDA. Following conservative treatment the duct closed in all neonates (100%), and none required ductal ligation or medical treatment. The rates of major complications were no higher than those reported by the Vermont Oxford Network (www.vrtoxford.org)[220] and in the literature. Hence, for a selected subgroup of VLBW preterm infants, conservative treatment consisting of fluid restriction (not exceeding 130 ml/kg/day beyond day 3) and ventilator adjustment may be an alternative treatment, although its efficiency should be studied in larger randomization controlled trials.

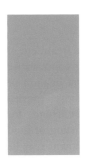

Persistent pulmonary hypertension of the newborn (PPHN)

Georg Hansmann

Definition

Persistent pulmonary hypertension of the newborn (PPHN) is a syndrome resulting from maladaptation to extrauterine life without a sustained normalization of pulmonary vascular resistance (PVR). PPHN is characterized by an elevation in PVR with resultant hypoxemia due to right-to-left shunting at the ductal and/or atrial level. PPHN may be confused with, or may coexist with, congenital heart disease: PPHN is frequently idiopathic but may be associated with respiratory failure/alveolar hypoxia (e.g., meconium aspiration syndrome, congenital pneumonia, sepsis, birth asphyxia, respiratory distress syndrome (RDS)), lung hypoplasia (e.g., congenital diaphragmatic hernia, alveolar capillary dysplasia) and maternal medication (e.g., late gestational use of selective serotonin reuptake inhibitors (SSRI); see Table 3.8).

Syndrome

Persistent fetal circulation (PFC) is used rarely.

Epidemiology

Incidence 0.67/1000[175] to 1.9/1000[224] live births. The risk of PPHN is about sixfold increased in newborns whose mothers used antidepressants of the SSRI class (e.g., Prozac®) after 20 weeks of gestation[161], with an overall incidence of approx. 6 to 12 per 1000 exposed women. However, the latter risk increase is based on a retrospective case controlled study with a very small effect size, i.e., 99% of women exposed to SSRI will have a baby not affected by PPHN. The incidence of "idiopathic" PPHN in neonates with Down syndrome (trisomy 21) is high ($\approx$12/1000)[225], but in the absence of associated conditions there is resolution of PPHN[226].

Etiology/pathophysiology

- See also p. 63 "Postnatal cardiopulmonary adaptation"
- PVR is high immediately after birth and increased even further in PPHN due to various reasons (Table 3.8). If the PVR is greater than the systemic vascular resistance (SVR) *right-to-left shunting across the ductus arteriosus (PA → DA → aorta) occurs. RV failure or tricuspid regurgitation directed towards the atrial septum results in a right-to-left shunt at the atrial level (RA → PFO/ASD → LA).* Both right-to-left shunts lead to *cyanosis of the newborn* (see pp. 124–7).
- PPHN often results when structurally normal pulmonary vessels constrict in response to acute alveolar hypoxia and hypoventilation, or parenchymal disorders ("*vascular*

Neonatal Emergencies: A Practical Guide for Resuscitation, Transport and Critical Care, ed. Georg Hansmann. Published by Cambridge University Press. © Cambridge University Press 2009.

Table 3.8 Persistent pulmonary hypertension of the newborn (PPHN)

Persistent pulmonary hypertension of the newborn (PPHN)

	Acute pulmonary vasoconstriction	Primary pulmonary vascular disease	Parenchymal lung disease
Etiology	• Alveolar hypoxia (MAS, RDS, pneumothorax, pneumonia), p. 269, p. 231, p. 410	• Idiopathic PPHN ("black lung" = "clear lung" PPHN)	• Congenital diaphragmatic hernia (CDH), p. 404
	• Sepsis (e.g., GBS), p. 280	• Chronic intrauterine hypoxia (e.g., placental insufficiency)	• Primary pulmonary hypoplasia, p. 404
	• Birth asphyxia, p. 304, p. 310	• Maternal intake of prostaglandin blockers (ASA, indomethacin, ibuprofen) may lead to a premature closure of the arterial duct and (imminent) death of the fetus especially during the last trimester	• Very rare cases of neurological hypoventilation (e.g., spinal muscular atrophy/Werdnig–Hoffmann disease, phrenic/nerve agenesis/aplasia of the diaphragm → pulmonary hypoplasia)
	• LV dysfunction/cardiogenic shock		• Alveolar capillary dysplasia
	• Hyperviscosity syndrome (polycythemia)		• Acinar dysplasia
	• Hypoglycemia	• Antepartum therapy with certain psychoactive substances (e.g., lithium, SSRI)	• Congenital cystic adenomatoid malformation (rarely associated with PPHN), p. 417
	• Hypocalcemia		• Hydrops fetalis, p. 427, anhydramnios
	• Hypothermia	• High pulmonary blood flow states, e.g., AV shunts/malformations (→ shear stress)	• Congenital surfactant disorders (e.g., SP-B deficiency or ABCA3 deficiency)
Pathophysiology	• Pulmonary vasoconstriction of the histologically normal pulmonary vasculature (structurally normal vasculature)	• Vascular media hypertrophy of pulmonary arterioles (structurally abnormal vasculature, i.e., peripheral and excessive PA muscularization)	• Abnormal development of pulmonary arterioles → total surface area and number of pulmonary vessels decreased (hypoplastic vasculature)

Table 3.8 (cont.)

Persistent pulmonary hypertension of the newborn (PPHN)

	Acute pulmonary vasoconstriction	*Primary pulmonary vascular disease*	*Parenchymal lung disease*
Etiology			
Outcome	• Varies, up to 95% survive • Survival is highest in ECMO centers	• Varies; mortality rate 10%–50%	• Poor
Note	• Early surfactant administration, particularly in MAS, is reasonable • iNO therapy improves oxygenation and reduces the frequency of ECMO treatment	• iNO therapy improves oxygenation and reduces the frequency of ECMO treatment.	• Primary surfactant treatment especially in the newborn with pulmonary hypoplasia is reasonable • iNO therapy improves oxygenation and reduces the frequency of ECMO treatment • iNO therapy does not seem to improve the outcome of infants with congenital diaphragmatic hernia[79]

ASA, acetylsalicylic acid (e.g., aspirin); ECMO, extracorporeal membrane oxygenation; GBS, group B streptococci; iNO, inhalative nitric oxide; MAS, meconium aspiration syndrome; PPHN, persistent pulmonary hypertension of the newborn; SSRI, selective serotonin reuptake inhibitor.

hyperreactivity", e.g., meconium aspiration syndrome, congenital pneumonia, sepsis, birth asphyxia)

- However, PPHN can also occur in the absence of underlying parenchymal disease. In these cases, the syndrome is thought to be the result of abnormal vascular remodeling in utero in response to prolonged fetal stress, hypoxia, high flow states (e.g., AV malformations) and/ or "idiopathic" pulmonary hypertension (*J Am Coll Cardiol* 2009; 54: s43–54). *Excessive and peripheral muscularization* of pulmonary arterioles can be seen in these cases
- Moreover, PPHN is commonly associated with lung hypoplasia, as seen in congenital diaphragmatic hernia, where the total *number of pulmonary vessels is decreased* (Table 3.8)
- With inadequate pulmonary perfusion, newborns develop refractory hypoxemia, respiratory distress, and acidosis. Hemodynamics and cyanosis/hypoxia are aggravated by systemic hypotension (e.g., hypovolemia, low cardiac output, sepsis). Further worsening of pulmonary vasoconstriction and right-to-left-shunting is caused by the hyperreactivity of neonatal pulmonary vessels, which are regulated by vasoactive substances such as endothelin-1, angiotensin II, nitric oxide (NO), prostaglandins, leukotrienes, bradykinin, histamine, adenosine, and nucleotides
- The *Euler-Liljestrand mechanism*, i.e., local decrease in ventilation in the smallest areas of the lung leads to *hypoxic pulmonary vasoconstriction* (HPV) and locally decreased lung perfusion, is an important regulatory process in all situations where ventilation perfusion (*V/Q*) mismatch occurs. To be effective, HPV needs normal pulmonary areas into which blood flow can be redirected ("normoxic pulmonary vasodilatation"). When most of the lung is hypoxic, there is no significant normoxic region to which the hypoxic region can divert flow. In this situation, HPV becomes a rather detrimental mechanism as it increases pulmonary artery pressure (PAP). At a certain turning point of severe (generalized) alveolar hypoxia, the gain in P_aO_2 is lost due to an increase in right ventricular afterload (i.e., PVR), leading to a decrease in cardiac output and RV failure
- A decrease in endogenous NO production and a genetically determined malfunction of the urea cycle may play a role in the pathophysiology of PPHN[227]
- Impaired VEGF–NO signaling within endothelial cells appears to contribute to abnormal vascular growth in utero[228]
- Exposure of fetal pulmonary artery smooth muscle cells to high levels of oxygen for 24 h leads to decreased responsiveness to exogenous NO, as determined by a decreased intracellular cGMP response, increased phosphodiesterase 5 (PDE5) expression, as well as increased PDE5 cGMP hydrolytic activity. PDE5 seems to play a critical role in modulating neonatal pulmonary vascular tone in response to common clinical treatments for PPHN, such as oxygen and inhaled NO[229]

Clinical presentation

- Usually a term or postterm newborn infant. The pale or cyanotic infant reveals tachypnea, jitteriness, circulatory depression, and sometimes hypothermia
- Signs and symptoms become obvious approx. 6–12 h after birth. Cyanosis is usually noticed outside the delivery room, e.g., in the nursery
- Auscultatory signs: cardiac gallop (optional) and holosystolic murmur (tricuspid regurgitation)
- In preterm infants, a combination of RDS and PPHN is possible, but not typical
- Duration of PPHN symptoms is approx. 3–5 days

> **!** Cyanosis may be absent in severe anemia pp. 124–7.

DDx.

Cyanotic heart disease (p. 124, p. 340), sepsis of the newborn (p. 280), RDS or pneumonia without PPHN, anemia

Diagnosis in the delivery room/nursery

- S_aO_2 monitoring (pulse oximetry) on the right arm and one leg. On the rare occasion of an aberrant right subclavian artery (originating postductally from the aorta), the only location for reliable preductal S_pO_2 measurements is the right ear lobe
  - An S_pO_2 difference of 10 percent points is significant if the peripheral blood flow is not reduced
  - In acrocyanosis or poor systemic perfusion, it may be necessary to confirm both the S_aO_2 and P_aO_2 difference by obtaining pre- and postductal arterial blood gases (ABGs) simultaneously (e.g., right radial artery and umbilical artery (or posterior tibial artery))
  - A *"differential cyanosis"* may become apparent between the upper (right) and lower extremities, when there is a large right-to-left shunt across the ductus arteriosus
  - Even though a "differential cyanosis" may not be clinically obvious, a P_aO_2 difference of 10–15 mmHg between the upper and lower extremities must be considered a significant ductal right-to-left shunt

> There is no large S_aO_2 and/or P_aO_2 difference or "differential diagnosis" if the right-to-left shunt across the PFO/ASD outweighs the ductal shunting.

- Obtain ABG (acidosis), blood glucose (hypoglycemia is common), and if possible electrolytes including calcium and magnesium (reliable ≈6 h after birth), and lactate. Further laboratory work-up might include coagulation panel, blood culture and smears
- Perform echocardiography, if necessary in the delivery room/nursery, otherwise as soon as possible in the ICU
- A hyperoxia test may be necessary if echocardiography is not rapidly available (p. 126)

DDx PPHN versus cyanotic heart disease

- If S_aO_2 and P_aO_2 rise significantly after oxygen supplementation/intubation/PPV and a loud PDA-like murmur is present, PPHN is a possible differential diagnosis. However, even HLHS or CoA may present with a P_aO_2 of 150–200 mmHg in 100% oxygen, and other congenital heart diseases such as truncus arteriosus and TAPVR may even have a higher P_aO_2 in 100% oxygen
- A S_aO_2 and P_aO_2 difference (*"ductal split"*) between the upper (right arm) and lower part of the body increases the likelihood of PPHN. However, a ductal split may be absent in PPHN with dominant atrial right-to-left shunt, in PPHN with an aberrant right subclavian artery (if preductal S_pO_2 is falsely measured at the right hand), and in PPHN with d-TGA
- Echocardiography usually confirms the diagnosis

Therapy in the delivery room/nursery

Resuscitative (ABCD) measures (ILCOR) as necessary (p. 153), especially suctioning and oxygen supplementation. If peripheral perfusion or the respiratory condition is critical, intubation/PPV and volume substitution may be necessary. Primary, rapid intubation without initial bag-and-mask ventilation in patients with congenital diaphragmatic hernia (CDH) or meconium aspiration syndrome (MAS). Catecholamines are rarely needed in the delivery room, but may be indicated in the NICU. Early surfactant administration may be considered (see under "Therapy in the NICU"). Normoventilation

> **!** **Avoid the "7 Hs"**: hypoxia, hypercarbia, hypocarbia, hypoglycemia, hypothermia, hyperthermia, systemic hypotension.
>
> **!** When the newborn is stable, **transfer the patient to the NICU** as soon as possible.
>
> **!** Volume expansions can aggravate ductal right-to-left shunts, but may also temporarily improve pulmonary blood flow. In PPHN, **blood pressure goals** are mean arterial pressure (MAP) approx. 45–50 mmHg (upper range for infant's weight) or $\geq$ gestational age in weeks, diastolic BP >25–30 mmHg or approx. 15 mmHg above the mean airway pressure ($\bar{P}_{aw}$).

Monitoring

Pre- (right arm) and postductal (leg) S_pO_2, and BP monitoring, temperature; ECG, if indicated. Arterial line (UAC and/or radial artery).

Diagnosis in the NICU

History, clinical presentation and echocardiography lead to the diagnosis of PPHN:

- ABG, lactate, laboratory work-up, if necessary blood culture
- Arterial and central venous line. Pre- and postductal S_aO_2 and BP monitoring (right arm/leg)
- Consider continuous transcutaneous P_aO_2 and P_aCO_2 measurement (tcPO$_2$ and tcPCO$_2$) in the NICU if the measurements are reliable and validated by intermittent arterial blood gas analysis (applicable mainly for small infants)
- Continuous temperature measurement
- Chest X-ray (vascular markings/transparency and heart size depend on underlying cause). Frequently, there is a discrepancy between "good chest X-ray" and poor clinical status
- Echocardiography: rule out any congenital heart disease. In PPHN, a right-to-left shunt across the arterial duct and PFO is present and dominant; right ventricular systolic pressure (RVSP) is increased due to high PAP; enhanced RV hypertrophy/dilatation and ventricular dysfunction may be present. Other findings may include septal wall flattening (D-sign), and tricuspid regurgitation (TR). Using TR jet velocity to estimate RV pressure (RVSP $= [4 \times v^2] +$ RAP) may help in guiding therapy
- Cardiac catheterization should be reserved for special circumstances
- Head ultrasound, especially prior to extracorporeal membrane oxygenation (ECMO)
- If the difference in pre- and postductal parameters (S_aO_2, P_aO_2 and BP) becomes smaller and is associated with both improvement of (preductal) ABG and echocardiography findings (fall of TR/RVSP/right-to-left shunt), one may assume better pulmonary blood flow (i.e., decreased PAP and PVR)! However, the same scenario may occur with

397

unchanged high PVR and a closing ductus arteriosus (echocardiogram). In the latter case, transient improvement in oxygenation may precede RV failure

Procedure/therapy in the NICU
Treatment goals (limited clinical data)

- *Supportive therapy:* minimal handling/avoid stressors (consider analgesia and sedation; arterial/central venous line). Optimize metabolism/parenteral nutrition, intravascular (blood) volume (maintain sufficient intravascular volume; avoid polycythemia; goal hematocrit 45%–50%) and hemostasis. Treat concomitant diseases
- *Reduction of PVR and PAP* by optimizing oxygenation ($F_iO_2 = 0.5–1.0$) and ventilation (P_aCO_2 goal 35–40 mmHg). In infants with PPHN, 100% O_2 has been considered a first-line therapy because of its rapid vasodilative action in the pulmonary circulation. However, postnatal exposure to high levels of oxygen may cause persistent lung injury, oxidative stress, and pulmonary vascular remodeling. Thus, the rationale for high inspired oxygen concentrations has come under question. One current hypothesis suggests that exposure to hyperoxia leads to increased production of reactive oxygen species (ROS), which increases PDE5 expression and activity. The increased PDE5 activity ultimately decreases the amount of available cGMP, leading to impaired vasorelaxation in response to exogenous NO. Aside from oxygen therapy, direct pulmonary vasodilatation (inhaled nitric oxide (iNO), sildenafil, etc.) and alkalinization (sodium bicarbonate, THAM IV) may be indicated (keep in mind that extreme alkalosis may compromise cardiac contractility). Analgesia, sedation, and muscle relaxation (optional) may also be necessary (avoid alkalosis but aim for high–normal pH; caution with hypertonic buffer solutions, especially in preterm infants!)
- *Treatment of myocardial dysfunction/arterial hypotension* with catecholamines (dopamine, rarely dobutamine, norepinephrine) and eventually diuretics may be indicated. Achieve and maintain sinus rhythm and sufficient cardiac output

Supportive therapy

- Monitoring vital parameters including temperature (36.6–37.2°C/97.9–99.0°F), perhaps tcPO$_2$, tcPCO$_2$.
- Minimal handling!
- An agitated neonate with PPHN needs analgesia/sedation; if peak inspiratory pressure (PIP)/mean airway pressure ($\bar{P}_{aw}$) is very high, administer additional muscle relaxant. These measures are not general recommendations and have to be applied and adjusted individually – especially when the infant is borderline hypotensive. With analgesia and sedation/relaxation, the respiratory situation (oxygenation, ventilation, decrease in PVR $\rightarrow$ larger ductal left-to-right shunting in theory) may improve; however, SVR may continue to fall, followed by enhanced right-to-left shunting across the patent ductus arteriosus ($\rightarrow$ central cyanosis, hypoxemia, worsening PPHN)
  - When analgesia/sedation is required: morphine (0.02–0.05 mg/kg/h IV) or 0.05–0.1 mg/kg/dose q 1–3 h PRN IV. Alternative: fentanyl/midazolam infusion. For disadvantages of midazolam in neonates see p. 82
  - When muscle relaxation is required: pancuronium 0.05–0.1 mg/kg/h or 0.1 mg/kg/dose q 1–3 h PRN IV. Good alternatives are: *cis*-atracurium (0.1–0.2 mg/kg/h IV; of special benefit in hepatic and renal insufficiency however, tachyphylaxis occurs)

or rocuronium (0.3–0.6 mg/kg/h IV). Muscle relaxant agents improve pulmonary complaints and slow down metabolism (beneficial in generalized hypoxia). However, paralysis may be associated with an increased risk of death[224] and sensorineural hearing loss in childhood survivors of CDH. *Check package insert and current drug approval for neonatal use!*

- Stabilize circulation with volume expansion and/or catecholamines (aim: MAP approx. 45–50 mmHg or ≥gestational age in weeks, diastolic BP >25–30 mmHg or approx. 15 mmHg above the mean $\bar{P}_{aw}$)
- Prevention of stress-induced erosive gastritis/gastric ulcer: proton pump inhibitors, e.g., omeprazole or pantoprazole, are more efficient and preferred over histamine receptor 2 antagonists (e.g., ranitidine) not least because histamine is a known pulmonary vasodilatator
- Recognition and treatment of metabolic crisis (monitor patient closely, especially blood glucose, calcium, magnesium, phosphate; maintain pH value >7.45, but keep pH <7.60)
- Treatment of anemia and polycythemia: goal is 14 g/dl < hemoglobin <18 g/dl (Hct goal 45%–50%)
- Use broad-spectrum antibiotics if indicated

Optimizing ventilation setting

Aim: preductal P_aCO_2 35–45 mmHg, preductal P_aO_2 90–100 mmHg (minimum >75 mmHg; F_iO_2 0.5–1.0, start with high F_iO_2 and titrate down); apply lowest possible PEEP; maintain pH in high – normal range or, in severe cases, between 7.45 and 7.55 by mild hyperventilation or alkalinization. Prolonged hyperventilation is associated with an increased prevalence of neurodevelopmental sequelae, including sensorineural hearing loss. Hence, many centers follow the guideline "avoid hypocarbia/hyperventilation in newborns with PPHN." See also pp. 193–209

- Adjust ventilator settings to maintain normal lung expansion (i.e., of approximately nine ribs) on chest radiography. Monitoring of tidal volume and pulmonary mechanics is frequently helpful in preventing overexpansion, which can elevate PVR and aggravate right-to-left shunting
- High-frequency oscillatory ventilation (HFOV) reduces the need for ECMO in patients with severe PPHN[175]. In newborns with severe airspace disease who require high PIP (i.e., >30 cmH$_2$O or mbar) or mean airway pressures (>15 cmH$_2$O or mbar), consider HFOV in order to reduce barotrauma. When HFOV is used, the goals remain: optimize lung expansion and functional residual capacity, and avoid overdistension

Pharmacotherapy

- *Surfactant administration*: aim to achieve/recruit optimum lung volume/FRC (caution: alveolar collapse vs. overdistension, i.e., atelectrauma vs. barotrauma). Consider early (i.e., before iNO) high-dose surfactant, especially in:
  - Preterm infants with PPHN
  - PPHN + MAS (surfactant lavage may be indicated)
  - PPHN + CDH[230]
- *Nitric oxide inhalation (iNO)*:
  - Improves oxygenation and reduces the need for ECMO treatment in near-term infants[80,231,232]

- In newborns with CDH, iNO does *not* improve outcome, in terms of oxygenation, ECMO indication or mortality rate (Cochrane metaanalysis, 2006)[80]! In these newborns, however, iNO may be used in non-ECMO centers to allow for acute stabilization, followed by immediate transfer to an ECMO center. Moreover, many centers still use iNO in CDH in an attempt to improve severe PPHN. Some intensivists use PGE$_1$ when the duct closes to prevent RV failure in severely affected infants (see box below) (not evidence-based)

Inhaled nitric oxide (iNO)

- Indicated in newborns (during transport, in NICU) with an oxygenation index (O.I.) >25 (indications may differ between centers and should be individualized for each patient). O.I. = (mean airway pressure $\times$ F_iO_2 $\times$ 100) $\div$ P_aO_2
- Start with 20 ppm[233] (some experts recommend 40 ppm)
- If systemic BP decreases under iNO, either reduce the iNO dose step by step or begin additional dopamine infusion; monitor methemoglobin (metHb) and NO_x
- Most newborns require iNO for 3–5 days. Reduce iNO gradually. In general, the dose can be weaned to 5 ppm after 6–24 h on iNO therapy. The dose is then weaned slowly and discontinued when the F_iO_2 is <0.6 and the iNO dose is 1 ppm. Sudden discontinuation should be avoided because it may cause abrupt rebound pulmonary hypertension
- *Rebound pulmonary hypertension* is a risk with cessation of iNO from even low doses (i.e., <5 ppm), after only a few hours of iNO therapy, and regardless of whether the infant initially responded to iNO (consider sildenafil)
- *Methemoglobinemia* (metHb >5%) occurs in approximately 10% of newborns treated with iNO and resolves with lowering the iNO dose. Daily metHb levels are indicated in infants receiving iNO therapy. MetHb can now be detected transcutaneously through a single finger probe (Masimo®: expanded spectrum analyzer to detect S_aO_2, metHb and carboxyhemoglobin)

Indications for and benefits of iNO may differ depending on the severity of illness and degree of prematurity. Barrington and Finer recently reviewed the controversial use of iNO for respiratory failure in *preterm* infants and conclude:

> "Inhaled nitric oxide as rescue therapy for very ill preterm infants undergoing ventilation does not seem to be effective and may increase severe intracranial hemorrhage. Later use of inhaled nitric oxide to prevent bronchopulmonary dysplasia does not seem to be effective. Early routine use of inhaled nitric oxide for mildly sick, preterm infants seems to decrease the risk of serious brain injury and may improve rates of survival without bronchopulmonary dysplasia." [234,235]

Prostaglandin E$_1$ (PGE$_1$)

- When the ductus arteriosus is about to close in newborns with PPHN and CDH, several centers use PGE$_1$ (50–100 ng/kg/min IV) to prevent RV failure (i.e., open ductus arteriosus is used as RV pop-off outlet in a clinical situation with very high PVR)
- Caution: if LV dysfunction is present, an effective iNO therapy may not only lead to an increase in pulmonary blood flow, but also to LV volume overload/failure with subsequent pulmonary edema. This can usually be prevented or treated with diuretics and/or by moderately decreasing SVR. However, if the ductus remains open, a decrease in SVR may worsen systemic hypoxia due to augmented right-to-left shunting

- Caution: under treatment with vasodilators (iNO, prostanoids, etc.), always ensure sufficient coronary perfusion pressure, i.e., for the coronary perfusion of the LV, maintain the diastolic BP >25–30 mmHg or approx. 15 mmHg above the mean $\bar{P}_{aw}$, and
  MAP >45–50 mmHg or $\geq$ gestational age in weeks p.m. Avoid tachycardia and hypovolemia
- *Future therapies*

Phosphodiesterase (PDE) inhibitors

- Sildenafil, which blocks PDE5 and other phosphodiesterases[236,237], enhances the effect of iNO inhalation and impairs the rebound vasospasm when iNO is discontinued[230]
- PDE inhibitors such as sildenafil PO/NG (1–2 mg/kg/dose q 6 h)[238] may be used when iNO is not available[238], in iNO non-responders or in infants to be weaned from iNO. PDE inhibitors (given via nebulizer[239], PO/NG[240–242] or IV) in combination with iNO may be a treatment option in the near future. However, the scarce data on PDE5 inhibitors in PPHN currently warrant against using sildenafil routinely for this indication until further data from RCT become available
- There are case reports on the beneficial effect of the PDE3 inhibitor milrinone in the treatment of neonates with PPHN not responding to iNO[243,244]
- Future therapies are under development, however their usefulness in PPHN will largely depend on a fast onset of action and lack of significant short- and long-term adverse effects[232,244]

- Additional vasodilators (which are not yet approved for neonatal use):
  - *Prostacyclin (PGI2)* – may be administered orally, IV (Flolan®: 5–20 ng/kg/min), by endotracheal instillation or inhalation (Iloprost®[245])
  - *Endothelin-1 receptor antagonists (ERA)*: may impair or prevent the pulmonary vascular crisis after weaning iNO (i.e., iNO rebound).[230,246] However, ERA have only minimal *acute* vasodilatory effects and there is currently insufficient clinical data (RCT) on the use of ERA to prevent iNO rebound
- For more information on pulmonary vasodilators and their adverse effects, see additional literature[82,230,232,246,247]

Catecholamines and diuretics: in myocardial dysfunction/persistent systemic hypotension.

Dopamine

- 5–10 (–20) µg/kg/min IV
- If systemic BP falls under treatment with iNO or prostanoids (IV, nebulizer), begin with dopamine (not primarily dobutamine) or increase initial dopamine dose (also consider IV volume)
- Disadvantage: high-dose dopamine may significantly increase PVR and PAP

Second-line catecholamines

Norepinephrine (noradrenaline)
- 0.05–0.1 (–1) µg/kg/min IV
- Use instead of dopamine when systemic arterial hypotension is the leading problem (consider IV volume as well)
- Disadvantage: may significantly increase PVR and PAP

Dobutamine
- 5–10 (–20) µg/kg/min IV
- Especially when LV dysfunction is evident

- Do not use dobutamine as monotherapy (may decrease SVR and diastotic BP), but in combination with dopamine or norepinephrine

Furosemide (may be indicated, e.g., in pulmonary edema)
- 0.5–1 mg/kg IV q 6–8 h

Goal: MAP approx. 45–50 mmHg (upper range for infant's weight), diastolic BP >25–30 mmHg or approx. 15 mmHg above the mean ventilation pressure (caution: decrease in diastolic BP and tachycardia, especially with dobutamine). Supportive treatment improves myocardial contractility (see above).

- Both dopamine and norepinephrine (noradrenaline) also increase PVR. *Dopamine and/or norepinephrine should be administered via a vein in the lower part of the body* (central venous line, e.g., umbilical vein), in order to bypass the lungs to some extent (via IVC → RA → PFO → LA) and to achieve higher drug levels in the systemic circulation/arterioles
- *Vasodilators such as prostacyclin IV (Flolan®) should be administered through a vein in the upper part of the body.* Hence, a high percentage of the drug dose will reach the PA (RA → RV → PA) and the pulmonary circulation, so that the total dose may be reduced to limit systemic adverse effects!

Extracorporeal membrane oxygenation (ECMO)
Indications for ECMO
Neonatal ECMO criteria may differ between large ECMO centers[81,82] (for detailed neonatal ECMO criteria, see also *chapter on MAS, p. 269*), and depend on the underlying cause (e.g., pulmonary vs. cardiac)[83].
- *Respiratory entry critera*[81a]
  - Alveolar–arterial oxygen gradient $(AaDO_2)$[b,c] >605–620 mmHg[c] for 4–12 h
  - Oxygenation index $(O.I.)$[d] >35–60 for 0.5–6 h
  - P_aO_2 <35 but <60 mmHg for 2–12 h
  - Acidosis and shock; pH <7.25 for 2 h or with hypotension
  - Acute deterioration in P_aO_2 <30 to <40 mmHg

Contraindications (ECMO)
Greater than second-degree ICH, severe HIE, severe concomitant malformations, GA <32 0/7 weeks p.m. (many centers consider GA <34 0/7 weeks a contraindication), body weight <1800 g (varies greatly between ECMO centers).

PPHN prevention
- *Primary prevention* is key: prevent the preventable causes of PPHN, thus
  - Avoid use of prostaglandin synthesis inhibitors (ASA/aspirin, indomethacin, ibuprofen), SSRI or lithium in pregnant women. However, women who are already

---

[a] 50% of ECMO centers use more than one respiratory entry criterion
[b] $P_{atm} = 760$ mmHg at sea level. F_iO_2 is 0.21–1.0. Normal $AaDO_2$ in room air is 5–20 mmHg
[c] $AaDO_2 = [(P_{atm} - 47) \times F_iO_2 - (P_aCO_2 \div 0.8)] - P_aO_2$
[d] O.I. = (mean airway pressure $\times F_iO_2 \times 100$) $\div P_aO_2$

on SSRI and/or lithium therapy and whose symptoms are well-controlled with these psychophamacological agents, are usually continued on their mediation during pregnancy

- Prevent (or detect early) acute or chronic pre/perinatal hypoxia/asphyxia, shock, (meconium) aspiration, severe infections (e.g., GBS), any form of perinatal stress, polycythemia, hypothermia, hypoglycemia, and hypocalcemia
- Secondary prevention
  - Screening for and early treatment of prenatal and perinatal infections (e.g., GBS screen)
  - Empiric broad-spectrum IV antibiotic treatment when neonatal infection is suspected.
  - Perform vaccination/prophylaxis for an infant s/p PPHN, although usually there is no residual pulmonary disease. Influenza vaccine in late fall; RSV immune prophylaxis (palivizumab; caution: adverse effects[234,235]) may be indicated for the newborn

Outcome

- Newborns with mild PPHN and an early response to therapy usually have a good prognosis
- If all available therapies including iNO and ECMO are utilized, the mortality rate appears to be less than 10%. However, the prevalence of major neurological disabilities among surviving newborns remains approximately 15%–20%
- Newborns s/p CDH and severe PPHN and need for prolonged (hyper-)ventilation with high F_iO_2 and high mean $\bar{P}_{aw}$ may develop chronic lung disease requiring home oxygen supplementation. PPHN morbidity is characterized by neurodevelopmental delay and neurological dysfunction, i.e., sensorineural hearing loss deafness, cerebral palsy, and EEG abnormalities. Therefore, CNS imaging (MRI brain), neurological/neurodevelopmental assessment and frequent hearing tests prior to discharge and during outpatient follow-up should be performed
- The oxygen index (O.I.) does not predict neurological and neurodevelopmental outcome
- Patients with an underdeveloped pulmonary vasculature (e.g., primary pulmonary hypoplasia or large congenital diaphragmatic hernia; p. 404) generally have a poor prognosis[175,231]

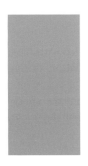

Congenital diaphragmatic hernia

Christoph Bührer and Andrea Zimmermann

Definition

Developmental defect in the diaphragm that allows abdominal viscera to protrude into the chest. Up to 90% of diaphragmatic defects are located on the left side. Right-sided congenital diaphragmatic hernia (CDH) has a morbidity and mortality pattern similar to that of left-sided CDH. Bilateral CDH is rare.

Epidemiology

- Incidence is 1:2200 (0.45/1000) live births
- The vast majority of CDH cases occur sporadically, but there are some familial cases with autosomal-recessive, autosomal-dominant, and X-linked inheritance patterns
- In the absence of a family history of CDH, the risk of recurrence of non-syndromic CDH for future siblings after one affected child is about 2%
- 50% of CDH cases are isolated, while the other 50% display karyotype abnormalities or further gross anatomical anomalies, such as neural tube defects, cardiac defects, cleft lip-cleft palate, and others

Etiology/pathophysiology

- Space limitation caused by protrusion of abdominal organs interferes with normal lung development leading to pulmonary hypoplasia (loss of pulmonary mass, decreased alveolar branching), and pulmonary hypertension (reduced total cross-sectional area of the pulmonary artery tree, muscular hyperplasia of remaining pulmonary arterioles)
- Prenatal diagnosis is based upon ultrasound. The principal findings include a chest mass (which may exhibit peristalsis), mediastinal shift, and malposition of stomach and liver
- Predictors of poor outcome:
  - Early prenatal diagnosis (<25 weeks)
  - Herniation of the liver into the thorax
  - Pulmonary hypoplasia (lung area to head circumfererence or lung-to-head ratio <1)
- In severe cases, which are easily diagnosed prenatally, and those with associated further anomalies, parents often opt for termination of pregnancy, leading to improved prognosis of the CDH infants born at referral centers[248–250]. About 60% (45%–75%) of these infants survive[249–252]

Neonatal Emergencies: A Practical Guide for Resuscitation, Transport and Critical Care, ed. Georg Hansmann. Published by Cambridge University Press. © Cambridge University Press 2009.

Clinical presentation

- Signs and symptoms range from severe respiratory failure that is fatal within less than 1 h after birth despite optimal treatment to accidental diagnosis by chest X-ray in children or even adults with non-specific respiratory or gastrointestinal symptoms[253,254]
- Infants with onset of respiratory distress later than 10 min after birth have an excellent prognosis with almost universal survival
- Features of more severe CDH:
  - Decline of Apgar values from 1 min to 10 min
  - Scaphoid (sunken) abdomen (abdominal organs translocated into the chest)
  - Breath sounds absent on the ipsilateral side. Bowel sounds may be audible on the ipsilateral chest
- Deviation of the tracheal axis to the unaffected side (observed during endotracheal intubation)
- Displacement of heart sounds to the right in most patients with CDH (CDH commonly on on left side → mediastinal shift to the right)

DDx.

- Respiratory distress syndrome (see p. 209, p. 231)
- Pneumothorax (see p. 410)
- Pleural effusion (see p. 419, p. 427)
- Pneumonia/sepsis
- Lung malformation (see p. 417)
- Tumor

> **!** A (typically left-sided) congenital diaphragmatic hernia can be differentiated from tension pneumothorax by palpating the spleen on the ipsilateral side. Infants with congenital diaphragmatic hernia present with a scaphoid (sunken) abdomen.

Diagnosis in the delivery room

- Auscultation, physical examination
- ABG

Monitoring in the delivery room

- Pre- and postductal S_pO_2, respiration, ABG, ECG (if possible, with low-voltage ECG monitoring), BP and ET tube position

Prenatal diagnosis and management

- Fetal ultrasound usually detects CDH, but small or late-occurring CDH may be missed
- Delivery in a tertiary center with on-site pediatric surgery
- Vaginal delivery following spontaneous onset of labor at term, at a specialized center (i.e., avoid postnatal transport of infants with CDH)
- Cesarean section in the absence of labor is not recommended unless there is a clear medical indication

Procedure/therapy in the delivery room

- Do not use bag-and-mask ventilation – this increases gastric and intestinal distension, and worsens mediastinal shift and respiratory distress. Instead, intubate the infant's trachea immediately, connect ET tube to ventilation device and perform PPV with 50%–100% oxygen. Use low PIP and low PEEP (2–3 cmH$_2$O). Infants with CDH do not tolerate higher PEEP levels
- Place pre- and post-ductal S_pO_2 probes. Use pre-ductal S_pO_2 to judge oxygenation
- Insert Replogle tube (large gastric tube) and set to suction to decompress stomach and small bowel
- Gas exchange: the aim of assisted ventilation should be to provide adequate oxygenation (preductal S_pO_2 ≥90%) and ventilation (P_aCO_2 ≤60 mmHg). Choose lowest ventilator settings to achieve these goals, and do not attempt to correct hypoxemia and hypercarbia rapidly. In large CDH, preductal S_pO_2 >75% might be acceptable if this allows decreasing high ventilator settings (PIP, $\bar{P}_{aw}$ = mean airway pressure). Oxygenation and ventilation frequently improve over the first few hours after birth. Lung recruitment is usually not needed but lung collapse may occur while weaning
- Ventilator setting: start with conventional ventilation settings, low to moderate rate (40 breaths/min), inspiratory time (T_{in}) 0.40 s and PEEP 2 cmH$_2$O (mode and settings may differ between institutions). If strategy fails, switch to higher frequency (80–100 breaths/min, T_{in} 0.30 s, PEEP 1 cm H$_2$O because of inadvertent PEEP). Use PIP monitoring (the benefits of volume monitoring must be weighed against increased dead space), and avoid PIP >25 cmH$_2$O. Choose low PEEP (2–3 cmH$_2$O) to increase pulmonary blood flow. See also "Mechanical ventilation" on pp. 193–209
- Change to high-frequency oscillatory ventilation (HFOV) if conventional ventilation fails (some centers may start with HFOV)
- Notify the pediatric surgeons immediately if there is a CDH

Additional procedures

- Establish venous access quickly (peripheral intravenous access (PIV), umbilical vein catheter (UVC)), obtain blood for routine laboratory and blood gas analysis
- Insert central venous line (UV catheter or peripherally inserted central catheter (PICC line))
- Consider volume expansion (e.g., normal saline 10 ml/kg/bolus IV) for low blood pressure
- Insert umbilical arterial catheter (or right radial artery catheter), for measurement of pH and P_aCO_2 (ABG). Capillary samples for pH, PCO_2 and PO_2 are not adequate
- Consider administration of morphine (0.1 mg/kg/dose IV) to facilitate assisted ventilation and prevent the infant from swallowing air

Diagnosis in the NICU

- Chest X-ray to confirm diagnosis, exclude air leaks, and verify position of the ET tube. The initial chest X-ray does not predict clinical outcome[255]
- Echocardiography to exclude congenital heart disease (e.g., transposition of the great arteries)[256], and to estimate right ventricular systolic pressure as an indicator of pulmonary hypertension. The ratio between postnatally assessed diameters of pulmonary

arteries and descending aorta (modified McGoon Index) is one of the best predictors of survival[257]

- Clinical examination to exclude additional anomalies. Consult a clinical geneticist when in doubt

Procedure/therapy in the NICU

- Minimal handling – any stress may increase pulmonary vascular resistance
- Sedation/analgesia, e.g., fentanyl 1–3 µg/kg/h IV
- Do not use muscle relaxing agents (e.g., pancuronium, vecuronium, rocuronium or cis-atracurium) if ventilator settings are acceptable. Prolonged pancuronium use may be associated with sensorineural hearing loss. Spontaneous breathing of infants with pulmonary hypoplasia (e.g., CDH) might facilitate postnatal lung growth and appears to be associated with improved survival[249]
- When using analgesia, sedation, and muscle relaxing drugs, one must keep in mind that both decrease systemic vascular resistance and may worsen right-to-left-shunting in PPHN ($\rightarrow$ systemic hypoxemia/postductal acidosis)
- Use echocardiography, CVP (if reliable), mixed venous SO_2 and lactate to guide circulatory support (additional intravenous volume; consider inotropes/vasopressors, and inhaled nitric oxide (iNO)). Pulmonary hypertension can be estimated by peak systolic regurgitation velocity across the tricuspid valve, interventricular septum movement, and ductal shunting. If there is good contractility of the right ventricle, vigorous attempts to reduce pulmonary vascular resistance do not provide additional benefit
- While iNO does not seem to improve the outcome for infants with diaphragmatic hernia in general[80], iNO may be attempted in PPHN associated with worsening gas exchange when other measures have failed. However, the combination of iNO and high F_iO_2 may be associated with significant pulmonary toxicity (radicals)
- Avoid precipitous changes in ventilator settings
- When gas exchange improves, prioritize weaning pressure over F_iO_2
- When gas exchange worsens, consider HFOV
- Limit PIP to $\leq 25\,cmH_2O$ (on conventional ventilation) or mean $\bar{P}_{aw}$ to $14\,cmH_2O$ (on HFOV). Outcome depends on judicious utilization of non-aggressive mechanical ventilation and permissive hypercapnea

Postnatal surgery

- Better outcomes by delaying surgical repair until hemodynamic and respiratory stability has been achieved for about 24–72 h. In many centers, surgical CDH repair is performed in the NICU
- There is little chance of surviving surgery for infants who never experienced a "honeymoon" during this time, i.e., those with persistently low preductal oxygen saturations despite ventilation with 100% oxygen or increased lactate concentrations
- Trans-abdominal repair using a subcostal incision is employed, allowing gentle reduction of liver, viscera, and spleen into the abdominal cavity with visualization of the diaphragmatic defect
- A true hernial sac is found only in a minority of patients
- If primary closure is not possible, the defect may be patched (prosthetic material)

- Minimally invasive techniques[258] require insufflation of CO_2 and are therefore reserved for stable infants with small CDHs
- After surgery of a large left-sided CDH, there will be an inevitable pneumothorax on the left side as the small left lung cannot fill the thoracic cavity. The small lung is also prone to air leak, turning pneumothorax ex vacuo to tension pneumothorax. While these two can be distinguished by manual aspiration from a drainage system placed during surgery but primarily not connected to suction, prophylactic pleural drain or chest tube placement has been abandoned by most centers. Pleural drainage is also required for CDH infants who develop chylothorax or non-chylous pleural effusion.

Prognosis

- Depends on the underlying disease, the degree of PPHN, and the sequelae of hypoxia/acidosis
- Re-herniation after several weeks to months may occur, especially with patches
- Major long-term morbidity in at least one-third of surviving infants includes sensori-neural hearing impairment[259], feeding difficulties requiring gastrostomy tube placement[260], respiratory problems[261], neurodevelopmental handicap[262], severe gastro-esophageal reflux disease (GERD), and scoliosis

Contentious issues[263]

- *Prenatal steroids*
  - No benefit according to a small randomized trial ($n = 32$) and a CDH registry[251]
- *Surfactant*
  - In surfactant-treated infants with CDH, use of ECMO and incidence of chronic lung disease are greater, and survival is lower[264]
- *Muscle paralysis*
  - Allowing spontaneous breathing appears to be associated with improved survival[249]
  - Early muscle paralysis and sedation to enhance compliance is emphasized in many protocols, but combined action of a ventilator and the infant's spontaneous breathing movements may be helpful for inflating lung tissue more evenly
  - Capillary leak and third-space fluid loss are increased by paralysis
  - Use of pancuronium in CDH infants is associated with a higher rate of the sensori-neural hearing loss[259]
- *HFOV*
  - Some reports suggest better survival in CDH with the use of HFOV[265,266]
  - HFOV strategy has never been tested in a randomized trial
  - Note that an infant who is stable on HFOV requires surgery in the ICU where it is being ventilated (HFOV precludes any transport, even small distances)
  - HFOV is no obstacle to surgery
- *Alkalinization* (using buffer solutions such as sodium bicarbonate or tris-hydroxymethyl aminomethane (THAM))
  - Unclear indication to buffer hypercapnia in infants with severe pulmonary compromise[267]
  - As sodium bicarbonate increases CO_2, buffering may be better achieved by THAM. THAM has been shown to modify the depressant effect of permissive hypercapnia

on myocardial contractility in patients with acute respiratory distress syndrome[268]. Some centers therefore use THAM early in the treatment of CDH (i.e., in the delivery room: THAM decreases PVR and may improve cardiac function)

- The use of THAM is limited by potentially serious adverse effects including hypoglycemia (dilute THAM in D_5W), hyperkalemia, extravasation-related necrosis, and hepatic necrosis when administered via an umbilical vein catheter[269]

- *iNO*
  - Slightly worsened outcome with iNO in a meta-analysis of randomized trials in human infants with CDH[80]
  - Increased survival rates in newborn rats with CDH[270]
- *Vasodilators*
  - Some case reports suggest that the phosphodiesterase inhibitor sildenafil and the prostanoid epoprostenol have the potential to reduce pulmonary vascular resistance in infants with CDH[271] (for sildenafil, see NCT00133679 under http://clinicaltrials.gov)
- *ECMO*
  - Varying results in infants with CDH, questioning the usefulness of ECMO in this setting[272]
  - While ECMO offers short-term benefits, the overall effect of employing ECMO in CDH infants is not clear[273]
  - Trend to use less ECMO and more iNO in high-risk infants with CDH[251]
  - ECMO survivors have a 25% risk of sensorineural hearing impairment[274] and impaired psychomotor development[262]
  - ECMO – if at all – should only be performed in an experienced, "high volume" center (see chapters on meconium aspiration syndrome and PPHN, p. 278, p. 402). If the decision for ECMO has been made (e.g., large CDH/significant lung hypoplasia and poor clinical status), contact ECMO team/center immediately
- *Fetal surgery*
  - Appears physiologically sound and technically feasible but is associated with a high rate of very preterm delivery
  - Sobering results in randomized trials: neither open (in utero) repair of CDH[275] nor fetal endoscopic tracheal occlusion[276] appears to improve survival when compared to standard postnatal treatment
  - Although fetal tracheal occlusion is no longer used for most cases of CDH, it is occasionally considered for the most severe cases of CDH for whom estimated survival is less than 10%. Fetuses with tracheal occlusion must be delivered by the EXIT procedure (partial delivery of the fetus, removal of the tracheal occlusion, administration of surfactant and institution of assisted ventilation while the infant is still on placental support)

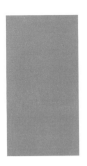

Pneumothorax

Andrea Zimmermann

Definition

Air in pleural cavity leading to total or partial collapse of one lung. Pneumothorax and pulmonary interstitial emphysema (PIE) are the most common forms of air leak syndrome. Less common air leak syndromes are pneumomediastinum, pneumopericardium, pneumo-peritoneum, and subcutaneous emphysema.

Epidemiology

Spontaneous asymptomatic pneumothoraces occur in 0.5%–2% of term infants; 10% of these are symptomatic. The rate of pneumothoraces in preterm infants with respiratory distress syndrome (RDS) is 3%–10%[277]. Upon positive pressure ventilation (PPV) more than 10% of newborn infants may develop a pneumothorax of variable degree.

Etiology/pathophysiology

- Rupture of alveoli leads to air entry into the perivascular connective tissue (interstitial emphysema), the pleural cavity (pneumothorax), the pericardial sac (pneumopericardium) and/or mediastinum (pneumomediastinum), and, rarely, into the peritoneal space (pneumoperitoneum)
- Illnesses and conditions leading to pneumothorax[278] are:
  - RDS (see p. 209, p. 231)
  - Aspiration (especially meconium and blood; see p. 261)
  - Pulmonary hypoplasia, e.g., in Potter's sequence (bilateral renal agenesis) or in chronic oligohydramnios
  - Congenital diaphragmatic hernia (CDH, strongly associated with pulmonary hypoplasia; see p. 404)
  - Pneumonia (especially pneumonia caused by staphylococci; see p. 280)
  - Lobar pulmonary emphysema
  - Congenital cystic adenomatoid malformation (CCAM, syn.: CAM, CAML; see p. 417)
  - Transient tachypnea of the newborn (TTN; also called: wet lung)
  - Immaturity (see p. 231)
- Pneumothorax may occur as a complication of certain therapeutic procedures[279]:
  - Resuscitation
  - Mechanical ventilation (especially high positive inspiratory pressure (PIP), long inspiratory time (T_{in}), breathing out of phase)[280]
  - Endotracheal suctioning

Neonatal Emergencies: A Practical Guide for Resuscitation, Transport and Critical Care, ed. Georg Hansmann.
Published by Cambridge University Press. © Cambridge University Press 2009.

> ❗Tension pneumothorax is a life-threatening EMERGENCY – due to restricted lung excursion and low cardiac output – and may lead to acute death if not treated promptly and properly.

Clinical presentation

- Small pneumothoraces are usually asymptomatic (and do not require drainage)
- Large pneumothoraces are associated with respiratory signs and symptoms of varying severity
- A tension pneumothorax (EMERGENCY) shows the following signs and symptoms:
  - Agitation
  - Dyspnea, tachypnea, retractions
  - Cyanosis or pallor
  - Bradycardia or tachycardia
  - Hypoxia, hypercarbia
  - Respiratory acidosis
  - Hypotension with a low pulse pressure (BP amplitude)
  - Shock
  - Breathing sounds weak or absent on the affected side
  - Asymmetrical chest movements
  - Diaphragmatic eventration and lung excursions absent on the affected side
  - In a left-sided pneumothorax, the heart sounds are shifted to the right side of the chest
  - Liver and spleen are displaced downwards; distended abdomen
  - Upper venous congestion and skin emphysema possible

Complications

Tension pneumothorax (air trapping, mediastinal shift to contralateral side, acutely lethal when not treated), intracranial hemorrhage (ICH), air embolism

> ❗Bradycardia, hypotension, hypercarbia, hypoxia, respiratory acidosis, and venous congestion due to (tension) pneumothorax are risk factors associated with cerebral hemorrhage, especially in preterm infants.

DDx.

- *Clinical:*
  - RDS (p. 209, p. 231)
  - Endotracheal tube obstruction
  - Aspiration (p. 269)
  - Congenital heart disease (p. 340)
  - Asphyxia (p. 310)
  - Congenital diaphragmatic hernia (CDH, p. 404)
  - Pleural effusion (p. 419, p. 427)

- Tumor
- Lung malformation (p. 417)
- *Radiological:*
  - Lobar emphysema
  - Large pulmonary cyst

> **!** Left-sided tension pneumothorax may be differentiated from (typically left-sided) CDH by palpating the spleen on the ipsilateral side (i.e., in left-sided CDH, the spleen is not palpable and abdomen is sunken).

Diagnosis in the delivery room

- Auscultation, physical examination
- ABG
- Transillumination of the chest (thoracal diaphanoscopy, cold light) – if rapidly available
- Blood glucose, and if necessary laboratory work-up

Monitoring

- S_pO_2, breathing, ECG (low voltage?), BP and ET tube position

Procedure/therapy in the delivery room

> **!** Pneumothorax can cause resuscitation failure (see standard algorithm, Figure 3.1, p. 222). If you cannot rule out (tension) pneumothorax by exam during prolonged resuscitation, empiric pleural puncture and chest tube placement are required.

For initial care and resuscitation follow the algorithm (Figure 3.1, p. 222); however, bag-and-mask ventilation is contraindicated when pneumothorax is suspected and immediate intubation is necessary.

What to do in an unstable neonate with possible tension pneumothorax

Does the infant have impaired breathing sounds on the contralateral side and are they failing to respond to cardiopulmonary resuscitation?

Yes:

- Rapid laryngoscopy to verify ET tube position
- Emergency decompression of the lungs by needle aspiration (Figure 3.34, p. 413) with a small gauge intracatheter or butterfly needle, or by chest tube placement (see pp. 413–16)
- Transillumination prior to emergency decompression is optional (depending on the newborn's clinical condition → no delays!)

(a)

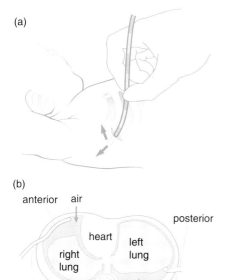

Figure 3.34 Chest tube placement. **(a)** Right-sided pneumothorax and tube placement (→ anterior pleural cavity). **(b)** Left-sided pleural effusion and tube placement (→ posterior pleural cavity). **(c)** Fixation of drainage. Note that the right lung is on the left side of the image (= CT view). Modified from: Cotten CM. Air leak syndromes. In: Spitzer A, ed. *Intensive Care of the Fetus and Neonate*, 2nd edn. Philadelphia: Elsevier Mosby, 2005.

(b)

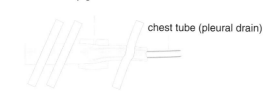

(c) y-gauze

chest tube (pleural drain)

Pleural puncture (pleurocentesis, thoracocentesis)

- Following skin disinfection (and infiltration with local anesthetic, no delays!) the pleural cavity is punctured with a 22- to 24-gauge intracatheter above the third rib in the midclavicular line. Alternatively a venous catheter (angiocath) or butterfly needle with tubing may be used[277]
- After the needle is removed (intracatheter, angiocatheter), attach a three-way stopcock that is connected to two 10- or 20-ml syringes to the tubing (intracatheter, angiocath or butterfly). Aspirate the air and turn the stop cock to discard the air. Repeat the procedure until no more air can be aspirated. Prepare for chest tube placement

Chest tube placement

- Sterile towels, gauze pads, scalpel, antiseptic solution, chest tube, sterile gloves, suction-drainage system, suture material and needle holder
- Advanced chest tube devices for neonatal use are now available (e.g., Intraspecial Catheters™)
- Option: sterile tape strips (12 × 100 mm) and adhesive tape to secure chest tube
- Tension pneumothorax is life-threatening – be focused and determined. To save time, work only with sterile gloves and skin disinfectant

- Place the patient in supine position
- *Local anesthesia:*
  - Chest tube may be placed without local anesthesia in an unconscious infant requiring resuscitation
  - If the child is awake and local anesthesia is readily available: infiltrate the site subcutaneously with lidocaine 1% (without epinephrine) and/or administer general analgesia with morphine; alternative option: fentanyl or piritramide
- Site of insertion:
  - Site for anterior placement: intersection of the second intercostal space and the midclavicular line
  - Site for antero-lateral and posterior placement: intersection of the fourth, fifth or sixth intercostal space and the anterior axillary line (stay above the intermammillary line)
  - Caution: bleeding may occur: Have sterile gauze handy!
- Make a small incision in the skin above the rib at the intersection of the fourth, fifth or sixth intercostal spaces with the anterior axillary line (0.5 cm beside the nipple, do not insert below the intermammillary line!). Alternatively, make the incision at the intersection of the second intercostal space with the midclavicular line
  - With a rotating movement insert the chest tube vertically to the surface of the thorax and penetrate the intercostal muscles to reach the pleural sac. Following penetration of the intercostal muscles, resistance fades promptly; in order not to "fall" into the pleural sac, support the hand on the chest while allowing an assistant to support the contralateral side of the chest
  - Alternatively insert a curved hemostat in the incision to spread the tissue down to the rib thereby creating a subcutaneous tunnel, then puncture the pleura and insert the tube through the opened hemostat into the pleural sac (rarely needed in neonates)
- As soon as the tube reaches the pleural cavity, remove the trocar to avoid perforation of the lung. Place the tip of the tube in the anterior pleural cavity (air anteriorly when patient supine)
- Connect the drain to a sterile syringe and advance the tube by approx. 2–3 cm (preterm infants) or 4–5 cm (term infants) towards the apex of the lung, then withdraw the air. The end of the tube can sometimes be palpated in the third intercostal space. If pneumothorax was the cause of clinical deterioration, there will be rapid improvement accompanied by an increase in heart rate and S_pO_2 and a change to rosy skin color
- The chest tube can be secured by suture or tape:
  - When secured by sutures, a suture is placed in the skin, which is followed by another knot (only one throw) leaving space between the knots; the tube is then secured at the level of 1 cm
  - When taped, the insertion is covered with sterile strips of tape and secured with adhesive tape
- Connect the tube to a water-seal drainage system, and use a negative (vacuum) suction pressure of -5 to -10 cm H_2O

Further procedures
- Placement of venous access, obtain blood gas analysis and withdraw blood (lab)
- Stabilize circulation: give volume: 10 ml/kg/bolus IV, repeat until adequate BP is reached

> **!** After successful pleural puncture/chest tube placement, inotropes generally are not required.

- Placement of UAC or other arterial line
- Consider correction of metabolic acidosis with buffer
- Placement of gastric tube
- Sufficient analgesia/sedation, e.g., diazepam, morphine/fentanyl IV
- If pneumothorax is suspected and the infant breathes spontaneously: maintain S_aO_2 >90% (warning: in preterm infants → oxygen-induced retinopathy of prematurity and BPD, P_aO_2 monitoring)

> **!** Do not administer surfactant when pneumothorax is suspected: unequal distribution may lead to overinflation of the contralateral lung.

Diagnosis in the NICU

- In an emergency, transillumination may be helpful (the chest will "light up" on the affected side)[281]
- If tension pneumothorax is likely and the patient is deteriorating, postpone chest X-ray and decompress immediately (pleura puncture and/or drainage). Obtain a chest X-ray when the patient is more stable
- Chest X-ray: verify diagnosis and position of the chest (and ET) tube.
  - Anteroposterior view will show mediastinal shift (with tension pneumothorax), ipsilateral depression of the diaphragm (with tension pneumothorax), and displacement of the lung on the affected side away from the chest wall (radiolucent band or air)
  - Cross-table lateral view may show rim of air around the lung but does not allow the affected side to be identified
  - Lateral decubitus view will detect even small pneumothoraces (infant should be positioned so that the suspected side of the pneumothorax is upper most, then X-ray is shot AP, i.e., chest to back)
- Optional: ultrasonography of the pleura: Effusion? Atelectasis?
- CT of the thorax should be performed only if indicated
- Consider echocardiography: Cardiovascular disease? Pulmonary hypertension?

Procedure/therapy in the NICU

- *Lungs/ventilation:*
  - SIPPV/SIMV: normoventilation, preferably with low PIP, short inspiration time (T_{in}), high rate (to reduce barotrauma); aim for P_aO_2 50–80 mmHg, S_aO_2 85%–95%; permissive hypercapnia depending on pH value and PVR (avoid high P_aCO_2 in PPHN) may be advantageous (Cochrane meta-analysis, 2006)[282]
  - The benefit of rescue high-frequency oscillatory ventilation (HFOV) is not yet established[283] (see p. 193)

- Use suction pressure of -5 to -10 mbar. Warning: begin with gentle suction especially after surgical correction of a diaphragmatic hernia to avoid mediastinal shift towards the tube (many centers do not place prophylactic chest tubes in CDH)
- Do chest X-ray 24 h after the chest tube has been clamped. Remove the tube if air is resolved
- In preterm/term infants with spontaneous breathing, supplement oxygen (S_pO_2 >90%) under $tcPO_2/P_aO_2$ monitoring (goal: S_pO_2 >90%, but caution: risk for retinopathy of prematurity and bronchopulmonary dysplasia in preterm infants), sedate cautiously (see below)
- *Additional procedures:*
  - Analgesia/sedation: e.g., with morphine 0.05–0.1 mg/kg/dose IV, or benzodiazepine (lorazepam, midazolam; 0.05–0.1 mg/kg/dose IV) plus fentanyl (1–3 µg/kg/h IV)
  - When muscle relaxation is indicated[284]: pancuronium, *cis*-atracurium, rocuronium or mivacurium as continuous infusion
  - Avoid unnecessary stimulation (minimal handling)
  - If needed, establish UVC/central venous line and arterial line
  - Blood pressure monitoring: sufficient systemic pressure, i.e., strive for MAP $\geq$40 mmHg in term infants or MAP $\geq$ GA in weeks in preterm infants. Give volume IV as needed. Inotropes are very rarely required (and indicate an unsolved problem, i.e., insufficient pleural decompression)

Prognosis

- Depends on the underlying (lung) disease, the degree of PPHN (if at all) and the sequelae of hypoxia/acidosis
- Depends on complications, such as intracranial hemorrhage or PVL
- Risk of recurrent pneumothorax

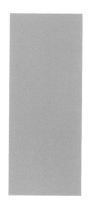

Congenital cystic adenomatoid malformation of the lung (CAM, CCAM)

Andrea Zimmermann

Syndrome

- Cystic adenomatoid malformation of the lung (CAML)

Definition

CCAM is a pulmonary hamartoma of the lung resulting from excessive growth of the terminal bronchioli leading to alveolar growth arrest. The lesion tends to be unilateral. The hamartoma may contain air or liquid and is connected to the bronchial system. Blood supply comes from the pulmonary circulation. In up to 20% CCAM is associated with malformations such as congenital diaphragmatic hernia (CDH), hydrocephalus, malformation of the bones, kidney, and small intestines.

Epidemiology

- Incidence approx. 1:30 000 (0.33/1000)

Pathophysiology

- Compression of surrounding organs, heart failure, hydrops, and lung hypoplasia are possible
- Possible decrease or increase of mass
- Poor prognosis in CCAM with fetal hydrops and polyhydramnios

Prenatal diagnosis

- Ultrasound: macrocystic (diameter >5 mm) and microcystic (diameter <5 mm) forms[285]

Prenatal DDx

- Sequestrated lung, tumour, CDH (see pp. 404–9), lobar pulmonary emphysema, bronchogenic cyst

---

! A congenital cystic adenomatoid malformation (CCAM) can be diagnosed prenatally. The expectant mother must be transferred to a tertiary perinatal center prior to delivery.

Neonatal Emergencies: A Practical Guide for Resuscitation, Transport and Critical Care, ed. Georg Hansmann. Published by Cambridge University Press. © Cambridge University Press 2009.

Prenatal therapy

- Puncture of a macrocystic malformation may be required
- In specific cases thoracoamniotic shunting may be considered[285]
- Prenatal surgical treatment is not yet established

Clinical presentation

- (Tachy) dyspnea
- Pallor/cyanosis
- O_2 requirement varies
- Hydrops fetalis and PPHN are possible[286]

Postnatal DDx

- Without a prenatal diagnosis: RDS, pneumothorax, aspiration, CDH, pleural effusion

Diagnosis in the delivery room

- Auscultation: faint breathing sounds on the affected side
- Blood gas analysis and blood glucose, laboratory work-up, and if necessary blood culture
- HIV/hepatitis serology, blood type and screen/cross

Procedure/therapy in the delivery room

- Symptomatic treatment: endotracheal intubation (start with high F_iO_2: 0.8–1.0) and cardiopulmonary resuscitation, if indicated
- Peripheral venous access; umbilical vein catheter/peripherally inserted central catheter line placement, as indicated
- If oxygenation is insufficient (and no pneumothorax present), administer surfactant
- In arterial hypotension with MAP $\ll$ GA in weeks: volume expansion with normal saline (10 ml/kg/bolus IV), repeat if indicated. Vasopressors/inotropes are rarely required (dopamine, norepinephrine, epinephrine, dobutamine)

Monitoring

- S_pO_2, ECG, BP monitoring, blood gas analysis, blood glucose

Diagnosis in the NICU

- Chest X-ray: mass containing air-filled cysts – may show air-fluid levels
- Ultrasonography of the thorax to rule out fluid in the cysts, and pleural effusions
- Consult pediatric radiology and pediatric surgery

Procedure/therapy in the NICU

- Generous indication for high-frequency oscillatory ventilation (HFOV)
- Treatment of PPHN is sometimes indicated prior to or after surgery
- Early thoracotomy in symptomatic infants and excision of significant lesions after preoperative imaging (CT)[285]
- Surgical treatment of small and asymptomatic lesions should be discussed on a case-by-case basis[287]

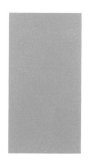

Chylothorax

Andrea Zimmermann

Definition

• Accumulation of chyle in the pleural space

Epidemiology

Incidence approx. 1:10 000 (0.1/1000) births[2]. Chylothorax is the most common cause of unilateral congenital pleural effusion and is more frequent in boys than in girls (2:1). It occurs in ≈50% of cases on the right side, and in 50% either on the left side or on both sides.

Etiology/pathophysiology[288,289]

• *Embryological disorder:*
  • Malformation of the lymphatic system:
    • Permeability of the thoracic duct
    • Absence of lymphatic-venous anastomosis
  • Malformation of the lungs
• *Traumatic/postoperative shift or rupture of the thoracic duct*
  • Birth injury (overextension, increased intrathoracic pressure) or tumors
  • Intrathoracic surgery
  • Thrombosis of the superior vena cava or subclavian vein
• *Additional causes:*
  • Cause or result of hydrops fetalis (see p. 427)
  • Association with syndromes: Down syndrome, Noonan or Turner syndrome[2] and infections (connatal or secondary acquired infections)
• *Idiopathic:* in up to 25%

Prenatal diagnosis

• Is possible by ultrasonography. Consider pleuro-amniotic shunting[290]

> *!* When pleural effusion is diagnosed prenatally, delivery of the infant must occur in a tertiary perinatal center.

Neonatal Emergencies: A Practical Guide for Resuscitation, Transport and Critical Care, ed. Georg Hansmann. Published by Cambridge University Press. © Cambridge University Press 2009.

Pathophysiology/sequelae

- *Prenatal:*
  - Absence of fetal breathing movements → lung hypoplasia is possible
  - Non-immunological hydrops fetalis
  - Further risks: see below
- *Postnatal:*
  - Dyspnea
  - Cardiac insufficiency
  - Mediastinal shift
  - Intravascular volume deficit
  - Obstruction of central venous return/venous congestion
  - Loss of protein, fats and lymphocytes
  - Anasarca (extreme generalized edema)

Clinical presentation

Depending on the severity of the effusion, affected newborns present with:
- Pulmonary insufficiency with dyspnea/tachypnea, cyanosis or pallor
- Weak or absent breath sounds on the affected side
- Brady- or tachycardia
- Arterial hypotension
- Skin edema
- Hydrops fetalis

DDx.

- RDS (p. 209, p. 231), asphyxia (p. 304 and p. 310), pneumothorax (p. 410), tumor, malformation of the lungs (CCAM=CAML, p. 417)

Diagnosis in the delivery room

- Auscultation
- ABG, blood glucose, Hct, CBC (further diagnostic work-up in the NICU)

Monitoring

Pulse oximetry (S_aO_2, HR), ECG, BP, temperature. Check ET tube position, if intubated. Obtain arterial blood gas/blood glucose before departure.

Therapy in the delivery room

- Clear and secure airway (in hydrops fetalis, oral intubation with a stylet may be necessary)
- If indicated: cardiopulmonary resuscitation
- If the respiratory function of the infant cannot be stabilized or resuscitation is unsuccessful and breathing sounds are absent on the contralateral or on both sides: → chest tube insertion on one or both sides and drainage of effusion until chest movements are seen and breathing sounds are heard (Figure 3.34, p. 413)

- Place peripheral intravenous catheter or umbilical venous catheter (UVC); obtain ABG/blood glucose; draw blood for further diagnostic work-up
- Substitute the volume of pleural effusion that was removed, e.g., with serum protein solution (e.g., human albumin 5%, fresh frozen plasma (FFP), packed red blood cells (different ratios for volume distribution may be used)
- Collect pleural fluid sample
- If oxygenation is inefficient despite positive pressure ventilation with F_iO_2 1.0 and pneumothorax is ruled out → administer surfactant 100 (–200) mg/kg/dose ET, as indicated
- Stabilize circulation:
  - Give volume 10 ml/kg/bolus IV, repeat, as necessary
  - After volume expansion, catecholamines are rarely required (dopamine, norepinephrine, dobutamine). Place UVC and administer dopamine 2–20 μg/kg/min or norepinephrine 0.05–0.1 (–1) μg/kg/min via central venous line and regulate volume substitution according to central venous pressure (CVP) and BP
- Place gastric tube
- Analgesia/sedation: morphine or fentanyl, diazepam/lorazepam IV

Diagnosis in the NICU
- Chest X-ray
- Analysis of pleural fluid:
  - Pleural chyle before enteral feeding is usually yellowish and becomes milky-turbid with oral feeding (breast milk, formula)
  - Pleural effusion is probably chyle when it contains a high cell count (>1000/μl) with $>80\%$ lymphocytes and triglyceride content >100 mg/dl (>1.1 mmol/l)[291]
- ABG, blood glucose, laboratory work-up (including total protein, albumin, triglyceride, transaminase, coagulation panel); if necessary blood culture, HIV/hepatitis serology, blood type and screen/cross
- Head, pleural and abdominal ultrasonography
- Echocardiography
- Chest CT, if indicated
- Chromosomal analysis (as indicated) and exclusion of further malformations

Procedure/therapy in the NICU
- If pleural effusions impair chest movements and chyle production is plenty and continuous: repeat pleural punctures or place *chest tube* with low suction (–1 to –2 cmH$_2$O).[289] Consider first or second generation cephalosporin IV (e.g., cefazolin) as long as chest tube is in place
- Replenish depleted protein (including immunoglobulins) and lipids (partial parenteral nutrition)
- Begin *enteral nutrition with medium-chain triglycerides (MCT)* to reduce production of chyle (MCT are absorbed in the portal system and not transported by chylomicrons into the lymph channels/thoracic duct). Do not feed long-chain fatty acids and breast milk PO^2
- If pleural effusion production is continuous (>2 weeks) in spite of an MCT diet, switch to *total parenteral nutrition*

- MCT formulas (Portagen™) have been shown to produce resolution of chylothorax in approximately one-third of patients after 2 weeks, while total parenteral nutrition typically results in resolution in 75%–80% of cases by that time
- Within 2–4 weeks consider *surgical treatment* (pleurodesis, ligature of thoracic duct, pleurectomy or pleuroperitoneal shunting)
- *Octreotide* (=long-acting synthetic analog of endogenous somatostatin) is a relatively new treatment option for congenital, spontaneous or postsurgical chylothorax[292–297]. Begin at 1 μg/kg/h IV. Titrate dose upward as necessary (maximum dose 7 μg/kg/h); chyle production should decrease within 24 h.[103] Although the exact mechanism by which the drug exerts its effects has not been defined, it is believed that the multiple effects of octreotide on the gastrointestinal tract and the reduction in splanchnic blood flow decrease thoracic duct flow and the triglyceride content of chyle
  - *Adverse effects:* changes in blood glucose levels, transient abdominal distension, and emesis have been associated with octreotide treatment. Octreotide seems to have fewer side-effects than somatostatin. However, Mohseni-Bod et al.[298] recently reported on a neonate with coarctation of the aorta: the baby developed necrotizing enterocolitis on postoperative day 16 while on octreotide. Hence, when using octreotide, caution should be exercised in infants with vascular compromise such as impaired systemic perfusion before or after cardiovascular surgery. Further studies on the use of octreotide are warranted

Clinical course of chylothorax

- Risk of chronicity due to loss of protein, immunoglobulins, and lymphocytes
- Production of chyle can last 10 weeks or longer

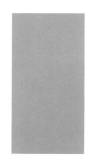

Hemolytic disease of the newborn

Shannon E. G. Hamrick

Syndrome/definition/pathophysiology/epidemiology

- Hemolytic disease of the newborn (HDN) is also known as erythroblastosis fetalis, isoimmunization, or blood group incompatibility
- HDN occurs when fetal red blood cells (RBCs), which possess an antigen that the mother lacks, cross the placenta into the maternal circulation, where they stimulate antibody production. The antibodies return to the fetal circulation and result in RBC destruction
- Rhesus positive (+) denotes presence of the D antigen. The number of antigenic sites on RBCs varies with the genotype, and the prevalence of the genotype varies with the population. In the USA, Rhesus-negative (d/d) individuals comprise 15% of Whites, 5.5% of African Americans, and <1% of Asians. A sensitized Rhesus-negative mother produces anti-Rh IgG antibodies which cross the placenta. Risk factors for antibody production include prior miscarriage or abortion, second (or later) pregnancies, maternal toxemia, paternal zygosity (D/D rather than D/d), and amount of antigen load[299]
- With maternal blood types A and B, isoimmunization does not occur because the naturally occurring antibodies (anti-A and -B) are IgM, not IgG. In type-O mothers, the antibodies are predominantly IgG, cross the placenta, and can cause hemolysis in the fetus. The association of a type-A or B fetus with a type-O mother occurs in ~15% of pregnancies. However, HDN occurs in only 3%, is severe in only 1%, and <1:1000 require exchange transfusion. Unlike Rh, ABO disease can occur in first pregnancies, because anti-A and anti-B antibodies are found early in life from exposure to A- or B-like antigens present in many foods and bacteria

Prenatal diagnosis

- RhoGAM (anti-D) was licensed in 1968 and since then the rate of HDM has plummeted. It is given to Rhesus-negative women at 28 weeks' gestation and following delivery and any procedures
- Poor correlation between antibody titers and neonatal disease: the spectrophotometric determination of amniotic fluid bilirubin concentration can be plotted on a "Liley curve" as a function of gestational age. Zone 3 is an indication for delivery[300,301]
- Fetal middle cerebral artery (MCA) Doppler measurements are a non-invasive, though user-dependent, method of estimating fetal anemia[302]

Prenatal therapy

- Intra uterine transfusion (IUT): with severe iso-immunization, IUTs are given to the fetus to prevent hydrops fetalis and fetal death[300]. After multiple IUTs, most of the

Neonatal Emergencies: A Practical Guide for Resuscitation, Transport and Critical Care, ed. Georg Hansmann.
Published by Cambridge University Press. © Cambridge University Press 2009.

baby's blood will be Rhesus-negative donor blood. Therefore, the direct antiglobulin test will be negative, but the indirect antiglobulin test will be positive
- Intravenous immunoglobulin: role in intrauterine management is unclear at this time

Clinical presentation/diagnosis in the delivery room/nursery

- *Clinical presentation of HDN* varies from mild jaundice and anemia to hydrops fetalis (with ascites, pleural, and pericardial effusions). Because the placenta clears bilirubin, the major risk to the fetus is anemia. Extramedullary hematopoiesis (due to anemia) results in hepatosplenomegaly
- *Risks during labor and delivery* include asphyxia and splenic rupture
- *Postnatal problems include:*
  - Asphyxia
  - Pulmonary hypertension
  - Pallor
  - Edema (hydrops, due to low serum albumin)
  - Respiratory distress – coagulopathies (platelets and clotting factors)
  - Jaundice – kernicterus
  - Hypoglycemia (due to hyperinsulinemia from islet cell hyperplasia)[299]
- *Laboratory findings vary with severity of HDN and include:*
  - Anemia
  - Reticulocytosis (6%–40%)[301]
  - Hyperbilirubinemia
  - Increased nucleated RBC count (>10/100 WBCs)
  - Positive direct antiglobulin Test[a]
  - Hypoalbuminemia
  - Rhesus-negative blood type[a] – smear: polychromasia, anisocytosis, no spherocytes

ABO incompatibility

- Generally less severe than Rh disease
- Laboratory findings for ABO incompatibility that differ from those of Rh disease:
  - Smear: microspherocytosis
  - MCV <95 fl, microcytic for a newborn (normal for adult)
  - Direct Coombs test is often weakly positive

Minor blood group incompatibility

- Uncommon, occurs in ~0.8% of pregnant women and usually with E, c, Kell, Kidd or Duffy incompatibility
- Clinical presentation may be similar to that of Rh disease. Anti-Kell disease may be severe due to hemolysis or erythroid suppression. Lewis antigen stimulates only IgM production, so maternal antibody screen may be positive, but fetus is not affected

---

[a] With severe HDN, high quantities of antibody may block the Rh antigen sites resulting in a Rhesus-positive infant typing as Rhesus-negative and having a negative direct antiglobulin test.

Procedure/therapy in the delivery room

- *Preparation prior to delivery should include:*
  - Blood: type-O Rhesus-negative packed RBCs, cross-matched against the mother. For severe HDN, have blood in the resuscitation room to correct severe anemia immediately after birth by partial exchange transfusion (ETX)
  - Surfactant ET, if infant is preterm
  - Catheters for immediate drainage of hydropic fluid
- *Resuscitation:* at birth, the major problems are cardiopulmonary and relate to effects of severe anemia, hydrops, and prematurity. Effective resuscitation requires several skilled individuals.
  - Obtain cord blood for bilirubin (total and direct), albumin, blood type and Rh, direct Coombs test, CBC, platelets, reticulocyte count, and nucleated RBCs
  - If the infant is hydropic, intubate immediately and begin assisted ventilation with oxygen. If ventilation is difficult, drain pleural and ascitic fluid; during paracentesis avoid puncturing the enlarged liver and spleen
  - Insert umbilical arterial (UAC) and venous catheters (UVC) and immediately measure blood pressures, arterial pH and blood gases, hematocrit (Hct) and blood sugar
  - Correct metabolic acidosis with alkali if giving assisted ventilation
  - Correct anemia, essential for effective resuscitation
    - If arterial blood pressure is low, give simple transfusion of packed RBCs (e.g., for Hct of 30%, push 10 ml/kg over 5 min; for Hct of 20%, push 10 ml/kg over 5 min, then repeat)
    - Do not infuse packed RBCs or blood through UAC because of risk of damage to spinal cord from emboli
    - With normal blood pressure, elevated central venous pressure, metabolic acidosis or hydrops, correct anemia by partial ETX (exchange 20 ml/kg, then repeat Hct)
  - Measure blood sugar frequently and correct hypoglycemia

Diagnosis/procedure/therapy in the NICU

- Measure bilirubin in cord blood and at least q4 h for the first 12–24 h. Plot bilirubin concentrations over time. After IUTs, the cord bilirubin is not an accurate indicator of rate of hemolysis or of the likelihood of the need for postnatal exchange transfusion. Cord blood bilirubin >4 mg/dl indicates severe iso-immunization
- Hyperbilirubinemia results from continued hemolysis and inability of the neonatal liver to handle a large bilirubin load. Kernicterus (bilirubin encephalopathy) results from high levels of indirect bilirubin (>20 mg/dl in a term infant with HDN). Kernicterus occurs at lower levels of bilirubin in the presence of acidosis, hypoalbuminemia, prematurity, and certain drugs (e.g., sulfonamides)
- Begin *phototherapy* shortly after birth. Although phototherapy may not eliminate the need for ETX, it may delay ETX and decrease the number of ETX required
- *IVIG* (0.5 to 1 g/kg), as an adjunct to phototherapy, reduced the need for ETX and reduced hospital stay in a recent systematic review[303]
- Use *exchange transfusion (ETX)* for hyperbilirubinemia not controlled by phototherapy
  - Indications depend upon absolute serum concentration of bilirubin, the rate of rise of bilirubin, gestational age, albumin concentration, and acid-base status. In general,

perform ETX for cord bilirubin >5 mg/dl, for a rate of rise of bilirubin >0.5–1 mg/h, and to prevent bilirubin >20 mg/dl in a term infant, and lower levels in preterm infants (e.g., maintain serum bilirubin <10× the birthweight in kg)

- Blood should be reconstituted (to Hct ~40%–50%) from fresh, O-negative packed RBCs cross-matched against the mother and type-specific fresh frozen plasma
- Technique: about 30 min before ETX, give albumin 1 g/kg to increase the bilirubin bound to albumin in the circulation and make the ETX more effective. Exchange 2× the blood volume (estimate blood volume at 85 ml/kg). Preferred technique is isovolumic ETX, withdrawing blood from UAC and infusing through UVC (with tip in inferior vena cava (IVC) or low right atrium). Do not infuse blood through UVC if tip is in portal circulation. Alternatively, ETX can be done through a single catheter (UAC or UVC) using aliquots <5% of the infant's blood volume (e.g., 5 ml/kg). The blood should be warmed and the bag agitated every few minutes (to prevent settling of the RBCs)
- *Complications of ETX:*
  - Hypocalcemia due to Ca^{2+} binding by citrate. Give calcium gluconate 100 mg after every 100 ml of blood exchanged
  - Hypoglycemia, particularly after the ETX, due to hyperinsulinism in HDN and rebound effect of exposure to dextrose in the blood
  - Thrombocytopenia and granulocytopenia due to washout with the ETX. Follow platelet counts; consider platelet transfusion for counts <50 000/μl
  - Hyperkalemia, especially with older units of blood
  - Hypothermia, associated with inadequate warming of blood

Outcome

- Late anemia: antibodies persist for weeks, cause continued hemolysis and can cause anemia as late as age 6 months (especially in infants who had received IUTs). After discharge, follow Hct weekly. Erythropoietin will help prevent severe anemia and further transfusions
- Neurological prognosis is good[301]. Most frequent problem is sensorineural hearing loss

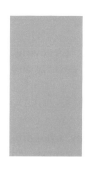

Hydrops fetalis

Andrea Zimmermann

Definition
Generalized edema (anasarca) and accumulation of fluid in one or two visceral cavities. Pleural/pericardial effusion(s) or ascites alone is insufficient to establish the diagnosis "hydrops fetalis." Hydrops may have an immunological (IHF) or a non-immunological (NIHF) cause. See also chapters on "hemolytic disease of the newborn" (HDN, p. 423) and "twin–twin (feto–fetal) transfusion syndrome" (TTTS, p. 240).

Epidemiology
NIHF occurs in approx. 1:1500 to 1:4000 (0.25–0.67/1000) pregnancies[304].

Etiology/pathophysiology
Immunological hydrops fetalis (IHF)
- Feto–maternal Rhesus incompatibility leads to fetal anemia due to hemolytic antibodies and results in hypoxia (central apnea), heart failure, and capillary leak syndrome causing generalized edema, fluid accumulation in visceral cavities, hypoproteinemia, and hepatomegaly of various degrees. Hemolysis and anemia induce or enhance extramedullary erythropoiesis ($\rightarrow$ hepatosplenomegaly)

Non-immunological hydrops fetalis (NIHF)
- Fetal anemia, hypoxia, hypoproteinemia, and/or heart failure due to multiple possible etiologies lead to generalized edema and effusions[305]
  - *Anemia (hemolytic, non-hemolytic)*: virus infection (e.g., parvovirus B 19); α-thalassemia; glucose-6-phosphate-dehydrogenase deficiency (G6PDD), fetal leukemia, aplastic anemia, feto–maternal or twin–twin (=feto–fetal) transfusion in monochorial twin pregnancies (p. 240)
  - *Pulmonary causes*: chylothorax (p. 419), hydrothorax, congenital diaphragmatic hernia (CDH; p. 404), congenital cystic adenomatoid malformation (CCAM; p. 417), lymphangiectasia, and tumor
  - *Cardiac causes*: fetal tachycardia or bradycardia (p. 325), heart failure associated with congenital cardiovascular malformations (p. 340) or myocardial disease (e.g., myocarditis, mitochondrial defects, endomyocardial fibrosis), arteriovenous (AV) and other cardiovascular malformations (p. 340), premature closure of the foramen ovale, thrombosis, and tumor

Neonatal Emergencies: A Practical Guide for Resuscitation, Transport and Critical Care, ed. Georg Hansmann.
Published by Cambridge University Press. © Cambridge University Press 2009.

- *Infections*: toxoplasmosis, rubella, cytomegalovirus, syphilis, hepatitis, adenovirus, leptospirosis, respiratory syncytial virus (RSV), Coxsackie virus, and possibly also hepatitis viruses and HIV (see Table 3.5)
- *Hepatic causes*: fibrosis, cysts, hepatic dysfunction (hypoalbuminemia)
- *Renal causes*: nephrotic syndrome, renal venous thrombosis
- *Chromosomal abnormalities and syndromes*: trisomy 13, 18, 21, triploidy, achondroplasia, Turner syndrome, Noonan syndrome (includes pulmonary valve stenosis, left ventricular hypertrophy, hypertelorism, down-slanting eyes, webbed neck, and chest deformity, and other signs)
- *Others*: meconium peritonitis, volvulus, intestinal atresia, tumors, chorioangioma, metabolic disorders: Gaucher's disease, mucopolysaccharidosis, osteopetrosis
- *Idiopathic*: in approx. 30% of cases no cause can be found

---

! Fetal hydrops can be diagnosed prenatally. Fetal treatment is possible in some cases (supraventricular tachycardia, fetal anemia, complete heart block). The expectant mother must be transferred in a timely fashion to a perinatal center if there is no urgent indication for delivery! If severe pleural effusion is present (prenatal diagnosis), the obstetricians (intrapartum) and neonatologists (postnatally) should attempt to drain pleural fluid before and immediately after delivery. Resuscitation of newborns with hydrops requires at least four highly skilled health care providers in the resuscitation room.

Preparing for advanced neonatal resuscitation

- Coordinate and gather the teams:
    - Delivery time
    - Assign responsibilities to team members (including two neonatologists)
    - Inform NICU
- Equipment
    - Endotracheal tube with and without stylets (various sizes), laryngoscope, straight blades size no. 0 and 1 (bulb working?)
    - Angiocatheter, butterfly needles (with tubing) and kits for pleural (chest tube, thoracocentesis) and abdominal (ascites) drainage (complete kit with stopcocks and connection tubes)
    - Umbilical catheterization kit/tray (UAC and UVC)
    - Disposable exchange transfusion tray; if not available, use two three-way stopcocks and syringes of different sizes
    - Surfactant
    - Inotropic drugs (first choice: epinephrine, dopamine; second choice: dobutamine)
    - Sodium bicarbonate 4.2%, or 8.4% diluted 1:1 with sterile water
    - Furosemide IV (vials)
    - RBCs (200 ml): type-O, Rhesus-negative, lysine-free, cross-matched with maternal serum, radiated, CMV-seronegative
    - Fresh frozen plasma (FFP), blood type "AB"

Clinical presentation

- Generalized edema
- Severe RDS, decreased chest excursions
- Tachy- or bradycardia
- Abdominal distension due to ascites and hepatomegaly
- Cyanosis or pale grayish skin color
- Hypoglycemia is likely
- Arterial hypotension is likely

Diagnosis in the delivery room

- Oscillometric BP measurement (measurement often unreliable due to edema), aim for immediate placement of arterial line (UAC or radial artery) to monitor BP
- Estimation of CVP using a measuring tape while holding the UVC vertically. Be aware of the risk of air embolism! CVP measurement is only accurate if the UVC can be advanced close to the right atrium (IVC/RA junction), and should be considered an estimate until the correct position is confirmed by chest X-ray. Normal CVP is 3–8 mmHg (= 2.2–5.9 cmH$_2$O) depending on newborn's cardiopulmonary condition
- Weight assessment: for treatment, do not use measured weight or calculated weight; rather use gestational age-related weight according to the 50th percentile
- ABG, blood glucose, Hct, baby's blood type; lactate, and further diagnostic work-up (blood draw)
- For further diagnostic work-up, save samples of pleural fluid or ascites (microbiology, cell count, cell differentiation, protein, and triglyceride content)

Monitoring

Verify position of ET tube, measure S$_a$O$_2$, BP, ECG, temperature, and ABG/blood glucose after birth, during resuscitation, and before leaving the resuscitation room.

Therapy in the delivery room

> *!* Generally, all newborns with hydrops fetalis should be resuscitated. Make every effort to establish the diagnosis for future counseling of the parents.

- Rapid intubation, ventilation with high PIP and PEEP, F_iO$_2$ 1.0 or according to S$_a$O$_2$
- Intubation may be problematic because of edema of the larynx, trachea, and soft tissue. Prepare ET tube size at least 0.5 mm smaller (internal diameter) than usual, and use stylet for intubation
- HR <60 bpm? → chest compressions, epinephrine (1:10 000) 0.3–1 ml/kg/single dose ET (= 0.03–0.1 mg/kg/dose); after placement of venous/IO access (UVC, PIV, IO) 0.1–0.3 ml/kg/dose IV/IO (= 0.01–0.03 mg/kg/dose IV/IO; UVC is the preferred access)
- If significant effusions are present (i.e., not drained in utero) and postnatal oxygenation is insufficient in spite of PPV with F_iO$_2$ 1.0, perform thoracentesis (unilateral, bilateral) with a small-gauge angiocath, butterfly or easy-to-use pleural drain (e.g., Intraspecial

429

Catheters™) and drain fluid from the pleural cavity. If the newborn is fairly stable, insert a *chest tube* (Figure 3.34). Drain ascites in the left lower abdomen (best under ultrasound guidance) if a high-standing diaphragm is suspected of causing ventilation/oxygenation problems. Caution: 10–20 ml/kg *pleural effusion* or *ascites* should be *substituted* with FFP and/or serum protein solutions (e.g., human albumin 5%). Send a sample of the pleural fluid for diagnostic purposes

- Prepare surfactant: approx. 100–200 mg/kg/dose ET, when oxygenation is insufficient
- Establish (second) peripheral venous access. Do not waste time with peripheral intra-venous (PIV) attempts but go straight to UVC placement if PIV access appears to be very difficult
- Pursue early placement of UVC/CVC (if necessary IO) by an experienced team, administer volume expansion, and measure central venous pressure (CVP) (normal 2–8 cmH$_2$O). Regulate volume expansion (10 ml/kg in 30–60 min IV) according to CVP and BP
- Use weight of the 50th percentile for gestational age, then run maintenance infusion with D$_{10}$W 30 ml/kg/h IV (=5 µg/kg/min); increase or decrease as per blood glucose
- Furosemide 1–2 mg/kg/dose IV
- Sodium bicarbonate 4.2% (or 8.4% diluted 1:1 in sterile water) to correct metabolic acidosis if pH <7.15
- Inotropes are rarely indicated after sufficient volume expansion. In persistent arterial hypotension where mean arterial pressure (MAP) is less than the number of weeks of gestation: dopamine 2–20 µg/kg/min, epinephrine and/or norepinephrine 0.05–0.5–1 µg/kg/min via UVC, other central venous line or IO access. Dopamine can be given via peripheral venous access until central access is established

Is the newborn stable (i.e., MAP > GA in weeks, sufficient oxygenation, Hct >30%)?

Yes
- Quick and careful transport to the nearest NICU
- In case of immunological hydrops fetalis with increased serum bilirubin >6 mg/dl and anemia with Hct <30%: inform NICU beforehand that exchange transfusion (with a negative fluid balance) is to be performed urgently

No
- Blood transfusion
  - If Hct is <30% and CVP is normal: transfuse with type-O Rhesus-negative PRBC 10 ml/kg; administer half of the volume by slow IV push in 5–10 min and the other half over 1 h (see p. 173)
- Isovolumetric partial exchange transfusion
  - Aim for negative fluid balance if CVP is increased
  - Withdraw 3–5 ml/kg in single portions (approx. 10–15) from the newborn and transfuse exchange blood (40 ml/kg type-O Rhesus-negative PRBC and blood-type-AB FFP over the same time period) to achieve a Hct of 40%–50%
  - Monitor CVP, BP, and HR closely

Be ready to transfer the newborn with hydrops fetalis if . . .

- HR persistently >100 bpm
- Arterial MAP > gestational age in weeks
- Adequate oxygenation
- HCT >30%

Diagnosis in the NICU

- Laboratory work-up (ABG, lactate, CBC, coagulation panel, protein, albumin, LDH, ALT/AST, bilirubin direct/indirect, blood type and cross, direct Coombs test, and, if necessary, microbiological diagnostics such as blood culture)
- Chest and abdominal X-ray
- Echocardiography. Congenital heart disease? Ventricular function? Pericardial effusion? Pulmonary hypertension?
- Pleural, abdominal, and cranial ultrasonography
- Send for chromosome analysis, if indicated also FISH diagnostics, and samples for advanced metabolic work-up

Procedure/therapy in the NICU

- Placement of UVC/other central venous catheter and arterial line (umbilical artery, radial artery), if not achieved or misplaced in delivery room
- Transfusion/partial or total exchange transfusion (as above)[305]
- Complete diagnostic tests, establish diagnosis
- Thoracocentesis with angiocath, butterfly or easy-to-use pleural drain (e.g., Intraspecial Catheters™), then place chest tube if indicated; drain ascites (both thoracocentesis and abdominal drain placement should be guided by ultrasonography); withdraw pleural fluid and ascites as needed
- Substitute pleural effusion and/or ascites with serum protein solution or FFP
- Mechanical ventilation and oxygenation may be complicated by pulmonary hypertension, pulmonary hypoplasia or lung edema. If so, consider inhaled nitric oxide (iNO)
- Correction of metabolic acidosis according to ABG
- Administration of digitalis (not in bradycardia or hypokalemia, or if patient receives calcium IV)
- Continuous phototherapy
- Fluid balancing (check input and output)
- Administration of diuretics, e.g., furosemide 1–2 mg/kg/dose IV
- In persistent arterial hypotension/poor ventricular function, catecholamines may be indicated (dopamine, norepinephrine, and/or epinephrine)

Prognosis

- Prognosis is poor, especially for immature infants, those with pleural effusions, pulmonary hypoplasia, in utero diagnosis before 24 weeks of gestation, and in the presence of chromosomal abnormalities, congenital heart disease and other malformations, as well as severe anemia[306]
- Mortality is up to 80% depending on etiology[304]

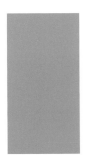

Choanal atresia

Andrea Zimmermann

Epidemiology
Incidence 1:5000 newborns[307]. The ratio of bilateral to unilateral atresia is 2:1.

Etiology/pathophysiology
- Unilateral or bilateral choanal obstruction by bony (90%) or soft (10%), tissue
- Single or combined anomaly, e.g., *CHARGE* association (**c** for coloboma, **h** for heart disease, **a** for choanal atresia, **r** for retarded growth and development, **g** for genital hypoplasia, **e** for ear malformation and/or deafness)[308]

Clinical presentation
- Infants are nose-breathers; obstruction of the upper airways and dyspnea are signs of bilateral choanal atresia
- An infant crying immediately after birth may not show any symptoms (pink when crying, blue when calm/feeding)
- Unilateral atresia may not be detected until later (partial airway obstruction)
- Viscous mucous plug in the atretic nares

Diagnosis in the delivery room
- Physical examination:
  - Dyspnea due to obstructed nose-breathing when the mouth is closed
  - No condensation forms on a mirror or polished scissors
  - No air movement is detected on holding wisp of cotton in front of nostril
  - Stethoscope held in front of the nostrils (breathing sounds?)
- Failure to pass a gastric tube or even a small suction catheter (Ch 6, Ch 4) through the nasal cavity
- Caution: unilateral atresia with only mild symptoms

Therapy in the delivery room
- Keep airways open with oral airway (Guedel tube)
- Laryngeal mask airway (LMA) placement or orotracheal intubation is rarely indicated

Neonatal Emergencies: A Practical Guide for Resuscitation, Transport and Critical Care, ed. Georg Hansmann.
Published by Cambridge University Press. © Cambridge University Press 2009.

Diagnosis/procedure/therapy in the NICU

- Rule out additional malformations:
  - Physical examination
  - Hearing tests (otoacoustic emissions = OAE, acoustic evoked potentials = AEP)
  - Referral to otolaryngologist (ENT) for consultation
  - Referral to pediatric cardiologist for consultation
  - Referral to ophthalmologist for consultation
  - Ultrasonography of abdomen, genital tract, etc.
- CT may be indicated to rule out nasal tumors, a septal deviation or other anatomical features
- Transnasal endoscopic treatment: usually stenting

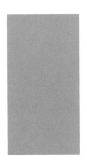

Esophageal atresia

Andrea Zimmermann

Definition
- Congenital atresia of the esophagus (EA)
  - With or without tracheoesophageal fistula (TEF)
- Distal TEF to the blind distal esophageal pouch in approx. 86% (type Vogt 3B = Gross C)[309]
- Up to 50% of patients with EA/TEF have associated anomalies[309], including:
  - Urogenital abnormalities
  - Intestinal malrotation
  - Chromosomal aberrations
  - Congenital heart disease
  - *VACTERL association* (**v** for vertebral malformation; **a** for atresia, especially ano-rectal malformations (e.g., anal atresia); **c** for cardiac, i.e., congenital heart disease, vascular malformation; **t** for tracheal malformation; **e** for esophageal, esophageal atresia; **r** for renal malformation; **l** for limbs, malformation of the extremities)
- Association with prematurity and low birth weight

Epidemiology
- 1:3500 (0.29/1000)[309]

Etiology/pathophysiology
- Incomplete separation of esophagus and trachea during embryogenesis

Prenatal diagnosis
- Polyhydramnios
- Fetal gastric bubble can be either present or absent by ultrasonography

Clinical presentation
- Excessive oral secretions and regurgitation of saliva[310]
- Choking, coughing, and risk of aspiration
- Possible abdominal extension
- Unable to pass gastric tube after birth; tip of tube curls and appears in the mouth

Neonatal Emergencies: A Practical Guide for Resuscitation, Transport and Critical Care, ed. Georg Hansmann.
Published by Cambridge University Press. © Cambridge University Press 2009.

Caution: The gastric tube can coil up in the pouch and thus give the appearance of having been passed through the esophagus. Therefore, large gastric tubes that cannot coil up should be used. To determine the correct location of the tube, auscultate the stomach during suctioning! If suction sounds are absent, inject air into the tube: it is recommended to auscultate the rush of air between the shoulders and not over the stomach region, because in esophageal atresia the air will easily escape through the nostrils. Get chest X-ray/abdominal X-ray (KUB) to verify clinical findings, and in any baby with gastric tube in place.

Diagnosis in the delivery room

- Physical examination (with special attention given to the spinal column, anus, kidneys and extremities, and auscultation of the heart and lungs)
- Auscultate the left subcostal region while suctioning the stomach
- Blood gas analysis (arterial, capillary)
- Blood glucose

Monitoring

- Pulse oximetry (S_pO_2)
- ECG
- BP
- Temperature

Therapy in the delivery room

- Frequent suctioning, avoid bag-and-mask ventilation, no pharyngeal CPAP
- Try to avoid endotracheal intubation
- Keep patient prone to avoid aspiration of gastric secretions
- When strongly indicated, i.e., respiratory failure: endotracheal intubation (caution: gastric and abdominal distension with mechanical ventilation likely), then frequent tracheal suctioning, ventilation with high rate and low PIP to avoid gastric and abdominal distension
- Double-lumen suction tube (Replogle catheter and continuous suctioning) with a suction pressure of -100 mbar
- If a Replogle catheter is not available, use a large gastric tube and suction intermittently
- Venous access: administer $D_{10}W$ 3–4 ml/kg/h (maintenance); if indicated, give volume (normal saline) 10–20 ml/kg/bolus IV

Transport

- Elevate upper part of the body (45°), or achieve prone position with head elevated[311]
- Place Replogle catheter or large gastric tube to secure outflow of secretions (see above)
- No oral feeding
- If indicated, treat drooling/hypersalivation with atropine (0.02 mg/kg/dose IV)
- Standard monitoring (S_pO_2, BP, temperature, ECG)

Diagnosis in the NICU

- Chest X-ray, abdominal X-ray (KUB):
  - Gastric tube is shown in the proximal esophageal pouch that is filled with air
  - If a distal TEF is present, a stomach bubble is seen (not if the fistula is proximal)
- Rule out further malformations (echocardiography, renal ultrasound, long bones and spine X-ray/skeletal survey, spine ultrasound to rule out tethered cord)

Procedure/therapy in the NICU

- Consider administration of broad-spectrum antibiotics IV
- Individual timing of ligation of the TEF and esophageal anastomosis[312]
- After surgery, leakage and strictures may occur at the site of anastomosis
- Gastroesophageal reflux disease (GERD) may occur immediately after surgery and lead to respiratory distress
- Another reason for respiratory difficulty post surgery is a missed proximal TEF
- Late complications include recurrence of TEF, esophageal stricture, and GERD (35%–58%). These complications may lead to chronic cough, dysphagia, recurrent pneumonia, obstructive and restrictive ventilatory defects, and airway hyperreactivity[313]
- Tracheomalacia is a coincident anomaly rather than a complication of surgery
- Prognosis depends on concomitant malformations, immaturity, birth weight, and occurrence and severity of aspiration pneumonia[312]

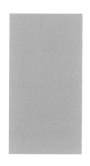

Gastrointestinal obstruction

Andrea Zimmermann

Ileus

Etiology/pathophysiology

- *Paralytic functional ileus (acute, intermittent or chronic; primary or secondary)* due to:
    - Necrotizing enterocolitis (NEC)/bacterial enteritis/perinatal enterovirus infection
    - Extraperitoneal infections (omphalitis, pneumonia, sepsis)
    - Peritonitis
    - Mesenteric hypoperfusion (hypovolemia, patent ductus arteriosus (PDA) with steal phenomenon, embolism (air, clot), thrombosis)
    - Renal vein thrombosis
    - Adrenal bleeding
    - Adverse effects of drugs that cross the placenta (opioids/heroin, neuroleptics, antidepressants, magnesium)
    - Hypokalemia, hypermagnesemia, hypercalcemia
    - Medications such as opiates and theophylline administered to the newborn
    - Endocrinopathies: hypothyroidism, diabetes mellitus, hyperparathyroidism, adrenal insufficiency
    - Gastrointestinal perforation
    - Abdominal surgery or trauma
    - Prematurity
- *Mechanical ileus due to:*
    - Obstruction/occlusion (intraluminal, bowel wall, extrinsic), i.e., intestinal stenosis, intestinal atresia, meconium plug, meconium ileus, Hirschsprung's disease, tumors, invagination, Meckel's diverticulum (presents more frequently as rectal bleeding and diverticulitis)
    - Strangulation. i.e., malrotation and volvulus, hernia (inguinal hernia, congenital diaphragmatic hernia, gastroschisis), adhesions, strangulation by a ligament (e.g., a cord remnant of the omphalomesenteric duct may allow for an internal hernia), intussusception (rare in the neonate)

Clinical presentation

Symptoms depend on the underlying cause, intestinal segments affected/level of obstruction, associated infection, and/or perforation:

Neonatal Emergencies: A Practical Guide for Resuscitation, Transport and Critical Care, ed. Georg Hansmann.
Published by Cambridge University Press. © Cambridge University Press 2009.

- Poor feeding, poor general condition, crying, moaning/whimpering, "unhappy facial expression"
- Vomiting or gastric residuals: may be clear or bile-stained, or contain partially digested food[314]
  - The beginning of symptoms and nature of emesis (non-bilious, bilious, feculent) depend on the level of obstruction (in small bowel ileus, expect symptoms after 8–10 h)
- Vital signs. In advanced stages: hypotension, tachycardia, shock
- Physical exam:
  - Distended abdomen
  - Abdominal wall may show edema, erythema, visible distended bowel loops, or greenish skin color
  - Absent or increased bowel sounds (paralytic vs. mechanical)
  - Abdominal tenderness
  - Dehydration: depressed fontanelle, reduced skin turgor, sluggish capillary refill, lethargy
- Stools:
  - No stool per rectum after initial meconium passage has been observed, or
  - Delayed stool >48 h after birth or none since birth
  - Mucous and/or bloody stools
  - Discolored/white viscous stool, mucous plug
- Laboratory: electrolyte imbalance with drop or rise in serum potassium (also sodium, chloride), acid-base disturbance (metabolic acidosis, possibly lactate acidosis; hypokalemic hypochloremic metabolic alkalosis in pyloric stenosis)

! DDx: Paralytic and mechanical ileus may be differentiated through auscultation:

- *Paralytic ileus* → bowel sounds absent
- *Mechanical ileus* → often loud, high-pitched, tinkling bowel sounds (hyperperistalsis), but may also present with absent or few bowel sounds (paralytic component of mechanical ileus)
- An **acute abdomen** is (at least intermittently) associated with signs and symptoms of paralytic ileus. Therefore, **mechanical ileus, especially bowel ischemia following strangulation (e.g., volvulus), should be first and urgently ruled out, if required by means of a surgical consultation and possible exploratory laparotomy**
- Acute abdominal symptoms in the neonate[315] due to intestinal obstruction, hypoperfusion or infection are mostly caused by:
  - Intestinal atresia or stenosis
  - Volvulus (→ strangulation → ileus and bowel ischemia)
  - Delayed meconium passage: meconium ileus, meconium plug
  - Necrotizing enterocolitis (NEC)
  - Hirschsprung's disease
- Depending on the nature of the obstruction, urgent laparotomy may or may not be indicated (most postsurgical adhesive bowel obstructions resolve with bowel rest, nasogastric decompression, and IV fluids)
- **"Bilious emesis" indicates a surgical emergency until proven otherwise** (need to rule out malrotation/volvulus because of the potential devastation of necrosing the entire midgut: → STAT upper GI study)

- **Volvulus and NEC are accompanied by fulminant symptoms (i.e., shock) and are surgical emergencies!**
- **Transfer**: transfer the newborn with ileus to a Pediatric Surgical ICU or a NICU collaborating with experienced pediatric surgeons. Inform the admitting ICU well in advance

Gastrointestinal atresias

! Colonic atresia (1:100 000) and pyloric atresia (1:1 000 000) are very rare. Other gastrointestinal atresias occur in approximately 1 to 3 of 10 000 births.

Pyloric atresia

Definition/pathophysiology/epidemiology
Congenital pyloric atresia (CPA) is a very rare anomaly that constitutes fewer than 1% of all upper gastrointestinal atresias. The estimated incidence is 1 per million newborns; its etiology is not well understood. Although CPA can occur in isolation, not uncommonly it is seen in association with either gastrointestinal atresias or epidermolysis bullosa (EB) and/or aplasia cutis congenita (ACC).

Prenatal diagnosis
- Polyhydramnios
- Possible associated malformations include Down syndrome, multiple intestinal atresias, congenital heart disease, cleft palate[316]
- Prepartal treatment of the mother with erythromycin increases the risk of pyloric atresia in the infant[317]

Clinical presentation
- Vomiting of clear (non-bilious) fluid, poor feeding

Diagnosis in the delivery room or nursery
- Palpable distended stomach
- Dehydration, weight loss
- CBC, blood gas analysis, lactate, blood glucose, electrolytes, CRP/IL-6

Procedure/therapy in the delivery room/nursery
- Placement of orogastric (or nasogastric) tube and venous access
- Transfer to pediatric center with associated pediatric surgery

DDx.
- Gastric volvulus[318]
- Hypertrophic pyloric stenosis: usually in male infants 2 weeks of age and older[319]
- Presentation (mottled skin color, hypotension, tachycardia, shock) may be similar in newborns with sepsis or congenital adrenal hyperplasia (CAH) = adrenogenital syndrome (AGS)

Diagnosis/procedure/therapy in the NICU

- Radiological imaging: chest X-ray, abdominal X-ray (KUB), barium swallow study/ fluoroscopy[320]
- Ultrasonography
- Placement of gastric tube (see above)
- Replacement of electrolytes
- Surgery when stable

Duodenal atresia/stenosis

Definition/epidemiology/etiology/pathophysiology

- Duodenal obstruction may be due to duodenal atresia (e.g., duodenal membrane) or duodenal stenosis, annular pancreas, preduodenal portal vein
- Small intestinal atresia occurs in approx. 2–3 per 10 000 births[321] (incidence decreases for more distal locations). Duodenal atresia is the most common intestinal atresia[322]
- Patients are frequently premature infants

Prenatal diagnosis

- Ultrasonography: double bubble sign[323]
- Polyhydramnios
- Association with chromosomal abnormalities in about 30%, especially trisomy 21[324]
- Often associated with congenital heart disease, vascular malformations, malrotation, annular pancreas, biliary malformations, additional atresia[321]
- May be a concomitant finding with the *VACTERL association* (for definition see p. 434)

Clinical presentation

- Distended stomach
- Emesis or gastric residuals, either bile-stained or clear
- Poor feeding
- Abdomen usually not distended (high obstruction)
- No meconium after normal-appearing initial meconium passage

Diagnosis/procedure/therapy in the nursery

- Physical examination
- Placement of orogastric (or nasogastric) tube and venous access
- CBC, blood gas analysis, lactate, blood glucose, electrolytes, CRP/IL-6
- Transfer to a pediatric surgical ward or NICU

DDx.

- Small intestinal obstruction: malrotation/volvulus (especially if emesis is green)

Diagnosis/procedure/therapy in the NICU

- Plain abdominal X-ray: two double-bubble or three air-fluid levels, lack of distal intestinal gas (this usually rules out malrotation)
- Abdominal ultrasonography
- Rule out additional malformations/VACTERL association
- Early non-emergent surgery unless malrotation cannot be ruled out

Jejunal and ileal atresia/stenosis

Definition/epidemiology/etiology/pathophysiology
- Affects jejunum and ileum in equal proportions
- May be associated with gastroschisis
- Multiple atresias may occur
- Estimated incidence is 2–10 per 10 000 births (similar to duodenal atresia)
- May be caused by intrauterine vascular accident due to intestinal volvulus, intussusception, vasoconstrictor drugs[325]

Prenatal diagnosis
- Polyhydramnios
- Dilated fetal bowel
- Frequent association with cystic fibrosis[326]
- Association with additional malformations[327]
- Birth weight lower than average

Clinical presentation
- Poor feeding
- Bile-stained emesis or gastric residuals
- Vomiting begins within 1 or 2 days after birth
- The higher the atresia the earlier the vomiting
- Distended abdomen with palpable bowel loops
- Failure to pass normal stools or no stools per rectum
- Signs of peritonitis

DDx.
- Meconium ileus
- Meconium plug syndrome
- Volvulus
- Hirschsprung's disease

Diagnosis and therapy in the nursery
- Physical examination
- Placement of orogastric (or nasogastric) tube and venous access
- CBC, blood gas analysis, lactate, blood glucose, electrolytes, CRP/IL-6
- Transfer to a pediatric surgical ward or NICU

Diagnosis/procedure/therapy in the NICU
- Plain abdominal X-ray (KUB): usually dilated gas-filled loops with no distal gas; intestinal air-fluid levels or calcifications possible
- Gastrointestinal contrast study
- Abdominal ultrasonography
- Rule out additional malformations
- Urgent surgical correction on the day of diagnosis[326]

Imperforate anus

Definition
- Defect in the formation of the urorectal septum
- Classification in relation to the levator ani muscles:
  - High, supralevator lesions
  - Intermediate, translevator lesions
  - Low, infralevator lesions

Epidemiology
- Approx. 2:10 000 live births (0.2/1000)

Pathophysiology/associated malformations
- In up to 75% of cases associated fistula to perineum, vulva, vagina, urethra, bladder. True rectovaginal fistula is actually extremely rare (approx. 1% of anorectal malformations). Rectofourchette fistula (i.e., the intestinal opening is located between the mucosa of the vestibule and the perineal skin) is usually what is meant by the term "rectovaginal fistula"
- In association with oesophageal atresia part of the *VACTERL association* (for definition, see p. 434)
- Associated gastrointestinal (e.g., Hirschsprung's disease), genito-urinary, skeletal, cardiovascular or spinal cord malformations[328]
- Part of syndromes such as VACTERL[328]

Clinical presentation
- First physical examination reveals imperforate anus
- In newborn females who have stooled it is still important to document the presence of an anus; a female with only one perineal opening technically has a persistent cloaca, i.e., one of the variants of imperforate anus

Diagnosis and therapy in the nursery
- Placement of orogastric (or nasogastric) tube and venous access
- CBC, blood gas analysis, lactate, blood glucose, electrolytes, CRP/IL-6
- Transfer to a pediatric surgical ward

Diagnosis/procedure/therapy in the NICU
- Thorough check-up to rule out additional malformations
- *VACTERL association* and additional anomalies ought to be investigated:
  - Passage of nasogastric tube into the stomach possible?
  - Is a normal anus present? Meconium/stool? Fistula?
- Abdominal and perineal ultrasonography
- Echocardiography
- X-ray/ultrasonography of the spine and extremities
- If indicated: further X-ray studies, i.e., prone cross-table lateral abdominal X-ray with hips raised (this causes air in the rectum to define the caudal extent of the gastrointestinal tract and helps to identify the lesion as "high" or "low")

- Surgical correction: primary pull-through procedure or diverting colostomy with definitive surgery in 3–6 months

Intestinal malrotation with volvulus (EMERGENCY)

Definition/etiology/pathophysiology

Acute or chronic intermittent torsion of the small intestine (less commonly torsion of the stomach or large intestine occurs) resulting in acute ischemia and hemorrhagic infarction of the affected bowel segment:

- Gastric volvulus – usually associated with congenital diaphragmatic hernia or anomaly of ligaments
- Primary small intestinal volvulus – often associated with Ladd's bands
- Secondary small bowel volvulus with abdominal tumors
- Other congenital anomalies

Epidemiology

- Approx. 1.7:10 000 (0.17/1000) live births

Clinical presentation

- Symptoms of obstruction may be intermittent and incomplete
- *Gastric volvulus:*
  - Symptoms of an upper intestinal obstruction with sudden pain and vomiting (DDx: may be confused or coexistent with gastroesophageal reflux disease)
  - Signs of peritonitis
  - Shock
- *Small intestine volvulus:* after normal meconium, acute symptoms develop:
  - Poor feeding
  - Bilious vomiting
  - Distended abdomen and tenderness
  - Bloody stool
  - Signs of peritonitis
  - Shock

Diagnosis and therapy in the nursery

Emergent[329]

- Physical examination
- Stabilize vital parameters
- Placement of orogastric (or nasogastric) tube and venous access
- Volume expansion (normal saline) 10–20 ml/kg/bolus IV, repeat bolus if indicated
- CBC, blood gas analysis, lactate, blood glucose, electrolytes, CRP/IL-6
- Urgent transfer to a pediatric surgery ward or NICU collaborating with pediatric surgical department
- Inform admitting NICU team well in advance

> **Delayed diagnosis and treatment of neonates with volvulus results in extensive necrosis of the gastrointestinal tract, and eventually death.**

443

DDx.
- Gastrointestinal atresia, NEC

Diagnosis/procedure/therapy in the NICU
- STAT upper GI study (contrast study): need to see the duodenum cross the midline and travel superiorly to approximately the same level as the pylorus; also need to see a lateral view that shows the second/third portion of the duodenum travelling posteriorly
- Abdominal ultrasonography with color Doppler[330]
- Correct electrolyte imbalance
- Emergent surgery

Prognosis
- Good, if surgery is performed early
- Risk of hemorrhagic infarction of the twisted bowel segment
- Midgut strangulation may occur
- (Postoperatively) short bowel syndrome

Hirschsprung's disease

Definition/cause/pathophysiology
Aganglionosis of the rectum and a segment of variable length of large (and rarely contiguous small) intestine resulting in tonic contraction of the affected bowel segment.

Epidemiology
- Approx. 1:5000 (0.2/1000)[331], common in trisomy 21 (Down syndrome)

Clinical presentation
- Symptoms may begin during or after the first week after birth: vomiting, poor feeding
- Delayed meconium, distended abdomen, prominent bowel loops
- Symptoms of infection and peritonitis may be present ("Hirschsprung's enterocolitis")

Diagnosis and therapy in the nursery
- Physical examination, check for imperforate anus
- Placement of oro- or nasogastric tube and venous access
- CBC, blood gas analysis, lactate, blood glucose, electrolytes, CRP/IL-6
- Volume expansion (crystalloids) 10 ml/kg IV if indicated
- Transfer to a pediatric surgical ward or NICU with collaborating pediatric surgical department

DDx.
- Intestinal atresia, NEC, meconium plug/meconium ileus, small left colon syndrome[332]

Diagnosis/procedure/therapy in the NICU
- Plain abdominal radiographs: dilated bowel loops, rectal gas absent
- Abdominal ultrasonography
- Rectal biopsy (gold standard: can be done at bedside with no anesthesia with biopsy gun)
- Only in older patients (not in neonates): consider rectosigmoidoscopy, anorectal manometry

- Correction of electrolyte abnormalities, IV antibiotics
- Surgical correction: resection of the aganglionic bowel (primary pull-through or leveling colostomy followed by definitive procedure in 3–6 months)

Bowel obstruction caused by meconium (problem: no stools in 48 h; see also DDx below)

Meconium plug

Definition/etiology/pathophysiology
- Obstruction of the lower colon or rectum caused by inspissated, viscous meconium plug

Epidemiology
- Rare in term neonates, more frequent in premature infants[333]

Clinical presentation
- Poor feeding
- Failure to pass stool (75% of premature infants pass stool by 24 h, and 99% by 48 h)
- Distended abdomen, prominent bowel loops
- Hyperperistalsis
- Vomiting

Diagnosis and therapy in the nursery
- Physical examination
- Placement of orogastric (or nasogastric) tube and venous access
- CBC, blood gas analysis, lactate, blood glucose, electrolytes, CRP/IL-6
- Transfer to a pediatric surgical ward or NICU with collaborating pediatric surgical department

DDx.
- Hirschsprung's disease, meconium ileus (e.g., in cystic fibrosis), small left colon syndrome (this is most likely a temporary motility disorder that will resolve in a few days)[334], colonic stenosis or atresia, imperforate anus

Diagnosis/procedure/therapy in the NICU
- (Rectal) contrast enema with hyperosmolar solutions often induces the passage of meconium (small-caliber, soft, rubber catheter (10–14 F) to be inserted into the rectum using minimal lubricant); may need to be repeated several times to clear meconium plugs (caution: do not inject large volume of contrast dye: iatrogenic bowel perforation and hypothermia during the procedure are described)
- Abdominal ultrasonography
- Adjustment of electrolytes, antibiotics if indicated
- Abdominal X-ray (KUB): lower intestinal ileus
- Surgical decompression and possible diversion, if indicated.

Meconium ileus

Definition/etiology/pathophysiology
- Obstruction of the terminal ileum due to intraluminal inspissated (thickened) meconium
- Associated with cystic fibrosis[334]
- Complications must be anticipated in 50% of cases:
  - Perforation with peritonitis/sepsis
  - Secondary bowel atresia
  - Bowel strangulation
  - Calcifications

Clinical presentation
- Soon after birth: poor feeding, clear or bilious vomiting
- No stool, or small pellets of pale material per rectum
- Visible bowel loops, hyperperistalsis
- Distended abdomen
- Signs of peritonitis

Diagnosis and therapy in the nursery
- Physical examination (imperforate anus?)
- Placement of orogastric (or nasogastric) tube and venous access
- CBC, blood gas analysis, lactate, blood glucose, electrolytes, CRP/IL-6
- Volume expansion (crystalloids) 10 ml/kg/bolus IV, repeat bolus if indicated
- Transfer to a pediatric surgical ward or NICU with collaborating pediatric surgical department

DDx.
- Intestinal atresia, NEC, colonic aganglionosis

Diagnosis/procedure/therapy in the NICU
- Rectal enema with or without contrast can induce stool (see above under "meconium ileus")
- Abdominal ultrasonography and X-ray
- Consult pediatric surgery
- Correction of electrolytes, prophylactic antibiotics
- Surgical decompression and possible diversion, if indicated

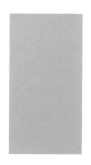

Necrotizing enterocolitis (NEC)

Andrea Zimmermann

Definition
- Hemorrhagic necrotizing inflammation of the small and large bowels

Epidemiology
Most common gastrointestinal emergency in the neonatal period:
- NEC occurs in 1–3/1000 live births[335]
- NEC occurs in up to 10% of preterm infants <1500 g (VLBW)[336]
- 5%–25% of affected neonates are term infants[337]

Etiology/pathophysiology
- Etiology remains unclear
- Known risk factors are bacterial colonization, intestinal ischemia or hypoxia, formula feeding,[336] prematurity, hyperviscosity, exchange transfusion, cocaine exposure

Clinical presentation
In term infants, symptoms usually start in the first days after birth; preterm infants might develop symptoms in the first weeks after birth (i.e., usually associated with feeding). Signs and symptoms may develop slowly and discretely or illness progresses rapidly.

NEC staging (modified Bell staging criteria[335])

Stage I: Suspected NEC
Clinical presentation: temperature instability, apnea, bradycardia
Intestinal signs: gastric residuals, mild abdominal distension, occult blood in stools
Abdominal X-ray, ultrasound: non-specific findings, normal or mild ileus, mildly distended bowel loops

Stage IIa: Mild NEC
Clinical presentation: similar to stage I
Intestinal signs: prominent abdominal distension ± tenderness, absent bowel sounds, grossly bloody stools
Abdominal X-ray, ultrasound: ileus, dilated bowel loops with pneumatosis

Stage IIb: Moderate NEC
Clinical presentation: mild acidosis and thrombocytopenia
Intestinal signs: abdominal wall edema and tenderness ± palpable mass
Abdominal X-ray, ultrasound: extensive pneumatosis intestinalis ± portal venous gas

Neonatal Emergencies: A Practical Guide for Resuscitation, Transport and Critical Care, ed. Georg Hansmann.
Published by Cambridge University Press. © Cambridge University Press 2009.

Stage IIIa: Advanced NEC, intact bowel
Clinical presentation: Respiratory and metabolic acidosis, mechanical ventilation, hypotension, oliguria, disseminated intravascular coagulation (DIC)
Intestinal signs: worsening wall edema and erythema with induration
Abdominal X-ray, ultrasound: persistent ascites, persistent bowel loops, no free air

Stage IIIb: Advanced NEC, perforated bowel
Clinical presentation: vital sign and laboratory evidence of deterioration, shock
Intestinal signs: evidence of perforation
Abdominal X-ray, ultrasound: pneumoperitoneum

Diagnosis/therapy in the nursery
- Physical examination (auscultation; brief and gentle palpation of the abdomen in suspected NEC)
- CBC, blood gas analysis, lactate, blood glucose, electrolytes, CRP/IL-6, coagulation panel, blood type and screen/cross
- If indicated, intubation and ventilation
- Placement of orogastric (or nasogastric) tube and venous access
- Start IV antibiotics in the nursery STAT when general condition is poor:
  - Ampicillin and cefotaxime and aminoglycoside (slow IV)
- When BP is insufficient:
  - Volume expansion (normal saline) 10 ml/kg/bolus IV, repeat if necessary
  - If mean arterial pressure (MAP) is persistently $\ll 40$ mmHg in term neonates or $\ll$ GA in weeks in preterm infants, dopamine infusion, if necessary via peripheral IV, other via central venous line. Transfuse PRBC early in persistent arterial hypotension (10–20 ml/kg/dose)
- Urgent transfer to a pediatric surgery ward or NICU with collaborating, experienced pediatric surgical department

> ! When NEC is suspected, do not perform repeated abdominal exams (palpation) and do not administer pharyngeal CPAP or pharyngeal PPV (intubate early instead).

DDx.
- Isolated intestinal perforation (IP), volvulus, intestinal atresia, sepsis with abdominal infection, septic ileus

Diagnosis/procedure/therapy in the NICU
- Gastric drainage tube, absolute bowel rest (nothing per mouth)
- Urgent consultation of pediatric surgery
- Abdominal ultrasonography and X-ray (AP = KUB and lateral decubitus views):
  - Intestinal dilatation, ascites, pneumatosis intestinalis and/or hepatis, portal venous gas or pneumoperitoneum?
  - In stage IIb repeat abdominal lateral decubitus X-ray views q 4 to 6 h (many centers recommend serial abdominal X-rays even in the earlier stages for 1–2 days until neonate improves clinically)
- Color Doppler sonography: increase in resistance index (RI), i.e., decreased diastolic flow, in the superior mesenteric artery

- Monitor abdominal girth every 2 h
- CBC (with differential/platelets), arterial blood gas analysis, lactate, blood glucose, electrolytes, CRP/IL-6, coagulation panel, blood type and screen/cross
- Parenteral nutrition, if necessary transfusion of blood and platelets
- Volume expansion (e.g., normal saline) 10 ml/kg/bolus IV, repeat if necessary
- In persistent hypotension, transfuse packed red blood cells (PRBC) 10–20 ml/kg/dose early
- Correction of significant coagulation disorder with fresh frozen plasma (FFP) and cryoprecipitate. Consider vitamin K IV
- Be aware that DIC may occur, requiring platelet transfusions
- Continue antibiotic therapy with:
  - Ampicillin + aminoglycoside (e.g., gentamicin) + cefotaxime (for dosing see p. 41; see chapter, "Chorioamnionitis and early-onset sepsis of the newborn infant," p. 280)
  - Anaerobic coverage with metronidazole IV (7.5 mg/kg/dose IV, interval 4; p. 41) or imipenem or meropenem IV (20 mg/kg/dose IV q 8–12h; p. 41) or clindamycin (5–7.5 mg/kg/dose IV q 6–12h; p. 41)
  - When there is no improvement with the initial empiric antibiotic therapy, re-evaluate antibiotic regimen (e.g., consider clindamycin), and always adjust selection and dosing according to antibiogram and drug levels. Consult Infectious Diseases in difficult cases
- Prepare for surgery (at the latest) during stage IIb; immediate exploratory laparatomy in stage III (see below)
- **Depending on the presentation and the surgical opinion, peritoneal drain may be advocated instead of primary surgery, particularly if the baby is very unstable and unlikely to survive an operation.** If the baby is very stable and has a large amount of pneumoperitoneum, suspect isolated intestinal perforation (IP, may be related to indomethacin use); these babies often do well with surgery because the disease is focal, not diffuse as in NEC
- A recent outcome study (initial peritoneal drain vs. surgery) from the NICHD Neonatal Research Network on ELBW infants with either isolated intestinal perforation or NEC showed the following[338]:
  - Laparotomy was never performed in 78% (28 of 36) of drain-treated survivors with NEC or isolated intestinal perforation. Among patients who underwent initial laparotomy, 40 of 76 infants (53%) either died before discharge or received prolonged parenteral nutrition compared with 53 (66%) of 80 infants in the initial drainage group. Mortality before discharge in the initial laparotomy group was 43% (33 of 76); 7 (9%) survivors had prolonged parenteral nutrition. Among initial drainage patients, 43 (54%) infants died before hospital discharge and 10 (12.5%) survivors had prolonged parenteral nutrition. However, clinical data on the best approach (peritoneal drain vs. surgery) are currently sparse and ambiguous, and warrant more information from future randomized controlled trials[338]

Prognosis
- Outcome is worse for NEC than for isolated intestinal perforation[338]
- Mortality for NEC remains high (approx. 35%–50% for perforated NEC[335,337,338]) and has improved little over the last few decades. Therefore, primary prevention remains crucial in order to decrease the incidence of NEC

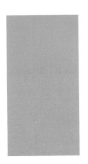

Omphalocele and gastroschisis

Andrea Zimmermann

Definition/etiology/pathophysiology

- *Omphalocele* (syn. exomphalos):
    - Is a failed closure of the abdominal wall with incomplete restoration of the herniation of the midgut (midgut herniation during the first 12 weeks of gestation is normal; in omphalocele bowel and often additional organs such as liver and spleen herniate through the abdominal wall and do not return to the peritoneal cavity)
    - Stomach, intestines, liver, several small parts of the bowel, and also bladder and spleen may protrude into the base of the umbilical cord depending on the size of the hernial sac (i.e., peritoneum and amnion)
    - Associated with intrauterine growth retardation (IUGR)
    - In very large omphaloceles, pulmonary hypoplasia may occur
    - *Complications:* rupture of hernial sac → unprotected intestine: infection, peritonitis, secondary intestinal atresia
    - *Associated anomalies occur in up to 70% of cases:* chromosomal aberrations, congenital heart disease, congenital diaphragmatic hernia, Beckwith–Wiedemann syndrome (exomphalos-macroglossia-gigantism syndrome)[339]
    - *DDx:* Umbilical cord hernia: some experts define this as a fascial defect of less than 4 cm. It does not carry the coexistent anomalies commonly present in omphalocele
- *Gastroschisis* (syn.: laparoschisis):
    - Defect in the development of the abdominal wall, usually to the right of the umbilical cord without surrounding membrane to protect the bowel loops in utero
    - Open prolapse of parts of the intestine, the whole intestine and/or rarely solid abdominal organs (one should suspect ruptured omphalocele in cases of solid organ prolapse and look for other anomalies)
    - Prolapsed bowel is edematous, swollen, inflamed/fibrinous and usually twisted
    - 20%–30% of cases lead to intestinal atresia, possibly due to ischemic infarction or strangulation, adhesions and stenosis
    - Associated with IUGR[340]
    - *Concomitant defects:* rare[339]

Epidemiology

- Omphalocele: incidence 2–3:10 000 (0.23/1000) births[339]
- Gastroschisis: incidence 1–2:10 000 (0.1/1000) births[340] (incidence increasing)

Neonatal Emergencies: A Practical Guide for Resuscitation, Transport and Critical Care, ed. Georg Hansmann.
Published by Cambridge University Press. © Cambridge University Press 2009.

Prenatal diagnosis
- Fetal sonography (U/S) detects both gastroschisis and omphalocele in up to 80% of cases. Fetal U/S can usually distinguish between the two by the presence or absence of the membrane; high false-positive results occur early in gestation due to normal gut evisceration during development (see above)
- Delivery in a center that collaborates with experienced pediatric surgeons

Mode of delivery
- There are ongoing controversies over the best obstetric management:
  - Vaginal delivery may be safe in isolated ventral wall defects[341]
  - Elective cesarean section may be of advantage (e.g., large omphalocele in which solid organs could be contused/lacerated)[342]

Clinical presentation
Omphalocele:
- Hernial sac, which may contain parts of the intestine or the whole bowel and abdominal organs; varies in size; the umbilical cord is attached to/inserts onto the hernial sac
- Postnatal adaptation is affected and depends on the immaturity and on the occurrence of further malformations
- Neonate may transition without any problem when the omphalocele is small omphalo-celes (<4-cm-diameter defect) with no additional malformations

Gastroschisis:
- Abdominal wall defect lateral/to the right of the umbilical cord, which reveals unpro-tected bowel; bowel may show livid discoloration, edema and fibrin coating, depending on possible strangulations and obstructions as well as exposure to inflammatory agents in amniotic fluid (Figure 3.35 and color plate section)
- Other organs may herniate through the abdominal wall/out of the peritoneal cavity (extremely rare, see above)

Diagnosis in the delivery room
- Extensive physical examination is usually not possible, especially when prenatal diag-nosis is established and the newborn infant is placed in a sterile and clear plastic bag immediately after delivery
- Estimate size and contents of hernia through the bag
- ABG, blood glucose, lactate, presurgical laboratory screen including coagulation panel, blood type and cross matching

DDx.
- Prenatally ruptured omphalocele
- Gastroschisis
- Vesicointestinal fissures
- Exstrophy of the bladder or cloaca
- Persistent allantois membrane

Monitoring

Pulse oximetry (HR, S_aO_2), BP, ECG, and, if intubated, ET tube position

Procedure/therapy in the delivery room

- Initial care under sterile conditions to avoid superinfection of the unprotected abdominal organs
- Place newborn infant in a sterile and transparent plastic bag to protect against cold (Figure 3.35a). For cesarean sections, this should be done by the obstetrician/OR staff

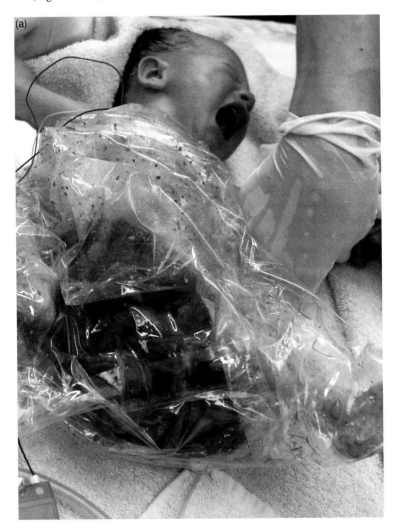

Figure 3.35a–c Gastroschisis. (a). Initial care of a preterm infant (35 + 5 weeks of gestation) with large gastroschisis after primary cesarean section. Umbilical artery pH 7.30, Apgar 9/10/10. Lower extremities and trunk have already been placed in a sterile plastic bag, no bag-and-mask ventilation, no nasal continuous positive airways pressure (CPAP). Later management included elective nasotracheal intubation 10 min postnatally, volume IV for arterial hypotension, surgery during the first hours of life. (b). Gastroschisis, surgical field right before surgery: abdominal hernia with eventration of the whole small bowel and large bowel including parts of the sigma. The bowel wall is massively swollen and partly fibrinous. Intestinal non-rotation. (c). Status post abdominal surgery with two GoreTex® patches (Schuster's plastic). See color plate section for full color version.

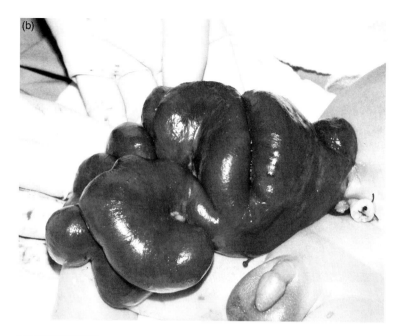

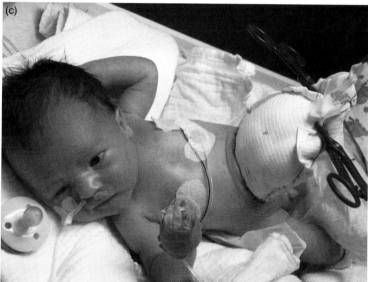

Figure 3.35 a–c *(cont.)* See color plate section for full color version.

- Stimulation and oxygen supplementation; immediate intubation in cases of respiratory insufficiency, otherwise early elective intubation
- To avoid abdominal distension: *no bag-and-mask ventilation*
- Orogastric (or nasogastric) tube to decompress GI tract; set tube to low suction
- To secure adequate blood supply to the intestine, avoid any kinking of mesentery over the edge of the defect: *Keep the baby on the side* with the intestines under no tension (see below under purple discoloration)

453

- *Avoid hypothermia.* If unprotected intestinal parts are kept moist with saline compresses, infant runs the risk of hypothermia (use plastic bag instead)
- A urine bag may be attached to the newborn while they are wrapped (will likely fall off)
- Establish IV access; $D_{10}W$ 3 ml/kg/h during transport and, if necessary, volume (normal saline) 10–20 ml/kg/bolus IV (repeat as indicated)
- *If purple discoloration of the bowels* ± torsion is seen in gastroschisis, carefully untangle the bowel loops. In case of strangulation hernia, orifice may require surgical widening right away in the delivery room. Temperature control

Transport
- *Omphalocele:* when the liver is herniated, patient is placed in a right semiprone position to avoid compression of the inferior vena cava
- *Gastroschisis:* lateral decubitus position (some recommend positioning the baby onto their right side)

Diagnosis/procedure/therapy in the NICU
- Supportive treatment (see above), early elective intubation in most cases (if not done yet)
- Chest and abdominal X-ray (AP view)
- Rule out additional malformations (exam, echocardiography, renal U/S)
- Broad-spectrum antibiotic, e.g., piperacillin (150–220 mg/kg/day) + cefotaxime (150–200 mg/kg/day) + possible metronidazol (15 mg/kg/day) IV (for exact dosing see 41, p. 280)
- Surgical correction:
  - Primary or staged closure of the abdominal wall defect, depending on its size[343]
  - Large omphalocele and gastroschisis (Figure 3.35b): protective prosthetic silo with, e.g., Gore-Tex™ patches (Figure 3.35c) or pre-fabricated wire-coil silo (Bentec bag)
  - Giant omphalocele: cover with silver sulfadiazine and perform delayed closure[344]

Prognosis
- *Omphalocele:* Prognosis depends on size and concomitant defects (especially congenital heart disease, chromosomal aberration). Midgut volvulus and intestinal obstruction may occur
- *Gastroschisis:* Prognosis depends on infectious reaction, peritonitis, intestinal atresia, and stenosis
- Both gastroschisis and omphalocele usually occur with intestinal malrotation/nonrotation and therefore patients are at risk for midgut volvulus

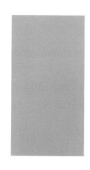

Neural tube defects

Christoph Bührer and Andrea Zimmermann

Definition

Spina bifida, encephalocele and anencephaly are the most common neural tube defects (NTD). Defective closure of the caudal neural tube in the third or fourth week of gestation results in anomalies of the lumbar and sacral vertebrae or spinal cord called spina bifida (Latin: "split spine"). Spina bifida malformations fall into three categories: *spina bifida occulta*, *spina bifida cystica (meningomyelocele)*, and *meningocele*. These anomalies range in severity from clinically insignificant defects of the L5 or S1 vertebral arches (spina bifida occulta) to major malformations of the thoracic spinal cord that lies uncovered by skin or bone on the baby's back. Spina bifida cystica, or meningomyelocele (MMC), is a sac-like casing filled with cerebrospinal fluid (CSF), spinal cord, and nerve roots that have herniated through a defect in the vertebral arches and dura. *Anencephaly and rachischisis are extremely severe forms of NTD* in which an extensive opening in the cranial and vertebral bone exists with an absence of variable amounts of the brain, spinal cord, nerve roots, and meninges.

Epidemiology

Incidence highly variable across regions, with highest rates being reported from Ireland, Great Britain, Hungary, Pakistan, India, and Egypt. In the USA, incidence is about 5.5, 3.7 and 1.4 per 10 000 live births for spina bifida (0.55/1000), anencephaly (0.37/1000), and encephalocele (0.14/1000), respectively[345]. The incidence of spina bifida, but not encephalocele or anencephaly, has been decreasing after the introduction of periconceptional folic acid supplementation.

Pathophysiology

- Genetic factors:
  - High NTD concordance rate in monozygotic twins. NTD is also more frequent among siblings (the risk for NTD is increased 10-fold with one affected sibling or parent, and 30-fold with two affected siblings)
  - NTD is more common in females compared to males
  - High prevalence of karyotypic abnormalities among infants with NTD, especially in the presence of other congenital anomalies
- Environmental factors:
  - Diabetes (NTD risk highly correlated with periconceptional blood glucose control: even a slightly impaired glucose tolerance associated with maternal obesity increases the risk of neural tube defects)

Neonatal Emergencies: A Practical Guide for Resuscitation, Transport and Critical Care, ed. Georg Hansmann.
Published by Cambridge University Press. © Cambridge University Press 2009.

- Valproate (strongly increased risk for NTD), and other common anticonvulsants (carbamazepine, phenytoin, phenobarbital, primidone)
- Folic acid deficiency (nutritive or folic acid antagonists such as trimethoprim and sulfasalazine). Periconceptional folic acid supplementation reduces NTD risk

Prenatal diagnosis

- Detection of NTD is usually possible well before delivery: increased α-fetoprotein (AFP) in amniotic fluid or maternal serum, and ultrasound examination in the second trimester. Hydrocephalus may be the leading sonographic sign
- Increased AFP is also observed in several non-neural "leaky" fetal abnormalities (ventral wall defects, tumors, dermatological disorders, congenital nephrosis, aneuploidy)
- Fetuses with spina bifida occulta have normal maternal AFP concentrations
- Cesarean section before the onset of labor is the desired mode of delivery since this has been associated with improved neurological outcome in a retrospective analysis[346]. No randomized controlled trials (RCTs) have been performed to date to prove this concept
- A select group of patients are being evaluated for inclusion in a randomized trial between conventional postnatal MMC repair and fetal surgery

---

! Once the diagnosis of spina bifida has been made and the parents opt against termination of pregnancy, refer to a specialized center where specialists experienced in dealing with these lesions can start discussing treatment options with the parents.

Clinical presentation diagnosis in the delivery room

- Neural plate appears as a raw, red, fleshy plaque through a defect in the vertebral column (known as spina bifida) and skin
- A protruding membranous sac containing meninges, CSF, nerve roots, and dysplastic spinal cord often protrudes through the defect
- The vertebral defect usually involves the lumbar or lumbosacral regions, although any segment may be involved. In most cases, a series of vertebrae distal to the most proximal malformed vertebra are affected, giving an open zipper-like appearance
- Approximately 10% of patients with spina bifida have a meningocele, in which only the meninges of the spinal cord herniate through the vertebral defect. In less severe forms, the lesion is covered by skin
- Spina bifida occulta features split vertebrae, but intact neural structures and dural sac
- *Arnold-Chiari II malformation* is a complex congenital malformation of the brain that is, nearly always associated with meningomyelocele. It is characterized by inferior displacement of the medulla, fourth ventricle, and cerebellum through the foramen magnum into the upper cervical canal, as well as elongation of the pons and fourth ventricle, probably due to a relatively small posterior fossa. This results in obstruction of CSF outflow from the fourth ventricle and through the posterior fossa and causes hydrocephalus in about 90% of infants with myelomeningocele
- At birth, cerebral ventricular dilatation is common but the patient usually lacks increased head circumference or signs of increased intracranial pressure.

Hydrocephalus frequently develops after surgical repair of the back lesion, which then stops leaking CSF

- Other brain abnormalities include cerebral cortical dysplasia and agenesis of the corpus callosum

Procedure/therapy in the delivery room

- Use sterile, non-latex gloves
- After birth, position the infant on the side or on the abdomen. Resuscitate as needed. Although nearly all MMC patients have a Chiari II malformation visualized on prenatal ultrasound or MRI, only a minority will be symptomatic at birth (e.g., stridor, upper airway obstruction)
- Carefully examine MMC to estimate the anatomical level of the lesion and to determine whether the sac is intact. A small amount of CSF usually "weeps" from the translucent edges of the neural placode. If the sac ruptures, it usually decompresses and retracts to the level of the back
- Cover the defect with sterile transparent non-adherent plastic dressing to prevent heat loss and infection
- In most cases, only the neurosurgeon should remove the dressing – if at all. Once the dressing is in place and if repair is planned within 24–48 h, do not change dressing unless it is soiled. If closure is delayed for more than 48 h, change the dressing twice a day and keep it moist with bacitracin solution
- Avoid contamination of site and dressing with stool and urine
- If the sac is open, the use of gauze or cotton towels is contraindicated, as they adhere to the neural tissue, are difficult to remove and cause granulomas
- Placement of the infant should be in the prone or lateral position to avoid pressure on the lesion
- Peripheral venous access is required to provide fluids and antibiotics

If the neonate did undergo prenatal surgical treatment of MMC, follow the guidelines of the surgical center.

Monitoring

- S_pO_2, ECG, frequent neurological checks, urine output, bowel sounds

Diagnosis in the NICU

- Perform physical examination and ultrasound, and look for:
  - Spontaneous activity, muscle weakness and level of paralysis
  - Flexion or extension contractures of hips, knees, and ankles
  - Sensation (response to touch)
  - Deep tendon reflexes
  - Anocutaneous reflex (anal wink)
  - Clubfeet
  - Hydrocephalus and brain malformations (U/S)
  - Congenital heart disease (echocardiography)
  - Renal malformations, ureteral dilatations, and reflux (U/S)
  - Hip dysplasia (U/S)

- Monitor infant closely for signs of meningitis
- Consult neurosurgeons regarding further work-up (e.g., cranial and abdominal U/S, radiograph of spine), timing of surgical repair and whether feedings can be started

Procedure/therapy in the NICU
Surgery

- Back lesion – closure should be performed within the first 24–72 h after birth by a neurosurgeon experienced in this type of repair, to reduce the rate of cicatrical tethered cord formation[347]
- Prophylaxis with broad-spectrum antibiotics until the back is closed reduces the risk of CNS infection[348]

Treatment of hydrocephalus

- Ventricular size should be evaluated by serial U/S studies
- Progressive hydrocephalus, occurring in about 90% of infants with meningomyelocele, is treated by insertion of a ventriculoperitoneal (VP) shunt
- Usually a VP shunt is placed several days after the initial repair. In some infants, simultaneous MMC repair and VP shunt placement may be appropriate[349]

> **!** In general, symptomatic hydrocephalus, progressive increase in head size, or leakage of CSF from the repaired defect site are indications for central shunt placement.

Post-operative management

- Observe carefully for signs of wound infection or CSF leak
- Discuss orders with neurosurgeon regarding positioning of infant, dressing changes, antibiotics, feeding, and timing of post-operative cranial U/S
- Obtain abdominal and hip U/S and request urology and orthopedics consults for evaluation of urinary function and associated orthopedic abnormalities

Prognosis

- For patients with MMC, prognosis depends upon decisions regarding their care, the level of the lesion, and the presence and severity of neurological deficits, hydrocephalus, and other CNS anomalies
- Clinical presentations and follow-up of patients with NTD require attention to various end organs besides the nervous system
- For most of these conditions, long-term follow-up is necessary regardless of the initial treatment
- The vast majority of infants with MMC survive beyond the neonatal period, and most have normal or near-normal cognitive development. Factors associated with poor neurodevelopment are brain malformations and repeated VP shunt infections
- As the entire spinal cord distal to the site of the lesion is usually non-functional, severe motor and sensory deficits in the trunk and legs result in complete paralysis and absence of sensation. There is urinary and fecal incontinence. Since the introduction of

prophylactic sterile intermittent catheterization and anticholinergic medication, repeated urinary tract infections rarely progress to end-stage renal failure

- Brainstem dysfunction due to the Chiari malformation occurs in some patients with myelomeningocele. This results in clinical problems such as swallowing difficulties, vocal cord paresis causing stridor, and apneic episodes, and is associated with a high mortality rate throughout childhood and adolescence

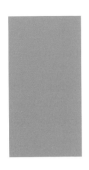

Cleft palate

Christoph Bührer and Andrea Zimmermann

Definition

- *Anterior* orofacial clefts, termed *cleft lip-cleft palate*, are lateral clefts of the lip through the philtrum with a variable degree of extension through the palatal shelves
- A *posterior* palate cleft, located in the midline, is part of the *Pierre Robin sequence*, which also features micrognathia (small retruded mandible) and glossoptosis (posterior displacement of the tongue into the pharyngeal airway), frequently leading to neonatal respiratory distress[350]

Epidemiology

Asians 1:500 live births (2/1000), Caucasians 1:900 live births (1.1/1000), African Americans 1:2000 live births (0.5/1000). The incidence of Pierre Robin sequence (as determined in a retrospective population-based epidemiological study of all Danish live births from 1990 through 1999) is at least 1 in 14 000 live births[350]

Etiology/pathophysiology

- *Most cases are isolated entities (both anterior and posterior palate clefts)*, but a considerable number present as part of a syndrome with multiple congenital anomalies
- *Cleft lip-cleft palate*
  - Syndromic in about 15% of cleft lip-cleft palate cases
  - Is a feature in at least 171 syndromes[351], including trisomy 13 and trisomy 18. About one-third of infants with cleft lip-cleft palate have some associated malformations
  - Non-syndromic cleft lip-cleft palate is a heterogeneous disease entity with candidate loci on eight chromosomes. Hereditary transmission rarely occurs in a simple Mendelian fashion, and most cases are sporadic. Concordance rates in monozygotic twins are 30%–60%, compared to 1.0%–4.7% in dizygotic twins. The risk of a second infant with cleft lip-cleft palate being born in a family with one affected child is 3%–4%, and 9% with two already affected children
  - Environmental associated factors include maternal alcohol consumption, corticosteroids, anticonvulsants (phenytoin, valproate), cigarette smoking, and residential proximity to waste sites and industrial facilities
  - Protective effect of periconceptional folic acid supplementation is controversial
- *Pierre Robin sequence*
  - One or several additional malformations occur in over one-third of infants with Pierre Robin sequence

Neonatal Emergencies: A Practical Guide for Resuscitation, Transport and Critical Care, ed. Georg Hansmann. Published by Cambridge University Press. © Cambridge University Press 2009.

- In 10% of cases, the triad of Pierre Robin is a minor feature of a complex syndrome[350]
- Stickler syndrome is the most common non-complex syndrome

Clinical presentation
- *Cleft lip-cleft palate*
  - Normal postnatal adaptation without respiratory problems
  - Most cases are diagnosed antenatally, including potentially associated anomalies
- *Pierre Robin sequence*
  - Sometimes severe obstructive apnea in the supine position due to posterior displacement of the tongue that is fixed to the small mandible
  - Symptoms such as choking attacks and cyanotic spells, especially during feeds, may become apparent in the first 2–3 weeks of life
  - Regurgitation of milk through the nose may be the leading symptom of a posterior palate cleft

Diagnosis in the delivery room
- Cleft lip-cleft palate is obvious in most cases
- The diagnosis of Pierre Robin sequence sometimes requires a high grade of clinical suspicion
  - Classical "bird-like" face with a small receding chin and a flattened nasal base is easily missed unless the infant is being viewed laterally
  - Difficulties with feeding may lead to the diagnosis later on

> **!** Perform digital or visual examination of the posterior palate in all newborns.

Monitoring
No specific monitoring for infants with cleft lip-cleft palate unless mandated by associated anomalies. Pulse oximetry is required for infants with Pierre Robin sequence.

Therapy in the delivery room
- *Cleft lip-cleft palate*
  - Enhance maternal – infant bonding and maximize the opportunity to stimulate milk flow by putting the infant prone onto the mother's belly close to the breasts for skin-to-skin contact
  - If cleft antenatally diagnosed and discussed with parents, do not disturb at this stage
  - If everybody has been surprised, talk quietly at the mother's bed, avoid separating the baby from the mother
- *Pierre Robin sequence*
  - Prone position. If persistent dyspnea is present, insert a simple oral airway (Guedel tube)
  - Alternatively, a nasopharyngeal tube may be inserted such that the tip is behind the tongue base just above the epiglottis (approx. 6–8 cm in term newborn infants)

- Endotracheal intubation is a difficult procedure in infants with Pierre Robin sequence, as visualization of the vocal cords may be impossible unless fiber optic techniques are employed
- A laryngeal mask airway (LMA) is a very useful alternative[352] (see p. 95)

Procedure/therapy in the NICU

- *Cleft lip-cleft palate*
  - Infant should remain with the mother, preferably on the maternity ward
  - Examine infant for additional anomalies
  - Consult lactation consultant urgently to establish feeding regimen. Details will depend on the extent of clefts, maternal wishes, and the lactation specialist's experience of clefts.
  - The sucking efficiency of an infant with cleft palate is reduced at both bottle and breast
  - Breast feeding an infant with cleft palate is demanding, and the baby is at risk for failure to thrive as oral intake is reduced and the baby fatigues during lengthy feedings
  - A top-up with expressed breast milk via a supply line or squeezable bottle equipped with a Haberman feeder or Pigeon teat may be required
  - Breast feeding an infant with an incomplete cleft lip can be achieved by sealing the cleft with the breast pressed into the cleft. Nasal regurgitation can be minimized by holding the infant in a semi-upright position
  - Although an artificial palatal plate will not enable the infant to seal the oral cavity effectively and generate more suction, a firm palatal surface may assist the infant to stabilize and compress the nipple
  - Staged surgery, to be performed in specialized centers, will usually commence around 3 months of age, and be completed as late as by age 16–18 years
- *Pierre Robin sequence*
  - Transfer the infant to NICU for proper monitoring
  - Examine the infant to rule out or find additional anomalies
  - The infant should be nursed prone with the head to one side
  - Level positioning is important – a head-up tilt may aggravate the tendency to glossoptosis, while head-down can stimulate gastroesophageal reflux and aspiration
  - All nursing procedures such as bathing, feeding, and changing diapers can be performed with the infant in this position
  - Have an oral airway (Guedel tube) and an LMA always ready at the cot side
  - If a nasopharyngeal airway has been inserted, confirmation of its position may be obtained by lateral X-ray
  - In most infants upper airway obstruction will resolve with time and mandibular catch-up growth
  - Approaches advocated for the treatment of severe, refractory airway obstruction include tongue-lip adhesion, mandibular distraction[353], and tracheotomy (as a last resort)
  - There are no scientifically established guidelines on which approach will provide the best solution for a particular patient and situation

Prognosis

- Strongly influenced by the presence of additional anomalies
- Good functional and cosmetic results after staged surgery in cleft lip-cleft palate
- Increased risk of otitis media/effusions, dental and speech problems
- Pierre Robin sequence: upper airway obstruction mostly resolves with mandibular catch-up growth

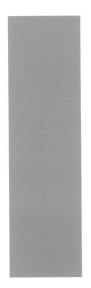

Birth trauma: brachial plexus palsy, facial nerve palsy, clavicular fracture, skull fracture, intracranial and subperiosteal hemorrhage (cephalohematoma)

Andrea Zimmermann

Epidemiology

- Incidence of birth injuries is about 2–7/1000 live births:
  - Duchenne-Erb's palsy (upper brachial plexus)
  - Klumpke's palsy (lower brachial plexus): rare; usually combined with Duchenne-Erb's palsy
  - Facial nerve palsy
  - Clavicular fracture
  - Skull fracture
  - Cephalohematoma

Etiology/pathophysiology

- *Brachial palsy*
  - Overexpansion, rupture or tearing of the nerve root of the brachial plexus due to traumatic delivery
  - Damage involving the roots of C5–C6 causes Duchenne-Erb's (upper brachial plexus) palsy
  - Damage involving the roots of C7–Th1 causes Klumpke's (lower brachial plexus) palsy
  - Risk factors: shoulder dystocia, macrosomia, operative vaginal delivery, fetal abnormal presentation
  - Not predictable before delivery[354]
- *Facial nerve palsy*
  - Especially after forceps delivery
  - Rare due to a compression of the head while passing the promontory of the mother in a prolonged delivery

Neonatal Emergencies: A Practical Guide for Resuscitation, Transport and Critical Care, ed. Georg Hansmann.
Published by Cambridge University Press. © Cambridge University Press 2009.

- *Clavicular fracture*
  - The most common bone fracture during delivery
  - Associated with shoulder dystocia and macrosomy (large for gestational age)
  - No risk factors are found in >50% of cases
  - Duchenne-Erb`s palsy may be associated
- *Skull fracture*
  - Thought to be uncommon in neonates but incidence may be underestimated
  - May occur perinatally in situations of "impacted head," or postnatally in the nursery or at home (e.g., drop from table, car seat)
  - Skull fracture after vacuum extraction is rare
  - May be associated with intracranial or subperiosteal (cephalohematoma) hemorrhage
- *Cephalohematoma*
  - Subperiosteal bleeding caused by a traumatic delivery
  - Associated with operative vaginal delivery (especially vacuum extraction)

Clinical presentation

- *Brachial palsy*
  - Upper brachial plexus palsy (Erb's palsy, C5–C6): lack of movement on the affected side; the arm is adducted, internally rotated and pronated, and the elbow extended (leading to a flaccid paralysis known as waiter's tip posture, while finger motor skills remain intact). No upward extension of the affected arm; absent Moro reflex; absent biceps and radial reflex; paralysis of the diaphragm is possible (C3–C5; ultrasound, phrenic nerve; chest X-ray: elevated hemidiaphragm?)
  - Lower plexus palsy (Klumpke, C7–Th1): fingers and wrist do not move (dropped hand), absent grasp reflex. If a sympathetic lesion is involved, Horner's syndrome (miosis, ptosis, and enophthalmos) can be observed
  - DDx: epiphyseolysis or fractured humerus
- *Facial nerve palsy*
  - Infant's eye is open on the affected side
  - Mouth is drawn to the normal side while crying
  - Nasolabial fold is missing on the affected side
  - Damage of the superficial temporal branch of the facial nerve (N. VII1) may lead to paralysis on the ipsilateral side, although this is quite rare
- *Clavicular fracture*
  - May be discovered postnatally or during the first days after birth[355]
  - Affected side is swollen and tender on palpation
  - Absent arm movements
  - Examination may reveal crepitus or a bone irregularity
  - Infant may cry during manipulation "for no reason"
- *Skull fracture*
  - May occur perinatally in situations of "impacted head"/vaccum- or forceps-assisted, difficult deliveries, or postnatally in the nursery/at home (e.g., drop from table, car seat)

- Most are linear and associated with cephalohematoma
- Fractures at the base of the skull may result in shock
- *Intracranial hemorrhage*
  - In large, progressing hematoma, inotropic and ventilatory support are indicated
  - Seizures and apnea may occur. May be associated with spinal hematoma.
- *Cephalohematoma*
  - Fluctuant and tender mass which does not cross the suture lines (DDx.: caput succedaneum or subgaleal hematoma)
  - Rarely results in hemorrhagic anemia

Monitoring
- Pulse oximetry (HR, S_aO_2), BP, temperature, and if necessary ECG

Transfer
- Indication for transfer may depend upon degree of perinatal stress, but not on the birth trauma itself. NICU admission for depressed skull fracture, intracranial hemorrhage, and any cerebrospinal injury
- Clavicular fracture: place infant in supine position and not on the affected side
- Brachial palsy (Duchenne-Erb, Klumpke): place infant in supine position and turn their head to the affected side
- Cephalohematoma: infant's head should not lie on the hematoma (painful)

Diagnosis in the NICU
- *Brachial palsy*
  - Ultrasonography to rule out capital humeral epiphyseolysis and phrenic nerve palsy
  - If necessary, X-ray to rule out fractures (humerus or clavicular fracture) and to evaluate for elevated hemidiaphragm (C3–C5, phrenic nerve palsy → paralysis of the diaphragm; U/S of fluoroscopy may be indicated)
  - Assessment of neurological status (depending on the general condition)
- *Clavicular fracture*
  - Rule out brachial palsy
  - Assess neurological status
  - X-ray is rarely indicated
- *Skull fracture*
  - X-ray (Ap, lateral), U/S, CT
  - Laboratory studies: spun hematocrit, CBC, eventually coagulation panel, blood type and screen/cross, serum bilirubin
- *Intracranial hemorrhage*
  - U/S, CT
  - Laboratory studies: spun hematocrit, CBC, coagulation panel, blood type and cross, serum bilirubin
- *Cephalohematoma*
  - Laboratory studies: spun hematocrit, CBC, serum bilirubin
  - Screen for skull fracture

Procedure/therapy/prognosis

- *Brachial palsy*[356]
    - Careful adduction of the arm and flexion of the elbow without traction on the nerve bundle
    - Physiotherapy is required if no recovery within 3 weeks
    - Lack of biceps function within 3 months: additional investigation in specialized centers is necessary
    - During the fourth and sixth months: plexus reconstruction
    - In 80%–90% recovery within the first year
    - If there is coexistent phrenic nerve palsy, treat based on symptoms – if infant is not in respiratory distress or needing only minimal respiratory support (nasal oxygen or low ventilator settings), observe. If respiratory status does not improve or worsens, refer to surgery for diaphragm plication
- *Facial nerve palsy*
    - To protect the eye from desiccation, apply synthetic tears/ointment
    - Recovery in 90% of the cases within months
- *Clavicular fracture*
    - Handle infants with care and avoid unnecessary manipulations that cause pain
    - X-ray is not routinely done
    - Callus formation and complete restitution without treatment[355]
- *Skull fracture*
    - Linear fractures: no treatement required if no intracranial hemorrhage (U/S, CT)
    - Depressed skull fracture: may require surgery, depending on size, progression and clinical condition
- *Intracranial hemorrhage*
    - Subarachnoid: usually resolution without treatment
    - Epidural: urgent surgical evacuation for large bleeds (U/S, CT: midline shift?)
    - Subdural: drainage of large hematoma may be indicated (U/S, CT: midline shift?)
- *Cephalohematoma*
    - Anemia and hyperbilirubinemia – due to resolving hematoma – may occur
    - Resolution occurs over a period of 2–3 weeks without complications (except in very rare cases)
    - Superinfection and residual calcification of the hematoma are rare but possible

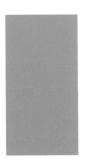

Sudden infant death syndrome (SIDS)

Andrea Zimmermann

Definition

- *SIDS* (sudden infant death syndrome): sudden and – with regard to the history – unexpected death of a healthy infant, that remains unexplained even after complete autopsy
- *ALTE* (apparent life-threatening event): a condition that is characterized by apnea, pallor, loss of muscle tone, non-responsiveness, periodic breathing and apnea; a condition that causes parents/guardians to consult a physician/hospital or to initiate cardiopulmonary resuscitative measures after calling the emergency line

Epidemiology

Estimated incidence is 7 of 10 000 live births (0.7/1000)[357]. The peak incidence of SIDS is between the second and fourth months of life. SIDS rarely occurs in the neonatal period or after the first year of life.

> **!** The most common cause of death beyond the neonatal period in the first year of life is SIDS.

Etiology

Remains unclear; possibly multifactorial[358]:

- Sweating during sleep can be a sign that an event is threatening
- Previously premature infants with low birth weight and bronchopulmonary dysplasia (BPD) are at higher risk
- Higher risk for children with prolonged QT interval in ECG[359]
- Siblings of infants who died of SIDS should be investigated thoroughly, even though a higher risk for SIDS is uncertain
- Frequent viral and bacterial infections and exposure to environmental tobacco smoke probably increase SIDS risk[360]
- Pathological obstructive sleep apnea[361]
- Previous ALTE episode ($\rightarrow$ home monitoring – controversial)
- Poor arousal (weakened response to stimulus while asleep)

Clinical presentation

- An infant who previously showed no unusual symptoms is found in bed with the key findings of pallor, pulselessness, and apnea
- 90% of the SIDS cases occur during sleep.

Neonatal Emergencies: A Practical Guide for Resuscitation, Transport and Critical Care, ed. Georg Hansmann.
Published by Cambridge University Press. © Cambridge University Press 2009.

DDx.

- Fulminant sepsis, critical congenital heart disease, accidental or non-accidental trauma (e.g., shaken baby syndrome) with or without cerebral hemorrhage, metabolic disorder

Diagnosis

- Diagnose cardiorespiratory arrest (apnea, no heart rate, no brachial or femoral pulse)
- Obtain blood glucose, blood gas analysis, electrolytes, CBC, coagulation panel
- Obtain a detailed history of events

Therapy

(See PALS algorithm for pulseless cardiac arrest; p. 330.)

- Rule out foreign body aspiration (if suspicion is high: back slaps and chest thrust)
- Begin cardiopulmonary resuscitation (CPR; do not start CPR if definite signs of death are present). The following sequence refers to infants >28 days old:
  - For lone, local first responders in unwittnessed SIDS: activate emergency response number after performing five cycles of CPR
  - Initial breaths: 2 effective breaths at 1 second/breath
  - Followed by 20–30 breaths per minute (approx. 1 breath every 3 seconds)
  - Ventilate with 100% oxygen (bag-and-mask), if oxygen available
  - Intubate (or place laryngeal mask airway) as soon as possible
  - Start chest compressions just below the nipple line (for lone rescuer: two-finger technique; for two rescuers two-thumb encircling hands technique). Compression: ventilation ratio is 30:2 with a single rescuer, and 15:2 with two rescuers. In young infants, you may use a 5:1 ratio of chest compressions (CC) to positive pressure ventilation (PPV); in neonates, you may use a 3:1 ratio. CC plus PPV = 100 (neonates: 120) events per minute. Compression depth is approximately one-half the depth of the chest
  - Attach defibrillator/monitor when available
  - Shockable rhythm? If ventricular fibrillation/ventricular tachycardia (VFib/VTach), defibrillate with pediatric system at 2 J/kg and resume CPR immediately (5 cycles), then re-check rhythm and pulse: if VFib/VTach, defibrillate again, this time at 4 J/kg, resume CPR immediately and give epinephrine q 3–5 min. If after 5 cycles of CPR there is still a shockable rhythm (VFib/VTach), defibrillate at 4 J/kg, resume CPR immediately and consider amiodarone (5 mg/kg/dose IV/IO). Consider magnesium 25–50 mg/kg/dose (max. 2 g) IV/IO for torsades de pointes
- Establish IV or IO access as soon as possible:
  - Epinephrine 0.01–0.03 mg/kg/dose IV/IO q 2–5 min
  - Volume: 10 ml/kg/bolus IV/IO, repeat bolus if indicated
  - If no response to epinephrine, consider sodium bicarbonate 1–2 mEq/kg/dose IV/IO
- Where there is a detectable heart rate with arterial hypotension and mean arterial pressure (MAP) ≪40–45 mmHg:
  - Place central venous line and administer dopamine 5–20 µg/kg/min, epinephrine 0.05–1 µg/kg/min (may be given through PIV or IO) or norepinephrine 0.05–1 µg/kg/min

> **!** If required, administer dopamine via peripheral venous or intraosseous access.

- Optional: dobutamine 5–20 µg/kg/min via peripheral or central venous line (caution: may lower diastolic BP and cause tachycardia)

Monitoring
- Pulse oximetry (HR, S_aO_2), BP, ECG (print ECG record if possible)

Procedure/therapy in the NICU/PICU
- If the patient responds to the CPR measures (i.e., pulse), do the following:
  - Continue ventilation
  - Inotropic support (see above)
  - Treatment of underlying cause (e.g., sepsis) and complications
- If indicated, make diagnosis of brain death according to published guidelines
- In case of SIDS death: death certificate should describe cause of death as "unknown"
- Talk with parents:
  - Offer support from crisis intervention team
  - Convey evaluation of medical findings and/or autopsy
  - Provide parents with number of local SIDS support groups
- Further diagnostics depend on the individual circumstances:
  - Laboratory work-up: CBC, blood gas analysis, blood glucose, lactate, ammonia, electrolytes with calcium, phosphate, magnesium, creatinine/BUN, AST/ALT
  - Toxicology screening tests (urine, serum, stool) to rule out toxic ingestion
  - Microbiological diagnosis: blood culture, lumbar puncture, urine culture
  - Cranial ultrasonography, amplitude-integrated EEG/EEG, fundoscopy, head or whole-body CT
  - Echocardiography, ECG to rule out long-QT syndrome
  - Diagnosis of metabolic disorder: serum amino acid analysis, serum long chain fatty acids, urine organic acids
  - Postmortem muscle and skin biopsy/histology
  - Rule out child abuse/shaken baby syndrome (head/C-spine CT/MRI)
  - In stable survivors: polysomnography (recording of electrophysiological signals during sleep: nasal airflow, periodic limb movements, ECG, S_aO_2)

SIDS – a difficult emotional and medical challenge for emergency physicians
- Emotions felt by health care professionals involved (helplessness, wish to leave the site of emergency)
- Hopelessness of the situation when definite signs of death are present
- Parents' insisting to continue resuscitative measures
- The need to explain to the parents that their child, who was completely normal the previous day, will never wake up again

- The need to explain to the parents that their child needs to be removed from the site of emergency despite ongoing grief, and that an autopsy is necessary (see below)

> *Call emergency psychologists, a crisis intervention support team and/or religious support to assist the family.

An autopsy should not only be offered but strongly recommended to the parents in order to (1) establish the cause of death, (2) eliminate potential accusations from others, and (3) minimize guilt on the part of the parents. In many countries, all SIDS cases are evaluated by the medical examiner (i.e., mandatory autopsy for any unwitnessed death of unknown cause). Qualified personnel (emergency physician, crisis intervention team) should assist the parents in these very difficult situations and decisions, including offering oral and written information on autopsy.

> - Diagnosis of death on the death certificate should read "cause unknown." Call to inform the local police/coroner; they usually collaborate with a funeral parlor. Usually the medical officer/examiner will arrange an autopsy with the department of forensic medicine
> - The parents should be given time to part with their child
> - The team present at the site should express an appropriate degree of sorrow and sympathy toward the parents
> - The term "child abuse" should not be uttered during any of these acute situations

Recommendations for the prevention of SIDS (AAP Task Force, 2005)[362]

- Supine sleeping position. The AAP no longer recognizes side sleeping as a reasonable alternative to fully supine sleeping
- Sleeping bag instead of blankets. Avoid the use of pillows and other soft objects in the infant's seleeping environment
- Allow the child to use a pacifier during sleep
- Sleeping room temperature at 16–18°C
- Adults should not sleep with an infant in the same bed
- Having infants and parents sleep in the same room reduces SIDS risk
- Breast feeding
- Both parents should give up smoking. Assure smoke-free environment. Maternal smoking in pregnancy is associated with an increased risk of SIDS

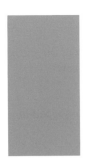

Questions for review

Georg Hansmann, Shannon E. G. Hamrick, Tilman Humpl, and Andrea Zimmermann

1. What are the initial steps in managing a vigorous term newborn infant – and which measures should be avoided? See p. 221.
2. When are advanced resuscitative measures indicated in newborns? Keywords: meconium, asphyxia, premature birth/prematurity, special events. See p. 227.
3. Why is endotracheal intubation in very small preterm infants difficult? Explain the anatomical features. See p. 236.
4. Estimate the birth weight for the following tube sizes (inner diameter) for endotracheal intubation: 2.0-, 2.5-, or 3.0-mm-ID tube. See p. 85, Table 2.2
5. What would you tell the parents: how high is the rate of brain damage (IVH, PVL) in preterm infants <1500g? See p. 238.
6. What could be the reasons for deterioration in spite of assuredly correct endotracheal intubation? See p. 222, p. 236, p. 340, p. 392, p. 410, p. 417.
7. Below which gestational age is viability of the fetus not probable? See pp. 185–6.
8. Is it legitimate to discontinue life-saving resuscitative measures once started in extreme prematurity? See p. 184, p. 235.
9. What are the possible complications of monochorial twin pregnancies? See p. 240.
10. What samples need to be collected prior to an emergency transfusion? See Table 3.1, p. 241.
11. What are the clinical signs of a twin–twin transfusion syndrome (TTTS)? See Table 3.1, p. 240.
12. What is in the differential diagnosis when the newborn presents with pallor and increased respiratory rate? See Table 3.2, p. 243.
13. When infection of the newborn is suspected what diagnostic tests should be performed in the delivery room? See Table 3.2, p. 244, p. 280.
14. You would like to obtain a blood gas analysis in a baby with decreased peripheral perfusion. Which parameters are valuable for clinical assessment (capillary, venous, arterial) ? See p. 124.
15. What needs to be done when an experienced nurse says "the baby does not look good today"? See p. 283.
16. What are the differences between home birth and hospital delivery in terms of perinatal monitoring? See p. 249.
17. When is a home birth contraindicated? See p. 249.
18. When should an antepartum transfer be considered in a pregnant woman after onset of uterine contractions? See p. 504.

Neonatal Emergencies: A Practical Guide for Resuscitation, Transport and Critical Care, ed. Georg Hansmann. Published by Cambridge University Press. © Cambridge University Press 2009.

19. When should a neonatologist/the neonatal transport team be called to a home birth? See p. 249.

20. What should the midwife keep in mind during and after a home birth? See p. 249.

21. What are "practical" low–normal blood glucose values (not evidence-based) for term neonates? → p. 260.

22. Which newborn infants bear a high risk for hypoglycemia? See p. 260.

23. What are typical symptoms of hypoglycemia in neonates and young infants! See p. 260.

24. What is the differential diagnosis of transient, recurrent or persistent hypoglycemia in neonates? See p. 260.

25. How do you manage borderline and low blood glucose levels? See p. 260 and Figure 3.4 (algorithm) on p. 261.

26. Describe the management of the newborn with meconium-stained amniotic fluid/skin? See p. 269, Figure 3.5 (algorithm) on p. 270.

27. What are the differences between managing a vigorous neonate born "merely out of meconium-stained amniotic fluid" and infants with meconium aspiration and meconium aspiration syndrome (MAS)? See Figure 3.5 (algorithm), p. 270, Table 3.4, pp. 271–3.

28. What is the decisive measure in resuscitating a depressed neonate with suspected meconium aspiration in the delivery room? See p. 269, Figure 3.5 (algorithm)

29. What are the key points for the medical treatment of meconium aspiration syndrome in the NICU? See p. 269.

30. Which factors increase the mortality rate in meconium aspiration syndrome? See p. 269, Table 3.4.

31. What is the difference between initial care/resuscitation of a depressed neonate with visible meconium and the standard initial care without meconium? Compare Figure 3.1 with Figure 3.5 (algorithms), p. 228 and p. 270.

32. Enumerate the maternal and fetal-neonatal risk factors for chorioamnionitis and early-onset sepsis in the newborn infant. What are the key points for prevention and treatment? → p. 280, Figure 3.6, p. 295.

33. When and which of the pregnant women who are colonized with GBS should receive intrapartum antibiotic prophylaxis to prevent neonatal sepsis? What are the diagnostic and therapeutic measures for those infants born to mothers who have received intrapartum antibiotic prophylaxis? → pp. 285–95, Figure 3.6

34. Describe the characteristics of neonatal infections. See p. 281, p. 283, Table 3.5, pp. 285–91.

35. Summarize the most important principles of antimicrobial treatment. See pp. 298–303, Table 3.6, Table 3.7.

36. What is the initial (empiric) therapy for suspected sepsis during the first week of life when a definite cause (blood culture, etc.) has not yet been identified? See p. 298.

37. What are possible causes of severe perinatal hypoxia-ischemia ("asphyxia")? See p. 304, p. 310.

38. Which events or conditions may be associated with severely depressed neonates not responding to resuscitative measures? See p. 171, see also standard algorithm p. 311, Figure 3.7, p. 305.

39. How has "birth asphyxia" been characterized (definition by Carter *et al.*, 1993)? See p. 310.

40. Does a low Apgar score (at 1, 5 and/or 10 min) predict poor neurodevelopmental outcome in neonates? See p. 310.

41. Is therapeutic whole-body hypothermia or selective head cooling effective in the treatment of hypoxic ischemic encephalopathy (HIE)? See p. 315.

42. Can infants have clinical seizures not documented on EEG, or have electrographic seizures not noted clinically? See p. 317.

43. Is the pharmacological treatment of neonatal seizures based on evidence of benefit? See p. 317.

44. Which drug is rarely useful in diagnosing and treating neonatal seizures, but worth trying under EEG monitoring? See p. 321.

45. What are the complications of intravenous phenytoin administration? What are the advantages of fosphenytoin vs. phenytoin ? See p. 41, p. 317.

46. Should naloxone be admistered in the delivery room? Give an explanation. See p. 35, p. 41, p. 164, p. 168, p. 323.

47. Which reliable methods are available for diagnosing fetal arrhythmias? See p. 325.

48. What is the most common arrhythmic disorder in infants and how is it treated? See p. 325, Figure 3.11

49. What causes bradycardia in infants? See p. 325.

50. Which conditions or events lead to cardiovascular emergencies in the newborn and young infants? See pp. 325–79.

51. Which congenital cardiovascular diseases have duct-dependent lung perfusion ("right heart obstructions"). Which lesions have duct-dependent systemic perfusion ("left heart obstructions")? See pp. 340–50, Figure 3.16 (algorithm)

52. What should be kept in mind when oxygen is supplemented to neonates with congenital heart disease ($F_iO_2 > 0.21$)? See p. 71, p. 161, pp. 342–6.

53. When is an empiric therapy with prostaglandin E_1 (as continuous intravenous drip) indicated, and what is a common starting dose? See p. 344, Figure 3.16 (algorithm), Table 2.1.

54. What is in the differential diagnoses of central and peripheral cyanosis? See p. 125.

55. Explain the pathophysiology of persistent pulmonary hypertension of the newborn (PPHN). See p. 392.

56. When PPHN (or congenital heart diseases with left heart obstruction, see p. X, p. X) is suspected, where should the pulse oximeter probe be placed and arterial S_aO_2 and P_aO_2 be obtained ("preductal sample")? Where should the S_pO_2 probe be placed when there is an aberrant left subclavian artery? See p. 392.

57. What are the key symptoms and aims of treatment in persistent pulmonary hypertension of the newborn? See p. 392.

58. What are the most important ICU treatment strategies when PPHN is evident? See p. 392.

59. When conventional treatment of PPHN has failed, which (ultimate) treatment option should be taken into consideration early (e.g., in meconium aspiration syndrome, congenital diaphragmatic hernia)? See pp. 278–9, p. 402.

60. Why is bag-and-mask ventilation a contraindication in the initial resuscitation of neonates with congenital diaphragmatic hernia (CDH)? See p. 404.

61. When is the optimal time point for surgical repair of a congenital diaphragmatic hernia? See p. 404.

62. Which factors determine the prognosis of patients with congenital diaphragmatic hernia? See p. 404.

63. How can tension pneumothorax (emergency) be relieved? See p. 410, see also Figure 3.34

64. Is anesthesia required for chest tube placement? See p. 410.

65. May bag-and-mask ventilation be applied in the delivery room when pneumothorax is suspected? See p. 410.

66. Describe the clinical presentation of congenital cystic adenomatoid malformation of the lung (syn.: CCAM, CAM CAML). See p. 417.

67. What are the resuscitative procedures in the delivery room for an infant with congenital cystic adenomatoid malformation of the lung? See p. 417.

68. What complications are to be expected in an infant when unilateral pleural effusion is diagnosed prenatally? See p. 419.

69. What are the possible causes of chylothorax? See p. 419.

70. Should chromosomal analysis be initiated in congenital chylothorax? See p. 419.

71. When and why are medium-chain triglycerides (MCT) suited for oral nutrition of an infant with chylothorax? What are alternative treatment options if changing to an MCT diet fails ? See p. 419.

72. Why does iso-immunization not occur with maternal blood types A and B? See p. 423.

73. Is the direct antiglobulin test (DAT = direct coombs test) reliable after an intrauterine transfusion? See p. 423.

74. What rate of rise of bilirubin suggests the need for an exchange transfusion? See pp. 425–6.

75. Which are the two forms of hydrops fetalis and how do their etiology and pathobiology differ? See p. XXX, p. 427.

76. What problems should health care providers expect when a newborn with hydrops needs to be intubated? See p. 427.

77. When and how are the symptoms of (unilateral vs. bilateral) choanal atresia recognized? See p. 432.

78. Which prenatal ultrasonography finding is consistent with esophageal atresia? See p. 434.

79. Which diagnostic procedure is useful to rule out esophageal atresia clinically? See p. 434.

80. What is a complication of esophageal atresia during mechanical ventilation of the newborn? See p. 434.

81. What are common causes of paralytic and mechanical ileus? See p. 437.

82. Can paralytic ileus be distinguished from mechanical ileus? See p. 437.

83. What are the most significant clinical signs and symptoms of (early) ileus? See p. 437.

84. Which causes of ileus accompany particular fulminant symptoms? See pp. 438–9.

85. How does a lower ileus and an upper ileus differ in their clinical presentation? Which diseases/malformations accompany bilious emesis indicating a surgical emergency? See pp. 437–9.

86. What are typical radiographic signs of duodenal atresia? See p. 440.

87. What is in the differential diagnosis and should be ruled out when meconium is not passed for more than 24 hours after birth? See p. 445.

88. What does VACTERL stand for? Should this syndrome be ruled out before surgery? See p. 434.

89. Who is at highest risk for the development of necrotizing enterocolitis (NEC)? What are the initial diagnostic and therapeutic measures when NEC is suspected? See p. 447.

90. Describe the clinical course and X-ray findings in necrotizing enterocolitis (NEC). Is there expert consent on when to place a peritoneal drain rather than perform primary explorative laparotomy in infants with NEC? See p. 447.

91. What are the differences between omphalocele and gastroschisis (review hernial orifice, associated malformations, etc.)? See p. 450.

92. What should be taken into account when providing initial care/resuscitation of newborns with gastroschisis or (large) omphalocele in the delivery room/the NICU? See p. 450.

93. Which factors determine the outcome of infants with congenital abdominal wall defects? See p. 450.

94. When is surgery indicated in a newborn with gastroschisis? See p. 450.

95. Which of the CNS malformations are summarized under "neural tube defects" (NTD)? See p. 455.

96. Which measures should be taken into consideration particularly during the initial care/ resuscitation of infants with neural tube defects (e.g., lumbosacral meningomyelocele; delivery room/NICU)? See p. 455.

97. What should be initiated when a baby is born with cleft lip-cleft palate? See p. 460.

98. Which problems can occur in Pierre Robin sequence, and how can they be managed in the delivery room? See p. 460.

99. Which additional diagnostic studies should be initiated in brachial plexus palsy? See p. 464.

100. At what age should the surgical reconstruction of perinatally acquired brachial plexus palsy be performed? See p. 467.

101. What should be monitored in a baby with cephalohematoma? See pp. 466–7.

102. What is the prognosis for infants with perinatally acquired brachial plexus palsy, facial nerve palsy, clavicular fracture or cephalohematoma? See p. 467.

103. Descibe the PALS algorithm for CPR of an infant (>28 days old) with pulseless cardiopulmonary arrest at home (SIDS). See p. 330 (Figure 3.10), p. 469.

104. What are the AAP Task Force recommendations for the prevention of sudden infant death syndrome (SIDS)? See p. 471.

References (Section 3)

1. Cordero L, Jr., Hon EH. Neonatal bradycardia following nasopharyngeal stimulation. *J Pediatr* 1971;**78**(3):441–7.

2. Rennie JM, Roberston NRC. *Roberston's Textbook of Neonatology*, 4th edn. Edinburgh: Churchill Livingstone, 2005.

3. Lippi G, Salvagno GL, Rugolotto S, *et al.* Routine coagulation tests in newborn and young infants. *J Thromb Thrombolysis* 2007;**24**(2):153–5.

4. Bührer C, Bahr S, Siebert J, Wettstein R, Geffers C, Obladen M. Use of 2% 2-phenoxyethanol and 0.1% octenidine as antiseptic in premature newborn infants of 23–26 weeks gestation. *J Hosp Infect* 2002;**51**(4):305–7.

5. Lokesh L, Kumar P, Murki S, Narang A. A randomized controlled trial of sodium bicarbonate in neonatal resuscitation – effect on immediate outcome. *Resuscitation* 2004;**60**(2):219–23.

6. Synnes AR, Chien LY, Peliowski A, Baboolal R, Lee SK. Variations in intraventricular hemorrhage incidence rates among Canadian neonatal intensive care units. *J Pediatr* 2001;**138**(4):525–31.

7. Vohra S, Roberts RS, Zhang B, Janes M, Schmidt B. Heat loss prevention (HeLP) in the delivery room: a randomized controlled trial of polyethylene occlusive skin wrapping in very preterm infants. *J Pediatr* 2004;**145**:750–3.

8. McCall EM, Alderdice FA, Halliday HL, Jenkins JG, Vohra S. Interventions to prevent hypothermia at birth in preterm and/or low birthweight babies. *Cochrane Database Syst Rev* 2005(1):CD004210.

9. Engle WA. Surfactant-replacement therapy for respiratory distress in the preterm and term neonate. *Pediatrics* 2008;**121**(2):419–32.

10. Aly H, Massaro AN, Patel K, El-Mohandes AA. Is it safer to intubate premature infants in the delivery room? *Pediatrics* 2005;**115**(6):1660–5.

11. Soll RF, Morley CJ. Prophylactic versus selective use of surfactant in preventing morbidity and mortality in preterm infants. *Cochrane Database Syst Rev* 2001(2):CD000510.

12. Booth C, Premkumar MH, Yannoulis A, Thomson M, Harrison M, Edwards AD. Sustainable use of continuous positive airway pressure in extremely preterm infants during the first week after delivery. *Arch Dis Child Fetal Neonatal Ed* 2006;**91**(6):F398–402.

13. Morley CJ, Davis PG, Doyle LW, Brion LP, Hascoet JM, Carlin JB. Nasal CPAP or intubation at birth for very preterm infants. *N Engl J Med* 2008;**358**(7):700–8.

14. Ammari A, Suri M, Milisavljevic V, *et al.* Variables associated with the early failure of nasal CPAP in very low birth weight infants. *J Pediatr* 2005;**147**(3):341–7.

15. Yost CC, Soll RF. Early versus delayed selective surfactant treatment for neonatal respiratory distress syndrome. *Cochrane Database Syst Rev* 2000(2):CD001456.

16. Verder H, Albertsen P, Ebbesen F, *et al.* Nasal continuous positive airway pressure and early surfactant therapy for respiratory distress syndrome in newborns of less than 30 weeks' gestation. *Pediatrics* 1999;**103**(2):E24.

17. Stevens TP, Harrington EW, Blennow M, Soll RF. Early surfactant administration with brief ventilation vs. selective surfactant and continued mechanical ventilation for preterm infants with or at risk for respiratory distress syndrome. *Cochrane Database Syst Rev* 2007(4):CD003063.

18. Kribs A. Is it safer to intubate premature infants in the delivery room? *Pediatrics* 2006;**117**(5):1858–9; author reply 1859.

19. Kribs A, Pillekamp F, Hunseler C, Vierzig A, Roth B. Early administration of surfactant in spontaneous breathing with nCPAP: feasibility and outcome in extremely premature infants (postmenstrual age ≤27 weeks). *Paediatr Anaesth* 2007;**17**(4):364–9.

20. 2005 American Heart Association (AHA) guidelines for cardiopulmonary resuscitation (CPR) and emergency cardiovascular care (ECC) of pediatric and neonatal patients: pediatric basic life support. *Pediatrics* 2006;**117**(5):e989–1004.

21. Hamrick SE, Miller SP, Leonard C, *et al.* Trends in severe brain injury and neurodevelopmental outcome in premature newborn infants: the role of cystic periventricular leukomalacia. *J Pediatr* 2004;**145**(5):593–9.

22. Bartels DB, Kreienbrock L, Dammann O, Wenzlaff P, Poets CF. Population based study on the outcome of small for

gestational age newborns. *Arch Dis Child Fetal Neonatal Ed* 2005;**90**(1):F53–9.

23. Ment LR, Allan WC, Makuch RW, Vohr B. Grade 3 to 4 intraventricular hemorrhage and Bayley scores predict outcome. *Pediatrics* 2005;**116**(6):1597–8; author reply 1598.

24. Heuchan AM, Evans N, Henderson Smart DJ, Simpson JM. Perinatal risk factors for major intraventricular haemorrhage in the Australian and New Zealand Neonatal Network, 1995–97. *Arch Dis Child Fetal Neonatal Ed* 2002;**86**(2):F86–90.

25. Ballabh P, Xu H, Hu F, *et al.* Angiogenic inhibition reduces germinal matrix hemorrhage. *Nat Med* 2007;**13**(4):477–85.

26. Rabe H, Reynolds G, Diaz-Rossello J. Early versus delayed umbilical cord clamping in preterm infants. *Cochrane Database Syst Rev* 2004(4):CD003248.

27. Kaiser JR, Gauss CH, Pont MM, Williams DK. Hypercapnia during the first 3 days of life is associated with severe intraventricular hemorrhage in very low birth weight infants. *J Perinatol* 2006;**26**(5):279–85.

28. Fabres J, Carlo WA, Phillips V, Howard G, Ambalavanan N. Both extremes of arterial carbon dioxide pressure and the magnitude of fluctuations in arterial carbon dioxide pressure are associated with severe intraventricular hemorrhage in preterm infants. *Pediatrics* 2007;**119**(2):299–305.

29. Osborn DA, Evans N, Kluckow M, Bowen JR, Rieger I. Low superior vena cava flow and effect of inotropes on neurodevelopment to 3 years in preterm infants. *Pediatrics* 2007; **120**(2):372–80.

30. Fowlie PW, Davis PG. Prophylactic indomethacin for preterm infants: a systematic review and meta-analysis. *Arch Dis Child Fetal Neonatal Ed* 2003;**88**(6):F464–6.

31. Ohlsson A, Roberts RS, Schmidt B, *et al.* Male/female differences in indomethacin effects in preterm infants. *J Pediatr* 2005; **147**(6):860–2.

32. Wu YW. Systematic review of chorioamnionitis and cerebral palsy. *Ment Retard Dev Disabil Res Rev* 2002;**8**(1):25–9.

33. Giannakopoulou C, Korakaki E, Manoura A, *et al.* Significance of hypocarbia in the development of periventricular leukomalacia in preterm infants. *Pediatr Int* 2004;**46** (3):268–73.

34. Resch B, Jammernegg A, Vollaard E, Maurer U, Mueller WD, Pertl B. Preterm twin gestation and cystic periventricular leucomalacia. *Arch Dis Child Fetal Neonatal Ed* 2004;**89**(4):F315–20.

35. Shankaran S, Langer JC, Kazzi SN, Laptook AR, Walsh M. Cumulative index of exposure to hypocarbia and hyperoxia as risk factors for periventricular leukomalacia in low birth weight infants. *Pediatrics* 2006;**118**(4):1654–9.

36. Meek JH, Tyszczuk L, Elwell CE, Wyatt JS. Low cerebral blood flow is a risk factor for severe intraventricular haemorrhage. *Arch Dis Child Fetal Neonatal Ed* 1999;**81**(1):F15–18.

37. Ment LR, Bada HS, Barnes P, *et al.* Practice parameter: neuroimaging of the neonate: report of the Quality Standards Subcommittee of the American Academy of Neurology and the Practice Committee of the Child Neurology Society. *Neurology* 2002;**58**(12):1726–38.

38. Ment LR, Duncan CC, Ehrenkranz RA, *et al.* Intraventricular hemorrhage in the preterm neonate: timing and cerebral blood flow changes. *J Pediatr* 1984;**104**(3):419–25.

39. Vohr BR, Wright LL, Poole WK, McDonald SA. Neurodevelopmental outcomes of extremely low birth weight infants <32 weeks' gestation between 1993 and 1998. *Pediatrics* 2005;**116**(3):635–43.

40. Vasileiadis GT, Gelman N, Han VK, *et al.* Uncomplicated intraventricular hemorrhage is followed by reduced cortical volume at near-term age. *Pediatrics* 2004;**114**(3):e367–72.

41. Patra K, Wilson-Costello D, Taylor HG, Mercuri-Minich N, Hack M. Grades I–II intraventricular hemorrhage in extremely low birth weight infants: effects on neurodevelopment. *J Pediatr* 2006;**149** (2):169–73.

42. Mercer JS, Vohr BR, McGrath MM, Padbury JF, Wallach M, Oh W. Delayed cord clamping in very preterm infants reduces the incidence of intraventricular hemorrhage and late-onset sepsis: a randomized, controlled trial. *Pediatrics* 2006;**117** (4):1235–42.

43. Wee LY, Fisk NM. The twin-twin transfusion syndrome. *Semin Neonatol* 2002;**7**(3):187–202.

44. Acosta-Rojas R, Becker J, Munoz-Abellana B, Ruiz C, Carreras E, Gratacos E. Twin chorionicity and the risk of adverse

perinatal outcome. *Int J Gynaecol Obstet* 2007;**96**(2):98–102.

45. Bagchi S, Salihu HM. Birth weight discordance in multiple gestations: occurrence and outcomes. *J Obstet Gynaecol* 2006;**26**(4):291–6.

46. Sperling L, Kiil C, Larsen LU, *et al.* Detection of chromosomal abnormalities, congenital abnormalities and transfusion syndrome in twins. *Ultrasound Obstet Gynecol* 2007;**29**(5):517–26.

47. Ruhmann O, Lazovic D, Bouklas P, Schmolke S, Flamme CH. Ultrasound examination of neonatal hip: correlation of twin pregnancy and congenital dysplasia. *Twin Res* 2000;**3**(1):7–11.

48. Sibai BM, Hauth J, Caritis S, *et al.* Hypertensive disorders in twin versus singleton gestations. National Institute of Child Health and Human Development Network of Maternal-Fetal Medicine Units. *Am J Obstet Gynecol* 2000;**182**(4):938–42.

49. Umur A, van Gemert MJ, Nikkels PG. Monoamniotic-versus diamniotic-monochorionic twin placentas: anastomoses and twin-twin transfusion syndrome. *Am J Obstet Gynecol* 2003;**189**(5):1325–9.

50. Roberts D, Neilson JP, Weindling AM. Interventions for the treatment of twin-twin transfusion syndrome. *Cochrane Database Syst Rev* 2001(1):CD002073.

51. Mari G, Roberts A, Detti L, *et al.* Perinatal morbidity and mortality rates in severe twin-twin transfusion syndrome: results of the International Amnioreduction Registry. *Am J Obstet Gynecol* 2001;**185**(3):708–15.

52. Gray PH, Cincotta R, Chan FY, Soong B. Perinatal outcomes with laser surgery for twin-twin transfusion syndrome. *Twin Res Hum Genet* 2006;**9**(3):438–43.

53. Ackermann-Liebrich U, Voegeli T, Gunter-Witt K, *et al.* Home versus hospital deliveries: follow up study of matched pairs for procedures and outcome. Zurich Study Team. *Br Med J* 1996;**313**(7068):1313–18.

54. Murphy PA, Fullerton J. Outcomes of intended home births in nurse-midwifery practice: a prospective descriptive study. *Obstet Gynecol* 1998;**92**(3):461–70.

55. Johnson KC, Daviss BA. Outcomes of planned home births with certified professional midwives: large prospective study in North America. *Br Med J* 2005;**330**(7505):1416.

56. Janssen PA, Lee SK, Ryan EM, *et al.* Outcomes of planned home births versus planned hospital births after regulation of midwifery in British Columbia. *CMAJ* 2002;**166**(3):315–23.

57. Janssen PA, Ryan EM, Etches DJ, Klein MC, Reime B. Outcomes of planned hospital birth attended by midwives compared with physicians in British Columbia. *Birth* 2007;**34**(2):140–7.

58. Fullerton JT, Navarro AM, Young SH. Outcomes of planned home birth: an integrative review. *J Midwifery Womens Health* 2007;**52**(4):323–33.

59. ACOG Practice Bulletin. Episiotomy. Clinical Management Guidelines for Obstetrician-Gynecologists. Number 71, April 2006. *Obstet Gynecol* 2006;**107**(4):957–62.

60. Cornblath M, Hawdon JM, Williams AF, *et al.* Controversies regarding definition of neonatal hypoglycemia: suggested operational thresholds. *Pediatrics* 2000;**105**(5):1141–5.

61. Cornblath M, Ichord R. Hypoglycemia in the neonate. *Semin Perinatol* 2000;**24**(2):136–49.

62. Stanley CA, Baker L. The causes of neonatal hypoglycemia. *N Engl J Med* 1999;**340**(15):1200–1.

63. World Health Organization: *Hypoglycaemia of the Newborn. Review of the Literature.* Geneva: World Health Organization, 1997.

64. Marcus C. How to measure and interpret glucose in neonates. *Acta Paediatr* 2001;**90**(9):963–4.

65. Williams AF. Hypoglycaemia of the newborn: a review. *Bull World Health Organ* 1997;**75**(3):261–90.

66. Dekelbab BH, Sperling MA. Hypoglycemia in newborns and infants. *Adv Pediatr* 2006;**53**:5–22.

67. Peters CJ, Hindmarsh PC. Management of neonatal endocrinopathies – best practice guidelines. *Early Hum Dev* 2007;**83**(9):553–61.

68. Boluyt N, van Kempen A, Offringa M. Neurodevelopment after neonatal hypoglycemia: a systematic review and

design of an optimal future study. *Pediatrics* 2006;**117**(6):2231–43.

69. Manganaro R, Mami C, Palmara A, Paolata A, Gemelli M. Incidence of meconium aspiration syndrome in term meconium-stained babies managed at birth with selective tracheal intubation. *J Perinat Med* 2001;**29**(6):465–8.

70. Wiswell TE. Handling the meconium-stained infant. *Semin Neonatol* 2001; **6**(3):225–31.

71. 2005 International Consensus on Cardiopulmonary Resuscitation and Emergency Cardiovascular Care Science with Treatment Recommendations. Part 7: Neonatal resuscitation. *Resuscitation* 2005;**67**(2–3):293–303.

72. 2005 American Heart Association (AHA) guidelines for cardiopulmonary resuscitation (CPR) and emergency cardiovascular care (ECC) of pediatric and neonatal patients: neonatal resuscitation guidelines. *Pediatrics* 2006; **117**(5):e1029–38.

73. Vain NE, Szyld EG, Prudent LM, Wiswell TE, Aguilar AM, Vivas NI. Oropharyngeal and nasopharyngeal suctioning of meconium-stained neonates before delivery of their shoulders: multicentre, randomised controlled trial. *Lancet* 2004; **364**(9434):597–602.

74. Saugstad OD, Rootwelt T, Aalen O. Resuscitation of asphyxiated newborn infants with room air or oxygen: an international controlled trial: the Resair 2 study. *Pediatrics* 1998;**102**:e1.

75. Wiswell TE, Knight GR, Finer NN, *et al.* A multicenter, randomized, controlled trial comparing Surfaxin (Lucinactant) lavage with standard care for treatment of meconium aspiration syndrome. *Pediatrics* 2002;**109**(6):1081–7.

76. Kattwinkel J. Surfactant lavage for meconium aspiration: a word of caution. *Pediatrics* 2002;**109**(6):1167–8.

77. Ng E, Taddio A, Ohlsson A. Intravenous midazolam infusion for sedation of infants in the neonatal intensive care unit. *Cochrane Database Syst Rev* 2003(1): CD002052.

78. Findlay RD, Taeusch HW, Walther FJ. Surfactant replacement therapy for meconium aspiration syndrome. *Pediatrics* 1996;**97**(1):48–52.

79. El Shahed A, Dargaville P, Ohlsson A, Soll R. Surfactant for meconium aspiration syndrome in full term/near term infants. *Cochrane Database Syst Rev* 2007(3):CD002054.

80. Finer NN, Barrington KJ. Nitric oxide for respiratory failure in infants born at or near term. *Cochrane Database Syst Rev* 2006(4): CD000399.

81. Bahrami KR, Van Meurs KP. ECMO for neonatal respiratory failure. *Semin Perinatol* 2005;**29**(1):15–23.

82. Wessel DL. Managing low cardiac output syndrome after congenital heart surgery. *Crit Care Med* 2001;**29**(10 Suppl): S220–30.

83. Allan CK, Thiagarajan RR, del Nido PJ, Roth SJ, Almodovar MC, Laussen PC. Indication for initiation of mechanical circulatory support impacts survival of infants with shunted single-ventricle circulation supported with extracorporeal membrane oxygenation. *J Thorac Cardiovasc Surg* 2007;**133**(3):660–7.

84. Hofmeyr GJ. Amnioinfusion for meconium-stained liquor in labour. *Cochrane Database Syst Rev* 2002(1):CD000014.

85. Xu H, Hofmeyr J, Roy C, Fraser WD. Intrapartum amnioinfusion for meconium-stained amniotic fluid: a systematic review of randomised controlled trials. *Br J Obstet Gynaecol* 2007;**114**(4):383–90.

86. Hagberg H, Wennerholm UB, Savman K. Sequelae of chorioamnionitis. *Curr Opin Infect Dis* 2002;**15**(3):301–6.

87. Kattwinkel J. *Neonatal Resuscitation*, 5th edn. Elk Grove Village: American Academy of Pediatrics and American Heart Association, 2006.

88. Kliegman R. Fetal and neonatal medicine. In: Behrman R, Kliegman R, eds. *Nelson Essentials of Pediatrics*, 4th edn. Philadelphia: W.R. Saunders Company. 2002;179–249.

89. Pickering LK. *Red Book: 2006 Report of the Committee on Infectious Diseases*, 27th edn. Washington, DC: American Academy of Pediatrics, 2006.

90. Berner R. Group B streptococci during pregnancy and infancy. *Curr Opin Infect Dis* 2002;**15**(3):307–13.

91. Behrmann R, Kliegman R. *Nelson Essentials of Pediatrics*, 4th edn. Philadelphia: W.B. Saunders Company, 2002.

92. Oddie S, Embleton ND. Risk factors for early onset neonatal group B streptococcal sepsis: case-control study. *Br Med J* 2002;**325**(7359):308.

93. Schrag SJ, Zywicki S, Farley MM, *et al.* Group B streptococcal disease in the era of intrapartum antibiotic prophylaxis. *N Engl J Med* 2000;**342**(1):15–20.

94. Schrag SJ, Zell ER, Lynfield R, *et al.* A population-based comparison of strategies to prevent early-onset group B streptococcal disease in neonates. *N Engl J Med* 2002;**347**(4):233–9.

95. Schrag SJ, Stoll BJ. Early-onset neonatal sepsis in the era of widespread intrapartum chemoprophylaxis. *Pediatr Infect Dis J* 2006;**25**(10):939–40.

96. Eschenbach DA. Prevention of neonatal group B streptococcal infection. *N Engl J Med* 2002;**347**(4):280–1.

97. Stoll BJ, Hansen N, Fanaroff AA, *et al.* Changes in pathogens causing early-onset sepsis in very-low-birth-weight infants. *N Engl J Med* 2002;**347**(4):240–7.

98. Benitz WE, Han MY, Madan A, Ramachandra P. Serial serum C-reactive protein levels in the diagnosis of neonatal infection. *Pediatrics* 1998;**102**(4):E41.

99. Harvey D, Holt DE, Bedford H. Bacterial meningitis in the newborn: a prospective study of mortality and morbidity. *Semin Perinatol* 1999;**23**(3):218–25.

100. Wiswell TE, Baumgart S, Gannon CM, Spitzer AR. No lumbar puncture in the evaluation for early neonatal sepsis: will meningitis be missed? *Pediatrics* 1995;**95**(6):803–6.

101. Kanegaye JT, Soliemanzadeh P, Bradley JS. Lumbar puncture in pediatric bacterial meningitis: defining the time interval for recovery of cerebrospinal fluid pathogens after parenteral antibiotic pretreatment. *Pediatrics* 2001;**108**(5):1169–74.

102. Nigrovic LE, Kuppermann N, Macias CG, *et al.* Clinical prediction rule for identifying children with cerebrospinal fluid pleocytosis at very low risk of bacterial meningitis. *J Am Med Assoc* 2007;**297**(1):52–60.

103. Young TE, Mangum B. *Neofax 2007*, 20th edn. London: Thomson PDR, 2007.

104. Taketomo CK, Hodding JH, Kraus DM. *Lexi Comp's Pediatric Dosage Handbook with International Index*, 13th edn. Hudson: Lexicomp, 2006.

105. Robertson J, Shilkofski N. *The Harriet Lane Handbook*, 17th edn. St. Louis: Mosby, 2005.

106. Gilbert D, Moellering R, Sande M. *The Sanford Guide to Antimicrobial Therapy.* Hyde Park, VT: Antimicrobial Therapy, Inc., 2001.

107. Carter BS, Haverkamp AD, Merenstein GB. The definition of acute perinatal asphyxia. *Clin Perinatol* 1993;**20**(2):287–304.

108. Gunn AJ, Gunn TR, de Haan HH, Williams CE, Gluckman PD. Dramatic neuronal rescue with prolonged selective head cooling after ischemia in fetal lambs. *J Clin Invest* 1997;**99**(2):248–56.

109. Azzopardi D, Edwards AD. Hypothermia. *Semin Fetal Neonatal Med* 2007;**12**(4):303–10.

110. Jacobs S, Hunt R, Tarnow-Mordi W, Inder T, Davis P. Cooling for newborns with hypoxic ischaemic encephalopathy. *Cochrane Database Syst Rev* 2007(4):CD003311.

111. ACOG Committee Opinion. Inappropriate use of the terms fetal distress and birth asphyxia. *Obstet Gynecol* 2005;**106**(6):1469–70.

112. ACOG Committee Opinion. The Apgar score. *Obstet Gynecol* 2006;**107**(5):1209–12.

113. Nelson KB, Emery ES, 3rd. Birth asphyxia and the neonatal brain: what do we know and when do we know it? *Clin Perinatol* 1993;**20**(2):327–44.

114. Vannucci RC, Perlman JM. Interventions for perinatal hypoxic-ischemic encephalopathy. *Pediatrics* 1997;**100**(6):1004–14.

115. The International Liaison Committee on Resuscitation (ILCOR) consensus on science with treatment recommendations for pediatric and neonatal patients: neonatal resuscitation. *Pediatrics* 2006;117(5):e978–88.

116. Hansmann G. Neonatal resuscitation on air: it is time to turn down the oxygen tanks [corrected]. *Lancet* 2004;**364**(9442):1293–4.

117. Vento M, Sastre J, Asensi MA, Vina J. Room-air resuscitation causes less damage to heart and kidney than 100% oxygen. *Am J Respir Crit Care Med* 2005;**172**(11): 1393–8.

118. Lundstrom KE, Pryds O, Greisen G. Oxygen at birth and prolonged cerebral vasoconstriction in preterm infants. *Arch Dis Child Fetal Neonatal Ed* 1995;**73**(2): F81–6.

119. Gluckman PD, Wyatt JS, Azzopardi D, *et al.* Selective head cooling with mild systemic hypothermia after neonatal encephalopathy: multicentre randomised trial. *Lancet* 2005;**365**(9460):663–70.

120. Eicher DJ, Wagner CL, Katikaneni LP, *et al.* Moderate hypothermia in neonatal encephalopathy: efficacy outcomes. *Pediatr Neurol* 2005;**32**(1):11–17.

121. Shankaran S, Laptook AR, Ehrenkranz RA, *et al.* Whole-body hypothermia for neonates with hypoxic-ischemic encephalopathy. *N Engl J Med* 2005;**353** (15):1574–84.

122. Edwards AD, Azzopardi DV. Therapeutic hypothermia following perinatal asphyxia. *Arch Dis Child Fetal Neonatal Ed* 2006; **91**(2):F127–31.

123. Wyatt JS, Gluckman PD, Liu PY, *et al.* Determinants of outcomes after head cooling for neonatal encephalopathy. *Pediatrics* 2007;**119**(5):912–21.

124. Rutherford MA, Azzopardi D, Whitelaw A, *et al.* Mild hypothermia and the distribution of cerebral lesions in neonates with hypoxic-ischemic encephalopathy. *Pediatrics* 2005;**116**(4):1001–6.

125. Gunn AJ, Hoehn T, Hansmann G, *et al.* Hypothermia, an evolving treatment for neonatal hypoxic ischemic encephalopathy. *Pediatrics* 2008;**121**:648–9.

126. Hoehn T, Hansmann G, Bührer C, *et al.* Therapeutic hypothermia in neonates. Review of current clinical data. ILCOR recommendations and suggestions for implementation in neonatal intensive care units. *Resuscitation* 2008; **78**(1):7–12.

127. Blackmon LR, Stark AR. Hypothermia: a neuroprotective therapy for neonatal hypoxic-ischemic encephalopathy. *Pediatrics* 2006;**117**(3):942–8.

128. Higgins RD, Raju TN, Perlman J, *et al.* Hypothermia and perinatal asphyxia: executive summary of the National Institute of Child Health and Human Development workshop. *J Pediatr* 2006;**148**(2):170–5.

129. Perlman JM. Intrapartum hypoxic-ischemic cerebral injury and subsequent cerebral palsy: medicolegal issues. *Pediatrics* 1997;**99** (6):851–9.

130. Volpe JJ. *Neurology of the Newborn*, 4th edn. Philadelphia: W.B. Saunders, 2001.

131. Dixon G, Badawi N, Kurinczuk JJ, *et al.* Early developmental outcomes after newborn encephalopathy. *Pediatrics* 2002;**109**(1):26–33.

132. Rutherford MA, Pennock JM, Counsell SJ, *et al.* Abnormal magnetic resonance signal in the internal capsule predicts poor neurodevelopmental outcome in infants with hypoxic-ischemic encephalopathy. *Pediatrics* 1998;**102**(2 Pt 1):323–8.

133. Miller SP, Newton N, Ferriero DM, *et al.* Predictors of 30-month outcome after perinatal depression: role of proton MRS and socioeconomic factors. *Pediatr Res* 2002;**52**(1):71–7.

134. Barkovich AJ, Baranski K, Vigneron D, *et al.* Proton MR spectroscopy for the evaluation of brain injury in asphyxiated, term neonates. *AJNR Am J Neuroradiol* 1999;**20**(8):1399–405.

135. Robertson C, Finer N. Term infants with hypoxic-ischemic encephalopathy: outcome at 3.5 years. *Dev Med Child Neurol* 1985; **27**(4):473–84.

136. Tharp BR. Neonatal seizures and syndromes. *Epilepsia* 2002;**43** (Suppl 3):2–10.

137. Jensen FE. The role of glutamate receptor maturation in perinatal seizures and brain injury. *Int J Dev Neurosci* 2002;**20**(3–5): 339–47.

138. Ben-Ari Y, Holmes GL. Effects of seizures on developmental processes in the immature brain. *Lancet Neurol* 2006;**5** (12):1055–63.

139. Sulzbacher S, Farwell JR, Temkin N, Lu AS, Hirtz DG. Late cognitive effects of early treatment with phenobarbital. *Clin Pediatr* 1999;**38**(7):387–94.

140. Calandre EP, Dominguez-Granados R, Gomez-Rubio M, Molina-Font JA. Cognitive effects of long-term treatment with phenobarbital and valproic acid in school children. *Acta Neurol Scand* 1990; **81**(6):504–6.

141. Mizrahi EM, Kellaway, P. Characterization and classification of neonatal seizures. *Neurology* 1987;**37**(12):1837–44.

142. Rennie J, Chorley G, Boylan G, Pressler R, Nguyen Y, Hooper R. Non-expert use of the cerebral function monitor for neonatal seizure detection. *Arch Dis Child Fetal Neonatal Ed* 2004;**89**(1):F37–40.

143. Toet MC, van der Meij W, de Vries LS, Uiterwaal CS, van Huffelen KC. Comparison between simultaneously recorded amplitude integrated electroencephalogram (cerebral function monitor) and standard electro-encephalogram in neonates. *Pediatrics* 2002;**109**(5):772–9.

144. de Vries LS, Toet MC. Amplitude integrated electroencephalography in the full-term newborn. *Clin Perinatol* 2006; **33**(3):619–32.

145. Miller SP, Weiss J, Barnwell A, *et al.* Seizure-associated brain injury in term newborns with perinatal asphyxia [see comment]. *Neurology* 2002;**58**(4):542–8.

146. Clancy RR. Summary proceedings from the neurology group on neonatal seizures. *Pediatrics* 2006;**117**(3 Pt 2):S23–7.

147. Bittigau P, Sifringer M, Genz K, *et al.* Antiepileptic drugs and apoptotic neurodegeneration in the developing brain. *Proc Nat Acad Sci USA* 2002;**99**(23):15089–94.

148. Diaz J, Schain RJ. Phenobarbital: effects of long-term administration on behavior and brain of artifically reared rats. *Science* 1978;**199**(4324):90–1.

149. Booth D, Evans DJ. Anticonvulsants for neonates with seizures. *Cochrane Database Syst Rev* 2004(4):CD004218.

150. Painter MJ, Scher MS, Stein AD, *et al.* Phenobarbital compared with phenytoin for the treatment of neonatal seizures. *New Engl J Med* 1999;**341**(7):485–9.

151. Wirrell EC. Neonatal seizures: to treat or not to treat? *Semin Pediatr Neurol* 2005; **12**(2):97–105.

152. Lanska MJ, Lanska DJ. Neonatal seizures in the United States: results of the National Hospital Discharge Survey, 1980–1991. *Neuroepidemiology* 1996;**15**(3):117–25.

153. Rennie JM. Neonatal seizures. *Eur J Pediatr* 1997;**156**(2):83–7.

154. Castro Conde JR, Hernandez Borges AA, Domenech Martinez E, Gonzalez Campo C, Perera Soler R. Midazolam in neonatal seizures with no response to phenobarbital [see comment]. *Neurology* 2005;**64**(5): 876–9.

155. Dzhala VI, Talos DM, Sdrulla DA, *et al.* NKCC1 transporter facilitates seizures in the developing brain [see comment]. *Nature Med* 2005;**11**(11):1205–13.

156. Manthey D, Asimiadou S, Stefovska V, *et al.* Sulthiame but not levetiracetam exerts neurotoxic effect in the developing rat brain. *Exp Neurol* 2005;**193**(2):497–503.

157. Sankar R, Painter MJ. Neonatal seizures: after all these years we still love what doesn't work. *Neurology* 2005;**64**(5):776–7.

158. Camfield CS, Chaplin S, Doyle AB, Shapiro SH, Cummings C, Camfield PR. Side effects of phenobarbital in toddlers; behavioral and cognitive aspects. *J Pediatr* 1979;**95**(3):361–5.

159. Oberlander TF, Warburton W, Misri S, Aghajanian J, Hertzman C. Neonatal outcomes after prenatal exposure to selective serotonin reuptake inhibitor antidepressants and maternal depression using population-based linked health data. *Arch Gen Psychiatry* 2006;**63**(8):898–906.

160. Cohen LS, Altshuler LL, Harlow BL, *et al.* Relapse of major depression during pregnancy in women who maintain or discontinue antidepressant treatment. *J Am Med Assoc* 2006;**295**(5):499–507.

161. Chambers CD, Hernandez-Diaz S, Van Marter LJ, *et al.* Selective serotonin-reuptake inhibitors and risk of persistent pulmonary hypertension of the newborn. *N Engl J Med* 2006;**354**(6):579–87.

162. Finnegan LP, Connaughton JF, Jr., Kron RE, Emich JP. Neonatal abstinence syndrome: assessment and management. *Addict Dis* 1975;**2**(1–2):141–58.

163. Lipsitz PJ. A proposed narcotic withdrawal score for use with newborn infants. A pragmatic evaluation of its efficacy. *Clin Pediatr (Phila)* 1975;**14**(6):592–4.

164. Zahorodny W, Rom C, Whitney W, *et al.* The neonatal withdrawal inventory: a simplified score of newborn withdrawal. *J Dev Behav Pediatr* 1998;**19**(2):89–93.

165. Osborn DA, Jeffery HE, Cole M. Opiate treatment for opiate withdrawal in newborn infants. *Cochrane Database Syst Rev* 2005 (3):CD002059.

166. Osborn DA, Jeffery HE, Cole MJ. Sedatives for opiate withdrawal in newborn infants. *Cochrane Database Syst Rev* 2005(3): CD002053.

167. Neonatal drug withdrawal. American Academy of Pediatrics Committee on Drugs. *Pediatrics* 1998;**101**(6):1079–88.

168. Levinson-Castiel R, Merlob P, Linder N, Sirota L, Klinger G. Neonatal abstinence syndrome after in utero exposure to selective serotonin reuptake inhibitors in term infants. *Arch Pediatr Adolesc Med* 2006;**160**(2):173–6.

169. Moses-Kolko EL, Bogen D, Perel J, *et al.* Neonatal signs after late in utero exposure to serotonin reuptake inhibitors: literature review and implications for clinical applications. *J Am Med Assoc* 2005;**293** (19):2372–83.

170. Strasburger JF. Fetal arrhythmias. *Prog Pediatr Cardiol* 2000;**11**(1):1–17.

171. Fasnacht M, Pfammatter JP, Ghisla R, *et al.* FETCH-Study: prospective fetal cardiology study in Switzerland. *40th Annual Meeting of the AEPC*, 2005. (Abstract) Card Young May 2005 Supplement 2, Vol. 15, p. 35.

172. Trappe HJ. Acute therapy of maternal and fetal arrhythmias during pregnancy. *J Intensive Care Med* 2006;**21**(5):305–15.

173. Strasburger JF. Prenatal diagnosis of fetal arrhythmias. *Clin Perinatol* 2005;**32** (4):891–912, viii.

174. Simpson JM. Fetal arrhythmias. *Ultrasound Obstet Gynecol* 2006;**27**(6):599–606.

175. Park MK. *Pediatric Cardiology for Practitioners*, 5th edn. St. Louis: Mosby, 2008.

176. Ralston M, Hazinski MF, Zaritsky AL, Schexnayder SM, Kleinman ME. *PALS Provider Manual*. Dallas: American Heart Association and American Academy of Pediatrics, 2006.

177. Izmirly PM, Rivera TL, Buyon JP. Neonatal lupus syndromes. *Rheum Dis Clin North Am* 2007;**33**(2):267–85, vi.

178. Johnson BA, Ades A. Delivery room and early postnatal management of neonates who have prenatally diagnosed congenital heart disease. *Clin Perinatol* 2005;**32** (4):921–46, ix.

179. Buyon JP, Hiebert R, Copel J, *et al.* Autoimmune-associated congenital heart block: demographics, mortality, morbidity and recurrence rates obtained from a national neonatal lupus registry. *J Am Coll Cardiol* 1998;**31**(7):1658–66.

180. Michaelsson M, Engle MA. Congenital complete heart block: an international study of the natural history. *Cardiovasc Clin* 1972;**4**(3):85–101.

181. Gordon PA. Congenital heart block: clinical features and therapeutic approaches. *Lupus* 2007;**16**(8):642–6.

182. Buyon JP, Rupel A, Clancy RM. Neonatal lupus syndromes. *Lupus* 2004;**13**(9):705–12.

183. Grifka RG. Cyanotic congenital heart disease with increased pulmonary blood flow. *Pediatr Clin North Am* 1999; **46**(2):405–25.

184. Waldman JD, Wernly JA. Cyanotic congenital heart disease with decreased pulmonary blood flow in children. *Pediatr Clin North Am* 1999;**46**(2):385–404.

185. Allen HD, Driscoll DJ, Shaddy RE, Feltes TF. *Moss and Adams' Heart Disease in Infants, Children, and Adolescents: Including the Fetus and Young Adult*, 7th edn. Philadelphia: Lippincott Williams and Wilkins, 2008.

186. Silberbach M, Hannon D. Presentation of congenital heart disease in the neonate and young infant. *Pediatr Rev* 2007;**28**(4):123–31.

187. Kovalchin JP, Silverman NH. The impact of fetal echocardiography. *Pediatr Cardiol* 2004;**25**(3):299–306.

188. Ades A, Johnson BA, Berger S. Management of low birth weight infants with congenital heart disease. *Clin Perinatol* 2005;**32**(4): 999–1015, x–xi.

189. Nichols DG, Ungerleider RM, Spevak PJ, *et al. Critical Heart Disease in Infants and Children*, 2nd edn. Philadelphia: Mosby, 2006.

190. De Wolf D, Vanderbruggen K, Verbist A, *et al.* Percutaneous interventions for congenital aortic stenosis. *Acta Cardiol* 2006;**61**(2):204–5.

191. Fyler DC. Report of the New England Regional Infant Cardiac Program. *Pediatrics* 1980;**65**(2 Pt 2):375–461.

192. Alsoufi B, Karamlou T, McCrindle BW, Caldarone CA. Management options in neonates and infants with critical left ventricular outflow tract obstruction. *Eur J Cardiothorac Surg* 2007;**31**(6):1013–21.

193. Alsoufi B, Bennetts J, Verma S, Caldarone CA. New developments in the treatment of hypoplastic left heart syndrome. *Pediatrics* 2007;**119**(1):109–17.

194. Ferencz C, Rubin JD, McCarter RJ, *et al.* Congenital heart disease: prevalence at livebirth. The Baltimore-Washington Infant Study. *Am J Epidemiol* 1985;**121**(1):31–6.

195. Pandey R, Jackson M, Ajab S, Gladman G, Pozzi M. Subclavian flap repair: review of 399 patients at median follow-up of fourteen years. *Ann Thorac Surg* 2006;**81**(4):1420–8.

196. Sudarshan CD, Cochrane AD, Jun ZH, Soto R, Brizard CP. Repair of coarctation of the aorta in infants weighing less than 2 kilograms. *Ann Thorac Surg* 2006;**82**(1):158–63.

197. Brown JW, Ruzmetov M, Okada Y, Vijay P, Rodefeld MD, Turrentine MW. Outcomes in patients with interrupted aortic arch and associated anomalies: a 20-year experience. *Eur J Cardiothorac Surg* 2006;**29**(5):666–73; discussion 673–4.

198. Cheung YF, Leung MP, Lee JW, Chau AK, Yung TC. Evolving management for critical pulmonary stenosis in neonates and young infants. *Cardiol Young* 2000;**10**(3):186–92.

199. Humpl T, Soderberg B, McCrindle BW, *et al.* Percutaneous balloon valvotomy in pulmonary atresia with intact ventricular septum: impact on patient care. *Circulation* 2003;**108**(7):826–32.

200. Derby CD, Pizarro C. Routine primary repair of tetralogy of Fallot in the neonate. *Expert Rev Cardiovasc Ther* 2005;**3**(5):857–63.

201. Karamlou T, Ashburn DA, Caldarone CA, *et al.* Matching procedure to morphology improves outcomes in neonates with tricuspid atresia. *J Thorac Cardiovasc Surg* 2005;**130**(6):1503–10.

202. DeBord S, Cherry C, Hickey C. The arterial switch procedure for transposition of the great arteries. *AORN J* 2007;**86**(2):211–26; quiz 227–30.

203. Singh RR, Warren PS, Reece TB, Ellman P, Peeler BB, Kron IL. Early repair of complete atrioventricular septal defect is safe and effective. *Ann Thorac Surg* 2006;**82**(5):1598–601; discussion 1602.

204. Hancock Friesen CL, Zurakowski D, Thiagarajan RR, *et al.* Total anomalous pulmonary venous connection: an analysis of current management strategies in a single institution. *Ann Thorac Surg* 2005;**79**(2):596–606.

205. Skinner J. Diagnosis of patent ductus arteriosus. *Semin Neonatol* 2001;**6**(1):49–61.

206. Clyman RI. Ibuprofen and patent ductus arteriosus. *N Engl J Med* 2000;**343**(10):728–30.

207. Thebaud B, Michelakis ED, Wu XC, *et al.* Oxygen-sensitive Kv channel gene transfer confers oxygen responsiveness to preterm rabbit and remodeled human ductus arteriosus: implications for infants with patent ductus arteriosus. *Circulation* 2004;**110**(11):1372–9.

208. Kajimoto H, Hashimoto K, Bonnet SN, *et al.* Oxygen activates the Rho/Rho-kinase pathway and induces RhoB and ROCK-1 expression in human and rabbit ductus arteriosus by increasing mitochondria-derived reactive oxygen species: a newly recognized mechanism for sustaining ductal constriction. *Circulation* 2007;**115**(13):1777–88.

209. Knight DB. The treatment of patent ductus arteriosus in preterm infants. A review and overview of randomized trials. *Semin Neonatol* 2001;**6**(1):63–73.

210. Ment LR, Oh W, Ehrenkranz RA, *et al.* Low-dose indomethacin and prevention of intraventricular hemorrhage: a multicenter randomized trial. *Pediatrics* 1994;**93**(4):543–50.

211. Schmidt B, Davis P, Moddemann D, *et al.* Long-term effects of indomethacin prophylaxis in extremely-low-birth-weight infants. *N Engl J Med* 2001;**344**(26):1966–72.

212. Clyman RI, Saha S, Jobe A, Oh W. Indomethacin prophylaxis for preterm infants: the impact of 2 multicentered randomized controlled trials on clinical practice. *J Pediatr* 2007;**150**(1):46–50, e2.

213. Ment LR, Vohr BR, Makuch RW, *et al.* Prevention of intraventricular hemorrhage by indomethacin in male preterm infants. *J Pediatr* 2004;**145**(6):832–4.

214. Ohlsson A, Walia R, Shah S. Ibuprofen for the treatment of patent ductus arteriosus in preterm and/or low birth weight infants. *Cochrane Database Syst Rev* 2005(4):CD003481.

215. Schmidt B, Roberts RS, Fanaroff A, *et al.* Indomethacin prophylaxis, patent ductus arteriosus, and the risk of broncho-pulmonary dysplasia: further analyses from the Trial of Indomethacin Prophylaxis in Preterms (TIPP). *J Pediatr* 2006; **148**(6):730–4.

216. Bose CL, Laughon M. Treatment to prevent patency of the ductus arteriosus: beneficial or harmful? *J Pediatr* 2006;**148**(6):713–14.

217. Bose CL, Laughon MM. Patent ductus arteriosus: lack of evidence for common treatments. *Arch Dis Child Fetal Neonatal Ed* 2007;**92**(6):F498–502.

218. Shah SS, Ohlsson A. Ibuprofen for the prevention of patent ductus arteriosus in preterm and/or low birth weight infants. *Cochrane Database Syst Rev* 2006(1): CD004213.

219. Herrera C, Holberton J, Davis P. Prolonged versus short course of indomethacin for the treatment of patent ductus arteriosus in preterm infants. *Cochrane Database Syst Rev* 2007(2):CD003480.

220. Van Overmeire B, Smets K, Lecoutere D, *et al.* A comparison of ibuprofen and indomethacin for closure of patent ductus arteriosus. *N Engl J Med* 2000;**343**(10):674–81.

221. Vanhaesebrouck S, Zonnenberg I, Vandervoort P, Bruneel E, Van Hoestenberghe MR, Theyskens C. Conservative treatment for patent ductus arteriosus in the preterm. *Arch Dis Child Fetal Neonatal Ed* 2007;**92**(4):F244–7.

222. Rennie JM, Cooke RW. Prolonged low dose indomethacin for persistent ductus arteriosus of prematurity. *Arch Dis Child* 1991;**66**(1 Spec No):55–8.

223. Jobe AH. Drug pricing in pediatrics: the egregious example of indomethacin. *Pediatrics* 2007;**119**(6):1197–8.

224. Walsh-Sukys MC, Tyson JE, Wright LL, *et al.* Persistent pulmonary hypertension of the newborn in the era before nitric oxide: practice variation and outcomes. *Pediatrics* 2000;**105**(1 Pt 1):14–20.

225. Cua CL, Blankenship A, North AL, Hayes J, Nelin LD. Increased incidence of idiopathic persistent pulmonary hypertension in down syndrome neonates. *Pediatr Cardiol* 2007;**28**(4):250–4.

226. Shah PS, Hellmann J, Adatia I. Clinical characteristics and follow up of Down syndrome infants without congenital heart disease who presented with persistent pulmonary hypertension of newborn. *J Perinat Med* 2004;**32**(2):168–70.

227. Pearson DL, Dawling S, Walsh WF, *et al.* Neonatal pulmonary hypertension – urea-cycle intermediates, nitric oxide production, and carbamoyl-phosphate synthetase function. *N Engl J Med* 2001; **344**(24):1832–8.

228. Gien J, Seedorf GJ, Balasubramaniam V, Markham N, Abman SH. Intrauterine pulmonary hypertension impairs angiogenesis in vitro: role of vascular endothelial growth factor nitric oxide signaling. *Am J Respir Crit Care Med* 2007;**176**(11):1146–53.

229. Farrow KN, Groh BS, Schumacker PT, *et al.* Hyperoxia increases phosphodiesterase 5 expression and activity in ovine fetal pulmonary artery smooth muscle cells. *Circ Res* 2008;**102**(2):226–33.

230. Weinberger B, Weiss K, Heck DE, Laskin DL, Laskin JD. Pharmacologic therapy of persistent pulmonary hypertension of the newborn. *Pharmacol Ther* 2001; **89**(1):67–79.

231. Rosenberg AA. Outcome in term infants treated with inhaled nitric oxide. *J Pediatr* 2002;**140**(3):284–7.

232. Hoehn T. Therapy of pulmonary hypertension in neonates and infants. *Pharmacol Ther* 2007;**114**(3):318–26.

233. Tworetzky W, Bristow J, Moore P, *et al.* Inhaled nitric oxide in neonates with persistent pulmonary hypertension. *Lancet* 2001;**357**(9250):118–20.

234. Barrington KJ, Finer NN. Inhaled nitric oxide for preterm infants: a systematic review. *Pediatrics* 2007;**120**(5):1088–99.

235. Barrington KJ, Finer NN. Inhaled nitric oxide for respiratory failure in preterm infants. *Cochrane Database Syst Rev* 2007 (3):CD000509.

236. Murray F, Patel HH, Suda RY, *et al.* Expression and activity of cAMP phosphodiesterase isoforms in pulmonary artery smooth muscle cells from patients with pulmonary hypertension: role for PDE1. *Am J Physiol Lung Cell Mol Physiol* 2007;**292**(1):L294–303.

237. Schermuly RT, Pullamsetti SS, Kwapiszewska G, *et al.* Phosphodiesterase 1

upregulation in pulmonary arterial hypertension: target for reverse-remodeling therapy. *Circulation* 2007;**115**(17):2331–9.

238. Baquero H, Soliz A, Neira F, Venegas ME, Sola A. Oral sildenafil in infants with persistent pulmonary hypertension of the newborn: a pilot randomized blinded study. *Pediatrics* 2006;**117**(4):1077–83.

239. Ichinose F, Erana-Garcia J, Hromi J, *et al.* Nebulized sildenafil is a selective pulmonary vasodilator in lambs with acute pulmonary hypertension. *Crit Care Med* 2001;**29**(5):1000–5.

240. Zhao L, Mason NA, Morrell NW, *et al.* Sildenafil inhibits hypoxia-induced pulmonary hypertension. *Circulation* 2001;**104**(4):424–8.

241. Humpl T, Reyes JT, Holtby H, Stephens D, Adatia I. Beneficial effect of oral sildenafil therapy on childhood pulmonary arterial hypertension: twelve-month clinical trial of a single-drug, open-label, pilot study. *Circulation* 2005;**111**(24):3274–80.

242. Shah P, Ohlsson A. Sildenafil for pulmonary hypertension in neonates. *Cochrane Database Syst Rev* 2007(3): CD005494.

243. McNamara PJ, Laique F, Muang-In S, Whyte HE. Milrinone improves oxygenation in neonates with severe persistent pulmonary hypertension of the newborn. *J Crit Care* 2006;**21**(2):217–22.

244. Abman SH. Recent advances in the pathogenesis and treatment of persistent pulmonary hypertension of the newborn. *Neonatology* 2007;**91**(4):283–90.

245. Hoeper MM, Schwarze M, Ehlerding S, *et al.* Long-term treatment of primary pulmonary hypertension with aerosolized iloprost, a prostacyclin analogue. *N Engl J Med* 2000;**342**(25):1866–70.

246. Wedgwood S, McMullan DM, Bekker JM, Fineman JR, Black SM. Role for endothelin-1-induced superoxide and peroxynitrite production in rebound pulmonary hypertension associated with inhaled nitric oxide therapy. *Circ Res* 2001;**89**(4):357–64.

247. Moya MP, Gow AJ, Califf RM, Goldberg RN, Stamler JS. Inhaled ethyl nitrite gas for persistent pulmonary hypertension of the newborn. *Lancet* 2002;**360**(9327):141–3.

248. Stege G, Fenton A, Jaffray B. Nihilism in the 1990s: the true mortality of congenital diaphragmatic hernia. *Pediatrics* 2003; **112**(3 Pt 1):532–5.

249. Boloker J, Bateman DA, Wung JT, Stolar CJ. Congenital diaphragmatic hernia in 120 infants treated consecutively with permissive hypercapnea/spontaneous respiration/elective repair. *J Pediatr Surg* 2002;**37**(3):357–66.

250. Colvin J, Bower C, Dickinson JE, Sokol J. Outcomes of congenital diaphragmatic hernia: a population-based study in Western Australia. *Pediatrics* 2005;**116**(3): e356–63.

251. Lally KP, Lally PA, Van Meurs KP, *et al.* Treatment evolution in high-risk congenital diaphragmatic hernia: ten years' experience with diaphragmatic agenesis. *Ann Surg* 2006;**244**(4):505–13.

252. Levison J, Halliday R, Holland AJ, *et al.* A population-based study of congenital diaphragmatic hernia outcome in New South Wales and the Australian Capital Territory, Australia, 1992–2001. *J Pediatr Surg* 2006;**41**(6):1049–53.

253. Baglaj M. Late-presenting congenital diaphragmatic hernia in children: a clinical spectrum. *Pediatr Surg Int* 2004;**20**(9):658–69.

254. Mei-Zahav M, Solomon M, Trachsel D, Langer JC. Bochdalek diaphragmatic hernia: not only a neonatal disease. *Arch Dis Child* 2003;**88**(6):532–5.

255. Holt PD, Arkovitz MS, Berdon WE, Stolar CJ. Newborns with diaphragmatic hernia: initial chest radiography does not have a role in predicting clinical outcome. *Pediatr Radiol* 2004;**34**(6):462–4.

256. Hamrick SE, Brook MM, Farmer DL. Fetal surgery for congenital diaphragmatic hernia and pulmonary sequestration complicated by postnatal diagnosis of transposition of the great arteries. *Fetal Diagn Ther* 2004;**19**(1):40–2.

257. Casaccia G, Crescenzi F, Dotta A, *et al.* Birth weight and McGoon Index predict mortality in newborn infants with congenital diaphragmatic hernia. *J Pediatr Surg* 2006;**41**(1):25–8; discussion 25–8.

258. Nguyen TL, Le AD. Thoracoscopic repair for congenital diaphragmatic hernia: lessons from 45 cases. *J Pediatr Surg* 2006;**41**(10):1713–15.

259. Masumoto K, Nagata K, Uesugi T, Yamada T, Taguchi T. Risk factors for sensorineural

hearing loss in survivors with severe congenital diaphragmatic hernia. *Eur J Pediatr* 2007;**166**(6):607–12.

260. Chiu PP, Sauer C, Mihailovic A, *et al.* The price of success in the management of congenital diaphragmatic hernia: is improved survival accompanied by an increase in long-term morbidity? *J Pediatr Surg* 2006;**41**(5):888–92.

261. Trachsel D, Selvadurai H, Bohn D, Langer JC, Coates AL. Long-term pulmonary morbidity in survivors of congenital diaphragmatic hernia. *Pediatr Pulmonol* 2005;**39**(5):433–9.

262. Ahmad A, Gangitano E, Odell RM, Doran R, Durand M. Survival, intracranial lesions, and neurodevelopmental outcome in infants with congenital diaphragmatic hernia treated with extracorporeal membrane oxygenation. *J Perinatol* 1999; **19**(6 Pt 1):436–40.

263. Logan JW, Rice HE, Goldberg RN, Cotten CM. Congenital diaphragmatic hernia: a systematic review and summary of best-evidence practice strategies. *J Perinatol* 2007;**27**(9):535–49.

264. Van Meurs K. Is surfactant therapy beneficial in the treatment of the term newborn infant with congenital diaphragmatic hernia? *J Pediatr* 2004; **145**(3):312–16.

265. Reyes C, Chang LK, Waffarn F, Mir H, Warden MJ, Sills J. Delayed repair of congenital diaphragmatic hernia with early high-frequency oscillatory ventilation during preoperative stabilization. *J Pediatr Surg* 1998;**33**(7):1010–14.

266. Desfrere L, Jarreau PH, Dommergues M, *et al.* Impact of delayed repair and elective high-frequency oscillatory ventilation on survival of antenatally diagnosed congenital diaphragmatic hernia: first application of these strategies in the more "severe" subgroup of antenatally diagnosed newborns. *Intensive Care Med* 2000;**26** (7):934–41.

267. Gehlbach BK, Schmidt GA. Bench-to-bedside review: treating acid-base abnormalities in the intensive care unit – the role of buffers. *Crit Care* 2004;**8**(4):259–65.

268. Weber T, Tschernich H, Sitzwohl C, *et al.* Tromethamine buffer modifies the depressant effect of permissive hypercapnia on myocardial contractility in patients with acute respiratory distress syndrome. *Am J Respir Crit Care Med* 2000;**162** (4 Pt 1):1361–5.

269. Adrogue HJ, Madias NE. Management of life-threatening acid-base disorders. First of two parts. *N Engl J Med* 1998;**338**(1):26–34.

270. Kluth D, Bührer C, Nestoris S, Tander B, Werner C, Lambrecht W. Inhaled nitric oxide increases survival rates in newborn rats with congenital diaphragmatic hernia. *Eur J Pediatr Surg* 1997;**7**(2):90–2.

271. Noori S, Friedlich P, Wong P, Garingo A, Seri I. Cardiovascular effects of sildenafil in neonates and infants with congenital diaphragmatic hernia and pulmonary hypertension. *Neonatology* 2007;**91**(2): 92–100.

272. Khan AM, Lally KP. The role of extracorporeal membrane oxygenation in the management of infants with congenital diaphragmatic hernia. *Semin Perinatol* 2005;**29**(2):118–22.

273. Elbourne D, Field D, Mugford M. Extracorporeal membrane oxygenation for severe respiratory failure in newborn infants. *Cochrane Database Syst Rev* 2002 (1):CD001340.

274. Fligor BJ, Neault MW, Mullen CH, Feldman HA, Jones DT. Factors associated with sensorineural hearing loss among survivors of extracorporeal membrane oxygenation therapy. *Pediatrics* 2005; **115**(6):1519–28.

275. Harrison MR, Adzick NS, Bullard KM, *et al.* Correction of congenital diaphragmatic hernia in utero VII: a prospective trial. *J Pediatr Surg* 1997; **32**(11):1637–42.

276. Harrison MR, Keller RL, Hawgood SB, *et al.* A randomized trial of fetal endoscopic tracheal occlusion for severe fetal congenital diaphragmatic hernia. *N Engl J Med* 2003;**349**(20):1916–24.

277. Cotten CM, Goldberg RN. Air leak syndromes. In: Spitzer A, ed. *Intensive Care of the Fetus and Neonate*, 2nd edn. Philadelphia: Elsevier Mosby, 2005; p. 715–28.

278. deMello DE. Pulmonary pathology. *Semin Neonatol* 2004;**9**(4):311–29.

279. McIntosh N, Becher JC, Cunningham S, *et al.* Clinical diagnosis of pneumothorax is late: use of trend data and decision support

might allow preclinical detection. *Pediatr Res* 2000;**48**(3):408–15.

280. Greenough A, Sharma A. What is new in ventilation strategies for the neonate? *Eur J Pediatr* 2007;**166**(10):991–6.

281. Watkinson M, Tiron I. Events before the diagnosis of a pneumothorax in ventilated neonates. *Arch Dis Child Fetal Neonatal Ed* 2001;**85**(3):F201–3.

282. Woodgate PG, Davies MW. Permissive hypercapnia for the prevention of morbidity and mortality in mechanically ventilated newborn infants. *Cochrane Database Syst Rev* 2001(2):CD002061.

283. Bhuta T, Henderson-Smart DJ. Rescue high frequency oscillatory ventilation versus conventional ventilation for pulmonary dysfunction in preterm infants. *Cochrane Database Syst Rev* 2000(2):CD000438.

284. Cools F, Offringa M. Neuromuscular paralysis for newborn infants receiving mechanical ventilation. *Cochrane Database Syst Rev* 2005(2):CD002773.

285. Davenport M, Warne SA, Cacciaguerra S, Patel S, Greenough A, Nicolaides K. Current outcome of antenatally diagnosed cystic lung disease. *J Pediatr Surg* 2004;**39**(4):549–56.

286. Adzick NS. Management of fetal lung lesions. *Clin Perinatol* 2003;**30**(3):481–92.

287. Sauvat F, Michel JL, Benachi A, Emond S, Revillon Y. Management of asymptomatic neonatal cystic adenomatoid malformations. *J Pediatr Surg* 2003;**38**(4):548–52.

288. Beghetti M, La Scala G, Belli D, Bugmann P, Kalangos A, Le Coultre C. Etiology and management of pediatric chylothorax. *J Pediatr* 2000;**136**(5):653–8.

289. Gaede C. Congenital chylothorax: a case study. *Neonatal Netw* 2006;**25**(5):371–81.

290. Picone O, Benachi A, Mandelbrot L, Ruano R, Dumez Y, Dommergues M. Thoracoamniotic shunting for fetal pleural effusions with hydrops. *Am J Obstet Gynecol* 2004;**191**(6):2047–50.

291. Kallanagowdar C, Craver RD. Neonatal pleural effusion. Spontaneous chylothorax in a newborn with trisomy 21. *Arch Pathol Lab Med* 2006;**130**(2):e22–3.

292. Markham KM, Glover JL, Welsh RJ, Lucas RJ, Bendick PJ. Octreotide in the treatment of thoracic duct injuries. *Am Surg* 2000; **66**(12):1165–7.

293. Cheung Y, Leung MP, Yip M. Octreotide for treatment of postoperative chylothorax. *J Pediatr* 2001;**139**(1):157–9.

294. Chan SY, Lau W, Wong WH, Cheng LC, Chau AK, Cheung YF. Chylothorax in children after congenital heart surgery. *Ann Thorac Surg* 2006;**82**(5):1650–6.

295. Roehr CC, Jung A, Proquitte H, *et al.* Somatostatin or octreotide as treatment options for chylothorax in young children: a systematic review. *Intensive Care Med* 2006;**32**(5):650–7.

296. Stajich GV, Ashworth L. Octreotide. *Neonatal Netw* 2006;**25**(5):365–9.

297. Barili F, Polvani G, Topkara VK, *et al.* Administration of octreotide for management of postoperative high-flow chylothorax. *Ann Vasc Surg* 2007;**21**(1):90–2.

298. Mohseni-Bod H, Macrae D, Slavik Z. Somatostatin analog (octreotide) in management of neonatal postoperative chylothorax: is it safe? *Pediatr Crit Care Med* 2004;**5**(4):356–7.

299. Phibbs RH. Hemolytic disease of the newborn. In: Rudolph AM, ed. *Rudolph's Pediatrics*, 21 edn. Stamford: Appleton & Lange, 1996; 1193–200.

300. Moise KJ, Jr. Management of rhesus alloimmunization in pregnancy. *Obstet Gynecol* 2002;**100**(3):600–11.

301. Stockman JA, 3rd. Overview of the state of the art of Rh disease: history, current clinical management, and recent progress. *J Pediatr Hematol Oncol* 2001;**23**(6):385–93.

302. Bullock R, Martin WL, Coomarasamy A, Kilby MD. Prediction of fetal anemia in pregnancies with red-cell alloimmunization: comparison of middle cerebral artery peak systolic velocity and amniotic fluid OD450. *Ultrasound Obstet Gynecol* 2005;**25**(4):331–4.

303. Gottstein R, Cooke RW. Systematic review of intravenous immunoglobulin in haemolytic disease of the newborn. *Arch Dis Child Fetal Neonatal Ed* 2003;**88**(1):F6–10.

304. Henrich W, Heeger J, Schmider A, Dudenhausen JW. Complete spontaneous resolution of severe nonimmunological hydrops fetalis with unknown etiology in the second trimester – a case report. *J Perinat Med* 2002;**30**(6):522–7.

305. Coulter. *Hydrops fetalis*. In: Spitzer AR, ed. *Intensive Care of the Fetus and Neonate,*

2nd edn. Philadelphia: Mosby Elsevier, 2005; 149–55.

306. Ismail KM, Martin WL, Ghosh S, Whittle MJ, Kilby MD. Etiology and outcome of hydrops fetalis. *J Matern Fetal Med* 2001; **10**(3):175–81.

307. Solarin KO. *Differential Diagnosis of Neonatal Respiratory Disorders*, 2nd edn. Philadelphia: Elsevier Mosby, 2005.

308. Jongmans MC, Admiraal RJ, van der Donk KP, *et al.* CHARGE syndrome: the phenotypic spectrum of mutations in the CHD7 gene. *J Med Genet* 2006;**43**(4):306–14.

309. Shaw-Smith C. Oesophageal atresia, tracheo-oesophageal fistula, and the VACTERL association: review of genetics and epidemiology. *J Med Genet* 2006; **43**(7):545–54.

310. Hartman G. *Surgical Care of Conditions Presenting in the Newborn*, 6th edn. Philadelphia: Lippincott Williams and Wilkins, 2005.

311. Kalhan SC. *Nutrition and Selected Disorders of the Gastrointestinal Tract*, 5 edn. Philadelphia: W.B. Saunders Company, 2001.

312. Ein SH, Palder SB, Filler RM. Babies with esophageal and duodenal atresia: a 30-year review of a multifaceted problem. *J Pediatr Surg* 2006;**41**(3):530–2.

313. Kovesi T, Rubin S. Long-term complications of congenital esophageal atresia and/or tracheoesophageal fistula. *Chest* 2004;**126**(3):915–25.

314. Walker GM, Raine PA. Bilious vomiting in the newborn: how often is further investigation undertaken? *J Pediatr Surg* 2007;**42**(4):714–16.

315. de la Hunt MN. The acute abdomen in the newborn. *Semin Fetal Neonatal Med* 2006;**11**(3):191–7.

316. Al-Salem AH. Congenital pyloric atresia and associated anomalies. *Pediatr Surg Int* 2007;**23**(6):559–63.

317. Kallen BA, Otterblad Olausson P, Danielsson BR. Is erythromycin therapy teratogenic in humans? *Reprod Toxicol* 2005;**20**(2):209–14.

318. Munoz JJ, Mansul AJ, Malpas TJ, Steinbrecher HA. Intrathoracic gastric volvulus mimicking pyloric stenosis. *J Paediatr Child Health* 2003;**39**(2):149–51.

319. Bianca S, Barbagallo MA, Ingegnosi C, Ettore G. Isolated hypertrophic pyloric stenosis and perinatal factors. *Genet Couns* 2003;**14**(1):101–3.

320. Gupta AK, Guglani B. Imaging of congenital anomalies of the gastrointestinal tract. *Indian J Pediatr* 2005;**72**(5):403–14.

321. Hemming V, Rankin J. Small intestinal atresia in a defined population: occurrence, prenatal diagnosis and survival. *Prenat Diagn* 2007;**27**(13):1205–11.

322. Shawis R, Antao B. Prenatal bowel dilatation and the subsequent postnatal management. *Early Hum Dev* 2006; **82**(5):297–303.

323. Poki HO, Holland AJ, Pitkin J. Double bubble, double trouble. *Pediatr Surg Int* 2005;**21**(6):428–31.

324. Lawrence MJ, Ford WD, Furness ME, Hayward T, Wilson T. Congenital duodenal obstruction: early antenatal ultrasound diagnosis. *Pediatr Surg Int* 2000; **16**(5–6):342–5.

325. Kimber CP, MacMahon RA, Shekleton P, Yardley R. Antenatal intestinal vascular accident with subsequent small bowel atresia: case report. *Ultrasound Obstet Gynecol* 1997;**10**(3):212–14.

326. Kumaran N, Shankar KR, Lloyd DA, Losty PD. Trends in the management and outcome of jejuno-ileal atresia. *Eur J Pediatr Surg* 2002;**12**(3):163–7.

327. Sweeney B, Surana R, Puri P. Jejunoileal atresia and associated malformations: correlation with the timing of in utero insult. *J Pediatr Surg* 2001;**36**(5):774–6.

328. Stoll C, Alembik Y, Dott B, Roth MP. Associated malformations in patients with anorectal anomalies. *Eur J Med Genet* 2007;**50**(4):281–90.

329. Williams H. Green for danger! Intestinal malrotation and volvulus. *Arch Dis Child Educ Pract Ed* 2007;**92**(3):ep87–91.

330. Epelman M. The whirlpool sign. *Radiology* 2006;**240**(3):910–1.

331. Amiel J, Sproat-Emison E, Garcia-Barceo M, *et al.* Hirschsprung disease: associated syndromes and genetics. *J Med Genet* 2008;**45**(1):1–14.

332. Cowles RA, Berdon WE, Holt PD, Buonomo C, Stolar CJ. Neonatal intestinal obstruction simulating meconium ileus in

infants with long-segment intestinal aganglionosis: radiographic findings that prompt the need for rectal biopsy. *Pediatr Radiol* 2006;**36**(2):133–7.

333. Dimmitt RA, Moss RL. Meconium diseases in infants with very low birth weight. *Semin Pediatr Surg* 2000;**9**(2):79–83.

334. Burge D, Drewett M. Meconium plug obstruction. *Pediatr Surg Int* 2004;**20**(2):108–10.

335. Dimmitt RA, Moss RL. Clinical management of necrotizing enterocolitis. *NeoReviews* 2001;**2**:e110–e117.

336. Caplan MS, Jilling T. New concepts in necrotizing enterocolitis. *Curr Opin Pediatr* 2001;**13**(2):111–15.

337. Ng S. Necrotizing enterocolitis in the full-term neonate. *J Paediatr Child Health* 2001;**37**(1):1–4.

338. Blakely ML, Tyson JE, Lally KP, *et al.* Laparotomy versus peritoneal drainage for necrotizing enterocolitis or isolated intestinal perforation in extremely low birth weight infants: outcomes through 18 months adjusted age. *Pediatrics* 2006;**117**(4):e680–7.

339. Kitchanan S, Patole SK, Muller R, Whitehall JS. Neonatal outcome of gastroschisis and exomphalos: a 10-year review. *J Paediatr Child Health* 2000;**36**(5):428–30.

340. Wilson RD, Johnson MP. Congenital abdominal wall defects: an update. *Fetal Diagn Ther* 2004;**19**(5):385–98.

341. How HY, Harris BJ, Pietrantoni M, *et al.* Is vaginal delivery preferable to elective cesarean delivery in fetuses with a known ventral wall defect? *Am J Obstet Gynecol* 2000;**182**(6):1527–34.

342. Vegunta RK, Wallace LJ, Leonardi MR, *et al.* Perinatal management of gastroschisis: analysis of a newly established clinical pathway. *J Pediatr Surg* 2005;**40**(3):528–34.

343. McNair C, Hawes J, Urquhart H. Caring for the newborn with an omphalocele. *Neonatal Netw* 2006;**25**(5):319–27.

344. Lee SL, Beyer TD, Kim SS, *et al.* Initial nonoperative management and delayed closure for treatment of giant omphaloceles. *J Pediatr Surg* 2006;**41**(11):1846–9.

345. Rowland CA, Correa A, Cragan JD, Alverson CJ. Are encephaloceles neural tube defects? *Pediatrics* 2006;**118**(3):916–23.

346. Luthy DA, Wardinsky T, Shurtleff DB, *et al.* Cesarean section before the onset of labor and subsequent motor function in infants with meningomyelocele diagnosed antenatally. *N Engl J Med* 1991;**324**(10):662–6.

347. Hudgins RJ, Gilreath CL. Tethered spinal cord following repair of myelomeningocele. *Neurosurg Focus* 2004;**16**(2):E7.

348. Charney EB, Melchionni JB, Antonucci DL. Ventriculitis in newborns with myelomeningocele. *Am J Dis Child* 1991;**145**(3):287–90.

349. Miller PD, Pollack IF, Pang D, Albright AL. Comparison of simultaneous versus delayed ventriculoperitoneal shunt insertion in children undergoing myelomeningocele repair. *J Child Neurol* 1996;**11**(5):370–2.

350. Printzlau A, Andersen M. Pierre Robin sequence in Denmark: a retrospective population-based epidemiological study. *Cleft Palate Craniofac J* 2004;**41**(1):47–52.

351. Eppley BL, van Aalst JA, Robey A, Havlik RJ, Sadove AM. The spectrum of orofacial clefting. *Plast Reconstr Surg* 2005;**115**(7):101e–114e.

352. Trevisanuto D, Verghese C, Doglioni N, Ferrarese P, Zanardo V. Laryngeal mask airway for the interhospital transport of neonates. *Pediatrics* 2005;**115**(1):e109–11.

353. Denny A, Amm C. New technique for airway correction in neonates with severe Pierre Robin sequence. *J Pediatr* 2005;**147**(1):97–101.

354. Donnelly V, Foran A, Murphy J, McParland P, Keane D, O'Herlihy C. Neonatal brachial plexus palsy: an unpredictable injury. *Am J Obstet Gynecol* 2002;**187**(5):1209–12.

355. Hsu TY, Hung FC, Lu YJ, *et al.* Neonatal clavicular fracture: clinical analysis of incidence, predisposing factors, diagnosis, and outcome. *Am J Perinatol* 2002;**19**(1):17–21.

356. Anand P, Birch R. Restoration of sensory function and lack of long-term chronic pain syndromes after brachial plexus injury in human neonates. *Brain* 2002;**125**(Pt 1):113–22.

357. Halloran DR, Alexander GR. Preterm delivery and age of SIDS death. *Ann Epidemiol* 2006;**16**(8):600–6.

358. Vennemann MM, Bajanowski T, Butterfass-Bahloul T, *et al.* Do risk factors differ between explained sudden unexpected death in infancy (SUDI) and SIDS? *Arch Dis Child* 2005; **90**(5):520–2.

359. Quaglini S, Rognoni C, Spazzolini C, Priori SG, Mannarino S, Schwartz PJ. Cost-effectiveness of neonatal ECG screening for the long QT syndrome. *Eur Heart J* 2006;**27**(15):1824–32.

360. Kum-Nji P, Meloy L, Herrod HG. Environmental tobacco smoke exposure: prevalence and mechanisms of causation of infections in children. *Pediatrics* 2006;**117**(5):1745–54.

361. Thach BT. The role of respiratory control disorders in SIDS. *Respir Physiol Neurobiol* 2005;**149**(1–3):343–53.

362. AAP. The changing concept of sudden infant death syndrome: diagnostic coding shifts, controversies regarding the sleeping environment, and new variables to consider in reducing risk. *Pediatrics* 2005;**116**(5):1245–55.

363. Dempsey EM, Barrington K. Crystalloid or colloid for partial exchange transfusion in neonatal polycythemia: a systematic review and meta-analysis. *Acta Paediatr* 2005; **94**(11):1650–5.

364. Armentrout DC, Huseby V. Polycythemia in the newborn. *MCN Am J Matern Child Nurs* 2003;**28**(4):234–9; quiz 240–1.

365. Cordero L, Franco A, Joy SD. Monochorionic monoamniotic twins: neonatal outcome. *J Perinatol* 2006;**26**(3):170–5.

366. Wiswell TE, Tin W, Ohler K. Evidence-based use of adjunctive therapies to ventilation. *Clin Perinatol* 2007;**34**(1): 191–204, ix.

367. Connor JA, Thiagarajan R. Hypoplastic left heart syndrome. *Orphanet J Rare Dis* 2007;**2**:23.

368. Ostrea EM, Villanueva-Uy ET, Natarajan G, Uy HG. Persistent pulmonary hypertension of the newborn: pathogenesis, etiology, and management. *Paediatr Drugs* 2006; **8**(3):179–88.

369. Birdi K, Prasad AN, Prasad C, Chodirker B, Chudley AE. The floppy infant: retrospective analysis of clinical experience (1990–2000) in a tertiary care facility. *J Child Neurol* 2005;**20** (10):803–8.

370. Vasta I, Kinali M, Messina S, *et al.* Can clinical signs identify newborns with neuromuscular disorders? *J Pediatr* 2005;**146**(1):73–9.

371. Rao P. Neonatal gastrointestinal imaging. *Eur J Radiol* 2006;**60**(2):171–86.

372. Moghal NE, Embleton ND. Management of acute renal failure in the newborn. *Semin Fetal Neonatal Med* 2006;**11**(3): 207–13.

373. Volmink J, Siegfried NL, van der Merwe L, Brocklehurst P. Antiretrovirals for reducing the risk of mother-to-child transmission of HIV infection. *Cochrane Database Syst Rev* 2007(1):CD003510.

374. Grosch-Worner I, Schafer A, Obladen M, *et al.* An effective and safe protocol involving zidovudine and caesarean section to reduce vertical transmission of HIV-1 infection. *Aids* 2000;**14**(18): 2903–11.

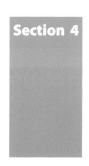

Section 4

Transport

Transport of preterm and term infants

Alan C. Fenton and Tilman Humpl

General aspects of neonatal transport

Neonatal emergency transport services (NETS) have evolved from single hospitals providing care for their immediate population to regionalized services, often operating as a managed clinical network, with designated centers providing tertiary care. Neonatal transfer services are key to the continued operation of these networks as they enable appropriate utilization of neonatal intensive care unit (NICU) beds: sick infants are moved to centers providing specialist intensive care and are subsequently returned for convalescent care.[1,2]

Neonatal transfer should be recognized as a **complex process** rather than a **single event**. It begins with the recognition of the need for transfer by a referring center and ends with the safe relocation of the patient to an appropriate facility. Key elements of any transfer service therefore must include[3]:

Organization and logistics

- Appropriately organized and coordinated transfer services
- Link to catchment area/population
- Operating with appropriate communication and liaison between all components of the service
- Agreed protocols and documentation and established quality control standards
- Direct affiliation to a particular neonatal unit
- Avoid transfers in an unplanned manner
- Avoid transfers using staff from the neonatal unit (depleting "in-house" staff establishment)

Communication

- Communication is essential and occurs between:
  - Referring and transport teams
  - Transport and accepting teams
  - Transport team and parents
- Ideally initiate the transfer process with a single call
- Provide initial advice whilst the appropriate specialists are contacted and a suitable facility is identified

Neonatal Emergencies: A Practical Guide for Resuscitation, Transport and Critical Care, ed. Georg Hansmann.
Published by Cambridge University Press. © Cambridge University Press 2009.

- Teleconferencing facility may be useful if more than one specialist is involved
- Record communications (paper-based or electronic means) to allow continuity of care and consistency of advice, and to enable subsequent review for quality improvement and risk management

Decision-making

- Recognition of a problem either in the patient or with the availability of facilities locally
- Patient assessment and stabilization begin at this point, i.e., well before the decision to dispatch the transfer team
- Establish clear guidelines for triaging referrals
- Senior staff are responsible for decision-making based on the most up-to-date information about the patient:
  - Understand the normal course of the patient's disease
  - Understand the logistics of transfer
  - Anticipate the duration of a transfer
  - Anticipate the potential adverse effects of transfer on the patient

Equipment considerations

- Conform to appropriate standards
- Should be adequately secured within the transport vehicle to prevent injury to staff or patients
- Appropriate certification for air transfers (i.e., radiofrequency interference)
- Functionality within the transfer environment (use of incubators in extreme ambient temperatures)
- Sufficient battery life and gas supplies for the entire transfer
- Staff must have appropriate competencies to enable them to use equipment safely and troubleshoot problems
- Daily checks should ensure equipment is functioning correctly
- Replace disposables immediately after each transfer
- Clear audit processes to monitor equipment preparation
- Routine protocols for infection control during and after neonatal transport (cleaning the incubators, diposable ventilation tubing, etc.)

Vehicles

- Familiarize transport team members with all vehicles used by their service
- Specific consideration to the safety considerations of air transport and the effects of altitude on patient physiology
- Choice of vehicle will be dictated by a combination of individual patient factors and availability
- The time gained by using aircraft (helicopter, fixed wing) is usually only of advantage when the ground-bound transport time exceeds 0.5–2 h (one-way).

Specifically trained staff

- Improves outcomes
- Team composition varies depending on the type of patient being transferred and illness severity (availability and cost considerations may play a part)

- Regular update of skills
  - Didactic teaching
  - Participation in Objective Structured Clinical Examination (OSCE)
  - Case scenario workshops
  - Review of particular cases/problems or practical skills

Resuscitation/stabilization of the patient before transfer

- Resuscitation must be commenced by the referring facility (pediatrician, anesthesiologist, obstetrician)
- May require input from the transfer team at the time of referral
- Focus on airway, breathing, and circulation (ABC)
  - Infants should be adequately stabilized prior to transfer unless they cannot be further improved or a delay in transfer would result in deterioration (for example in some infants referred for extracorporeal membrane oxygenation (ECMO))
  - Potential problems that might occur during transfer should be considered and appropriate interventions undertaken to minimize the likelihood of these problems actually occurring
- Establish adequate vascular access

Specific preparation of the patient for transport (pre-departure checklist)

- Is further stabilization required? (or possible?)
- Secure all vascular access, tubes and drains and attach sufficient monitoring equipment, (ECG leads, S_pO_2, etc.) before loading the patient into the transport incubator
- Check gas and power supplies (adequate for the return journey?)
- Complete documentation
- Ensure relevant communication with local and receiving staff and the infant's family

Delivery of care during transfer

- Interventions during transfer should be minimal (assuming that appropriate stabilization has been performed and potential problems anticipated)
- Mainstay of care is regular continuous monitoring
- All complications that may occur "in-house" may also occur during transfer
- If transferring a neonate by road ambulance: stop the vehicle before performing any intervention

Patient sign out

- Transfer of clinical responsibility for the patient to the receiving facility/physician
  - The infant's history
  - Interventions prior to and after the transfer team's arrival
  - Results of investigations
  - Information given to parents
  - Problems encountered during transfer
  - The infant's current status
- The sign-out process should be documented in the transfer protocol

Documentation

- Full, accurate and contemporaneous documentation is essential at each stage of the transfer ("If it isn't documented, it didn't happen")
- How often vitals signs, etc. may be documented will be dictated by the infant's condition (e.g., a ventilated patient should have vital signs documented every 15 min)
- The transfer protocol is part of the subsequent patient record
- Regular review of documentation should form part of the transfer service quality improvement program

Safety

- Transfer environment is potentially hostile (transport in winter conditions)
- Safety considerations include those related to team members and the patient in addition to operational and clinical protocols

Teaching, training, and outreach education

- Ensure that individual team members are properly trained
- Referring staff need to be able to recognize conditions that warrant transfer and should be able to initiate sufficient resuscitative measures pending the NETS arrival

Specific problems during neonatal transport
Temperature regulation

- Acceptable temperature range:
  - Axillary or rectally: 36.5–37.5°C (97.7–99.4°F)
  - Skin: 36–37°C (96.8–98.6°F)
- Very small preterm infants are especially susceptible to hypothermia:
  - Unfavorable relation between body surface and body weight
  - Underdeveloped subcutaneous fat
  - No chemical thermogenesis

Cold stress

- Causes
  - Loss of heat through convection and evaporation
    - Insufficient adjusted temperature (see Figure 2.10, p. 34)
    - Insufficient warmth protection (wet blankets, gauze, clothing, open incubator doors, air draft)
    - Transfer to the transport incubator
    - Procedures if incubator doors or portholes are left open
  - Move the transport incubator to, from, and between vehicles as quickly as possible (in extreme cold: use insulated incubator covers)
  - Polyethylene bags can greatly reduce heat loss following delivery in preterm infants – leave until after transfer is completed (do not use wet gauze or blankets!)
  - Infants with abdominal wall defects are also at risk for heat loss ($\rightarrow$ use bag)
- Symptoms
  - Poor peripheral perfusion (weak pulse, capillary refill >2 s)
  - Acrocyanosis

- Lethargia
- Apnea
- Bradycardia

! Hypothermia may have a protective effect on cell metabolism (e.g., reduction of hypoxic-ischemic brain damage after birth asphyxia, and therapeutic hypothermia may be applied to newborns s/p birth asphyxia during their transport from the delivery room to the NICU and beyond (i.e., for the next 72 h in the NICU)[4,5]. However, hypothermia should not be induced during transport of either stable or critically ill newborn infants who do not meet the criteria of hypoxic-ischemic brain damage, or by transport teams lacking experience in these measures! In any case, hyperthermia should be avoided during neonatal resuscitation, transports, and intensive care.

- Consequences
  - Hypoglycemia
  - Respiratory distress syndrome
  - Persistent acidosis
  - Hypoxemia
  - Shock
  - Death

Heat stress
- Causes
  - "Environmental" (e.g., incubator temperature set too high, over-wrapped infant, radiant heat, sunlight)
  - "Dressed" child in an improperly overheated incubator
- Symptoms
  - Tachycardia
  - Tachypnea
  - Peripheral vasodilatation

Breathing
- Monitoring with pulse oximetry
- Avoid hyperoxia!
- Avoid prophylactic oxygen therapy – especially in preterm infants
- Caution: in preterm infants with S_aO_2 values >92% → reduce F_iO_2
- Oxygen delivery (if indicated)
  - Flood incubator with oxygen (calibrate O_2 sensor)
  - Nasal prongs
  - Continuous positive airways pressure (CPAP) or endotracheal tube (ETT)

! In cases of sudden oxygen requirement: bag-and-mask system is more effective than flooding the incubator. Always connect a bag-and-mask system to oxygen tubing and the oxygen source.

- The indication for mechanical ventilation in a neonate is usually respiratory failure:
  - Central etiology (e.g., asphyxia with CNS depression)
  - Muscle fatigue
  - Inability to expand stiff lungs (e.g., poor lung compliance in RDS)

- Early use of *CPAP* may reduce the subsequent need for ventilation by maximizing functional residual capacity (FRC) and minimizing the work of breathing
- If there is any doubt as to whether an infant may be maintained on CPAP for the duration of the transfer, it is advisable to intubate and ventilate prior to departure
- Tendency to ET tube dislocation (unilateral intubation, spontaneous extubation) and ET tube obstruction. **A mechanically ventilated newborn who suffers from sudden respiratory decompensation during transport has ETT dislocation, ETT obstruction or pneumothorax unless proven otherwise (i.e., check for those emergencies immediately).** See "Pitfalls during neonatal transports", p. 499.
- Airways are not protected (aspiration, overdistension of the stomach is possible)
- Contraindications to the use of CPAP include the presence of intra-abdominal pathology due to the risks of bowel distension

---

Circulation (hemodynamics)

- **Assess the baby** by looking at peripheral perfusion, urine output, and metabolic acidosis
- Well babies with a "low BP" do not always require treatment whilst the same value in a "sick" baby may require intervention
- **Be aware that BP alone does not necessarily reflect cardiac output** (i.e., mean arterial pressure (MAP) may be normal for gestational age (GA) but mixed venous SO_2 might be low and lactate high)
- The method of choice used for arterial BP measurement will depend on the clinical condition of the baby and the access available
  - **Intra-arterial** measurement is the "gold standard." The transducer should be accurately calibrated and placed at the same level as the baby's right atrium. The waveform should be sufficiently undamped so that the dicrotic notch is clearly visible
  - **Doppler** measurement using a standard sphygmomanometer gives readings closest to intra-arterial measurements but may cause fluctuations in BP whilst it is being carried out. The cuff should be soft and the largest size that fits comfortably on the upper arm. The transducer should be placed over the radial artery
  - **Oscillometric** measurement (e.g., Dinamap®) is very useful in many babies because it allows frequent measurements to be made without much disturbance and, most of the time, gives readings that correlate closely with simultaneous intra-arterial values. *This method tends to overestimate BP if the limb is edematous or if the systemic circulation is poor, and should always be validated against a Doppler or arterial measurement*

Metabolism

Avoid hypoglycemia:

- During the transport provide continuous maintenance infusion
  - $D_{10}W$, glucose infusion rate (GIR) at 3 ml/kg/h ($=5$ mg/kg/min)
  - Use D_5W during the transport of preterm/term neonates with high normal or increased blood glucose levels (e.g., shortly after resuscitation)

- Term/preterm neonates with *blood glucose (D-stix) values <45 mg/dl*:
  2–5 ml $D_{10}W$/kg/dose IV. After $D_{10}W$ bolus, double maintenance fluids to $D_{10}W$ 6 ml/kg/h (=10 mg/kg/min) until arrival on NICU and documentation of two blood glucose levels in the normal range (60–120 mg/dl), then adjust GIR

! Newborn infants may be compromised by the key "*H's*": hyperthermia/hypothermia, hypotension, hyperoxia/hypoxia, hypercarbia/hypocarbia, and hypoglycemia.

Central nervous system

Avoid intraventricular hemorrhage caused by neonatal transport:

- Mechanical stress, hypothermia, hypoxia, blood pressure changes, acidosis, etc. can trigger intraventricular hemorrhage in preterm neonates (and also in term infants):
  - Lift the transport incubator when passing over expansion joints or other uneven ground
  - Move and turn the transport incubator carefully
  - Gently load and unload the transport incubator
  - Elevate the hydraulic stretcher in the ambulance
  - Drive carefully: avoid sudden acceleration and breaking maneuvers
  - Position the neonate on a mattress with liquid silicon ($\rightarrow$ prevents increase of oscillation arising during the transport); additional mini pillow, placed at the head-end of the inner incubator as additional protection

---

Pitfalls during neonatal transport: sudden clinical deterioration
- ET tube position?
- ET tube obstruction?
- ET tube twisted or kinked?
- Pneumothorax? (In emergency cases: use 18–20 G needle and aspirate)
- Continuous infusion disconnected or not intravascularly (prostaglandin E (PGE), inotropes, etc.)?
- Monitoring and symptoms do not match up

Typical scenarios in the neonatal emergency transport service (NETS)

Transport of preterm and term infants out of the delivery room
Indication
Sudden clinical deterioration, e.g. due to:
- Respiratory disorder (e.g., wet lung, RDS, pneumonia, pneumothorax)
- Infection
- CNS disorder (e.g., cerebral seizures, suspicion of intracranial hemorrhage (ICH))
- Cyanosis (e.g., congenital heart disease)
- Malformation (e.g., esophageal atresia $\rightarrow$ concern for aspiration)

Consider intubation and mechanical ventilation early (the transport incubator in the ambulance or aircraft is the worst place to perform an intubation or any other procedure).

Provide sedation and analgesia whenever needed (bumpy roads may cause discomfort for the ventilated infant). Muscle relaxant agents are rarely indicated.

Management

Depending on the regional circumstances and symptoms:

- ABCD measures and stabilization according to clinical diagnosis by the physicians/nurses in the delivery room/or by the transport team
- Transfer newborn in a transport incubator
- Transfer within a close distance to the NICU and in relatively stable condition:
  - ABCD measures
  - Supportive therapy (e.g., oxygen supplement, pharyngeal CPAP $D_{10}W$ infusion)
  - Care of term/preterm infants will be continued by the admitting NICU

Transport of preterm and term infants from NICU to NICU

Indications

- Adequate technical equipment is not available (e.g., inhaled nitric oxide (iNO), high-frequency oscillatory ventilation (HFOV), dialysis, etc.)
- Malformations (e.g., surgical intervention)
- Congenital heart disease
- Surgical closure of patent ductus arteriosus (PDA) and other indications

Before the transport

- Identification of risks and proper preparation, for example:
  - Secure IV access, consider extra IV access catheter for emergency drug or volume injection (connect with a three-way stopcock)
  - Secure connection for invasive arterial blood pressure monitoring
  - Assure whether the securely fixed ETT is in the correct position (exam, CXR)
  - Is reliable monitoring in place?
  - Estimate the duration of transport (Are the infusions sufficient? Blood glucose monitoring necessary?)
  - Know exact address of the admitting facility (city, ward, floor)
- Use the most appropriate transport vehicle (ambulance, helicopter, aircraft)
- Caring for the infant is a continuous process (from the initial resuscitation → transport → NICU)
- Consider needs of the parents and the child

> **!** The transfer of critically ill preterm and newborn infants between hospitals is not without risk and should only be performed if it will be of significant benefit for these patients.

Airborne transport of preterm and term infants (helicopter or fixed-wing aeroplane; Figure 4.1; Table 4.1)

Indications
- Rural areas
- Long-distance transport

Checklist for the departure of the NETS-team to the admitting hospital
Landing possibility has to be clarified: frequent transfers (e.g., ambulance – helicopter – ambulance) of the incubator and the transport team may delay the transport. Check availability of an ambulance at the landing area! Is transport with a helicopter or fixed-wing aircraft really indicated, or is the patient better off with a ground-bound transfer?
- *Decision-making process:*
  - Weather conditions?
  - Necessary stopovers (e.g., fuel? talk to pilot?)
  - Is the transport with an emergency helicopter justified under these conditions?

Disadvantages of a helicopter transport
- Limited space
- Darkness
- Decreased partial pressure of oxygen
- Noise
- Vibration
- Low temperatures
- Limited monitoring (auscultation during a flight is impossible), therefore:
  - Use visual alarms
  - End-tidal CO_2 (if available – indicator for correct ET tube position)
  - Observe chest movements

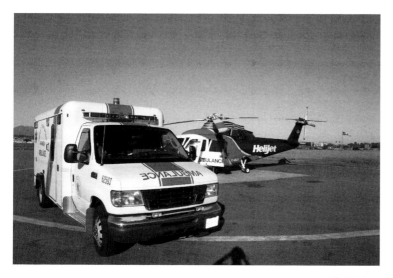

Figure 4.1
Ambulance and helicopter used in the neonatal emergency transport service (NETS).

Table 4.1 Comparison of ground and airborne transfers

Patient		Staff	
Advantages	**Disadvantages**	**Advantages**	**Disadvantages**
Ground transfer			
Easier monitoring	Safety	Patient access	Motion sickness
Acute emergencies	Speed (traffic)	Monitoring	Safety
Door to door		Space	Speed (traffic)
Rapid 'all-weather' availabilty		Cost	
Space			
Helicopter transfer			
Urban use	Safety	Urban use	Motion sickness
Immediate landing	Monitoring	Immediate landing	Safety
Speed	Altitude/temperature	Speed	Comfort
	Range/turbulence		Patient access
	Noise/vibration		Space
	Acute emergencies		Cost
	Weather limited		Landing zone availability
Fixed-wing transfer			
Range	Limited access	Comfort	Motion sickness
Weather	Monitoring	Speed	Safety
Speed	Altitude/temperature		Patient access
Safety	Vibration/noise		Ground transfer
	Ground transfer		Cost

- Limited communication (headphones, microphone)
- Limitation of resuscitation measures (intubation and venous access during the flight is very difficult! Landing is often necessary, but not always immediately feasible)
- Effects on the medical personnel:
  - Motion sickness (with dizziness and nausea)
  - Inhalation of potentially toxic gases (carbon monoxide, etc.)
  - Security (crash)

Problems of helicopter/or aircraft (fixed-wing) transport
- **Air-filled chambers (expansion of air according to Boyle's law):**
  - Within the patient:
    - Pneumothorax
    - Pneumomediastinum
    - Pneumopericardium

- Gastrointestinal obstruction (ileus)
- Air in balloons/cuffs (e.g., trapped air in the bladder catheter (Foley), rarely: cuffed ET tube)
- Outside the patient:
  - Blood pressure cuffs

> **!** Before transport by helicopter or aircraft: always place a gastric tube, even if the patient is not intubated, and confirm proper positioning.

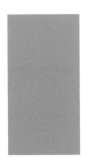

Acute antenatal transfer

Alan C. Fenton and Tilman Humpl

Acute antenatal transfer is an alternative (nearly always superior) to postnatal transfer in situations where local facilities are insufficient to provide the necessary care for sick or high-risk (e.g., preterm) infants or their mothers. This group does not include pregnancies where an antenatally detected problem (for example, congenital heart disease) results in the planned delivery of an infant in a specialist center. Rates of acute antenatal transfers vary considerably and may be influenced by the level of care configuration of neonatal intensive care services, local availability of staff, and distance to the referral center.

Indications for transfer

- Requirement for enhanced care for mother, fetus or neonate
- Local neonatal unit closed/full
- Lack of availability of neonatal cot of the appropriate level. The likelihood of the infant needing such a cot needs to be assessed using all available information, e.g., gestational age, intrauterine growth retardation (IUGR), etc.
- Neonatal team request – staffing/work load ratio
- Delivery suite capacity

The majority of antenatal transfers are performed primarily for fetal reasons:
- Anticipated or established preterm labor
- Imminent delivery is anticipated
- Preeclampsia or amniorrhexis

Other indications for antenatal transfer:
- Intrauterine infection
- Hemolytic disease of the newborn
- Fetal brady- and tachyarrhythmia
- Severe fetal growth retardation
- Oligohydramnios
- Fetal malformation
- Multiple gestation
- Chronic or acute maternal diseases:
  - Diabetes mellitus
  - Heart disease
  - Infections: HIV, HSV, CMV, toxoplasmosis
  - Current drug abuse

Neonatal Emergencies: A Practical Guide for Resuscitation, Transport and Critical Care, ed. Georg Hansmann.
Published by Cambridge University Press. © Cambridge University Press 2009.

- Potential risk for the child due to drug intake during pregnancy
- Condition after solid organ transplantation
- Hypo/hyperthyroidism
- Phenylketonuria
- Autoimmune disease

Several studies have reported lower neonatal mortality and morbidity (respiratory disease, patent ductus arteriosus, intraventricular hemorrhage, and nosocomial infection) in infants delivered after in-utero transfer compared to infants transferred postnatally.[6,7] However, confounding variables such as case selection, birth weight, and gestation at delivery or working practices may be responsible for these apparent differences.[8] Not all studies have reported significant differences in outcome between antenatal and postnatal transfers.[9] Antenatal transport of high-risk pregnant women to tertiary centers is nearly always the better alternative, given that the rate of prematurely delivered newborns is inversely correlated with the quality of care and neonatal outcomes in those non-level-III (non-tertiary) nurseries. Requirements for neonatal intensive care following antenatal transfer are difficult to predict, not least because many women remain undelivered. Only one study to date has related the likelihood of delivery to the reason for transfer.[10]

Potential maternal complications of antenatal transfer

- Hypertensive crisis
- Eclampsia
- Hemorrhage
- Delivery
- Social dislocation
- Vehicle accidents

Prior to transfer appropriate stabilization of the mother's medical condition must be undertaken. Cervical assessment immediately prior to transfer using translabial or trans-rectal ultrasonography may indicate the extent to which labor has progressed since referral. Tocolysis and delayed active management of the second stage of labor may also reduce the likelihood of delivery during transfer.

The selection of staff to accompany an antenatal transfer will vary with both the health care setting and general availability of personnel. In general, paramedics will often be present. In Europe the majority of antenatal transfers may be accompanied by a midwife. Additional obstetric staff may accompany these transfers if there are co-existent problems such as breech presentation or more than one fetus. The use of pediatric staff on this type of transport is not always mandatory.

In contrast to neonatal transfers, during which monitoring is an essential component of the care, the use of fetal heart rate monitoring during antenatal transfer is questionable. Whilst monitoring may enhance knowledge of the fetal condition, therapeutic strategies are limited to administration of oxygen, tocolysis, and change in maternal position.

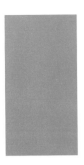

Questions for review

1. How may the likelihood of problems on transport be minimized? See pp. 493–503.
2. Under which conditions may stabilization before transfer be deferred? See pp. 493–503.
3. What steps are required in the specific preparation of a patient for transfer? See pp. 493–503.
4. What are the components of proper patient sign out to the NICU team following transfer? See pp. 493–503.
5. How may cold stress be minimized during infant transfer? See pp. 493–503. Figure 2.10, p. 34.
6. What methods are available to measure arterial blood pressure during transfer? See pp. 493–503.
7. What are the most common causes of infant deterioration during transfer? See pp. 493–503.
8. List the potential problems caused by gas within body compartments during transfer by aircraft. See pp. 493–503.
9. What are the most common indications for antenatal transfer? See p. 504.
10. What are the potential maternal complications of antenatal transfer? See p. 505.

Neonatal Emergencies: A Practical Guide for Resuscitation, Transport and Critical Care, ed. Georg Hansmann.
Published by Cambridge University Press. © Cambridge University Press 2009.

References (Section 4)

1. Mori R, Fujimura M, Shiraishi J, *et al.* Duration of inter-facility neonatal transport and neonatal mortality: systematic review and cohort study. *Pediatr Int* 2007;**49** (4):452–8.

2. Das UG, Leuthner SR. Preparing the neonate for transport. *Pediatr Clin North Am* 2004;**51**(3):581–98, vii.

3. Woodward GA, Insoft RM, Kleinman ME, Alexander SN. *Guidelines for Air and Ground Transport of Neonatal and Pediatric Patients*, 3rd edn. Elk Grove Village: Section on Transport Medicine, American Academy of Pediatrics, 2007.

4. Zanelli SA, Naylor M, Dobbins N, *et al.* Implementation of a "Hypothermia for HIE" program: 2-year experience in a single NICU. *J Perinatol* 2008;**28**(3):171–5.

5. Gunn AJ, Hoehn T, Hansmann G, *et al.* Hypothermia, an evolving treatment for neonatal hypoxic ischemic encephalopathy. *Pediatrics* 2008;**121**:648–9.

6. Kollee LA, Verloove-Vanhorick PP, Verwey RA, Brand R, Ruys JH. Maternal and neonatal transport: results of a national collaborative survey of preterm and very low birth weight infants in The Netherlands. *Obstet Gynecol* 1988;**72**(5):729–32.

7. Shlossman PA, Manley JS, Sciscione AC, Colmorgen GH. An analysis of neonatal morbidity and mortality in maternal (in utero) and neonatal transports at 24–34 weeks' gestation. *Am J Perinatol* 1997;**14** (8):449–56.

8. Field D, Draper ES. Survival and place of delivery following preterm birth: 1994–96. *Arch Dis Child Fetal Neonatal Ed* 1999;**80**(2): F111–14.

9. Beverley D, Foote K, Howel D, Congdon P. Effect of birthplace on infants with low birth weight. *Br Med J (Clin Res Ed)* 1986;**293** (6553):981–3.

10. Fenton AC, Ainsworth SB, Sturgiss SN. Population-based outcomes after acute antenatal transfer. *Paediatr Perinat Epidemiol* 2002;**16**(3):278–85.

Appendix

Training NICU nurses and paramedics in the neonatal emergency transport service (NETS)

Alan C. Fenton

Training programs for neonatal transport will in part depend on:
- The types of transfers to be undertaken
- The range of anticipated conditions in the patient population
- The background of team members

While training should focus on skill levels necessary to successfully transport patients rather than specific educational degrees, the recognition of transport as a specialist area within perinatal care has led to the establishment of academic courses for neonatal transport. Neonatal-trained nurses will in general have a large part of the requisite background knowledge and skills for neonatal transport. Paramedics will be familiar with working in a moving environment but will require intensive training to participate in "hands on" intensive care.

Basic training requirements should include

Organizational knowledge

An understanding of the logistics of the transfer process is essential. The best information about the infant's condition must be available to enable appropriate support to be given to the referring clinician and the appropriate decisions made regarding transfer.

- Models of transport
- Regional perinatal care
- Hospital vs. transport environment
- Principles of transport medicine
- Initiation of transport process
- Documentation
- Communication during transfer process
- Transport safety
- Medico-legal issues
- Viability
- Public relations

Neonatal Emergencies: A Practical Guide for Resuscitation, Transport and Critical Care, ed. Georg Hansmann. Published by Cambridge University Press. © Cambridge University Press 2009.

Practical knowledge

Team members must be able to diagnose and manage the infant's problem and to identify the most likely reasons for deterioration in their condition. This level of skill is generally achieved and maintained only through significant experience in caring for critically ill infants.

- Pathophysiology of congenital and acquired diseases of the newborn
- Common conditions of the newborn
- Normal/low-risk birth and neonates
- Abnormal/high-risk birth and neonates
- Transport physiology
- Air-medical physiology
- Stress management

Procedural skills (See pp. 511–12)

A very high level of expertise is necessary because practical procedures may be needed in the transfer environment.

- Resuscitation and advanced life support
- Physical examination/assessment
- Anatomy and physiology
- Equipment orientation
- Invasive monitoring
- Initiating intravenous infusions
- Arterial access
- Central venous lines
- Airway management and intubation
- Chest drain insertion
- Ventilator management

Miscellaneous

Extended training including didactic sessions on individual problems, case discussions, patient- or equipment-related scenarios and stress management may also be helpful in enabling staff to anticipate potential problems during the transfer process. A flexible approach is useful in dealing with problems outside the scope of established protocols, although it is essential that team members always operate within the scope of practice that they would use in their base hospital. Particular attention should be given to communication. Clearly team members must communicate well with each other in addition to communicating with:

- The referring facility
- The accepting facility
- The patient's family members who have to deal both with an acutely ill infant and the prospect of transfer away from home

All staff involved in neonatal transport should be able to critically appraise their performance and be involved in audit/quality improvement exercises. Regular updates of particular aspects of training will help maintain skills.

Training delivery room staff in the resuscitation of newborn infants

Sam Richmond

Resuscitating babies at birth, like resuscitation at other times of life, requires both theoretical knowledge and practical skills. Perhaps the most effective introduction to these is gained by attendance at a practical course designed for the purpose, ideally followed by a period of well supervised in-service training. Two such courses are currently in widespread use. The Newborn Life Support course[1], developed by the Resuscitation Council (UK) and endorsed by all relevant UK professional bodies, has been available in the UK since 1999 and has more recently become available in other countries in Europe under the auspices of the European Resuscitation Council. In the USA the Neonatal Resuscitation Program[2], first developed by the American Academy of Pediatrics in 1985, is very widely used and has spread to other countries. Members of the committees controlling the development of each of these courses also work together as members of the neonatal section of the International Liaison Committee on Resuscitation (ILCOR)[3], thus ensuring that a reasonably consistent approach is adopted by both courses. Whatever system is adopted for training doctors and other delivery room staff, it is important that those involved in teaching should themselves have not only significant practical experience of newborn resuscitation but also appropriate skills in teaching[4].

Theoretical knowledge

An understanding of the physiology of birth asphyxia (as outlined in the chapter on resuscitation of newborns at birth, p. 150) leads logically to the familiar ABCD approach (Airway, Breathing, Circulation, Drugs), which can be readily adapted to this situation. Such information is easy to impart using written materials and standard lecture techniques.

Practical skills

Successful resuscitation at birth is crucially dependent on establishing an open airway followed by effective lung inflation. The vast majority of babies in difficulty at birth will respond immediately to these simple measures with only a small minority appearing to require more invasive procedures such as chest compression, umbilical venous access and the administration of drugs. The skills required are amenable to teaching in groups using the standard four-stage technique. This technique involves the teacher first demonstrating the skill in question at the appropriate pace and without commentary. He or she then repeats the demonstration while providing a commentary, this time breaking the skill down into simple steps performed more slowly. The third stage involves one of the learners providing a commentary as the skill is demonstrated a third time, and in the fourth stage each of the learners demonstrates the skill while providing a commentary themselves. Given sufficient time this is then followed by further individual supervised practice.

Neonatal Emergencies: A Practical Guide for Resuscitation, Transport and Critical Care, ed. Georg Hansmann.
Published by Cambridge University Press. © Cambridge University Press 2009.

Scenario teaching

The information gleaned from the lectures and the skills gained from the small-group practical demonstrations can then be fused together by means of role play using standard resuscitation equipment and appropriate manikins. Situations can be presented and worked through by the candidates in small groups under the supervision of suitably trained instructors. Such a process can be fairly stressful for candidates but, as long as the instructors maintain a non-threatening environment where feedback is supportive but honest, this is a very powerful learning tool. It is also very useful for brief review sessions during quiet periods on the wards. Complex and expensive computerized neonatal manikins are in development which may enhance this process but the standard manikins currently available already provide very valuable experience.

Refining skills

The need for (advanced) resuscitation at birth is relatively uncommon. Skills therefore need to be maintained despite being only rarely needed. Regular scenario revision sessions as suggested above are useful, as are formal debriefing sessions after any significant resuscitation episode[5]. These debriefing sessions can be very significantly enhanced if video recording of the resuscitation episode is available for discussion, though various legal and ethical issues need to be addressed to allow this[6].

Web links: societies, hospitals, guidelines and learning programs

Georg Hansmann

Abnormal newborn neurologic exams, University of Utah: http://library.med.utah.edu/pedineurologicexam/html/home_exam.html

American Academy of Pediatrics (AAP homepage): www.aap.org

American Academy of Pediatrics (Neonatal Resuscitation Program) www.aap.org/nrp/nrpmain.html

American Heart Association (CPR & ECC): www.americanheart.org

Antiarrhythmic drug dosages and preparations for children, UCSF and Stanford University: http://pediep.stanford.edu/Drug_guide-2000.html#anchor419046

Bilirubin and indications for phototherapy. www.bilitool.com

Cardiovascular Disorders, Lucile Packard Children's Hospital, Stanford University: www.lpch.org/DiseaseHealthInfo/HealthLibrary/cardiac/chdhub.html

Center for Advanced Pediatric and Perinatal Education (CAPE), Stanford University: http://cape.lpch.org/index.html

Council On Medical Student Education in Pediatrics (COMSEP): www.comsep.org/EducationalResources/MultimediaTeaching.htm

Dermatology Atlas: http://dermatlas.med.jhmi.edu/derm/

Digital Library (Archives of Radiology): http://www.pediatricradiology.com

ECG library: www.ecglibrary.com/

General Pediatrics – one of the most complete sites for pediatric links: www.general pediatrics.com/

The Heart Center Encyclopedia – Cincinnati's Children's Hospital Medical Center: www.cincinnatichildrens.org/health/heart-encyclopedia/default.htm

The Hospital for Sick Children, Toronto: www.sickkids.ca

Hot Topics in Neonatology, Washington, DC: www.hottopics.org/

Maternal and Child Health Library: http://www.mchlibrary.info

MD consult: www.mdconsult.com

Multimedia Library, Children's Hospital Boston: www.childrenshospital.org/cfapps/mml/index.cfm

Neonatal Dermatology. Auckland City Hospital: www.adhb.govt.nz/newborn/Teaching Resources/Dermatology/OtherLesions.htm

Neonatal Handbook, NETS, Victoria, Australia. www.netsvic.org.au/nets/handbook

Neonatology on the web (Cedar Sinai Medical Center):http://www.neonatology.org/

NICHD Cochrane Neonatal Homepage (reviews): www.nichd.nih.gov/cochrane/default.cfm

NICU-Web – University of Washington, Seattle: http://neonatal.peds.washington.edu/

Pediatrics Center (Martindale's Health Science Guide; excellent): www.martindalecenter.com/MedicalPed.html

Neonatal Emergencies: A Practical Guide for Resuscitation, Transport and Critical Care, ed. Georg Hansmann.
Published by Cambridge University Press. © Cambridge University Press 2009.

Primary Care Dermatology Module Nomenclature of Skin Lesions – University of Wisconsin: www.pediatrics.wisc.edu/education/derm/tutorials.html

Radiology Cases in Neonatology (University of Hawaii): www.hawaii.edu/medicine/pediatrics/neoxray/neoxray.html

Radiology Education (Pediatric Radiology): www.radiologyeducation.com

Recommended Standards for Newborn ICU Design: www.nd.edu/~nicudes/

Royal Children's Hospital Melbourne (Clinical Practice Guidelines): www.rch.org.au/clinicalguide/

Transport of the Critically Ill Newborn, emedicine. www.emedicine.com/ped/topic2730.htm

UpToDate. http://www.uptodate.com/home/clinicians/index.html

Vermont Oxford Network: http://www.vtoxford.org

Virtual Pediatric Hospital: www.virtualpediatrichospital.org/

The Visible Embryo: www.visembryo.com

Growth charts (Figure 5.1)

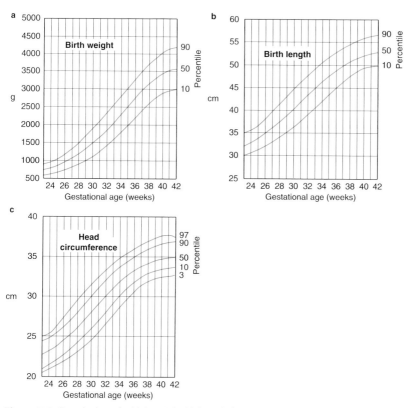

Figure 5.1 Growth charts for birth weight (a), length (b) and head circumference (c) in relation to gestational age.

Neonatal Emergencies: A Practical Guide for Resuscitation, Transport and Critical Care, ed. Georg Hansmann.
Published by Cambridge University Press. © Cambridge University Press 2009.

Bilirubin diagrams and transfusion exchange limits (Table 5.1, Figure 5.2)

Table 5.1 Therapeutic interventions in hyperbilirubinemia

Age (h)	Total bilirubin mg/dl (µmol/l)			
	Consider phototherapy	Phototherapy	Phototherapy 4–6h, if w/o success: exchange transfusion[a]	Exchange transfusion
25–48	≥12 (170)	≥15 (260)	≥20 (340)	≥25 (430)
49–72	≥15 (260)	≥18 (310)	≥25 (430)	≥30 (510)
>72	≥17 (290)	≥20 (340)	≥25 (430)	≥30 (510)

[a]Exchange transfusion, when bilirubin does not decrease by 1–2 mg/dl (20–30 µmol/l) within 4–6 h. Please note that newborn infants (e.g., VLBW, ELBW) with unconjugated bilirubin values >8–10 mg/dl in the first 24 h of life may require urgent phototherapy. For details, please refer to http://www.bilitool.com.

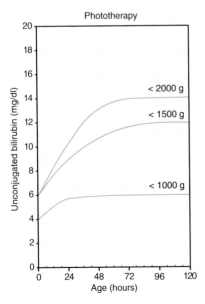

Figure 5.2 Phototherapy thresholds for preterm newborn infants and sick term newborn infants. For details, please refer to http://www.bilitool.com.

Neonatal Emergencies: A Practical Guide for Resuscitation, Transport and Critical Care, ed. Georg Hansmann. Published by Cambridge University Press. © Cambridge University Press 2009.

Aortic blood pressure during the first 12 h of life in infants with birth weight 610–4220 g (Figure 5.3)

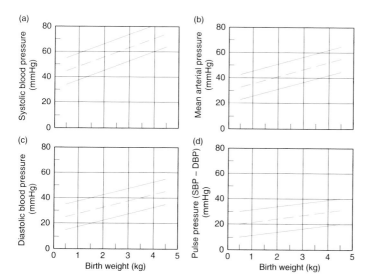

(a)

Systolic blood pressure (mmHg)

(b)

Mean arterial pressure (mmHg)

(c)

Diastolic blood pressure (mmHg)

Birth weight (kg)

(d)

Pulse pressure (SBP – DBP) (mmHg)

Birth weight (kg)

Fig. 5.3a–d Normogram of aortic blood pressure (mmHg) during the first 12 hours of life in infants with birth weight 610–4220 g. From Versmold HT, Kitterman JA, Phibbs RH, Gregory GA, Tooley WH. Aortic blood pressure during the first 12 hours of life in infants with birth weight 610 to 4220 grams. *Pediatrics* 1981; 67:607–13.

Neonatal Emergencies: A Practical Guide for Resuscitation, Transport and Critical Care, ed. Georg Hansmann. Published by Cambridge University Press. © Cambridge University Press 2009.

Laboratory: normal values (Tables 5.2–5.7)

Table 5.2 Normal laboratory values for blood, urine, and liquor analysis. Please note that normal values for very preterm infants are either not established or different than the ones given in the table below

Parameter	Age	SI units	Conventional units
Acid phosphatase, total 37°C			
Albumin		30–45 g/l	3.2–4.5 g/dl
Alkaline phosphatase, 37°C			
Ammonia		up to 150 µmol/l	up to 255 µg/dl
α-Amylase 37°C			
Antithrombin III		approx. 0.6–0.9 U/ml	approx. 38%–63%
α1-Antitrypsin		0.9–2.2 g/l	90–220 mg/dl
Bilirubin, total		see Figure 5.1 and Table 5.1 and also www.bilitool.com	
Bleeding time		2–7 min	2–7 min
Calcium, ionized	Term neonates	1.0–1.3 mmol/l	
	Preterm infants	0.9–1.3 mmol/l	
Calcium, total	Term neonates	1.75–2.7 mmol/l	7.0–10.8 mg/dl
	Preterm infants (aim)	2.1–2.8 mmol/l	8.4–11.2 mg/dl
Chloride		95–110 mmol/l	95–110 mval/l
Cholesterine		up to 5.0 mmol/l	up to 190 mg/dl
Cholinesterase, 37°C			
C-reactive protein (CRP)	day of life 1–3:	<20 mg/l	<2.0 mg/dl
	≥ 4 days old	<5 mg/l	<0.5 mg/dl
Creatinine[a]	age-dependent	Up to 58 µmol/l	Up to 0.6 mg/dl
Creatine kinase 37°C	1st–5th day of life	Up to 625 U/l	
	up to 6 months	Up to 295 U/l	
	7th–36 months	Up to 229 U/l	
Ferritin	0–7th day of life		90–770 µg/dl
	7th–14th day of life		250–950 µg/dl
	14th–21st day of life		160–770 µg/dl

Neonatal Emergencies: A Practical Guide for Resuscitation, Transport and Critical Care, ed. Georg Hansmann. Published by Cambridge University Press. © Cambridge University Press 2009.

Table 5.2 *(cont.)*

Parameter	Age	SI units	Conventional units
Glucose		2.8–5.6 mmol/l	50–100 mg/dl
Protein, total		46–68 g/l	4.6–6.8 g/dl
Protein fractions			
Albumin		57%–68%	57%–68%
Alpha₁ globulin		1%–6%	1%–6%
Alpha₂ globulin		5%–11%	5%–11%
Beta globulin		7%–13%	7%–13%
Gamma globulin		10%–18%	10%–18%
α-fetoprotein		<100 mg/l	<10 mg/dl
Fibrinogen		1.25–3.0 g/l	0.125–0.3 g/dl
Galactose		<0.4 mmol/l	<7.4 mg/dl
Gamma-glutamyl transpeptidase (γ-GT) 37°C	1st–5th day of life	Up to 194 U/l	
	Up to 6 months	up to 215 U/l	
	7th–12th month of life	up to 35 U/l	
Hemoglobin, total	1st–4th day of life	10.2–13.2 mmol/l	16.2–21.2 g/dl
	1st–2nd week of life	9.6–12.2 mmol/l	15.5–19.6 g/dl
	3rd–4th week of life	7.8–10.7 mmol/l	12.6–17.2 g/dl
	5th–12th week of life	6.5–7.8 mmol/l	10.5–12.6 g/dl
	≥12 weeks	6.8–8.9 mmol/l	11.0–14.4 g/dl
Hemoglobin, fetal (Hgbf)	Postnatal	70.0%–95.0% of the total Hgb	
		11.0%–33.0% of the total Hgb	
		0.2%–12.0% of the total Hgb	
Haptoglobin		0–0.4 g/l	0–40 mg/dl
17-Hydroxy-progesterone	2–10 days	0.7–12.4 µmol/l	0.13–2.8 µg/l

Immunoglobulins		IgG (g/l)	IgM (g/l)	IgA (g/l)
	Newborn	7.0–16	Undetectable	0.1–0.7
	1–3 months	2.5–7.5	0.05–0.5	0.1–0.7

Parameter	Age	SI units	Conventional units
Immunoglobulin E	Newborn	up to 1.5 IU/ml	Up to 3.6 ng/ml
Iron		7–33 µmol/l	40–184 µg/dl
Lipase 37°C			
Magnesium		0.7–1.5 mmol/l	1.7–3.7 mg/dl
Osmolality		260–295 mosmol/kg	260–295 mosmol/kg

Table 5.2 (*cont.*)

Parameter	Age	SI units	Conventional units
Phenylalanine		<121 µmol/l	<2 mg/dl
phosphorus		1.6–3.1 mmol/l	4.8–9.5 mg/dl (including preterm infants)
Potassium		3.6–6.0 mmol/l	3.6–6.0 mval/l
Pyruvate (fasting)		45–90 µmol/l	0.4–0.8 mg/dl
Renin		1.7–2.6 µg/l/h	
Sodium		135–145 mmol/l	130–145 mval/l
Thyroid-stimulating hormone (TSH)		<15 mU/l	<15 µU/ml
Thyroxine (T_4) Total	At birth	12.7 (5.9–19.5) µg/dl	163 (75–251) nmol/l
	24–48 h	16.5 (11.7–21.3) µg/dl	212 (150–274) nmol/l
	7 days	14.1 (8.1–20.1) µg/dl	181 (100–259) nmol/l
	1–12 months	10.8 (6.2–15.4) µg/dl	139 (78–199) nmol/l
Free tri-iodothyronine (fT_3)		2–8 pmol/l	2–8 pmol/l
Free thyroxine (fT_4)		9–23 pmol/l	9–23 pmol/l
Transaminases			
GOT (=AST), 37°C	1st–5th day of life up to 12 months	Up to 80 U/l	Up to 80 U/l
		Up to 67 U/l	Up to 67 U/l
GPT (=ALT), 37°C	1st–5th day of life up to 12 months	Up to 51 U/l	Up to 51 U/l
		Up to 59 U/l	
Transferrin		1.0–2.5 g/l	100–250 mg/dl 200–400 mg/dl
Transferrin saturation		30%–100%	30%–100%
Triglycerides	1st week of life	Up to 3.0 mmol/l	Up to 266 mg/dl
Urea nitrogen (BUN)		up to 7.1 mmol/l	up to 20 mg/dl
Uric acid		120–350 µmol/l	2–6 mg/dl

Table 5.2 (cont.)

Parameter	Age	SI units	Conventional units
Vitamin A	Up to 2 years	0.3–2.0 μmol/l	8.6–57 μg/dl
Zinc		9.8–16.8 μmol/l	64–110 μg/dl

[a]Creatinine concentration depends on chronological and gestational age.
Enzyme activities are now measured at 37°C (since 2003).
Enzyme activities are based upon a conversion of established old normal values at different temperature.
Unestablished normal values are left blank.
GOT, Glutamyl oxaloacetic transaminase; AST, aspartate aminotransferase.
GPT, Glutamyl pyruvic transaminase; ALT, alanine aminotransferase.

Table 5.3 Normal laboratory values of red blood cells (erythrocytes). Please note that normal values for very preterm infants are either not established or different than the ones given in the table below.

Age	Absolute number					
	RBC ($\times 10^3$/µl)	Reticulocytes (‰ RBC)	Hematocrit (%)	MCV (μm^3 = fl)	MCH (pg)	MCHC (%)
1st day of life	5.5 (4.5–6.5)	42 (15–65)		106 (99–113)	35.5 (33–38)	33.5 (31.8–35.2)
5th day of life	5.3 (4.4–6.1)	30 (10–50)	60 (58–62)			
7th day of life	5.2 (4.4–5.9)	10 (5–15)		103 (96–119)	35.3 (96–110)	34.5 (32.8–36.2)
2nd week	5.0 (3.0–5.5)	8 (3–13)	55 (53–58)			
4th week	4.7 (3.9–5.3)	8 (3–13)	44 (41–48)	100 (94–106)	33.5 (31.5–35.5)	34.2 (32.7–35.7)
2nd month	4.5 (3.7–5.0)	8 (3–15)	37 (34–39)			

RBC, Red blood cells; MCV, mean corpuscular volume; MCH = mean corpuscular hemoglobin; MCHC = mean corpuscular hemoglobin concentration. A normal range of value is given in parentheses.

Table 5.4 Normal laboratory values of white blood cells (leukocytes, $\times 10^3/\mu l$ or $\times 10^9/l$) and platelets. Please note that normal values for very preterm infants are either not established or different from the ones given in the table below.

	Absolute number	
WBC = Leukocytes ($\times 10^3/\mu l$ or $\times 10^9/l$)		
Directly after birth	18.1	(8.0–30.0)
12 h	22.8	(13.0–38.0)
1 week old	12.2	(9.4–34.0)
2 weeks old	11.4	(5.0–20.0)
4 weeks old	10.8	(5.0–19.5)
Granulocytes		%
Neutrophils	2250–9750/µl	25–65
Bands	0–1500/µl	0–10
Segmented neutrophils	2250–9750/µl	22–65
Eosinophils	90–1050/µl	1–7
Basophils	0–300/µl	0–2
Mononuclear leukocytes		
Monocytes	630–3000/µl	7–20
Lymphocytes	1800–10 500/µl	20–70
Platelets (thrombocytes)	100 000–250 000/µl	

Table 5.5 Normal laboratory values for blood coagulation tests. Please note that normal values for very preterm infants are either not established or different from the ones given in the table below. Numbers indicate mean (range) and depend on the assay used ($\rightarrow$ institutional reference values).

Coagulation test	Preterm infant	Full-term infant
Activated partial prothrombin time = APTT[a] (s)		day 1: 39 (34–45)
		day 3: 36 (30–42)
Prothrombin time = PT (s)		day 1: 16 (14–16)
		day 3: 15 (14–16)
International normalized ratio (INR)		day 1: 1.26 (1.15–1.35)
		day 3: 1.20 (1.05–1.35)
Fibrinogen		day 1: 280 (192–374)
		day 3: 330 (283–401)
Antithrombin III = AT III (%)		day 1: 76 (58–90)
		day 3: 74 (60–89)

[a]The STA-PTT-A assay reagent was used.

Table 5.6 Normal laboratory values of urine analysis. Please note that normal values for very preterm infants are either not established or different from the ones given in the table below.

Urine analysis

RBC (erythrocytes)	0–5/μl
Protein	<150 mg/m^2 of body surface area/day
Calcium^a	1–2 mmol/l; Ca^{2+}/creatinine = 0.28–1.12 or
	0.2–0.5 $\frac{mg/dl\ mg/\mu l}{mg/dl\ mg/dl}$
Copper	5–120 μmol Cu/mol creatinine
	(=3–67 μg Cu/g Creatinine) in morning urine
Leucocytes (WBC)	
Upper limit of normal	20/μl
Infection likely	20–50/μl
Sodium	0.5–4.9 mmol/kg/day
Creatinine	8–15 mg/kg/day
Phosphorus^b	1–2 mmol/l; P/Crea ratio = 0.8–8.03 or
	0.8–2.2 $\frac{mg/dl\ mg/\mu l}{mg/dl\ mg/dl}$
Osmolality	Up to 600 mosmol/l
pH	5.0–7.0

^{a}Calcium conversion factor: mg/dl × 0.2495 = mmol/l.
^{b}Phosphorus conversion factor: mg/dl × 0.3229 = mmol/l.

Table 5.7 Normal laboratory values of cerebrospinal fluid (CSF) analysis. Please note that normal values for very preterm infants are either not established or different from the ones given in the table below.

Cerebrospinal fluid (CSF)	SI unit	Conventional unit
Albumin	0.1–0.17 g/l	10–17 mg/dl
Protein, total		
Postnatally	Up to 1.0 g/l	Up to 100 (150) mg/dl
1st month	Up to 0.9 g/l	Up to 90 mg/dl
from the 2nd month	Up to 0.4 g/l	Up to 40 mg/dl
Glucose	45%–80% of blood glucose	
Immunoglobulins	IgG 6–64 mg/l	0.6–6.4 mg/dl
	IgA 4–6 mg/l	0.4–0.6 mg/dl
	IgM 0	0
WBC (leukocytes)		
Newborn	Up to 9 (–22)/μl	
Older children	Up to 5/μl	

Unit conversions

Pressure

$1\,\text{mbar} = 0.75\,\text{mmHg}$ (mbar $\times$ 0.750 28 = mmHg)

mbar $\simeq$ cmH$_2$O

$1\,\text{cmH}_2\text{O} \simeq 1\,\text{mbar} = 0.736\,\text{mmHg}$

$1\,\text{kPa} = 7.5\,\text{mmHg}$ (kPa $\times$ 7.5 = mmHg)

$1\,\text{kPa} = 10\,\text{cmH}_2\text{O} = 7.5\,\text{mmHg} = 10\,\text{mbar}$

$1\,\text{cmH}_2\text{O} = 98.0665\,\text{Pa} = 9.806\,65 \times 10^{-2}\,\text{KPa}$

kPa $\times$ 10 $\simeq$ cmH$_2$O

kPa $\times$ 7.5 = mmHg

Diameter

$1\text{F} = 1\,\text{Ch} = 0.33\,\text{mm}$

Neonatal Emergencies: A Practical Guide for Resuscitation, Transport and Critical Care, ed. Georg Hansmann.
Published by Cambridge University Press. © Cambridge University Press 2009.

References (Section 5)

1. Richmond S, ed. *Resuscitation at Birth*, 2nd edn. London: Resuscitation Council (UK), 2006.

2. Kattwinkel J. *Neonatal Resuscitation*, 5th edn. Elk Grove Village: American Academy of Pediatrics and American Heart Association, 2006.

3. 2005 International Consensus on Cardiopulmonary Resuscitation and Emergency Cardiovascular Care Science with Treatment Recommendations. Part 7: Neonatal Resuscitation. *Resuscitation* 2005; **67**(2–3):293–303.

4. Mackway-Jones K, Walker M. *Pocket Guide to Teaching for Medical Instructors*. London: BMJ Books, 1999.

5. Halamek LP. Teaching versus learning and the role of simulation-based training in pediatrics. *J Pediatr* 2007;**151**(4):329–30.

6. O'Donnell CP, Kamlin CO, Davis PG, Morley CJ. Ethical and legal aspects of video recording neonatal resuscitation. *Arch Dis Child Fetal Neonatal Ed* 2008;**93**(2):F82–4.

Index